Stem Cell Biology

Stem Cell Biology

Edited by **Rex Turner**

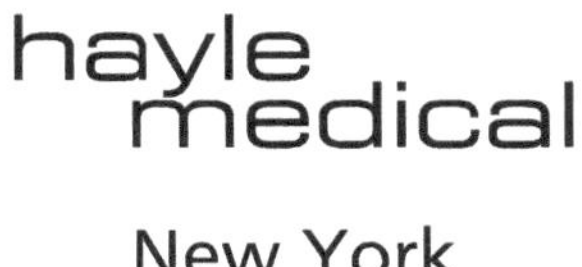

New York

Published by Hayle Medical,
30 West, 37th Street, Suite 612,
New York, NY 10018, USA
www.haylemedical.com

Stem Cell Biology
Edited by Rex Turner

International Standard Book Number: 978-1-63241-417-5 (Hardback)

Printed in the United States of America.

Contents

Preface

It is often said that books are a boon to mankind. They document every progress and pass on the knowledge from one generation to the other. They play a crucial role in our lives. Thus I was both excited and nervous while editing this book. I was pleased by the thought of being able to make a mark but I was also nervous to do it right because the future of students depends upon it. Hence, I took a few months to research further into the discipline, revise my knowledge and also explore some more aspects. Post this process, I began with the editing of this book.

This book provides comprehensive insights into the field of stem cell biology. Stem cells refer to the undifferentiated biological cells that can divide themselves through mitosis to form more stem cells. These cells are generally seen in multicellular organisms and are of two types, namely, embryonic stem cells and adult stem cells. They are found in embryos, fetuses and some adult tissues. This book unravels the recent studies in the field of stem cells. It will also provide interesting topics for research which readers can take up. From theories to research to practical applications, case studies from across the globe related to stem cell biology, have been included in this book. Students, scientists, biologists, doctors and other interested readers will benefit alike from this text.

I thank my publisher with all my heart for considering me worthy of this unparalleled opportunity and for showing unwavering faith in my skills. I would also like to thank the editorial team who worked closely with me at every step and contributed immensely towards the successful completion of this book. Last but not the least, I wish to thank my friends and colleagues for their support.

Editor

1

Human umbilical cord-derived mesenchymal stromal cells promote sensory recovery in a spinal cord injury rat model

Sachiko Takikawa[1], Akihito Yamamoto[2*], Kiyoshi Sakai[2], Ryutaro Shohara[2], Akira Iwase[1*], Fumitaka Kikkawa[1], Minoru Ueda[2]

[1]Department of Obstetrics and Gynecology, Nagoya University Graduate School of Medicine, Nagoya, Japan;
[*]Corresponding Author: akiwase@med.nagoya-u.ac.jp
[2]Department of Oral and Maxillofacial Surgery, Nagoya University Graduate School of Medicine, Nagoya, Japan;
[*]Corresponding Author: akihito@med.nagoya-u.ac.jp

ABSTRACT

While paralysis is widely appreciated to impact the quality-of-life after spinal cord injuries (SCIs), neuropathic chronic pain may also occur in many cases. In this study, we investigated whether human umbilical cord-derived mesenchymal stromal cells (hUCMSCs) possess the therapeutic potential to reduce neuropathic pain following SCI in rats. Spinal cord hemitransection, which was used as a rat SCI pain model, induced tactile hypersensitivity in the hind paw and hyperexcitability of wild dynamic range neurons in response to natural cutaneous stimuli. Following hemitransection, we transplanted hUCMSCs into the spinal cord. Attenuation of neuronal hyperexcitability was observed in the hUCMSC-treated group compared with that observed in the vehicle-treated group. Immunohistochemistry showed that the transplanted hUCMSCs retained the expression of gammaamino butyric acid (GABA). The results suggest that transplanted hUCMSCs ameliorate GABAergic inhibition in the spinal cord. In summary, the production of GABA plays a critical role in the plasticity of neuropathic pain after implantation of hUCMSCs.

Keywords: Human Umbilical Cord; Mesenchymal Stromal Cell; Mesenchymal Stem Cell; GABA

1. INTRODUCTION

Spinal cord injuries (SCIs) result in a severe impairment of the motor and sensory function below the level of the lesion. Stem cell therapy is a potential treatment for SCI, and the therapeutic benefits of a variety of different stem cell types have been evaluated in animal models and humans with SCI. The cellular sources of stem cells include human embryonic stem cells, induced pluripotent stem cells, fetal neural stem cells, adult bone marrow-derived mesenchymal stem cells (hBMMSCs) and dental pulp-derived stem cells [1-5]. It has been shown that the umbilical cord matrix (the Wharton's Jelly surrounding the umbilical vessels) contains a great number of fibroblastoid mesenchymal cells that have been characterized as exhibiting the properties of self-renewal and multipotent differentiation [6]. Recently, one group found that umbilical cord-derived mesenchymal stromal cells (hUCMSCs) can be induced to differentiate into neuron-like cells *in vitro* [6], while transplantation of hUCMSCs achieves improvement of the motor function in SCI animal models [7]. We have also reported remarkable benefits of hUCMSCs in wound treatment [8].

In many cases, SCIs are also accompanied by chronic pain syndrome, including allodynia (pain elicited by normally non-painful stimulation) and hyperalgesia (exaggerated pain evoked by noxious stimulation) [9]. Previous studies provide evidence that cell transplantation strategies that allow a long-term supply of gamma-aminobutyric acid (GABA) are a useful means of treating pain following injury to the peripheral and central nervous system [10,11]. We focused on the neural stem-like characteristics of hUCMSCs, in particular, the expressions of basic herix-loop-herix (bHLH) transcription factors known to function during mammalian neurogenesis. HES/HEY-like transcription factor (Helt) is coexpressed with achaete-scute complex homolog 1 (Ascl1, also known as Mash1) in brain regions that give rise to GABAergic neurons [12,13]. In addition, pancreas transcription factor 1 subunit alpha (Ptf1a) has been found to be involved in driving neural precursors to differentiate into GABAergic neurons in the cerebellum and the dorsal horn of the spinal cord [14].

In the present study, we attempted to investigate the characteristics of hUCMSCs as GABAergic neurons for the treatment of SCI-induced neuropathic pain. Hucmscs, which combine several advantages of fetal stem cells and adult stem cells, have been proposed to be an appropriate source of self-renewal with a high growth rate and multipotent differentiation properties for transplantation [6,15]. We transplanted hUCMSCs into the spinal cord-to examine the effects of implanted cells. After transplantation, we examined behavioral tests to investigate whether SCI-induced hypersensitivity is attenuated. Thereafter, a histological analysis was performed to confirm the survival of engrafted hUCMSCs in lesions. We investigated the characteristics of hUCMSCs in vitro, in particular, with respect to differences from hBMMSCs, and found that hUCMSCs possess the potential for GABA production.

2. MATERIALS AND METHODS

2.1. Isolation and Culture of HUCMSCs

Human umbilical cords were obtained from Nagoya University Hospital after full-term elective Caesarian sections. hUCMSCs were extracted as previously described [8,16,17]. The umbilical vein was pulled away with the surrounding tissue and placed into low-glucose Dulbecco's modified Eagle medium (DMEM-LG; Life Technologies, Carlsbad, CA) containing 0.075% collagenase type II (Sigma, St. Louis, MO) and 1 mM of L-glutamine (Life Technologies) with 100 U/mL of penicillin, 0.1 mg/mL of streptomycin and 0.25 μg/mL of amphotericin B. After performing enzymatic dissociation for six hours at 37°C, the centrifuged cell pellets were suspended in DMEM culture medium supplemented with 10% fetal bovine serum (FBS; Life Technologies) and 1 mM of L-glutamine. The cells and medium were seeded into 6-well plates (Becton, Dickinson and Company, Franklin Lakes, NJ) at a density of 10,000 cells/cm^2 and maintained in a cell incubator (37°C, 5% CO_2, 1% O_2 and 90% humidity). When the cells reached 80% confluence in approximately 4 - 5 days, the monolayers were split at a ratio of 1:3 using trypsin-EDTA (TryLE Express, Life Technologies). In this study, cells of passage two to five were used.

2.2. Immunophenotyping

For the immunocytochemical procedure, hUCMSCs of passage three were permeabilized with 0.1% Triton X-100 in PBS. After a subsequent rinse with PBS, the cells were blocked with 1% FBS in PBS and incubated for two hours with the primary antibodies: anti-nestin (mouse, 1:1000; Becton, Dickinson and Company), anti-glial fibrillary acidic protein (GFAP; mouse, 1:500; Cell Signaling Technology, Inc, Danvers, MA), antidoublecortin (goat, 1:500, Becton, Dickinson and Company), anti-neuronal nuclei (NeuN; mouse, 1:500, Becton, Dickinson and Company), anti-neuron-specific class III β-tubulin (Tuj-1; rabbit, 1:500; Millipore Corporation, Billerica, MA), anti-CNPase (mouse, 1:500; Cell Signaling Technology, Inc.) or anti-CD11b-FITC-conjugated (mouse, 1:500; Becton, Dickinson and Company). Following two rinses in PBS, unconjugated markers were reacted for one hour with secondary antibodies: Alexa Fluor 488 goat anti-mouse IgG (Life Technologies), Alexa Fluor 488 goat anti-rabbit IgG (Life Technologies) or PE rabbit anti-goat IgG (Abcam, Kenbridge, UK). A total of 10,000 labeled cells were analyzed using a FACS Calibur flow cytometer (Becton, Dickinson and Company).

2.3. Sphere Formation of HUCMSCs

For the suspension culture, dissociated hUCMSCs were placed on ultra low-attachment culture dishes (Corning, Tewksbury, MA) at a concentration of 2×10^5 cells/cm^2 at 37°C in 5% CO_2 and 1% O_2. This sphere formation procedure was modified from the method of the sphere assay protocol [17,18]. The protocols were as follows: hUCMSCs were treated in serum-free DMEM supplemented with 20 ng/mL of epidermal growth factor (EGF; Pepro-Tech, Rocky Hill, NJ), 20 ng/mL of basic fibroblast growth factor (FGF-2; Pepro-Tech), 20 mM of GlutaMAX (Life Technologies) and an N_2 supplement (1:100, Life Technologies). After 48 hours, sphere formation was observed.

2.4. Qualitative and Quantitative Real-Time RT-PCR Analyses

Total RNA from hBMMSCs (Lonza, Basal, Switzerland) and hUCMSCs was extracted using the RNeasy Mini Kit (QIAGEN GmbH, Hilden, Germany). The total RNA yield was determined using the NanoDrop^{TM} 1000 (Thermo Fisher Scientific Inc, Waltham, MA), and the RNA integrity was evaluated and used for subsequent experiments only if the A_{260}/A_{280} ratio exceeded 1.8. An RT reaction with 1 μg of total RNA was carried out using a first-strand cDNA synthesis kit (ReverTra Ace α; Toyobo Co. Ltd. Osaka, Japan). Thereafter, qualitative PCR was performed by mixing 1 μg of cDNA and 10 μM of specific primers at 94°C for two minutes, followed by 35 cycles of 94°C/15 sec, 60°C/30 sec and 72°C/60 sec, with a final extension of 72°C/10 min.

Quantitative real-time PCR was performed in 96-well 0.2-mL thin-wall PCR plates using the Thermal Cycler Dice (Takara Bio Inc., Tokyo, Japan) and SYBR Premix Ex Taq II (Takara Bio). The real-time PCR mixture contained 2 × SYBR Premix Ex Taq II, 10 µM of specific primers and 100 ng of cDNA in a total volume of 25 µL. The PCR profile included an initial incubation at 95°C/10 sec, then 40 cycles of 95°C/5 sec and 60°C/30 sec followed by dissociation at 95°C/15 sec, 60°C/30 sec and 95°C/15 sec. The primer pairs used in this study are listed in **Table 1**.

2.5. SCI Rat Model

Eight-week-old Female Sprague-Dawley rats (250 - 300 g body weight) were obtained from the Animal Center of Chubu Kagaku Shizai, Japan. All animal procedures were performed under protocols that conformed to the National Institutes of Health Guidelines. For different treatments, the rats were divided into three experimental groups: 1) the hUCMSC-treated hemitransection group (n = 8), 2) the PBS-treated hemitransection group (n = 8) and 3) the Sham (control) group (n = 5).

2.6. Transplantation of HUCMSCs

The animals were anesthetized with sodium pentobarbital (3 mg/100 g). After performing laminectomy at the 7 - 9th thoracic vertebral levels, the dura was opened and the spinal cord (T9-T10) was left-half transected using a surgical blade and a 27-gauge needle. Before administration, we triturated hUCMSC-spheres into single cell suspension. Immediately following hemitransection, 10 µl of PBS containing 1 × 10^6 hUCMSCs was implanted into the severed spinal cord using a 10-µl Hamilton syringe (Hamilton, Reno, NV) with an automatic microinjection pump (model KDS-310; Muromachi Kikai Co. Tokyo, Japan). The cells were deposited into three injection sites at the ipsilateral side of the rostral and caudal stumps, 2 mm from the lesion and 1 mm lateral to the midline at a depth of 1 mm. 6 µl of fibrin glue was injected into the gap to fill the lesion site in the severed spinal cord. For the control groups, only 10 µl of PBS was injected. All animals received daily cyclosporine A at a dose of 10 mg/kg for eight weeks after transplantation.

Table 1. List of PCR primers used in the present study.

Gene name	Accession number	Product size	Sequences
Sox2	NM_003106.2	109	F: 5'-TACAGCATGTCCTACTCGCAG-3'
			R: 5'-GAGGAAGAGGTAACCACAGGG-3'
NeuroD1	NM_002500	141	F: 5'-ATGACCAAATCGTACAGCGAG-3'
			R: 5'-GTTCATGGCTTCGAGGTCGT-3'
Neurogenin 1	NM_006161	107	F: 5'-GCTCTCTGACCCCAGTAGC-3'
			R: 5'-GCGTTGTGTGGAGCAAGTC-3'
Neurogenin 2	NM_024019	125	F: 5'-TCCTCCGTGTCCTCCAATTC-3'
			R:5'-AGGTGAGGTGCATAGCGGT-3'
GAD65	NM_001134366	234	F: 5'-GGCTTTGGTCTTTCGGGTC-3'
			R: 5'-TTCTCGGCGTCTCCGTAGAG-3'
Acsl1	NM_004316	142	F: 5'-TCTTCGCCCGAACTGATGC-3'
			R: 5'-CAAAGCCCAGGTTGACCAACT-3'
Helt	NM_001029887.1	131	F: 5'-AGATCCTCGAGATGACCGTTCAGTA-3'
			R: 5'-TTCATGCACTCGTGGTAGCCATA-3'
Ptf1a	NM_178161	140	F: 5'-CAGGACACTCTCTCTCATGGA-3'
			R:5'-TGGTGGTTCGTTTTCTATGTTGT-3'
GAPDH	NM_002406	102	F: 5'-AAGGTGAAGGTCGGAGTCAAC-3'
			R: 5'-GGGGTCATTGATGGCAACAATA-5'

2.7. Assessment of the Sensory Function after SCI

2.7.1. Tail Dip Test

For the studies of thermal nociception, a tail-immersiontest was used in which the last 3.5 cm of the tail was dipped into a water bath at 55°C and the latency to flutter the tail was taken as the end-point. The maximal latency allowed was 15 seconds to avoid potential tissue damage.

2.7.2. Von Frey Test

The left hind paw withdrawal threshold was determined using von Frey filaments and was expressed in grams. Seven filaments ranging from 4.0 to 60.0 g were used. The protocol used in this study was a variation of that described by Pitcher *et al.* [19]. A series of von Frey filaments was applied from below the wire mesh to the plantar surface of the left hind paw in ascending order beginning with the lowest filament (4.0 g). A trial consisted of the application of a von Frey filament to the hind paw five times at 5 second intervals or as soon as the hind paw was placed appropriately on the platform. When the hind paw was withdrawn from a particular hair either four or five times out of the five applications, the value of that hair in grams was considered to be the withdrawal threshold.

2.8. Immunohistochemistry

The procedure used in this study was modified from the method described by Zhang *et al* [20]. The animals were sacrificed and fixed transcardially with ice-cold PBS and 4% paraformaldehyde. 20-mm transverse segments of the SCI lesions were dissected and stored in the same fixative overnight. The tissue specimens were frozen and cryosectioned as 20-μm thick longitudinal sections of the transected sites via a cryomicrotome (Microcom/ HM500V, Walldorf, Germany). Individual sections were immunostained overnight with primary antibodies: anti-glutamate decarboxylase (GAD) 65 (rabbit, 1:50; abcam, Cambridge, UK), anti-human nuclei (HuN; mouse. 1:250; Millipore), anti-NeuN (1:500), anti-GFAP (1:500) or anti-CNPase (1:500). The sections were then incubated with secondary antibodies for one hour, washed and mounted on glass slides with fluorescent mounting medium (Vectorshield, Vector Laboratories, Burlingame, CA). The samples were examined using a fluorescent microscope (Leica Microsystems, Wetzlar, Germany) and an IM50 imaging system.

2.9. Ethics Statement

The Nagoya University Ethical Committee approved this study, and all participants gave their written informed consent. The animal research protocol was approved by the Nagoya University Institutional Animal Care and Use Committee (IACUC Protocol 21352). All surgeries were performed under anesthesia, and all efforts were made to minimize suffering.

3. RESULTS

3.1. Neural Markers of HUCMSCs

To verify the culture homology of hUCMSCs, third-passage cultures were analyzed for their presentation of neural stem cell markers and markers that characterize neuronal and glial cells and precursors (**Figure 1**). As revealed by flow cytometry, the hUCMSCs expressed nestin, GFAP, doublecortin, NeuN, Tuj-1 and CNPase, whereas the microglia marker CD11b was negative. However, the NeuN expression was low (1.04%), and the hUCMSCs contained a heterogeneous mixture of stem

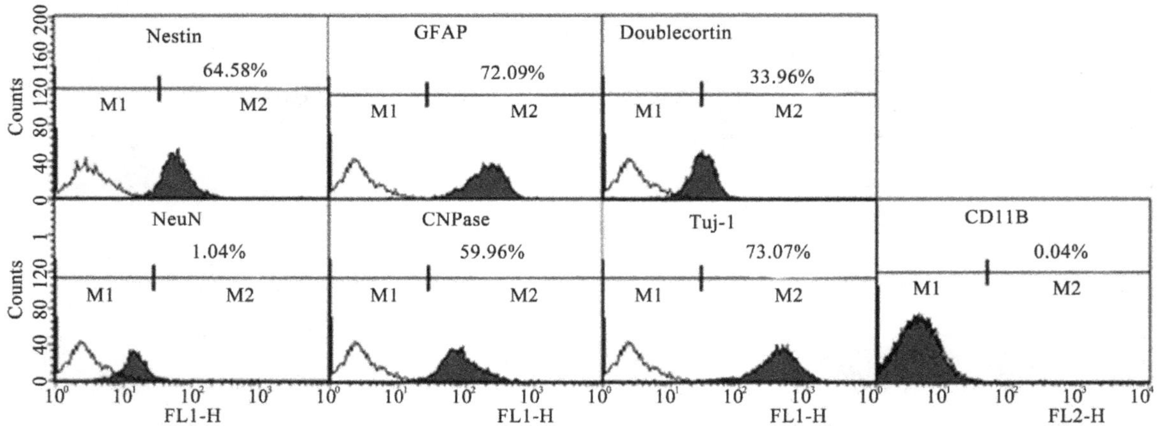

Figure 1. Flow cytometric histograms of hUCMSCs. hUCMSCs of passage three were stained with antibodies specific to neural stem cell markers and markers that characterize neuronal and glial cells and precursors. The cell debris was gated-out and histogram charts were plotted. Nestin: 64.6%, GFAP: 72.1%, doublecortin: 34.0%, NeuN: 1.04%, CNPase: 60.0% and Tuj-1: 73.1%.

and progenitor cells at different lineage commitment stages.

3.2. Expression of Neural Stem Cell Transcription Factors in HUCMSC Spheres

To investigate the potential effects of forming floating colonies, we cultured hUCMSCs in suspension with EGF and FGF on ultra low-attachment culture dishes. After 48 hours, aggregated hUCMSCs were collected. To determine whether the hUCMSC spheres increased neurogenesis, quantitative real-time PCR was performed to confirm the changes in the expressions of genes that have been implicated in neural stem cell transcription factors. As shown in **Figure 2**, Sox2 and NeuroD1 in plate cultured hUCMSCs were expressed at similar levels as those observed in hBMMSCs. However, the expression levels of hUCMSCs were increased in sphere formation. In addition, neurogenin 1 and neurogenin 2 in the hUCMSC spheres were expressed at higher levels in comparison with those observed in hBMMSCs, whereas the expressions in hUCMSCs were very low.

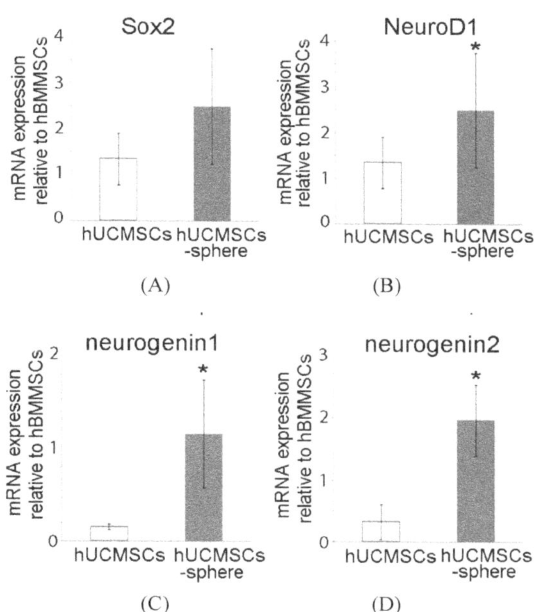

Figure 2. Effects of sphere formation of hUCMSCs on the Sox2, NeuroD1, neurogenin 1 and neurohenin 2 gene expression. The values are expressed as the mean ± SD relative to the internal control housekeeping gene GAPDH. As compared with hBMMSCs, the hUCMSCs exhibited 1.3-((A): Sox2), 1.1-((B): NeuroD1), 0.18-((C): neurogenin 1) and 0.12 ((D): neurogenin 2)-fold expressions. After performing a suspension culture, the hUCMSC spheres exhibited 2.5-((A): Sox2), 2.8-((B): NeuroD1), 1.2-((C): neruogenin 1) and 2.0 ((D): neurogenin 2)-fold expressions. Student's *t*-test was performed to detect significant alterations in the gene expression, where *, $p < 0.05$.

3.3. Functional Recovery after Transplantation of HUCMSC Spheres

Single cell suspensions of hUCMSC spheres were transplanted into hemitransected spinal cords (**Figure 3(A)**). The tail dip test and the von Frey test were performed to demonstrate improvements in sensory hypersensitivity against thermal and mechanical stimulation in the sham operation group (control), the hUCMSC-sphere transplantation group and the PBS-treated hemitransection group. In **Figure 3(B)**, prolongation of latency was observed from two weeks after transplantation onward. A similar trend was observed in the von Frey test (**Figure 3(C)**). These results suggest that hUCMSC transplantation significantly affects recovery from hypersensitivity.

3.4. Survival of Engrafted HUCMSCs

Eight weeks after transplantation, a histological examination was performed. Double-staining of HuN and NeuN antigens revealed that most hUCMSCs did not

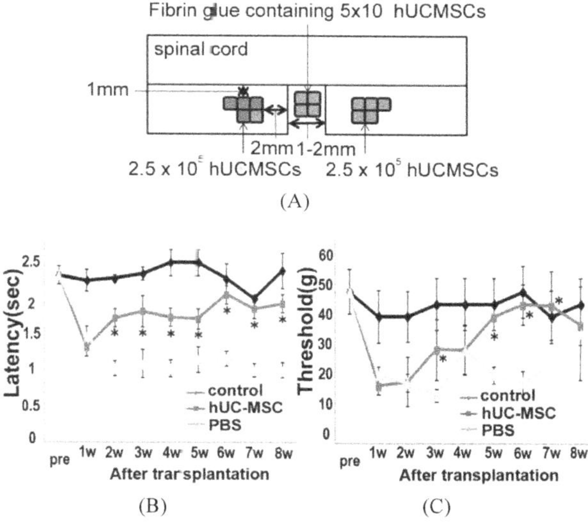

Figure 3. Sensory recovery after transplantation of hUCMSCs. (A) Experimental design for cell grafting after hemitransection of the spinal cord at the Th 9 - 10th level. (B) Tail immersion test: the latency to flick the tail after immersion in a 55°C water bath for the assessment of thermal hypersensitivity. The results are expressed as the mean ± SEM. The hUCMSCs group exhibited elongation of latency after two weeks post-transplantation. One-way ANOVA with the HolmSidak Test was used to analyze the differences in the lstency, where *, $p < 0.05$ between the PBS group and the hUC-MSC group. (C) von Frey test: the tactile sensitivity threshold of the ipsilateral hind paw of SCI for the assessment of mechanical hypersensitivity. The hUCMSCs group exhibited elevation of the threshold after two weeks post-transplantation. The results are expressed as the mean ± SEM. One-way ANOVA with the Holm-Sidak Test was used to analyze the differences in the threshold, where *, $p < 0.05$ between the PBS group and the hUC-MSC group.

differentiate into neurons (data not shown). The majority of HuN-positive hUCMSCs expressed GAD65, suggesting that these cells remained undifferentiated (**Figure 4(A)**). A few HuN-positive grafted cells in the hUCMSCs group survived in the hemitransected spinal cords. Most of the surviving cells were located at the periphery of the lesion site next to unaffected tissue. At the rostral and caudal stumps of the injured epicenter, surviving neural and glial cells were labeled with anti-NeuN, GFAP and CNPase antibodies in the hUCMSCs group (**Figures 4(B)-(D)**). On the other hand, there were few surviving cells in the PBS-treated hemitransection group, and imnmunostaining showed negligible signals (data not shown). The percentage of HuNpositive neural-like cells was small; however, many neural cells remained in the hUCMSCs group.

3.5. GABA Production in the HUCMSC Culture

We measured the concentrations of neurotransmitters in the culture media of hUCMSCs and hBMMSCs incubated with 1×10^6 cells for 48 hours using high performance liquid chromatography (**Figure 5(A)**). The hUCMSCs secreted GABA at the level of 1038 pmol/mL, while the hBMMSCs secreted GABA at the level of 665 pmol/mL. To determine whether hUCMSCs exhibit the characteristics of GABAergic neurons compared to hBMMSCs, we examined the expressions of mRNAs known to be associated with GABAergic neuron differentiation. GABAergic neurons are classically identified by their expression of GAD65, the rate-limiting enzyme that functions in the biosynthesis of GABA. Approximately 80% of the hUCMSCs were positive for GAD65 immunostaining (**Figure 5(B)**), which was a higher rate than that observed for hBMMSCs (**Figure 5(C)**). As shown in **Figure 5(D)**, semiquantitative RT-PCR analyses also revealed that hUCMSCs express a high level of GAD65. **Figures 5(E)-(G)** present the quantitative real-time RT-PCR results for genes involved in GABA ergic neuron differentiation *in vivo*, including Ascl1, Helt and Ptf1a. In the hUCMSCs, the gene expressions of Ascl1, Helt and Ptf1a exhibited 4.8-, 5.4-and 3.2-fold increases compared with those observed in the hBMMSCs, respectively.

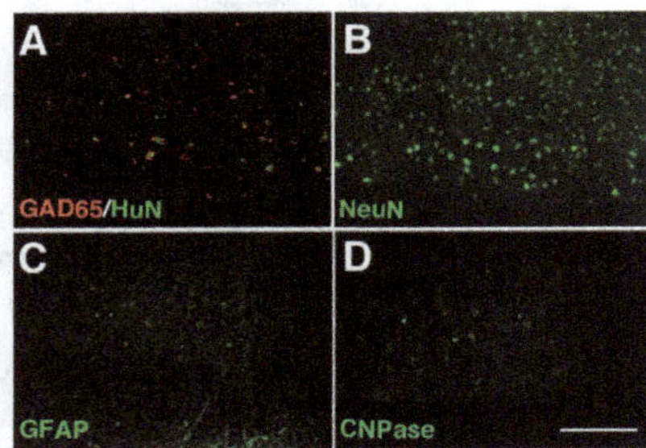

Figure 4. Engraftment of GAD-positive hUCMSCs and neuroprotection around the lesion site with hUCMSC transplantation. Eight weeks after transplantation, a pathological analysis was performed. Most of the surviving HuN-positive hUCMSCs (green; (A)) were double-labeled with anti-GAD65 antibodies (red; (A)), whereas there were few GAD-positive cells in the PBS group (data not shown). In the hUCMSCs group (B)-(D), a few neural and glial cells survived. The scale bar indicates 100 μm in (D).

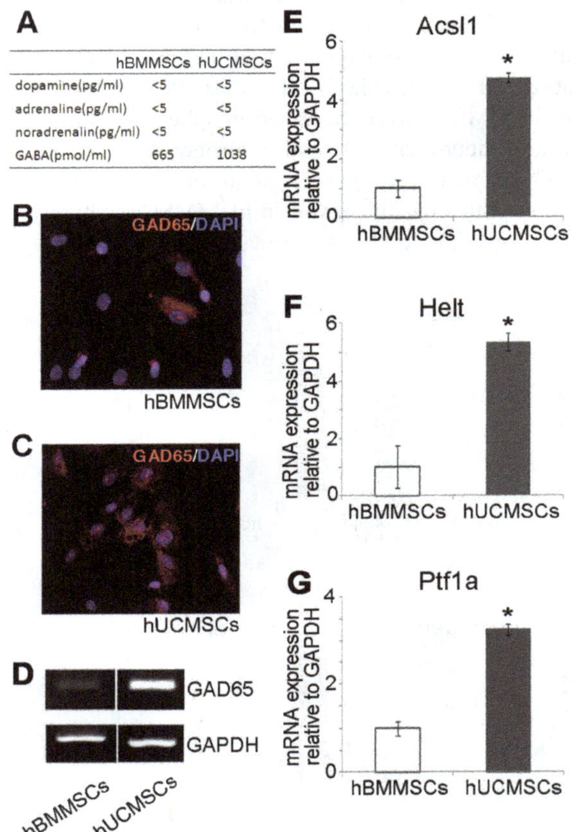
A

	hBMMSCs	hUCMSCs
dopamine(pg/ml)	<5	<5
adrenaline(pg/ml)	<5	<5
noradrenalin(pg/ml)	<5	<5
GABA(pmol/ml)	665	1038

Figure 5. Expression of GAD65 in hUCMSCs. (A) The concentrations of dopamine, adrenaline, noradrenalin and GABA in the culture media of hUCMSCs and hBMMSCs were measured using high performance liquid chromatography. The hUCMSCs of passage three (B) and hBMMSCs (C) were stained with anti-GAD65 antibodies. Approximately 80% of the hUCMSCs expressed GAD65, while only 30% of the hBMMSCs expressed GAD65. (D) An RT-PCR analysis showed an enhanced expression of GAD65 in the hUCMSCs compared with that observed in the hBMMSCs. (E)-(G) A quantitative real-time PCR analysis demonstrated the expressions of markers involved in GABA synthesis (Ascl1, Helt and Ptf1a). Student's *t*-test was performed to detect significant alterations in the gene expression, where *, $p < 0.05$.

4. DISCUSSION

In this study using an animal model of SCI, we focused on determining whether transplantation of hUCMSCs as GABAergic neurons effectively reduces pain-like responses induced by SCI in order to verify the possibility of cell replacement therapy using hUCMSCs for the treatment of SCI-induced neuropathic pain. hUCMSCs can provide a potentially unlimited supply of GABA following grafting intraspinal administration as a practical cell based-therapy. In previous studies, cell-based therapies for neuropathic pain that deposited GABAergic cells onto the subarachnoid space [21] or into the spinal cord [22] produced reductions in mechanical allodynia within one week post-transplantation. The present study shows that transplantation of hUCMSCs directly into the spinal cord improves hypersensitivity against tactile and thermal stimulation within two weeks after transplantation, with a peak reduction in allodynia observed at four weeks that persisted even eight weeks following transplantation.

There is some evidence indicating that the spinal GABAergic system plays a critical role in the development and maintenance of chronic pain states following injury of the central and peripheral nerves [23]. The increased expression of P2X4 receptors, which are induced in hyperactive microglia after nerve injury, promotes GABA-induced membrane depolarization at sensory terminals [24,25]. In our study, infiltration of activated microglia was suppressed 72 hours after hUCMSC transplantation. This decrease in inflammation might be caused by the neuroprotective effects of surviving hUCMSCs on spinal cord inhibitory interneurons. GABA-mediated neuroprotective effects have been demonstrated in various animal models of ischemia [26].

In the present study, the PBS group exhibited more obvious apoptosis and demyelination in peri-injured areas compared with the hUCMSCs group. We found that hUCMSCs prevented myelin and neural cell apoptosis and further improved the motor and sensory functions. Recently, the paracrine effects of MSC have been emphasized. It has been reported that MSCs provide protection via paracrine mechanisms involving the release of a wide array of cytokines (such as vascular endothelial growth factor, hepatocyte growth factor and insulin-like growth factor-1) that exert their effects on surrounding cells [27,28]. Other studies have hypothesized that trophic factors secreted by transplanted cells contribute to behavioral improvement by protecting or limiting the death of cells affected by endogenous cord injury [29,30]. Neural stem and precursor cells have also been shown to secrete trophic factors that regulate the fate determination of neighboring cells [31,32]. The underlying reasons may be that surviving hUCMSCs secrete cytokines, while paracrine effects may contribute to profound anti-apoptotic potency and reduction of injury.

We herein demonstrated improvement of neuropathic pain following transplantation of hUCMSCs. The underlying mechanism is thought to involve hUCMSCs that act as GABAergic cells and play neurotrophic and neuroprotective roles. Although this effect may be related to the GABAergic effects of restoration of GABA immunoreactivity in the spinal cord, it is also thought to be related to the secretion of non-GABAergic substances. The use of a transplantation strategy may be necessary to achieve more complete amelioration of nociception that occurs using neurotransmitter systems in addition to GABA.

5. CONCLUSION

Our data suggest that the use of intraspinal transplantation of hUCMSCs as GABAergic cells is a novel strategy to attenuate the pain induced by SCI. The use of cell-based therapies will require further investigation to ensure that the behavioral effects are persistent and without adverse effects over the long term. The development of transplantation strategies to relieve SCI-induced pain will increase the possibility of the therapeutic application of hUCMSCs, as well as ES and iPS cells.

REFERENCES

[1] Baker, D.E., Harrison, N.J., Maltby, E., Smith, K., Moore, H.D., *et al.* (2007) Adaptation to culture of human embryonic stem cells and oncogenesis *in vivo*. *Nature Biotechnology*, **25**, 207-215. doi:10.1038/nbt1285

[2] Erceg, S., Ronaghi, M., Oria, M., Rosello, M.G., Arago, M.A., *et al.* (2010) Transplanted oligodendrocytes and motoneuron progenitors generated from human embryonic stem cells promote locomotor recovery after spinal cord transection. *Stem Cells*, **28**, 1541-1549. doi:10.1002/stem.489

[3] Ronaghi, M., Erceg, S., Moreno-Manzano, V. and Stojkovic, M. (2010) Challenges of stem cell therapy for spinal cord injury: Human embryonic stem cells, endogenous neural stem cells, or induced pluripotent stem cells? *Stem Cells*, **28**, 93-99.

[4] Sasaki, M., Radtke, C., Tan, A.M., Zhao, P., Hamada, H., *et al.* (2009) BDNF-hypersecreting human mesenchymal stem cells promote functional recovery, axonal sprouting, and protection of corticospinal neurons after spinal cord injury. *The Journal of Neuroscience*, **29**, 14932-14941. doi:10.1523/JNEUROSCI.2769-09.2009

[5] Sakai, K., Yamamoto, A., Matsubara, K., Nakamura, S., Naruse, M., *et al.* (2012) Human dental pulp-derived stem cells promote locomotor recovery after complete transection of the rat spinal cord by multiple neuro-regenerative mechanisms. *Journal of Clinical Investigation*, **122**, 80-90.

[6] Mitchell, K.E., Weiss, M.L., Mitchell, B.M., Martin, P.,

Davis, D., *et al.* (2003) Matrix cells from Wharton's jelly form neurons and glia. *Stem Cells*, **21**, 50-60. doi:10.1634/stemcells.21-1-50

[7] Hu, S.L., Luo, H.S., Li, J.T., Xia, Y.Z., Li, L., *et al.* (2010) Functional recovery in acute traumatic spinal cord injury after transplantation of human umbilical cord mesenchymal stem cells. *Critical Care Medicine*, **38**, 2181-2189. doi:10.1097/CCM.0b013e3181f17c0e

[8] Shohara, R., Yamamoto, A., Takikawa, S., Iwase, A., Hibi, H., *et al.* (2012) Mesenchymal stromal cells of human umbilical cord Wharton's jelly accelerate wound healing by paracrine mechanisms. *Cytotherapy*, **14**, 1171-1181. doi:10.3109/14653249.2012.706705

[9] Yezierski, R.P. (1996) Pain following spinal cord injury: The clinical problem and experimental studies. *Pain*, **68**, 185-194. doi:10.1016/S0304-3959(96)03178-8

[10] Kim, D.S., Jung, S.J., Nam, T.S., Jeon, Y.H., Lee, D.R., *et al.* (2010) Transplantation of GABAergic neurons from ESCs attenuates tactile hypersensitivity following spinal cord injury. *Stem Cells*, **28**, 2099-2108. doi:10.1002/stem.526

[11] Stubley, L.A., Martinez, M.A., Karmally, S., Lopez, T., Cejas, P., *et al.* (2001) Only early intervention with gamma-aminobutyric acid cell therapy is able to reverse neuropathic pain after partial nerve injury. *Journal of Neurotrauma*, **18**, 471-477. doi:10.1089/089771501750171092

[12] Fode, C., Ma, Q., Casarosa, S., Ang, S.L., Anderson, D.J., *et al.* (2000) A role for neural determination genes in specifying the dorsoventral identity of telencephalic neurons. *Genes & Development*, **14**, 67-80.

[13] Miyoshi, G., Bessho, Y., Yamada, S. and Kageyama, R. (2004) Identification of a novel basic helix-loop-helix gene, Heslike, and its role in GABAergic neurogenesis. *The Journal of Neuroscience*, **24**, 3672-3682. doi:10.1523/JNEUROSCI.5327-03.2004

[14] Glasgow, S.M., Henke, R.M., Macdonald, R.J., Wright, C.V. and Johnson, J.E. (2005) Ptf1a determines GABAergic over glutamatergic neuronal cell fate in the spinal cord dorsal horn. *Development*, **132**, 5461-5469. doi:10.1242/dev.02167

[15] Karahuseyinoglu, S., Cinar, O., Kilic, E., Kara, F., Akay, G.G., *et al.* (2007) Biology of stem cells in human umbilical cord stroma: *In situ* and *in vitro* surveys. *Stem Cells*, **25**, 319-331. doi:10.1634/stemcells.2006-0286

[16] Sarugaser, R., Lickorish, D., Baksh, D., Hosseini, M.M. and Davies, J.E. (2005) Human umbilical cord perivascular (HUCPV) cells: A source of mesenchymal progenitors. *Stem Cells*, **23**, 220-229. doi:10.1634/stemcells.2004-0166

[17] Weiss, S., Dunne, C., Hewson, J., Wohl, C., Wheatley, M., *et al.* (1996) Multipotent CNS stem cells are present in the adult mammalian spinal cord and ventricular neuroaxis. *The Journal of Neuroscience*, **16**, 7599-7609.

[18] Pastrana, E., Silva-Vargas, V. and Doetsch, F. (2011) Eyes wide open: A critical review of sphere-formation as an assay for stem cells. *Cell Stem Cell*, **8**, 486-498. doi:10.1016/j.stem.2011.04.007

[19] Pitcher, G.M., Ritchie, J. and Henry, J.L. (1999) Paw withdrawal threshold in the von Frey hair test is influenced by the surface on which the rat stands. *Journal of Neuroscience Methods*, **87**, 185-193. doi:10.1016/S0165-0270(99)00004-7

[20] Zhang, L., Zhang, H.T., Hong, S.Q., Ma, X., Jiang, X.D., *et al.* (2009) Cografted Wharton's jelly cells-derived neurospheres and BDNF promote functional recovery after rat spinal cord transection. *Neurochemical Research*, **34**, 2030-2039. doi:10.1007/s11064-009-9992-x

[21] Eaton, M.J., Plunkett, J.A., Martinez, M.A., Lopez, T., Karmally, S., *et al.* (1999) Transplants of neuronal cells bioengineered to synthesize GABA alleviate chronic neuropathic pain. *Cell Transplant*, **8**, 87-101.

[22] Mukhida, K., Mendez, I., McLeod, M., Kobayashi, N., Haughn, C., *et al.* (2007) Spinal GABAergic transplants attenuate mechanical allodynia in a rat model of neuropathic pain. *Stem Cells*, **25**, 2874-2885. doi:10.1634/stemcells.2007-0326

[23] Coull, J.A., Boudreau, D., Bachand, K., Prescott, S.A., Nault, F., *et al.* (2003) Trans-synaptic shift in anion gradient in spinal lamina I neurons as a mechanism of neuropathic pain. *Nature*, **424**, 938-942. doi:10.1038/nature01868

[24] Coull, J.A., Beggs, S., Boudreau, D., Boivin, D., Tsuda, M., *et al.* (2005) BDNF from microglia causes the shift in neuronal anion gradient underlying neuropathic pain. *Nature*, **438**, 1017-1021. doi:10.1038/nature04223

[25] Tsuda, M., Shigemoto-Mogami, Y., Koizumi, S., Mizokoshi, A., Kohsaka, S., *et al.* (2003) P2X4 receptors induced in spinal microglia gate tactile allodynia after nerve injury. *Nature*, **424**, 778-783. doi:10.1038/nature01786

[26] Lyden, P.D. and Lonzo, L. (1994) Combination therapy protects ischemic brain in rats. A glutamate antagonist plus a gamma-aminobutyric acid agonist. *Stroke*, **25**, 189-196. doi:10.1161/01.STR.25.1.189

[27] Dai, W., Hale, S.L., Martin, B.J., Kuang, J.Q., Dow, J.S., *et al.* (2005) Allogeneic mesenchymal stem cell transplantation in postinfarcted rat myocardium: Short- and long-term effects. *Circulation*, **112**, 214-223. doi:10.1161/CIRCULATIONAHA.104.527937

[28] Kinnaird, T., Stabile, E., Burnett, M.S., Shou, M., Lee, C.W., *et al.* (2004) Local delivery of marrow-derived stromal cells augments collateral perfusion through paracrine mechanisms. *Circulation*, **109**, 1543-1549. doi:10.1161/01.CIR.0000124062.31102.57

[29] Cejas, P.J., Martinez, M., Karmally, S., McKillop, M., McKillop, J., *et al.* (2000) Lumbar transplant of neurons genetically modified to secrete brain-derived neurotrophic factor attenuates allodynia and hyperalgesia after sciatic nerve constriction. *Pain*, **86**, 195-210. doi:10.1016/S0304-3959(00)00245-1

[30] Eaton, M.J., Plunkett, J.A., Karmally, S., Martinez, M.A. and Montanez, K. (1998) Changes in GAD- and GABA-immunoreactivity in the spinal dorsal horn after peripheral nerve injury and promotion of recovery by lumbar transplant of immortalized serotonergic precursors. *Journal of Chemical Neuroanatomy*, **16**, 57-72. doi:10.1016/S0891-0618(98)00062-3

[31] Llado, J., Haenggeli, C., Maragakis, N.J., Snyder, E.Y.

and Rothstein, J.D. (2004) Neural stem cells protect against glutamate-induced excitotoxicity and promote survival of injured motor neurons through the secretion of neurotrophic factors. *Molecular and Cellular Neuroscience*, **27**, 322-331. doi:10.1016/j.mcn.2004.07.010

[32] Rafuse, V.F., Soundararajan, P., Leopold, C., Robertson, H.A. (2005) Neuroprotective properties of cultured neural progenitor cells are associated with the production of sonic hedgehog. *Neuroscience*, **131**, 899-916. doi:10.1016/j.neuroscience.2004.11.048

2

The combination of epidermal growth factor and glycogen synthase kinase 3 inhibitor support long-term self-renewal of Sca-1 positive hepatic progenitor cells from normal adult mice

Cai-Xia Jin[1,2], Lisa Samuelson[1], Cai-Bin Cui[1], Yang-Zhong Sun[1], David A. Gerber[1,3*]

[1]Department of Surgery, University of North Carolina at Chapel Hill, Chapel Hill, USA;
[*]Corresponding Author: david_gerber@med.unc.edu
[2]Department of Regenerative Medicine and Huadong Stem Cell Bank, Tongji University School of Medicine, Shanghai, China
[3]Lineberger Cancer Center, University of North Carolina at Chapel Hill, Chapel Hill, USA

ABSTRACT

Isolation and long-term maintenance of hepatic progenitor cells (HPCs) from healthy, non-injured adult livers remains challenging due to the lack of specific surface markers for selection and a limited understanding of the mechanisms for maintaining self-renewal. Previously, we identified a Sca-1 positive, bipotent HPC population in the peri-portal region of adult liver, and found MAPK/ERK and Wnt/β-Catenin pathways to be synergistically involved in their proliferation. In this study, we report the long-term culture of Sca-1 positive HPCs with epidermal growth factor (EGF) and CHIR99021, a small molecule inhibitor of glycogen synthase kinase 3 (GSK-3). Sca-1+ HPCs remain non-tumorigenic when passaged 35 times *in vitro* over 1 year. Flow cytometric analysis indicates that HPCs are positive for Sca-1 and putative liver progenitor cell markers, including CD13, CD24 and Prominin-1, but negative for hematopoietic/endothelial cell markers CD31, CD34, CD45, CD90 and CD117. Immunocyto-chemistry and RT-PCR indicate Sca-1+ HPCs express albumin (ALB), α-fetoprotein (AFP), cytokeratin19 (CK19), Sox9 and a panel of special hepatic progenitor transcriptional factors. Moreover, Sca-1+ HPCs are able to differentiate into hepatocyte-like and cholangiocyte-like cells under appropriate culture conditions *in vitro* and can take part in liver repopulation in an acetaminophen (APAP) induced liver injury mouse model. This study provides a paradigm to capture and maintain HPCs from naïve liver tissue and offers a valuable cell model for investigating the molecular mechanisms underlying the cell lineage relationship in normal liver.

Keywords: Liver Progenitor Cell; Stem Cell Antigen 1; Liver Disease; Hematopoietic Stem Cell

1. INTRODUCTION

The liver's post-injury regenerative capability is well described. Previous studies suggest that self-duplication of mature hepatocytes is enough to maintain physiological tissue homeostasis and regenerate the liver after injury, such as 2/3 hepatectomy. However, when the proliferative ability of mature hepatocytes is inhibited, "oval cells" are induced and participate in liver regeneration by differentiating into both hepatocytes and cholangiocytes [1-6]. Oval cells are not present in normal liver and are thought to be the descendant of putative endogenous hepatic progenitor cells (HPCs). However, despite extensive investigation of oval cells and ductal reaction after liver injury [5-9], there is limited knowledge about the naïve HPCs and their role in physiological and pathological liver regeneration.

Unique and discriminative surface markers that can be utilized for HPC isolation and identification have yet to be definitively reconciled. Several stem cell associated markers have generated interest in non-hematopoietic stem cell research. The murine stem cell antigen, Sca-1, is highly expressed on hematopoietic stem cells (HSC). Interestingly, Petersen *et al.* demonstrated Sca-1 expression on murine oval cells in the 3,5-diethoxycarbonyl-1, 4-dihydrocollidine (DDC) liver injury model [10]. Previously, we identified a Sca-1 positive, bipotent HPC population in the peri-portal region of mouse liver [4]. By magnetic activated cell sorting (MACS), these Sca-1 positive HPC cells can be purified and demonstrate bipotent differentiation [4]. Recently, we found that MAPK/ERK and Wnt/β-Catenin pathways are synergistically involved in proliferation of Sca-1 positive HPCs [11]. In the current study we report the long-term maintenance and culture of Sca-1 positive HPCs with epidermal growth factor (EGF) and CHIR99021, a small molecule inhibitor of glycogen synthase kinase 3 (GSK-3). CHIR99021 works via activation of the canonical Wnt pathway by inhibiting GSK-3β-dependent phosphorylation of β-Catenin [12]. Sca-1+ HPCs can be maintained for over 30 passages *in vitro* >1 year under such conditions while remaining non-tumorigenic. Even after long-term *in vitro* culture, HPCs remain bipotent and can generate functional hepatocytes *in vivo*.

Our study provides a new thread to molecular identification of HPCs from naïve mature liver tissue using Sca-1 as a marker. These Sca-1+ HPCs could be a useful cell model to investigate physiological liver regeneration and the self-renewal mechanisms of naïve HPCs.

2. MATERIALS AND METHODS

2.1. Mice

C57BL/6 mice and Rag2-/-γ-/- mice were purchased from Jackson Laboratory (Bar Harbor, ME) and used for all of the experiments. All animal care and use protocols were approved by the Institutional Animal Care and Use Committee at the University of North Carolina at Chapel Hill in accordance with principles and procedures outlined in the National Institutes of Health Guide for the Care and Use of Laboratory Animals.

2.2. Sca-1$^+$ HPCs Isolation and Culture

Sca-1+ HPCs were isolated from 6 - 8 week old C57BL/6 mice using a modification of the 2-stage liver perfusion technique as described [4,11,13]. Enrichment of Sca-1+ HPCs was performed using a Sca-1 antibody conjugated to mini-magnetic beads (Miltenyi Biotec, Inc.; Auburn, CA) according to the manufacturer's instructions. The cells were regularly maintained in Dulbecco's modified Eagle medium (DMEM) (Gibco; Carlsbad, California) with 10% fetal bovine serum (FBS) (PAA Laboratories, Inc.; Dartmouth, MA), 20 mM hepes (Sigma Chemical Co.; St. Louis, MO), 10 mM nicotinamide (Sigma), 1 mM ascorbic acid 2-phosphate (Sigma), 30 mg/L L-proline (Sigma), 10 ng/mL EGF (Sigma) and 2 μM CHIR99021 (Stemgent; San Diego, CA). The 9th passage Sca-1+ HPCs were serially diluted and plated onto 96-well plates for subcloning. Two weeks later, 10 isolated clones were selected, dissociated and expanded. Among these ten clonal lines, lines #2, #4, #8 and #10 demonstrated homogeneous epithelial cells, while the other lines expressed a mixed cellular morphology. All ten cultures have been stably cultured *in vitro* for more than 30 passages without a decrease in proliferation. Two clones were selected for extensive analysis in this study. They were labeled Clone 9-1, clone 9-8 and they were compared with the heterogeneous initial population of mixed HPCs.

2.3. Cell Surface Markers and Cell Proliferation Analysis by Flow Cytometry

Cells were dissociated into a single cell suspension with 0.25% trypsin (Sigma) and stained with primary antibodies labeled with relevant fluoroprobes for 20 min at room temperature at 1 μg antibody per 1,000,000 cells in DPBS. After three washes with DPBS, cells were resuspended in cold DPBS buffer containing 1% FBS at 1×10^6 cells/ml. Unstained cells and cells stained with isotype control antibody were used as blank and negative controls. The directly conjugated primary antibodies included phycoerythrin (PE)-conjugated Sca-1, CD31, CD45 and CD117 (BD Pharmingen™, San Diego, CA) and Prominin-1 (Miltenyi Biotec, Inc.), PE-Cy7-conjugated EpCAM (eBiosciences; San Diego, CA), fluorescein isothiocyanate (FITC)-conjugated CD13, CD24, CD34, CD90 (Pharmingen). The fluorescence-labeled cells were analyzed with Cyan ADP (Dako) or LSR II flow cytometer (Beckman Coulter, Inc. Brea, CA). Debris and doublets were excluded by forward scatter and side scatter manipulation. Gating was implemented based on isotype control staining profiles. All data were analyzed with Summit 4.3 Software (Dako).

2.4. RNA Isolation and RT-PCR

Total RNA was extracted from HPCs, 9-1 HPCs and 9-8 HPCs by RNeasy Plus Mini Kit (Qiagen, Inc., Valencia, CA). One microgram of total RNA were reverse-transcribed using the RETRO script Reverse Transcription Kit (Ambion; Austin, TX). PCR conditions were 95°C for 5 min, 94°C for 30 sec, annealing temperature for 40 sec, and 72°C for 60 sec, 35-40 cycles, and then 72°C for 10 min.

2.5. Western Blot Analysis

Cells were harvested and homogenized in RIPA buffer (Sigma Aldrich; St Louis, MO) containing 1 ml protease inhibitor cocktail and 1ml phosphatase inhibitor per 100 ml. Lysates were centrifuged at 14,000 g for 2 min. Protein concentrations of supernatants were determined by using a standard Bradford assay on a BioTek microplate reader. Equivalent amounts of 50 μg protein were heating at 95°C for 10 min and ran on SDS-PAGE, transferred to nitrocellulose membrane, incubated with 5% nonfat milk blocking buffer for 2 h at room temperature and probed with primary antibodies overnight at 4°C. After incubation with peroxidase-conjugated secondary antibodies at room temperature for 1 h, activity was detected by ECL™ Western Blotting Detection Reagents (Amersham). The primary antibodies of β-Actin and AFP were purchased from Sigma, ALB and CK19 were purchased from Dako (Carpinteria, CA), E-Cadherin was purchased from Cell Signaling Technology (Beverly, MA). Horseradish Peroxidase conjugated secondary antibodies were purchased from Dako.

2.6. Immunofluorescence Assay

Cells were fixed in 4% paraformaldehyde for 30 min at room temperature (RT) and washed in PBS with 0.05% Tween-20 (T-PBS) three times, followed by blocking with 5% normal goat serum for 30 min, then incubated with primary antibodies at 4°C overnight, washed three times in T-PBS, then incubated with second antibody for 30 min. The following primary antibodies were used: Rat anti-Sca-1 (1:100) (BD Pharmingen™; San Jose, CA), Rabbit polyclonal anti-ALB (1:200) (DAKO), Rabbit anti-CK19 (1:200) (Abcam; Cambridge, MA), Rabbit anti-E-Cadherin (1:200) (Cell Signaling Technology) and Rabbit anti-Sox9 (1:400) (Abcam). Then the cells were stained with AlexaFlour conjugated secondary antibodies from Invitrogen. All images were recorded with a Nikon Microphot-FXA microscope equipped with an Optronics DEI 750 3-chip CCD camera or a Zeiss AxioCarvert fluorescence microscope system with an Axiocam digital camera. Images were acquired and processed using Q imaging and AxioVision software.

2.7. *In Vitro* Differentiation of Sca-1+ HPCs

To analyze the hepatic differentiation capacity of single HPCs, cells were plated at a density of 100 cells per 35 mm dish and cultured in 10% FBS-supplemented medium overnight before being changed into chemically defined medium, CDM, which is defined as DMEM/F-12 supplemented with 2 mM L-glutamine, 0.11 mM 2-mercaptoethanol, 1 mM non-essential amino acids, 0.5 mg/ml BSA (fraction V)]. HPCs were cultured in CDM with 20 ng/mL hepatocyte growth factor (HGF, R&D Systems, Minneapolis, MN), 10 ng/mL oncostatin M (OSM, Sigma), 0.5 mg/L insulin-transferring-selenium (ITS, Sigma) and 1 μM dexamethasone (Sigma). The medium was changed every 2 - 3 days. The total RNA was extracted after 10, 15 and 20 days of induction.

To induce cholangiocytic differentiation, 0.5 ml matrigel (Invitrogen) mixed with 0.5 ml serum free DMEM/F12 medium supplement was added into 35 mm dishes. After incubation in 37°C for 2 h, 5×10^3 cells were plated onto the matrigel and medium was replaced with fresh CDM supplement containing 2% matrigel and 2 mg/ml laminin with 10 ng/ml HGF every 3 days [14]. Total RNA was extracted after a 20 day incubation. First, confirm that you have the correct template for your paper size. This template has been tailored for output on the custom paper size (21 cm*28.5 cm).

2.8. Tumor Formation Assay and Cell Transplantation

For tumor formation assays, up to 5×10^6 cells suspended in 100 μl PBS were subcutaneously injected into the right and left lower flanks of 6 - 8 week old Rag2-/-γ-/-mice (n = 10). HepG2 cells were injected as a control and mice were observed over 6 months.

To assess the differentiation capacity of Sca-1+ HPCs *in vivo*, 1×10^6 pMX-IRES-EGFP-transduced HPCs were injected into the spleens of C57BL/6 mice (n = 12, 8 - 10 week old). Acute liver damage was induced by intraperitoneal injection of 250 mg/kg body weight acetaminophen (APAP, Sigma) in sterile PBS eight to twelve hours before transplantation. Mice were euthanized at four weeks or six weeks after cell implantation. Recipient livers were fixed in 4% phosphate-buffered paraformaldehyde overnight at 4°C and embedded in paraffin. Frozen livers were cut to 10 μm cryosections and observed under fluorescence microscope for EGFP expression. Paraffin-embedded liver sections in 5 μm were stained with anti-GFP (EMD Millipore, Billerica, MA) and anti-ALB antibodies.

3. RESULTS

3.1. Isolation and Characterization of HPCs from Normal Adult Mouse Liver

Previously, we identified a Sca-1 positive, bipotent HPC population in the periportal region of normal mouse liver tissue. By two-step liver perfusion with collagenase and subsequent cell enrichment by MACS using Sca-1 antibody conjugated mini-magnetic beads, the Sca-1 positive HPC populations were purified [4]. The cells are routinely cultured with EGF and CHIR99021. The primary cultures consist of mainly epithelial-shaped cells mixed with fewer fibroblast-like cells. However, during a series of subpassage cultures, the Sca-1+ HPCs appear morphologically homogenous with epithelial shaped cells (**Figures 1(A)** and **(B)**). The 9th passage Sca-1+ HPCs were serially diluted and plated onto two 96-well tissue culture plates (one cell in 100 μl culture medium per well) and 10 clones then selected and named numerically as: clone 9-1-HPC, 9-2-HPC, 9-3-HPC, ··· 9-10-HPC.

Cells were cultured in a humidified 5% CO_2 atmosphere at 37˚C and the medium changed at regular time intervals. Two clones 9-1-HPC (**Figures 1(C)** and **(D)**), 9-8-HPC (**Figures 1(E)** and **(F)**), and mixture HPCs were characterized in the present studies. RT-PCR shows that the HPCs express Sca-1, liver related genes (including AFP, ALB, Transferrin, TAT, CK19, GGT, ApoAII, ApoCII and ApoE) and liver-enriched transcription factors (including GATA-4, HNF-1α, HNF-3α, HNF-6, HNF-4, HNF-1β, HNF-3β and C/EBP-γ) (**Figure 1(G)**).

To fully characterize the Sca-1+ HPCs and distinguish them from other cell fractions in the adult liver, cell surface profiles were analyzed using specific antibodies for hepatic progenitor cells (Sca-1, CD13 and Prominin-1), oval cells/biliary epithelial cells (CD24/EpCAM) and hematopoietic/endothelial cells (CD31, CD34, CD45, CD90 and CD117) by flow cytometry. The flow cytometric data of 9-8-HPCs at the 18th, 26th and 31st passages indicate that a majority of cells are continuously positive for Sca-1 (61% ± 0.12%); along with CD13 (12.7% ± 0.02%), CD24 (22.8% ± 0.95%), Prominin-1 (16.4% ± 0.19%) and EpCAM (12.6% ± 1.05%) but do not express the endothelial cell and hematopoietic cell markers CD31, CD34, CD45, CD90 and CD117 (**Figure 2**). 9-1-HPC at the 16th, 22nd and 25th passages have similar expression patterns with 9-8 HPCs but are negative for EpCAM. Mixed HPCs at the 20th, 26th and 30th passages have similar expression pattern with 9-8 HPCs but with a lower percentage of cells expressing Sca-1 (34% ± 0.06%) (**Table 1**).

We further examined the Sca-1+ HPCs using immunocytochemistry (ICC) and western blot analysis. ICC analysis shows that HPCs are positive for Sca-1, AFP, ALB and CK19 (**Figure 3(A)**). Western blot analysis confirms the expression of AFP, ALB and CK19 (**Figure 3(B)**). Meanwhile, we find that Sca-1+ HPCs also express E-Cadherin and Sox9 by ICC (**Figures 3(C)** and **(D)**) and RT-PCR (**Figure 3(E)**), markers which have been used as liver progenitor cell markers [15,16]. These results strongly suggest that Sca-1+ HPCs can be stably maintained during long-term *in vitro* culture.

3.2. *In Vitro* Differentiation Potential of Sca-1+ HPCs

To evaluate the potential of Sca-1+ HPCs to differentiate into hepatocyte-like cells, we used HGF, OSM, ITS and dexamethasone to promote maturation of HPCs. Sca-1+ HPCs were plated at ultra-low density(100 cells per 35 mm dish) and cultured with HGF for 5 days, followed by another 2 weeks of OSM, ITS and dexamethasone treatment in CDM. We analyzed colony-constituent cells after 10, 15 and 20 days of induction for expression of albumin and CK19. Sca-1+ HPCs coexpress albumin and CK19 before induction (**Figure 4(A)**). After 10 days of induction, half (50%) of HPCs are only albumin-positive (**Figure 4(B)**). By 15 days of induction 90% of HPCs are albumin positive only, while 10% are

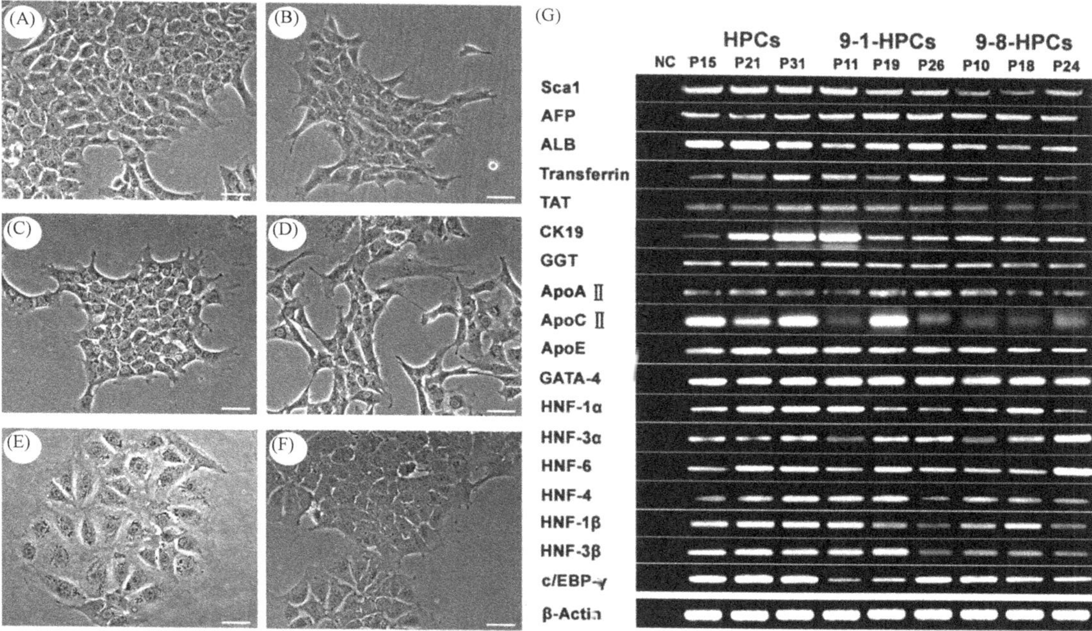

Figure 1. Establishment of HPC cell lines from wild type C57BL/6 mice. Phase contrast photographs of HPCs in passage 8 and 28, 9-1-HPCs in passage 7 and 18, 9-8-HPCs in passage 12 and 22 (Magnification, 200×) (A)-(F). Bars, 50 μm. RT-PCR analysis of selected transcription factors and liver-related genes in HPCs, 9-1-HPCs and 9-8-HPCs (G). NC, negative control.

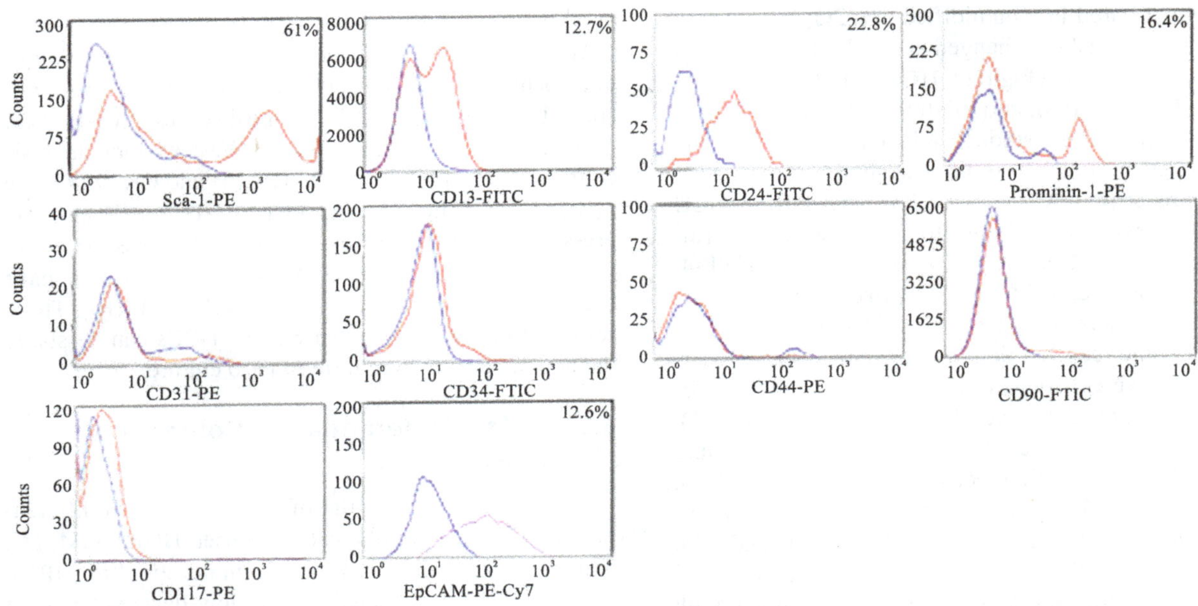

Figure 2. Identification of surface markers in HPCs by flow cytometry. Histograms represent the analyzed markers versus their corresponding isotype controls. Blue curve: fluorescence of isotype controls; Red/Purple curve: fluorescently labeled cells. The data shown represent the experiments using 9-8 HPCs.

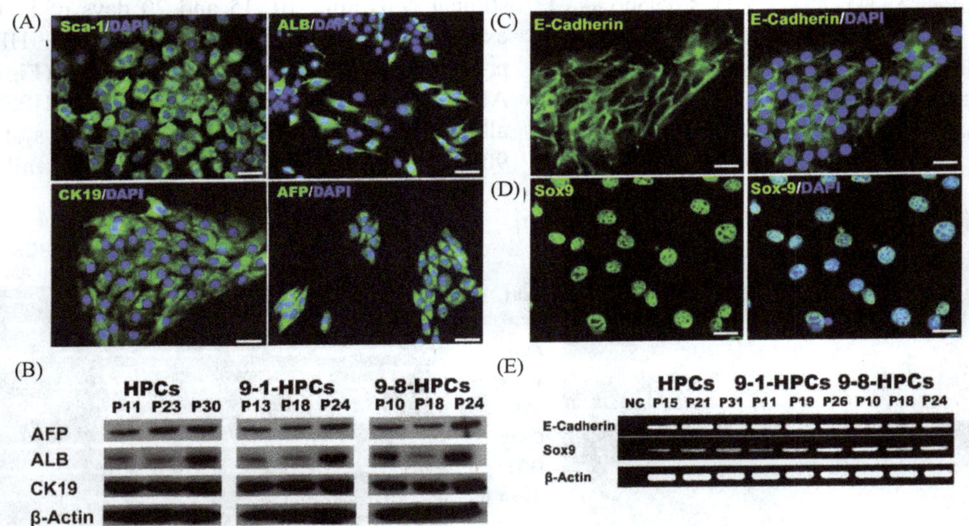

Figure 3. Phenotypic analysis of HPCs. Immunofluorescence analysis for Sca-1, ALB, CK19 and AFP (A). Protein was collected from different passage cells and analyzed for expression of AFP, ALB and CK19 (B). Immunofluorescence analysis of E-Cadherin and Sox9 (C) and (D). RT-PCR analysis of E-Cadherin and Sox9 (E). Data are from one representative of at least three independent experiments. Magnification: (A) 200×; (C) and (D) 400×. Bars: 50 μm. The nucleus was stained with DAPI.

only positive for CK19 (**Figure 4(C)**). Almost all HPCs are albumin-positive and CK19-negative after 20 days of induction (**Figure 4(D)**), which suggests that HPCs can differentiate into hepatocyte-like cells. Periodic acid-Schiff staining of HPCs shows very weak staining before induction (**Figure 4(E)**) but become strongly positive after 20 days of induction (**Figure 4(F)**), indicating that HPCs can differentiate into mature hepatocytic cells with sufficient glycogen expression after 20 days of induction in culture. RNA analysis of the HPCs in hepatic induction medium for 20 days confirms up-regulation of hepatic lineage marker ALB, with a 10-fold increase after 20 days of induction. However, the expression of CK19 decreases slightly compared to initial control levels (**Figures 4(G)** and **(H)**).

When HPCs are cultured on Matrigel in CDM with 10

Table 1. Expression of surface markers in HPCs, 9-1 HPCs and 9-8 HPCs.

	HPCs	9-1-HPCs	9-8-HPCs
Sca-1	34 ± 0.06	57 ± 0.18	61 ± 0.12
CD13	29.6 ± 0.17	13.6 ± 2.26	12.7 ± 0.02
CD24	27.8 ± 0.75	37.4 ± 1.69	22.8 ± 0.95
Prominin-1	11.5 ± 0.65	11.4 ± 0.4	16.4 ± 0.19
EpCAM	19.4 ± 0.25	negative	12.6 ± 1.05
CD31	negative	negative	negative
CD34	negative	negative	negative
CD45	negative	negative	negative
CD90	negative	negative	negative
CD117	negative	negative	negative

ng/ml HGF, tubule-like branching morphogenesis appears after 10 days of plating (**Figure 5(A)**) and bile duct-like structures form 20 days latter (**Figure 5(B)**). While HPCs cultured on Matrigel in CDM without HGF do not form any branching or bile duct-like structures and most cells die after 20 days of plating (**Figure 5(C)**). Immunofluoresence analysis shows that bile duct-like structures are strongly positive for CK19 (**Figure 5(D)**) with a concomitant decrease in hepatocyte marker ALB expression after 20 days of plating (**Figure 5(E)**). RNA analysis of the HPCs in 3D Matrigel culture for 20 days reveals increased expression of biliary lineage marker CK19, aquaporin-1 (Aqp1), cystic fibrosis transmembrane conductance regulator (CFTR) and hairy and enhancer of split 1 (Hes1), and decreased expression of hepatocyte marker ALB (**Figure 5(F)**). These results indicate that HPCs have the capacity to differentiate into both hepatocyte-like cells and cholangiocyte-like cells.

Importantly, after transplantation of 20th passage HPCs into Rag2-/-γ-/-mice, no tumors are detected in the mice after 6 months (n = 5) of continuous observation. Three control mice (n = 5) transplanted with HepG2 cells formed tumors 3 weeks post injection, suggesting HPCs are non-tumorigenic.

3.3. *In Vivo* Differentiation Potential of Sca-1+ HPCs

To investigate the potential of HPCs to engraft and to differentiate within the microenvironment of the liver *in vivo*, we prepared recipient mice by using acetaminophen to injure the liver prior to cell transplantation [17]. HPCs labeled with EGFP were transplanted into APAP-treated mice. The mice were euthanized at 4 weeks (n = 6) or six weeks (n = 6) after implantation to detect transplanted cells. EGFP+ HPCs were detected in the recipient livers by fluorescent stereoscopic microscopy (**Figure 6(A)**). Immunofluorescence analysis showed that HPCs differentiate into parenchymal heaptocytes that produce both EGFP and ALB (**Figure 6(B)**). The percentage of EGFP positive cell engraftment was 3.92% ± 0.52% (n = 6) at 4 weeks. There was no significant difference between 4-week and 6-week engraftment. The donor-derived cells were observed mainly in liver parenchyma near the per portal area. The results confirmed that HPCs can differentiate into hepatocyte lineage in vivo after transplantation into recipient animals.

4. DISCUSSION

Hepatocyte transplantation has long been recognized as a potential treatment for life-threatening liver diseases. However, considering the severe shortage of usable primary hepatocytes and the limited proliferative nature of these valuable cells, a renewable stem cell source of

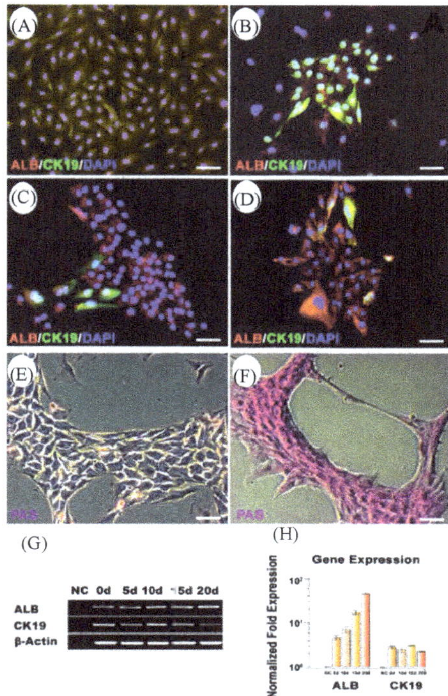

Figure 4. Hepatocyte differentiation of HPCs. Dual immunofluorescence stain of ALB and CK19 of HPCs before induction (A) and a single-cell source of HPCs cultured in chemical defined medium with 20 ng/mL HGF, 1 μM dexamethasone, 0.5 mg/L ITS and 10 ng/mL OSM for 10 days (B), 15 days (C) and 20 days (D), the nucleus was stained with DAPI (Magnification, 200×). Periodic Acid Schiff (PAS) staining of HPCs before induction (E) and after 20 days induction (F). All bars, 50 μm. (G) and (H) RT-PCR and Real-time PCR analysis of HPCs that cultured in medium same as described above for 5, 10, 15 and 20 days.

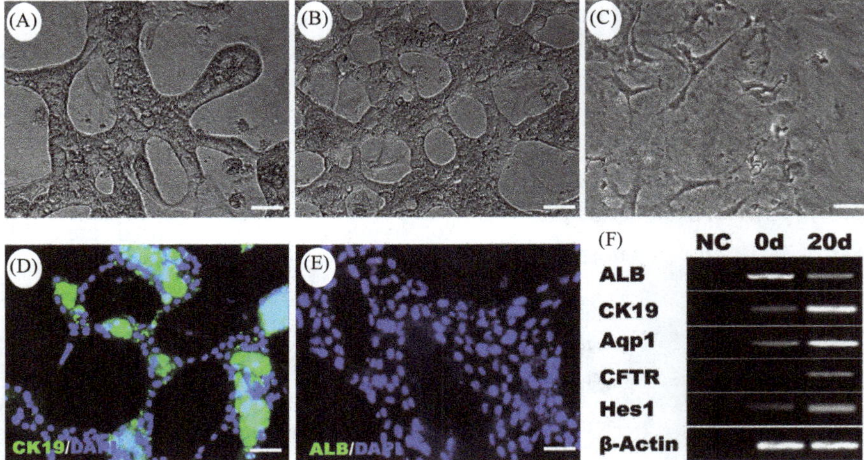

Figure 5. Differentiation of Sca-1+ HPCs into cholangiocyte-like cells. Sca-1+ HPCs showed branching morphogenesis (A) and bile duct-like structure (B) in 3-D matrigel culture after 10 and 20 days compared with control group (C). Immunofluorescence analysis for CK19 and ALB of HPCs cultured on 3D matrigel in CDM with 10 ng/mL HGF after 20 days, the nucleus was stained with DAPI (D)and (E). (F) RT-PCR analysis of cholangiocyte-related genes in HPCs after cultured on 3D matrigel for 20 days. Magnification, 200×; Bars, 50 μm.

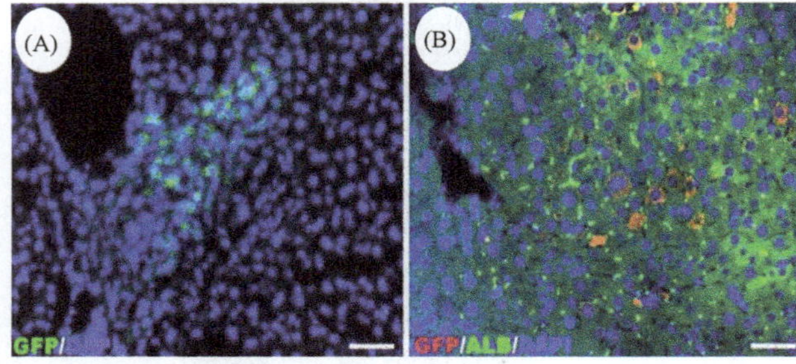

Figure 6. Differentiation of Sca-1+ HPCs in mice *in vivo*. (A) Fluorescent views of transplanted liver cryostat sections after 6 weeks of transplantation *in vivo*. (B) Immunofluorescence analysis of recipient liver sections. Transplanted Sca-1+ HPCs are positive for GFP (red) and ALB (green). The nucleus was stained with DAPI. Magnification, 200×; Bar, 50 μm.

hepatocytes is important for therapeutic transplant. Recent studies confirm that hepatic stem cells are resident in adult liver and play a critical role in mediating physiological and pathological liver regeneration [18]. However, despite extensive efforts, the isolation and maintenance of hepatic stem cells from liver has been hampered by the lack of specific surface markers and high efficiency culture systems.

Based on our previous studies with Sca-1, we further demonstrate in this study that Sca-1 can be utilized as a reliable surface marker to isolate liver progenitor cells from naïve murine adult liver tissues, and more importantly, these cells can be maintained in long-term culture using a combination of EGF and a small molecule GSK3 inhibitor CHIR99021. The proliferation of Sca-1+ HPCs is strictly dependent on the combination of EGF and CHIR99021. Cell survival and growth are significantly retarded after the removal of CHIR99021 or EGF from the medium. Remarkably, even after long term expansion, cells are still competent to differentiate into mature hepatocytes or cholangiocytes efficiently *in vitro* and generate hepatocytes *in vivo*, suggesting the bipotential differentiation capability of the cells. Our study represents a novel paradigm to self-renew of hepatic progenitor cells. The cells can be used as a promising cell model to understand the molecular mechanisms involved in liver progenitor cell proliferation and differentiation. Moreover, it would be useful to test if the same regimen could also be used to expand human liver progenitor cells in the future.

Although the cells were purified using Sca-1 labeled MACS, we found the cultured HPCs do not homogenously express Sca-1 and other liver stem cell markers even after single cell cloning. This suggests that HPCs cultured under such conditions are a hierarchical cell population. Whether Sca-1 positive cells are progenitor cells that are responsible for long-term self-renewal of the cell population remains to be determined. Interestingly, we found HPCs under this culture condition also express Sox9, a gene labeling a liver progenitor pool within the peri-portal region. This population has been shown through *in vivo* lineage tracing to physiologically supply hepatocytes and bile duct cells [16]. This supports the notion that Sca-1 positive HPCs may be the *in vitro* counterpart of naïve liver progenitors. However, further studies are required to depict the lineage relationship of Sca-1 positive and Sox9 positive liver progenitors in situ.

5. ACKNOWLEDGEMENTS

We thank Montserrat Caballero for providing cryostat, Carolyn Suitt for tissue section histology support, Barry Udis for flow cytometric analysis and the UNC Institutional Animal Care and Use Committee staff for help with animal work. We thank Microscopy Services Laboratory and Tissue Culture Facility for providing support.

REFERENCES

[1] Azuma, H., Hirose, T., Fujii, H., Oe, S., Yasuchika, K., Fujikawa, T. and Yamaoka, Y. (2003) Enrichment of hepatic progenitor cells from adult mouse liver. *Hepatology*, **37**, 1385-1394. doi:10.1053/jhep.2003.50210

[2] Fougere-Deschatrette, C., Imaizumi-Scherrer, T., Strick-Marchand, H., Morosan, S., Charneau, P., Kremsdorf, D., Faust, D.M. and Weiss, M.C. (2006) Plasticity of hepatic cell differentiation: Bipotential adult mouse liver clonal cell lines competent to differentiate *in vitro* and *in vivo*. *Stem Cells*, **24**, 2098-2109. doi:10.1634/stemcells.2006-0009

[3] Wang, J., Clark, J.B., Rhee, G.S., Fair, J.H., Reid, L.M. and Gerber, D.A. (2003) Proliferation and hepatic differentiation of adult-derived progenitor cells. *Cells Tissues Organs*, **173**, 193-203. doi:10.1159/000070375

[4] Wright, N., Samuelson, L., Walkup, M.H., Chandrasekaran, P. and Gerber, D.A. (2008) Enrichment of a bipotent hepatic progenitor cell from naive adult liver tissue. *Biochemical and Biophysical Research Communications*, **366**, 367-372. doi:10.1016/j.bbrc.2007.11.129

[5] Lazaro, C.A., Croager, E.J., Mitchell, C., Campbell, J.S., Yu, C., Foraker, J., Rhim, J.A., Yeoh, G.C. and Fausto, N. (2003) Establishment, characterization, and long-term maintenance of cultures of human fetal hepatocytes. *Hepatology*, **38**, 1095-106. doi:10.1053/jhep.2003.50448

[6] Kamiya, A., Kakinuma, S., Yamazaki, Y. and Nakauchi, H. (2009) Enrichment and clonal culture of progenitor cells during mouse postnatal liver development in mice. *Gastroenterology*, **137**, 1114-1126, 1126 e1-e14.

[7] Dabeva, M.D., Alpini, G., Hurston, E. and Shafritz, D.A. (1993) Models for hepatic progenitor cell activation. *Proceedings of the Society for Experimental Biology and Medicine*, **204**, 242-252. doi:10.3181/00379727-204-43660

[8] Wang, X., Foster, M., Al-Dhalimy, M., Lagasse, E., Finegold, M. and Grompe, M. (2003) The origin and liver repopulating capacity of murine oval cells. *Proceedings of the National Academy of Sciences of USA*, **100**, 11881-11888. doi:10.1073/pnas.1734199100

[9] Theise, N.D., Saxena, R., Portmann, B.C., Thung, S.N., Yee, H., Chiriboga, L., Kumar, A. and Crawford, J.M. (1999) The canals of Hering and hepatic stem cells in humans. *Hepatology*, **30**, 1425-1433. doi:10.1002/hep.510300614

[10] Jelnes, P., Santoni-Rugiu, E., Rasmussen, M., Friis, S.L., Nielsen, J.H., Tygstrup, N. and Bisgaard, H.C. (2007) Remarkable heterogeneity displayed by oval cells in rat and mouse models of stem cell-mediated liver regeneration. *Hepatology*, **45**, 1462-1470. doi:10.1002/hep.21569

[11] Jin, C., Samuelson, L., Cui, C.B., Sun, Y. and Gerber, D.A. (2011) MAPK/ERK and Wnt/beta-Catenin pathways are synergistically involved in proliferation of Sca-1 positive hepatic progenitor cells. *Biochemical and Biophysical Research Communications*, **409**, 803-807. doi:10.1016/j.bbrc.2011.05.094

[12] Ring, D.B., Johnson, K.W., Henriksen, E.J., Nuss, J.M., Goff, D., Kinnick, T.R., Ma, S.T., Reeder, J.W., Samuels, I., Slabiak, T., Wagman, A.S., Hammond, M.E. and Harrison, S.D. (2003) Selective glycogen synthase kinase 3 inhibitors potentiate insulin activation of glucose transport and utilization *in vitro* and *in vivo*. *Diabetes*, **52**, 588-595. doi:10.2337/diabetes.52.3.588

[13] Seglen, P.O. (1976) Preparation of isolated rat liver cells. *Methods in Cell Biology*, **13**, 29-83. doi:10.1016/S0091-679X(08)61797-5

[14] O'Brien, L.E., Yu, W., Tang, K., Jou, T.S., Zegers, M.M. and Mostov, K.E. (2006) Morphological and biochemical analysis of Rac1 in three-dimensional epithelial cell cultures. *Methods in Enzymology*, **406**, 676-691.

[15] Furuyama, K., Kawaguchi, Y., Akiyama, H., Horiguchi, M., Kodama, S., Kuhara, T., Hosokawa, S., Elbahrawy, A., Soeda, T., Koizumi, M., Masui, T., Kawaguchi, M., Takaori, K., Doi, R., Nishi, E., Kakinoki, R., Deng, J.M., Behringer, R.R., Nakamura, T. and Uemoto, S. (2011) Continuous cell supply from a Sox9-expressing progenitor zone in adult liver, exocrine pancreas and intestine. *Nature Genetics*, **43**, 34-41. doi:10.1038/ng.722

[16] Nierhoff, D., Ogawa, A., Oertel, M., Chen, Y.Q. and Shafritz, D.A. (2005) Purification and characterization of mouse fetal liver epithelial cells with high *in vivo* repopulation capacity. *Hepatology*, **42**, 130-139. doi:10.1002/hep.20735

[17] Quintana-Bustamante, O., Alvarez-Barrientos, A., Kofman, A.V., Fabregat, I., Bueren, J.A., Theise, N.D. and Segovia, J.C. (2006) Hematopoietic mobilization in mice increases the presence of bone marrow-derived hepatocytes via *in vivo* cell fusion. *Hepatology*, **43**, 108-116. doi:10.1002/hep.21005

[18] Fukuda, A., Kawaguchi, Y., Furuyama, K., Kodama, S., Horiguchi, M., Kuhara, T., Koizumi, M., Boyer, D.F., Fujimoto, K., Doi, R., Kageyama, R., Wright, C.V. and Chiba, T. (2006) Ectopic pancreas formation in Hes1-knockout mice reveals plasticity of endodermal progenitors of the gut, bile duct, and pancreas. *Journal of Clinical Investigation*, **116**, 1484-1493. doi:10.1172/JCI27704

3

Embryonic-like stem cells derived from postpartum placenta delivered after spotaneous labor emerging as universal prophylactic cancer vaccine

Manole Corocleanu

Private, Brasov, Romania; corocleanu@yahoo.com

ABSTRACT

In the eighth decade of the last century extensive clinical delayed-type hypersensitivity (DTH) skin tests to an intradermal injection of a pharmaceutical allogeneic human Placenta Suspension (phPS) performed in obstetrical, gynecological and control group patients have shown positive reaction in 239 patients with clinical conditions having been as histopatrhological substratum, a hypoxia-induced adaptive/reactive epithelial cell proliferation, e.g. syncytiotrophoblastic cell hyperplasia, endometrial cell hyperplasia, or different gynecological cancers. Because the immune response against phPS has shown antigenc similarities between normal placental and endometrial hyperplastic cells and different kinds of cancer cells and because many cancers adopt an embryonic stem-like gene expression pattern, it is suggested that the profile of hypoxia-promoting placental and endometrial stem cell proliferation is more embryonic-like, and that the immune respose against phPS is expected to cross-react with tumor cells *in vivo*. In the process of persistent growth and accelerated oxygen consumption by hyperplastic cytotrophoblastic cells and neoplastic cells in a hypoxic microenvironment, a basic shift in energy metabolism is accompanied by appearance of heat shock proteins (HSPs), of fetal isoenzymes and of membrane glycoproteins (reappearance of oncofetal antigens, OFAs), which, as result of their overexpression/amplification may induce a host immunological response. Thus, it is assumed that phPS prepared from full-term human placentas delivered after a spontaneous labor comprises stem/progenitor cells reverted to a proliferative embryonic stem cell-like-state upon exposure to labor-inducing intrmittent placental hypoxia and that by expressing HSP/OFAs could immunize to generate immune response againjst a variety of antigens that are shared by different kinds of epithelial cancers. This immunological feature of phPS qualifies is as a vaccine-related product that may be used for a preventive cancer vaccine when mixed with a potent adjuvant (BCG-Vaccine) and given normal healthy individuals.

Keywords: Placenta; Embryonic-Like Stem Cells; Preventive Cancer Vaccine

1. INTRODUCTION

The field of tumor immunology has made great advancements in recent years. A retrospective analysis of our previous studies [1] and our proposed pharmaceutical allogeneic human Placenta-Lysates/BCG-vaccine strategy design for cancer prevention [2], based on the assumption that placenta shares identical growth mechanisms, antigenic determinants, and immune-escape properties with cancer cells, combined with present knowledges may provide additional insight in this vaccination approach.

Proteins that are expressed by both malignant and healthy fetal tissues (the placental-fetal complex) are recognized as oncofetal antigens (OFA). These antigens are associated with cell proliferation and differentiation and are produced in high concentrations in pregnancy and malignancy [3]. Their biological role in malignancy is the suppression of the host's immune system, while in pregnancy they affect the maternal immune response, generating maternal tolerance toward the embryo [4]. On the other hand, the involvement of oncofetal antigens in both embryonic and malignant development supports the concept that oncofetal antigens may intervene in the control of maternal immune responses during pregnancy, in the manner of the host defense to carcinogenesis [5].

1.1. Human Embryonic Genes Are Re-Expressed in Cancer Cells and Are Immunogenic

Marilyn Monk *et al.* [6] have shown that processes occurring during tumorigenesis may be similar to processes occurring in early development. Human preimplantation embryonic cells are similar in phenotype to cancer cells. Both types of cell undergo deprogramming to a proliferative stem cell state and become potentially immortal and invasive. The exact nature of the initiating event is unknown but, in both processes, development and tumorigenesis, the result is genome-wide demethylation. Therefore, it might be expected that cancer cells will express genes in common with these very early embryonic cells, especially genes specifically associated with deprogramming and return to the undifferentiated and proliferative stem cell state, and the maintenance of that state.

Recently several laboratories have demonstrated that introduction of just four active genes into a mature differentiated cell can convert it into a cell with embryonic stem cell characteristics [7].

Coggin Jr., J. H., *et al.* [8,9] has identified the OFA/iLRP protein and its role as a T-cell inducing and immuno-regulating factor in fetogenesis and oncogenesis. This protein was also detected in early to mid gestation fetal cells and emerging trophoblast, hence the term "Oncofetal Antigen". It is concluded that OFA/immature LRP, the 37 kDa fetal-restricted molecule, unlike mLRP (mature LRP, MW 67 kDa), is a true "immunogenic." In breast cancer patients, Rohrer *et al.* established several OFA/iLRP-specific CD4+ and cytotoxic as well as regulatory CD8+ T cell clones. This phenomenon caused by an excess of the T cell immunogenic, 37 - 44 kDaOFA, enables the immune system to suppress Tc-mediated immunity. In other words, it is an immuno-regulatory controlled measure that prevents overproduction of Tc cells to any Tc-antigen. This immuno-regulation prevents anti-self Tc-mediated immunity and other anti-self immunity. The IL-10 inhibited Tc activity and so these cells can dampen anti-tumor immunity of whatever specificity.

During tumor development in mice and humans, oncofetal 32 - 44 kDa Ag/immature laminin receptor (OFA/iLRP)-specific Th1, CTL, and IL-10-secreting T-suppressor cells (Ts) cells are induced. The presence of too many Ts or too few effector T cells appears to predict a poor prognosis [10,11].

1.2. The Human Discarded Placentas of Healthy Newborns Comprise Embryonic-Like Stem Cells

Researchers at the University of Pittsburgh (2005) have revealed findings that some placental cells of afterbirth placenta have many of the same characteristics of embryonic stem cells and thus, placenta may yield alternative to embryonic stem cells.

Myoung Woo Lee *et al.* [12] have shown that in addition to hematopoietic stem cells (HSCs), other potential stem cells (SCs), such as mesenchymal SCs (MSCs), unrestricted somatic SCs (USSCs), cord blood-derived embryonic-like SCs (CBEs), and umbilical cord blood (UCB)-derived multipotent progenitor cells (MPCs) have been isolated from Umbilical Cord Blood and characterized.

The newly discovered human cells, named "cord blood-derived embryonic-like stem cells" or CBEs, but also, multipotent non-hematopoietic stem cells are not quite as primitive as embryonic stem cells, which can give rise to any tissue type of the body, but they appear to be much more versatile than "adult stem cells", in that they express some but not all embryonic stem cell markers.

1.3. The Human Endometrium Comprises Endometrial Regenerative Cells (ERCs)

Zhong Z. *et al.* [13] have shown that Endometrial Regenerative Cells (ERCs) are a population of mesenchymal-like cells which possesse pluripotent differentiation capacity and are characterized by unique surface markers and growth factor production. They have some degree of pluripotency similar with bone marrow derived mesenchymal stem cells (MSC) positive for some proteins distinctive of embryonic stem cells. Also, these endometrial derived stem cells possess various characteristics similar to MSC including ability to immune modulate, to induce Treg production and to induce neoangiogenesis. Immunochemical assays of cultured menstrual blood reveal that endometrial cells express embryonic-like stem cell phenotype markers (Oct4, SSEA, Nanong).

1.4. Hypoxia, Hypoxia-Inducible Factor (HIF) and the Placenta

Adelman D. M. *et al.* [14] have shown that placental development is profoundly influenced by oxygen (O_2) tension. Human cytotrophoblasts proliferate *in vitro* under low O_2 conditions but differentiate at higher O_2 levels, mimicking the developmental transition they undergo as they invade the placental bed to establish the maternal-fetal circulation *in vivo*. Hypoxia-inducible factor-1 (HIF-1), consisting of HIF-1α and ARNT subunits, activates many genes involved in the cellular and organismal response to O_2 deprivation [15].

Placental development is initiated and regulated by the hypoxic uterine environment that is already a hypoxic, 3% - 5% O_2 versus normal physiologic oxygen tension (normoxia) of approximately 8%. O_2 and the added stress of the limited O_2 diffusion stimulates trophoblasts to proliferate, migrate, differentiate, and promote maternal and fetal vascular contribution to the placenta [16,17]. In the first trimester, establishment of blood flow into the intervillous space is associated with a burst of oxidative stress at a time when placental vascular development is occurring [18].

HIF-1 is a heterodimeric transcript factor that consist of two subunits. The HIF-1 beta subunit is constitutively expressed whereas HIF-1 alfa subunit is regulated by oxigen levels. It is stable under hypoxic conditions but is rapidily degraded under normoxic conditions. After stabilization or activation, HIF-1 translocates to the nucleus where it induces the transcription of numerous downstream genes via their hypoxia response elements. One of the target genes is vascular endothelial growth factor (VEGF).

Recent reports [19] suggest that preeclampsia (PE) is associated with a Th1 predominant profile and may be considered as a failure of the tolerance system allowing the second physiological trophoblastic invasion. This Th1 predominant immunity is closely related to inflamemation, endothelial dysfunction and poor placentation [10,20].

A deficiency of regulatory T cells may play a role in the pathophysiology of preeclampsia. Immunological data [21] have shown that the increased levels of T CD4 (+) 45RO (+) and T CD8 (+) CD25 (+) cells can suggest the activation of CD4 (+) and CD8 (+) T lymphocytes in pre-eclampsia. It seems possible that the activation of T lymphocytes is associated with the deficiency of T regulatory cells in PE. A decreased number of T (reg) cells were present in pre-eclampsia, and these changes might break the maternal tolerance to the fetus.

Tereza Cindrova-Davies *et al.* [22] have shown that labor is a powerful inducer of placental oxidative stress, inflammatory cytokines, angiogenic regulators, and heat shock proteins as result of acute hypoxia/reoxygenation process. These findings are consistent with intermittent perfusion being the initiating cause. Uterine contractions during labor are known to be associated with intermittent utero-placental perfusion. The oxidative stress is a potent inducer of placental synthesis and release of pro-inflammatory factors. At cellular level the transcripts changed in the same direction as observed in preeclampsia, suggesting that the placenta responds similarly to the oxidative stress induced during labor and in preeclampsia.

1.5. Heat Shock Proteins (HSP) and Immune Function

HSPs are evolutionarily ancient and highly conserved intracellular molecular chaperones. They are constitutively expressed in the cells, but are highly induced by different stresses such as heat, oxidative stress, oxygen radicals, or transformation. HSPs also perform immune functions. They have the inherent property of binding non-covalently to the peptides generated within cells as a result of degradation of cellular proteins, self and alien. HSP-peptide complexes are intracellular under normal conditions and have a protective function. On the other hand, extracellular located or membrane-bound HSPs mediate immunological functions [23]. It is becoming evident that oxidative stress is at the heart of the regulation mechanisms that maintain a balance between efficient regeneration and proper control of stem cell function. This activity of stem cells, however, has to be carefully controlled, as too much stem cell activity can cause diseases like cancer. Cellular stress may give rise to misfolded or mutated "self" proteins, which in turn result in the presentation of sequences being hidden from the immune system under normal healthy conditions. Such hidden cryptic epitopes of "self" proteins are considered as endogenous danger signal and also "nonself" or new peptides by the host's immune system because of the fact T cells were not exposed to these hidden epitopes during positive and negative selection in the thymus. A large variety of chaperoned antigenic peptides could be tumor antigens. Such HSPs are expected to carry a repertoire of tumor antigens, some of which would be subdominant or cryptic epitopes and seen by the host's immune system as nonself peptides.These consequences point to a key role of heat shock proteins in fundamental immunological phenomena such as activation of antigen presenting cells, indirect presentation (or cross-priming), and chaperoning of peptides during antigen presentation [24]. Yosino I. *et al.* [25] in their research conclude that HPS70-reactive CD4+ T cells exist in tumor tissue. These tumor-infiltrating lymphocytes (TIL) recgnize stressed cells and seem to play a Th1-like role that may support antitumor T cell responses at local tumor sites.

1.6. The Role of CD40/CD40L in Regulating Immune Response, Epithelial Cell Growth and Differentiation and in Induction of Cell Cycle Blockage and/or Apoptosis of Epithelial Cancer Cells

Young L. S. *et al.* [26] have shown that the wide expression of CD40 in normal epithelial cells and carcinoma cells suggests that this receptor has important, additional influences beyond that of regulating immune responses. The major ligand for the external domain of CD40 is CD154 (CD40L), a member of the TNF superfamily. The most abundant source of CD154 is activated T lymphocytes. While CD40-CD40 ligand interactions are known to regulate B cell proliferation and differenttiation, much less is known about the role this receptor plays on other cell types, especially those of nonhemopoietic origin. CD40 is expressed and functional on human epidermal basal cells and that, on these cells, CD40 ligation may be a signal for limitation of cell growth and induction of differentiation [27]. A direct growth-inhibitory effect can be found when ligated CD40 is on human breast, ovarian, cervical, bladder, non-small cell lung, and squamous epithelial carcinoma cells. This effect is related to the induction of cell cycle blockage and/or apoptosis. The CD40/CD154 couple plays a critical role both in humoral and cellular immune response. The CD40/CD40L system, a key regulator and amplifier of immune reactivity is required for antigen-presenting cell activation as it induces costimulatory molecules and cytokine synthesis. Thus, CD40-CD40L interactions are crucial in the delivery of T cell help for CTL priming. A natural antagonist of CD40/CD154 interaction is the soluble form of CD40 (sCD40) which has been shown to inhibit the binding of CD154 to CD40 *in vitro*.. High levels of sCD40 could compete for the ligation of membrane CD40 on CD154 thus resulting in inhibition of antibody production. The rapid up- and down-regulation of CD154 on the surface of T cells is an obvious and important way of control. In a first step, CD154 is quickly expressed upon T-cell receptor engagement and in a second step the CD40 itself contributes to down-regulating CD154 expression on T cells as sustained interaction between CD40/CD154 leads to endocytosis of the ligand. Although this mechanism is considered to be the major way the CD40/CD154 interaction is down-regulated, the production of a soluble form of CD40 (sCD40) could also be involved, demonstrating a potential antagonistic role for sCD40 in the immune response. However, little is known about the mechanism leading to sCD40 production. The process of shedding is important, as it up-regulates the production of soluble receptors that compete with the membrane receptor for ligand binding, and also reduces the amount of surface receptor, thus modulating the capacity of the cell to signal and thus, inducing immunosuppression. Given the antagonistic activity of sCD40 on the CD40/CD154 interaction, this shedding mechanism might represent an important negative feedback control of CD40 functions [28]. As CD40-CD154 (CD40L) pathway has been shown to attribute to the regulation of T-cell activation, both by independently costimulating T cells and at least in part by up-regulating CD80/CD86 molecules on APCs, suppression may be generated from fully differentiated Th1 effector cells by stimulation with antigen in the absence of costimulation.

In the light of the above studies, this paper provides further a review and a retrospective analysis in summary of our previous published [1] and unpublished investigations to answer the question whether Placenta Suspension prepared upon Filatov's method from the allogeneic human placenta-tissue after a live full-term delivery, expresses trophoblast cross-reactive antigens present on certain types of trophoblast cells and on transformed cells in the sense that both types of cells express embryonic-like features.

1.7. Preventive Cancer Vaccine Based on Placental Stem/Progenitor Embryonic-Like Cells of Full-Term Human Placentas Delivered after Spontaneous Labor

1.7.1. Background

Based on the assumption that developing placenta shares identical growth mechanisms, antigenic determinants, and immune-escape properties with cancer cells, immunological cross-reactivity between placental antigens and cancer antigens was investigated.

1.7.2. Methods Summary

In the eighth decade of the last century extensive clinical delayed-type hypersensitivity (DTH) skin tests to an intradermal injection in the 1/3 upper anterior surface of the forearm of 0.2 ml of a pharmaceutical allogeneic human Placenta Suspension (ph PS) (Suspensio Placentae pro injectionibus, Odesski zavod Hinfarmapreparatov, Odessa, former USSR), prepared upon Filatov's method from cryopreserved and mechanically disrupted of full term human placentas delvered after spontaneous labor were performed in obstetrical (150 pts.), gynecological (175 pts.) patients with different clinical conditions.

All tests were made under institutional approval and with documented informed consent.

DTH reaction is an immune function assessment that measures the presence of activated T-cells that recognise certain substances. Similar to the mantoux skin test for tuberculosis, a mononuclear cell response is mounted at the site of antigen challenge if the patient has preexisting T cell immunity.

1.7.3. Results

239 patients with different clinical conditions, such as hypertensive disorders during pregnancy (98 pts. with preexisting hypertension, gestational hypertension, preeclampsia, superimposed preeclampsia), abnormal perimenopausal and menopausal uterine bleeding (141 pts.) have shown positive cutaneous delayed-type hypersensitivity (DTH) reactions to phPS.

According to the clinical and histopathlogical diagnosis, two large groups have resulted in which obstetrical and gynecological patients with different clinical conditions have shown positive cutaneous DTH-response to phPS: a group of benign obstetrical and gynecological clinical conditions having as histopathological substratum adaptive syncytiotrophoblast-cell hyperplasia (98 pts.), or reactive/adaptive endometrial cell hyperplasia (76 pts.) and a group of different gynecological cancers (65 pts.).

2. CONCLUDING REMARKS

2.1. Hypertensive Disorders in Pregnancy Stimulates Proliferation of Cytotrophoblastic Stem Cells That Adopt an Embryonic-Like Stem Cell Antigenic Profile

Syncytiotrophoblast hyperplasia is commonly seen in patients with hypertension, preeclampsia and occasionally diabetes. Traditionally these clinical conditions have been associated with "placental insufficiency". A compromised maternal circulation in the intervillous space may create a state of true or relative hypoxia that stimulates proliferation of cytotrophoblast stem-like cells that differentiate into the syncytiotrophoblast on the villosities surface in order to increase the exchange area of the placenta. Hypoxic clinical conditions, such as arterial hypertension, diabetes, but also unopposed estrogen stimulation of endometrial growth are also seen in patients with perimenopausal or postmenopausal endometrial cell hyperplasia which have shown positive skin reaction to phPS.

Because the immune response against phPS have shown antigenc similarities between normal placental and endometrial hyperplastic cells and different kind of cancer cells and because many cancers adopt an embryonic stem-like gene expression pattern, it is suggested that the profile of hypoxia-promoting placental and endometrial stem cell proliferation is more embryonic-like. Thus it is assuming that the hyperplastic cells in cytotrophoblastic cell hyperplasia and in abundant endometrial growth, as result of perfusion-limited or diffusion-limited hypoxic clinical conditions, acquire characteristic traits by reactivating genes normally expressed in emerging trophoblast and in transforming cells. It is considered that the potentialities of regeneration of the cytotrophoblast are possible by remodeling the "cytotrophoblast stem-like cells" and that the presence of "adult stem cells" in the endometrial mesenchyme highlights their importance in the regenesis and remodeling of endometrial structures.

2.2. Labor Intermittent Hypoxia Shifts the Antigenic Profile of Induced Placental Proliferating Stem Cells to One That Is More Embryonic-Like

We hypothesized also that labor intermittent hypoxia-induced placental stem/progenitor embryonic-like cells of afterbirth placenta could immunize to generate immune response against a variety of antigens that are shared by different kind of epithelial cancers. This raises the exciting possibility of developing a prophylactic vaccine capable of preventing the appearance of various types of cancers in humans.

Hypoxia has shown to play an important role in favoring the stem cell state, but also in promoting stem cell proliferation as result of the ability of adult stem cells capable of genomic reprogramming upon exposure to a novel hypoxic environment to adopt the expression profile to one that is more embryonic-like and express some but not all embryonic stem cell markers (multipotent non-hematopoietic stem cells). Also, cancer transformation is intimately coupled with the appearance" of embryonic stem cell-like features, in that both overexpress oncofetal developmental antigens (OFA) and relay exclusively on glucose metabolism for their energy required for rapid cell growth and division.

Persistent growth and accelerated oxygen consumption by hyperplastic placental cells and hyperplastic endometrial cells in a hypoxic microenvironment, a basic shift in energy metabolism is accompanied by appearance of heat shock proteins (HSPs), increase of fetal isoenzymes and of membrane glycoproteins (oncofetal antigens, OFA), which, as result of their overexpression/amplification may induce a host immune response. Both types of cell undergo deprogramming to a embryonic-like stem cell state similar in phenptype to cancer cells. Together, these findings suggest that HIF targets may act as key inducers of a dynamic state of stemness in pathologic conditions and that tissue regeneration after injury appears to recapitulate the pathway of embryonic tissue development.

The up-modulation of OFA gene expression in hyperplastic placental and endometrial cells and in tumors might be related to the requirement of proliferating cells for increased protein synthesis to face the new growth needs of these cells closely related to cell proliferation, that classified it as oncogene and that by overexpression/amplification becomes immunogenic.

The mechanism by which overexpression converts a self proteine into an immunologically recognizable antigen has not been completely elucidated. Most likely the overexpressed protein either becomes more consistently presented to the immune system or the density of presentation crosses the threshold needed for T cell stimulation.

The abundance of HSPs in the hyperplastic placental and endometrial stem/progenitor embryonic-like cells in response to hypoxia, or in tumor cells may make overexpressed antigens in these proliferative cells intrinsically more cross-presentable to the host DCs for generating protective antitumor activity.

2.3. Preeclampsia Is Characterizeed by Hypoxia-Reactivated Placental Stem/Progenitor Cells Reverted to a Proliferative Embryonic Stem-Like State and a Prdominant Th1-Cell Immune Profile

Concerning the preeclampsia, reactivation of the cytotrophoblast as result of placental hypoxia and unusual immune response to self-antigens of the emerging trophoblast, suggests that proinflammatory cytokines and vascular oxidative stress play a role in causing hypertension by activating multiple neurohumoral and endothelial factors and that ligation of CD40 on proliferating extravillous trophoblast stem/progenitor embryonic-like cells, by CD40 ligand (CD154) on CD4+ T cells, may lead to limitation of cell growth and induction of incomplete differentiation and inadequate invasion of the trophoblast and thus, to ineffective vascular remodeling of the uterine spiral arteries that results in insufficient placental perfusion as well as widespread dysfunction of the maternal vascular endothelium [20].

In conclusion, it is assuming that CD4+ T cells frequently recognize nonmutated "self" antigens that are overexpressed by both hyperplastc cytotrophoblastic and endometrial stem cells, but also growing tumor cells. Since patients with positive skin DTH-reaction to phPS can harbor CD4+ T cells specific for non-mutated, differentiation antigens overexpressed by hyperplastic placental embryonic-like stem cells and neoplastic cells, vaccination might reasonably be expected to amplify the frequency and strength of these pre-exsiting responses or perhaps induce some *de novo* reactions.

2.4. Placental Embryonc-Like Stem Cells of Human Full-Term Placentas Delivered after Spontaneous Labor Shares Antigens in Common with Different Kind of Epithelial Cancer Cells and Thus PhPS Emerges as a Preventave Cancer Vaccine-Related Product

Labor-induced intermittent hypoxia promotes proliferation of placental stem/progenitor cells reverted to an embryonic-like stem cell state by expressing some but not all embryonic stem cell markers and thus, full-term human placenta delivered after spontaneous labor (afterbirth placenta) based on proliferating cord blood-derived embryonic-like stem cells, hypoxia-induced multipotent non-hematopoietic stem cells mixed with other proliferating placental matrix-stem cell populations could immunize to generate immune response againjst a variety of antigens that are shared by different kind of epithelial cancers. The abundance of HSPs in the undifferentiated state of proliferating placental embryonic-like stem cells may make overexpressed OFA antigens in these cells intrinsically more cross-presentable to the host DCs for generating protective antitumor activity both in mother and in newborn. Such a model, although attractive, remains speculative. However, together these findings suggest that the phPS could be considered as a placental embryonic-like stem cell vaccine and that the cutaneous DTH-reaction to phPS is a Th1-cell response to antigens expressed by these cells and which are also cross-reactive with antigens expressed by different epithelial cancer cells. This feature of phPS qualifies it as a multiepitope vaccine-related product that may be used as universal preventive cancer vaccine. Through imparting exogenous and activating endogenous anti-tumor mechanisms within normal healthy individuals by utilizing universal, non-mutated oncofetal antigen vaccines, e.g. phPS vaccine based on embryonic-like stem cells, the immune system is able to destroy nascent cancerous cells before accumulating mutational changes are occuring. The use of overexpressed proteins, as tumor-associated antigens yelds rational targets for specific immunoprevention.

In cancer prophylaxis, we need to destroy just a single cell—the one transformed cell that may give rise to malignancy. Among tumor associated antigens are antigens upregulated in malignant transformation e.g. oncofetal antigens-carcinoembryonic antigen (CEA), alphafetoprotein (AFP), growth factor receptors-Her2/neu, telomerase and p53. A prophylactic vaccination that involves a number of shared antigens may represent a strength of this vaccination approach in as much as immune recognition of multiple antigens would make it less likely for nascent tumor cells to escape immune detection and destruction.

3. DISCUSSIONS

3.1. A Novel Hypoxic Environment Shifts the Antigenic Profile of Adult Stem Cells to One That Is More Embryonic-Like

A corollary of the stem cell theory of the origin of cancer is that cancers contain the same functional cell populations as normal tissues: stem cells, transit-amplifying cells and mature cells. Cancer tissue differs from normal tissue in that the transit-amplifying cells that do not differentiate to mature cells (maturation arrest) accumulate in cancer, whereas in normal tissue differentiate so that they no longer divide (terminal differentiation) [29]. Unrestained growth and accelerated oxigen consumpton by proliferating stem/progenitor (transit-amplifying) cells of normal tissue, or at distance from blood vessels indicating a hypoxic microenvironment, displays gene expression signatures characteristic of human embryonic stem-like cells, or by prmoting genomic instabillity drives transformation of stem/progenitor cells also into a stable para-embryonal condition and thus, both may be recognized as dangerous by the immune system. The premise that cancer cells share the expression of oncofetal antigens with stem/progenitor embryonic-like cells and that the immune response against these antigens is cross-protective against cancer and that the disease only manifests if immune response are impeded in protecting against transformation, the use of overexpressed proteins of these stem/progenitor embryonic-like cells, as tumor-associated antigens yelds rational targets for specific cancer immunoprevention.

3.2. The Soluble Forms of Membrane Molecule CD40 (sCD40) May Have a Role in Modulating Antitumor Responses

Systemic immunity to some gynecological tumors and to syncytiotrophoblast hyperplasia as measured by skin delayed-type hypersensitivity response to phPS strongly support the notion that the host immune system, harboring specific CD40+ T cells, recognizes the presence of the reexpressed and overexpressed oncofetal antigens (OFAs) on transformed stem/progenitor cells, or on placental stem/progenitor cells reverted to a proliferative embryonic-like stem cell status as result of genomic reprogramming during labor exposure to a novel hypoxic environment, and that can remain alive for days after delivery.

Unfortunately, this proof that the immune system can recognize spontaneous tumors, is for no lasting benefit to the patient. It appears that it is the immune system itself that is hindering its own activity of defense through interference with inhibitory immunological checkpoints controlling T cell activation.

The ways tumors become unrecognizable to the immune system are various and numerous.

Darrasse-Jèze G., Bergot A-S., *et al.* [30] emphsize that the relative activation speed of self-specific memory Tregs (regulatorys) versus that of tumor-specific naive Teffs (effector) at the time of tumor emergence dictates tumor outcome. Thus, CD4+-cell responses can also elicit not only stimulatory but also suppressive immunity. It is becoming clear that T regs play a pivotal role in the tumor progression and the suppression of tumor immunity. Furthermore, effector/memory regulatory T cells increased as the primary tumor progressed. Data suggest that effector/memory Treg cells are responsible for the loss of concomitant tumor immunity associated with tumor progression [31].

Recently it was shown that T cell help for CTLs is critically dependent on interaction between CD40L expressed by Th cells and CD40 expressed by APCs.

CD40-CD154 interactions are of central importance and pivotal in the induction of cellular immune responses to many antigens [26]. Several lines of evidence indicate that CD40 signaling is part of an important pathway in T cell-dependent antigen presentig cell (APC or DC) activation. CD40 ligation on antigen-presenting cells (APCs) by CD40L (CD154) on CD4+ T cells was found to be necessary to induce CD8+ T cell priming by APC. This pathway play a critical role in the induction type-1 cytokine responses of protective immunity. Dendritic cell (DC) exist in two stages: Immature and mature. Mature DC cells prime T cells, whereas immature DC can induce tolerance to the presented antigens. The immature DCs are non immunologically quiescent; they have been shown to induce T cell tolerance *in vivo* through the induction of T cell anergy, direct depletion of T cells, or by generation of regulatory or suppressor cells that block the function of other T effector T cells. For full maturation and aquisition of T cell priming capacity DCs need to be "licensed", which can occur by receiving pro-inflammatory signals in the form of CD4 T cell "help" through CD40-CD40L interaction. Adequate activation of T cells requires multiple signals from the DC to the T cell. MHC-peptide recognised by the T cell recptor (TCR) on the T cell is crucial for initial activation, but will lead to anergy or non-responsiveness without appropriate additional costimulation provided by interaction between CD28 on the T cell and B7.1/B7.2 on the DC. Besides help in CD8+ T cell priming and maintenance, CD4 T cells have been shown to recruit and activate various cell populations into the tumor environment, provide bystander mediated killing and affect angiogenesis.

Natural killer (NK) and Natural Killer T (NKT) cells are innate immune cells critical for the first line of defense against tumorigenesis. Although NKT cells possess NK-like cytolytic activity, their activation results in rapid production of IFN-γ and expression of CD40L, thus providing help for activation of CD40-expressing APCs and generation of cellular and humoral immune responses.

Therefore, it has been shown that a dominant pathway of CD4+ help is via antigen-presenting cell (APC) activation through engagement of CD40 by CD40 ligand (CD154) on NKT cells and CD4+ T cells. CD40L is mainly expressed transiently on activated CD4+ helper T cells subsequent to recognition of MHC-peptide complexes. It is required for antigen-presenting cell activetion as it induces costimulatory molecules and cytokine synthesis. It has been suggested that in absence of a strong "danger" signal at this time contributes to the ability of newly forming tumors to avoid recognition by the host immune response. Finally, priming of CD8+ cytotoxic T lymphocytes generally requires help provided by CD4+, and the CD40-CD40L interaction was shown to be essential in the CTL priming via activated DCs.

Also, CD40 is expressed and functional on human epithelial cells, and on these cells, CD40 ligation may be a signal for limitation of cell growth and induction of differentiation [26,27]. Ligation of CD40 on cancer cells was also found to produce a direct growth-inhibitory effect through cell cycle blockage and/or apoptosis with no overt side effects on normal cells. But, the natural antagonist of CD40/CD154 interaction is the soluble form of CD40 (sCD40) which has been shown to inhibit the binding of CD154 to CD40 *in vitro*. High levels of sCD40, which are often over-expressed in tumors, could compete for the ligation of membrane CD40 on CD154, thus resulting in inhibition of antibody production, but also in impeding T cell activation and in limitation of growth-inhibitory effect of cancer cells by CD 154 on CD40 T cells. The rapid up- and down-regulation of CD154 on the surface of T cells is an obvious and important way of control. In a first step, CD154 is quickly expressed upon T-cell receptor engagement and in a second step the CD40 itself contributes to down-regulating CD154 expression on T cells as sustained interaction between CD40/CD154 leads to endocytosis of the ligand [7]. Given the antagonistic activity of sCD40 on the CD40/CD154 interaction, this shedding mechanism might represent an important negative feedback control of CD40 functions, and thus impairing of CD4 T cells in inducing memory-effector CD8 T cells (Tc). As all DC types are sensitive to T-cell feedback signals delivered by activated T cells through CD40 ligand (CD40L) and at least in part by up-regulating CD80/CD86 molecules on APCs, suppression may be generated from fully differentiated Th1 effector cells by stimulation with antigen in the absence of costimulation.

Barry D. Hock. *et al.* [32] have shown that CD40 plays a critical role in immunoregulation, suggesting that sCD40 may have a role in modulating antitumor responses and also may be a useful prognostic marker. The release of soluble forms of membrane molecules provides an important mechanism by which cells can either enhance or inhibit the signals delivered by their respective membrane-bound counterparts, suggesting that *in vivo* release of functional sCD40 would be immunomodulatory. The release of sCD40 by the immune system and/or by malignant cells provides a potentially powerful mechanism for regulating antitumor responses by modulating the interaction of mCD40 with its ligands.

On the other hand effective activation of T cells requires engagement of two separate T-cell receptors. The antigen-specific T-cell receptor (TCR) binds foreign peptide antigen-MHC complexes, and the CD28 receptor binds to the B7 (CD80/CD86) costimulatory molecules expressed on the surface of antigen-presenting cells (APC). The simultaneous triggering of these T-cell surface receptors with their specific ligands results in an activation of this cell. In contrast, CTLA-4 (CD152) is a distinct T-cell receptor that, upon binding to B7 molecules, sends an inhibitory signal to T cell activation. CD86 could be more important for initiating T-cell responses, while CD80 could be more significant for maintaining these immune responses [33].

This interpretation assumes that CD28 functions not as an "on-off" switch but rather as a kind of "rheostat" which, depending on the strength and/or duration of its engagement by B7 molecules, can display a degree of plasticity in the intracellular signals it generates [33].

Most $CD4^+$ T cells belong to either the Th1 or Th2 subsets. However ~10% of them do not. These so-called T-regulatory (Treg) cells. The CTLA-4 molecules on Treg cells bind very tightly to the B7 molecules on antigen-presenting dendritic cells and B cells. Once bound, they kill the target (by secreting perforins). Treg cells can also kill cytotoxic T lymphocytes (CTL) and natural killer (NK) cells.

Consistent with a B7 "competition model" because CTLA-4 has been estimated to have 50 - 100-fold higher affinity to B7 than CD28, it is conceivable that the T reg cells, are competitively engaging available B7 molecules on the APCs, thereby preventing CD28 signaling, and subsequent T cell activation in effector T cells. [34] The co-existence of tumor specific immunity with a progressing tumor is observed in a variety of experimental systems and remains one of the major paradoxes of tumor immunology. It appears that it is the immune system itself that is hindering its own activity of defense. This behavior marks a resemblance to that of the embryo and of cancer [35].

The above observations lead to the conclusion that re-expression and overexpression of the trophoblast cross-reactive antigens present on placental hyperplasic cells, but also on neoplastic cells and continuously shedding of CD40 (sCD40) represent an adaptive response of these cells to natural selection pressures as a biological response to resist immunological recognition and rejection by the host. Inhibition of the CD/E (expressing) 40 pathway by increased levels of soluble CD40 receptor (sCD40) which reduces availability, may impede the immune system from mounting appropriate humoral and cell-mediated responses against precancerous cells Given the antagonistic activity of sCD40 on the CD40/CD154 interaction, this shedding mechanism might represent an important negative feedback control of CD40 functions, suggesting that sCD40 may have a role in modulating a pre-existing or *de novo* anti-tumor responses through interference with inhibitory immunological check points controlling T cell activation.

3.3. Placental Stem/Progenitor Embryonic-Like Cells Based Cellular Vaccine an Efficient Immuno Preventive of Human Malignancies

To overcome these escape mechanisms and to acquire the goal of an optimal adaptive immune response particularly to reexpression of embryonic proteins that begin to be overexpressed in tumor cells early in their transformation and which can be considered as non-self by the immune system, it proposed a vaccination strategy design by intradermal injection of a pharmaceutical human allogeneic Placenta Suspension (phPS), prepared upon Filatov's method and admixed with BCG Vaccine ("danger" signal) in normal healthy individuals to induce activated/memory T effector cells (amTeffs). This cross-priming of the tumor cells overexpressed antigen-specific response by potent APC is a major mechanism of the developing integrated endogenous immune response, thereby shifting the balance from tolerance to activation induction, and/or rejuvenating functionally inferior responses of the exausted T cells.

Activated Th1 cells have longevity compared with other activated immune cells (APCs and CTL) and are conventionally viewed as responsible for immune memory, capable of revitalizing the immune response if a specific antigen is reencountered, including promtly function of CD40/CD40L interaction, prior to the release of sCD40 by the immune system and/or by transformed cells. The presence of activated/memory T effector cells (amTeffs) at the time of tumor emergence shifts the Treg/Teff balance toward efficient antitumor immune response. Alternatively, or in addition, the CD4 T cells may be required for activation of macrophages and dendritic cells, an event crucial for killing of transformed cells. This antisupressive approach reverses the host's immune factors that confer a survival advantage to tumor emergence and require an intact immune system to function.

The biological adjuvant Bacillus Calmette Guerin-Vaccine (BCG-Vaccine) takes advantage of the fact that it is an immunogenic compound, naturally recognized as foreign and known to induce migration of APCs to the site of delivery. APCs responding to the adjuvant stimulation are thus able to coincidentally capture and process placental antigens present in the inflammatory milieu.

Becker Th. *et al.* [36] have suggested that CD40 is a cochaperone-like receptor mediating the uptake of exogenous Hsp70-peptide complexes by macrophages and dendritic cells. For the generation of potent T cell immune responses against self-tumor Ags, Hsp70 Ag from Mycobacterium tuberculosis was shown to induce Th1-polarized cytokine responses and activate DCs via binding with CD40 (perhaps via promoting cross-talk between various inflammatory cells recruited at the vaccine site). Although the Ag targeting alone, without activation of dendritic cells (DCs), is proposed to induce tolerance, the vaccines expressing self-tumor Ags is rendered immunogenic if targeted to the APCs using mycobacterial Hsp70 Ag [36] and thus, eliciting long-term protective CD8+ T cell-mediated memory responses effective in killing the emerging tumor cells.

At the same time the immune response is mediated through the release of different cytokines which can influence the synthesis and actions of one another in the setting of an immunoregulating cytokine network, shaping an environment in which the presence of active/memory T effector cells (am Teffs) at the very time of tumor emergence, are able to bypass the tumor immunity mediated by self-specific memory regulatory T cells. These two aspects of a preventive vaccination with multiepitope phPS/BCG-Vaccine might be useful for generating an immune response against a broad-spectrum of cancers, thus serving as a universal cancer vaccine.

The possibility of inducing long-term protection against tumors by vaccination at the earliest signs of its development has the potential to cause a dramatic paradigm shift in the prevention of tumors.

The rationale for prevention is strong because, in that setting one deals with an immune system that is neither impaired by tumor- and treatment-induced suppression nor tolerant to tumor-associated antigens that have been encountered in the absence of correct presentation and costimulatory/danger signals. On the other hand, a future success of cancer prevention will depend on how effectively a preventive vaccination strategy simultaneously acts on emerging pretumor cells as well as on its microenvironment [37].

Conceptually, to avoid the regulatory T cells' immune suppression that develops in tumor-bearing patients, vaccination with a pharmaceutical allogenic human Placenta Suspension prepared upon Filatov's method, after a "danger signal" is added e.g. BCG-Vaccine, would be capable of eliciting immunological responses in normal healthy individuals, not only to marker antigens shared between the Placenta-Suspension preparation and neoplasia, but also by introducing a new environment of T-cell-induced cytokines, that provide a more "complete" immune response, to prevent tumor development far into future, by inhibition, or by elimination of transformed cells at their earliest manifestation. Thus, active immunoprevention uses the host's immune cells and requires an intact immune system to function.

Using of isolated labor intermittent hypoxia-induced placental stem/progenitor embryonic-like cells of afterbirth placenta per se, or of phPS prepared upon Filatov's method, as a vaccine-related product for a preventive cancer vaccine, warrants further investigation.

The above hypothesis is rising as a challenge to the scientific community in the hope that it will cause an examination of this matter.

REFERENCES

[1] Corocleanu, M. (1981) Humoral and cellular reactions to placental antigens in women with pathological pregnancies and cancer patients. *Revue Roumaine de Biochimie*, **18**, 7-13.

[2] Corocleanu, M. (2008) A possible "universal" cancer vaccine that might cause an immune response against emerging cancer cells that originate from any tissue. *Medical Hypothesis*, **70**, 381-383.

http://dx.doi.org/10.1016/j.mehy.2007.04.040

[3] Redman, C.W.G. (1986) Immunology of the placenta. *Clinical Obstetrics and Gynecology*, **16**, 469.

[4] Hamilton, M.S. (1983) Maternal immune responses to oncofetal antigens. *Journal of Reproductive Immunology*, **5**, 249. http://dx.doi.org/10.1016/0165-0378(83)90252-8

[5] Sarandakou, A., *et al.* (2007) Tumor markers in biological fluids associated with pregnancy. *Critical Reviews in Clinical Laboratory Sciences*, **44**, 151-178. http://dx.doi.org/10.1080/10408360601003143

[6] Marilyn, M., *et al.* (2001) Human embrionic genes re-expressed in cancer cells. *Oncogene*, **20**, 8085-8091. http://dx.doi.org/10.1038/sj.onc.1205088

[7] Yu, J.Y., *et al.* (2007) Induced pluripotent stem cell lines derived from human somatic cells. *Science*, **318**, 1917-1920. http://dx.doi.org/10.1126/science.1151526

[8] Coggin Jr., J.H., Barsoum, A.L., Rohrer, J.W., Tucker, J.A. and Dyess, D.L. (2001) Materno-fetal immunobiology hypothesis: Immature laminin receptor protein is a primitive, species conserved, universal embryonic T and B cell immunogenic providing both maternal and fetal protection. *Modern Aspects of Immunobiology*, **2**, 84-91.

[9] Coggin Jr., J.H. and Anderson, N.G. (1974) Cancer, differentiation and embryonic antigens: Some central problems. *Advances in Cancer Research*, **19**, 105-165. http://dx.doi.org/10.1016/S0065-230X(08)60053-6

[10] Siegel, S., *et al.* (2006) Identification of HLA-A*0201-presented T cell epitopes derived from the oncofetal antigen-immature laminin receptor protein in patients with hematological malignancies. *The Journal of Immunology*, **176**, 6935-6944.

[11] Rohrer, J.W., *et al.* (1999) Human breast carcinoma patients develop clonable oncofetal antigen-specific effector and regulatory T lymphocytes. *Journal of Immunology*, **162**, 6880-6892.

[12] Lee, M.W., *et al.* (2010) Stem and progenitor cells in human umbilical cord blood. *International Journal of Hematology*, **92**, 45-51. http://dx.doi.org/10.1007/s12185-010-0619-4

[13] Zhong, Z., *et al.* (2009) Feasibility investigation of allogeneic endometrial regenerative cells. *Journal of Translational Medicine*, **7**, 15. http://dx.doi.org/10.1186/1479-5876-7-15

[14] Adelman, D.M., *et al.* (2000) Placental cell fates are regulated *in vivo* by HIF-mediated hypoxia responses. *Genes & Development*, **14**, 3191-3203.

[15] Fryer, B.H., *et al.* (2006) Hypoxia, HIF and the placenta, *Cell Cycle*, **5**, 495-498. http://dx.doi.org/10.4161/cc.5.5.2497

[16] Pugh, C.W., *et al.* (2003) Regulation of angiogenesis by hypoxia, role of the HIF system. *Nature Medicine*, **9**, 677-684. http://dx.doi.org/10.1038/nm0603-677

[17] Myatt, L., *et al.* (2004) Oxidative stress in the placenta, *Histochemistry and Cell Biology*, **122**, 369-382. http://dx.doi.org/10.1007/s00418-004-0677-x

[18] Vaiman D. *et al.* (2005) Hypoxia-activated genes from early placenta are elevated in pre-eclampsia, but not in intra-uterine growth retardation. *BMC Genomics*, **6**, 111. http://dx.doi.org/10.1186/1471-2164-6-111

[19] Shigeru, S., *et al.* (2003) Th1/Th2 balance in preeclampsia. *Journal of Reproductive Immunology*, **59**, 161-173. http://dx.doi.org/10.1016/S0165-0378(03)00045-7

[20] Darmochwal-Kolarz, D., *et al.* (2007) Activated T lymphocytes in pre-eclampsia. *American Journal of Reproductive Immunology*, **58**, 39-45. http://dx.doi.org/10.1111/j.1600-0897.2007.00489.x

[21] Sasaki, Y., *et al.* (2007) Proportion of peripheral blood and decidual CD(4+) CD25(bright) regulatory T cells in pre-eclampsia. *Clinical & Experimental Immunology*, **149**, 139-145. http://dx.doi.org/10.1111/j.1365-2249.2007.03397.x

[22] Cindrova-Davies, T., *et al.* (2007) Oxidative stress, gene expression, and protein changes induced in the human placenta during labor. *American Journal of Pathology*, **171**, 1168-1179. http://dx.doi.org/10.2353/ajpath.2007.070528

[23] Schmitt, E., *et al.* (2007) Intracellular and extracellular functions of heat shock proteins: Repercussion in cancer therapy. *Journal of Leukocyte Biology*, **81**, 15-27. http://dx.doi.org/10.1189/jlb.0306167

[24] Srivastava, P. (2002) Interaction of heat shock proteins with peptides and antigen-presenting cells: Chaperoning of the innate and adaptive immune responses. *Annual Review of Immunology*, **20**, 395-425. http://dx.doi.org/10.1146/annurev.immunol.20.100301.064801

[25] Yoshino, I., *et al.* (1994) Human tumor-infiltrating CD4+ T cells react to B cell lines expressing heat sock protein 70. *The Journal of Immunology*, **153**, 4149-4158.

[26] Young, L.S., *et al.* (1998) CD40 and epithelial cells: Across the great divide. *Immunology Today*, **19**, 502. http://dx.doi.org/10.1016/S0167-5699(98)01340-1

[27] Peguet-Navarro, J., *et al.* (1997) CD40 ligation of human keratinocytes inhibits their proliferation and induces their differentiation. *The Journal of Immunology*, **158**, 144-152.

[28] Contin Cécile, J., *et al.* (2003) Membrane-anchored CD40 is processed by the tumor necrosis factor-α-converting enzyme. *Journal of Biological Chemistry*, **278**, 32801-32809. http://dx.doi.org/10.1074/jbc.M209993200

[29] Stewart, S. (2008) Alpa-fetoprotein, stem cells and cancer: How study of the production of alpha-fetoprotein during chemical hepatocarcinogenesis led to raffirmation of the stem cell theory of cancer. *Tumor Biology*, **29**, 161-180. http://dx.doi.org/10.1159/000143402

[30] Darrasse-Jèze, G., Bergot, A.-S., *et al.* (2009) Tumor emergence is sensed by self-specific CD44hi memory Tregs that create a dominant tolerogenic environment for tumors in mice. *Journal of Clinical Investigation*, **119**, 2648-2662.

[31] Goreliki, E. (1983) Concomitant immunity and the resistance to a second tumor challenge. *Advances in Cancer Research*, **39**, 71-120. http://dx.doi.org/10.1016/S0065-230X(08)61033-7

[32] Hock, B.D., *et al.* (2006) Circulating levels and clinical

significance of soluble CD40 in patients with hematological malignancies. *Oncology & Radiotherapy*, **106**, 2148-2157.

[33] Prilliman K.R., *et al.* (2002) Cutting edge: A crucial role for B7-CD28 in transmitting T help from APC to CTL. *The Journal of Immunology*, **169**, 4094-4097.

[34] Peggs Karl, S., *et al.* (2009) Blockade of CTLA-4 on both effector and regulatory T cell compartments contributes to the antitumor activity of anti-CTLA-4 antibodies. *Journal of Experimental Medicine*, **206**, 1717-1725. http://dx.doi.org/10.1084/jem.20082492

[35] Vasilevko, V., Ghochikyan, A., Holterman, M.J. and Agadjanyan, M.G. (2002) CD80 (B7-1) and CD86 (B7-2) are functionally equivalent in the initiation and maintenance of CD4+ T-cell proliferation after activation with suboptimal doses of PHA. *DNA and Cell Biology*, **21**, 137-149. http://dx.doi.org/10.1089/10445490252925404

[36] Becker, Th., *et al.* (2002) CD40, an extracellular receptor for binding and uptake of Hsp70-peptide complexes. *The Journal of Cell Biology*, **158**, 1277-1285. http://dx.doi.org/10.1083/jcb.200208083

[37] Finn, O.J., *et al.* (2002) Prophylactic cancer vaccines. *Current Opinion in Immunology*, **14**, 172-177. http://dx.doi.org/10.1016/S0952-7915(02)00317-5

4

Matrigel modulates a stem cell phenotype and promotes tumor formation in a mantle cell lymphoma cell line

Abigail Hielscher[1], Timothy McGuire[2], Dennis Weisenburger[3], John Graham Sharp[4*]

[1]Department of Chemical and Biomolecular Engineering, Johns Hopkins University, Baltimore, USA
[2]School of Pharmacy, University of Nebraska Medical Center, Omaha, USA
[3]Department of Pathology, City of Hope Medical Center, Duarte, USA
[4]Department of Cell Biology, Genetics and Anatomy, University of Nebraska Medical Center, Omaha, USA;
[*]Corresponding Author: jsharp@unmc.edu

ABSTRACT

Tumors may be maintained by subpopulations of cells possessing stem cell-like properties. We evaluated the stem cell-like and tumor-forming properties of side population (SP) and CD133$^+$/CD44$^+$ cells in Granta 519, a human mantle cell lymphoma cell line. The *in-vitro* Cobblestone Area Forming Cell (CAFC) assay, designed to detect stem and progenitor cells, revealed that SP cells contained the greatest proportion of stem cell-like cells. The addition of Matrigel to CAFC assays of SP and non-SP cells both increased their respective stem cell frequencies in comparison to those cultures without Matrigel, and additionally resulted in observed stem cell frequencies which were the same between SP and non-SP cells. Contrary, Matrigel decreased the stem cell frequencies of CD133$^+$/CD44$^+$ or CD133$^-$/CD44$^-$ cells. *In-vivo* assays revealed tumor formation from Matrigel-mixed SP and non-SP cells, and in one instance, occurred with as few as one Matrigel-mixed SP cell. Vehicle-mixed injections of SP and non-SP tumor cells resulted in tumor formation from SP cells only. Tumor formation did not occur from Matrigel nor hyaluronan (cellular substrate for CD44-expressing cells)-mixed populations of CD133$^+$/CD44$^+$ or CD133$^-$/CD44$^-$ cells. These data demonstrate that Matrigel modulates a stem cell phenotype and promotes tumor formation from SP and non-SP cells. The tumor micro-environmental niche and tumor cell to micro-environmental interactions may be important future targets for novel chemotherapeutic agents.

Keywords: Mantle Cell Lymphoma; Side Population; Tumor-Initiating Cells; Microenvironment

1. INTRODUCTION

Mantle cell lymphoma (MCL) is a type of non-Hodgkin's Lymphoma, characterized by an aberrant proliferation of mature B lymphocytes in the mantle zones of lymphoid follicles. The disease has an aggressive clinical course with a median patient survival of only 3 - 4 years following diagnosis [1,2]. This dismal outcome is due to the advanced stage of disease upon diagnosis with several extranodal sites typically involved including the spleen [3], bone marrow [4] and gastrointestinal tract [5]. Although a wide variety of chemotherapeutic agents are presently available to treat the disease, such therapeutic strategies have not significantly improved patient outcome [6-8] with patient relapse being a frequent occurrence [9,10]. Due to the aggressive nature of the disease and the high propensity for relapse, novel approaches for identifying the cell type(s) responsible for MCL initiation and progression are imperative for understanding and better combating the disease.

Increasing evidence has pointed to the existence of subsets of tumor cells proposed to be responsible for tumor initiation and propagation. Such tumor cells are referred to as tumor-initiating cells (TICs), rare subpopulations of tumor cells capable of tumor initiation when introduced in small numbers into immunocompromised mice, self-renewal upon serial transplantation into immunocompromised mice and differentiation into cells making up the bulk of the original tumor [11]. First described by Bonnet *et al* [12] in human leukemias, TICs have since been discovered in solid tumors including breast [13], prostate [14,15], colorectal [16], and liver carcinomas [17,18] amongst others. Regarding lymphomas, TICs have been identified in a mouse model of MCL [19] and have recently been prospectively identified in human MCL tumors [20]. In the latter study, it was reported that MCL cells lacking the mature B cell surface receptor CD19 were enriched for self-renewal and tumor-forming capabilities following xenotransplantation in immunodeficient animals [20]. Additional investigation is warranted to further define and characterize this population of putative MCL TICs so as to better identify and design chemotherapeutic agents aimed at eliminating these potentially rare and aggressive MCL subpopulations.

Validated methods, similar to those employed for tissue stem cells, are required for isolation and evaluation of putative MCL TICs. Such methods include the use of cell surface markers, aldehyde dehydrogenase activity, or the presence of a side population (SP). Of particular interest is the cell surface marker CD133, a hematopoietic stem cell (HSC) marker [21], and CD44, a cell surface adhesion receptor which facilitates cellular attachment to the extracellular matrix (ECM) [22,23]. Both CD133 and CD44, alone or in conjunction with other cell surface markers, have been assigned to cells having enhanced tumorigenic and stem cell-like properties [14-16,18,24]. The second cell population evaluated is the SP, a tail-shaped cell population visualized as a result of ABCG2-mediated efflux of the Hoechst 33342 dye [25]. First described by Goodell *et al.* [26] as a novel method for isolating HSCs from murine bone marrow, the SP has been employed to isolate both tissue stem cells [27] and putative TIC populations [11,17,19,20].

Tissue stem cells are known to reside in supportive niches or microenvironments, comprised of cellular and non-cellular components which together maintain stem cell homeostasis [28,29]. It is possible that the enhanced tumorigenicity and stem cell-like properties of TICs may be a result of their maintenance in supportive micro-environmental niches. Indeed, Vermeulen *et al.* [30] reported that the microenvironment was imperative for regulating Wnt activity, functionally assigned to colon TICs. Similarly, Calabrese *et al.* [31] discovered that brain TICs were localized to the brain vascular niche, which they demonstrated to be responsible for promoting self-renewal and accelerating tumor growth from brain TICs. Regarding lymphomas, it has been demonstrated that the lymph node microenvironment actively participates in the progression of follicular lymphoma [32].

In the present study, we sought to determine whether microenvironmental factors were necessary for accelerating self-renewal and tumor-formation capabilities of Granta MCL TICs isolated on the basis of either CD133/CD44 co-expression or the SP functional pheno-type. While the stem cell niche is comprised of numerous cellular and non-cellular entities, the ECM is of particular interest as it is known to play an important role in regulating stem cell self-renewal and differentiation [33-37]. As such, we elected to utilize Matrigel, a commercially available conglomerate of ECM proteins derived from a murine sarcoma. Matrigel served as a biological substrate to promote MCL TIC xenograft tumor formation, previously demonstrated by others [38-40]. We demonstrate that Matrigel, rather than cell phenotype differences, affect the enrichment of stem cell-like cells *in-vitro* and expedite tumor development *in-vivo* for both SP and non-SP cells. Elucidating the role whereby the tumor microenvironment influences proposed MCL TIC behaviors is imperative for implementation of better and/or novel therapeutics targeted toward both the tumor microenvironment and MCL to niche interactions.

2. MATERIALS AND METHOD

2.1. Cell Lines and Culture

Granta 519 (herein, Granta) cells were kindly obtained from Dr. Shantaram Joshi, UNMC and cultured in DMEM (Invitrogen; Grand Island, NY) containing 10% fetal bovine serum (FBS) and 1× penicillin/streptomycin (Invitrogen). Murine bone marrow stromal cells (MS5) [41] were kindly provided by Dr. John Jackson (Wake Forest Institute of Regenerative Medicine, Winston Salem, NC) and employed as described previously [42]. MS5 were cultured in RPMI (Invitrogen) containing 10% FBS, 1× penicillin/streptomycin and 1 μg/ml hydrocortisone (Sigma-Aldrich; Allentown, PA). MS5 cells were rendered non-adherent with 0.05% trypsin/EDTA (Invitrogen). Granta and MS5 cells were passaged every 2 - 3 days and were maintained at 37°C in a humidified air atmosphere containing 5% CO_2.

2.2. Flow Cytometry and Sorting

Granta cells were stained 1:11 with PE-CD133 (Miltenyi; Gergisch Gladbach, Germany) and 1:89 with APC-CD44 (e-Bioscience; San Diego, CA) for 20 minutes at 4°C. For SP analyses, Granta cells were re-suspended in 1 ml of Hoechst IMDM (Invitrogen; IMDM media supplemented with 2% FBS, 1μM Hepes, and 1x penicillin/streptomycin) for incubation at 4°C overnight, adjusted to 1.0×10^6 cells/ml and stained with 6μg/ml Hoechst 33342 (Sigma-Aldrich) at 37°C for 30 minutes. For confirmation of the SP, Granta cells were stained with 40 μM of verapamil (Sigma-Aldrich) for 15 minutes at 37°C prior to incubation with Hoechst 33342. Analyses were conducted in the cell analysis facilities at

UNMC and Creighton University, Omaha, NE. Data was analyzed using FlowJo™. Granta TIC and non-TIC cells were isolated using Fluorescence Activated Cell Sorting (FACS).

2.3. Cobblestone Area Forming Cells Assays

Granta populations were sorted in limiting dilutions into 96 well plates containing Murine Stromal 5 (MS5) cells. $CD133^+/CD44^+$ and $CD133^-/CD44^-$ populations were adjusted to six dilutions ranging from 407 to 1 cell/well. SP and non-SP populations were adjusted to 10 dilutions ranging from 33,300 to 1 cell/well. All dilutions were made at a factor of 3 with each dilution being conducted in a total of 20 or 30 wells. In some instances, Granta populations were overlaid with a final concentration of 275 μg/ml of Matrigel (BD Biosciences; San Jose, CA). The co-cultures were maintained for 5 weeks. Phase contrast microscopy was used to assess for the presence of phase dark cobblestones (groups of 3 or more cells growing in a colony beneath the stromal layer). Using a semi-logarithmic scale, the frequency of stem cell-like cells in each population was plotted and measured as the inverse of the number of seeded cells corresponding to 37% negative wells [43]. Images were captured at 10× magnification using a Nikon P5000 digital camera.

2.4. Tumorsphere Assays

Granta SP and non-SP fractions were sorted at dilutions of 1, 10, 100 and 1000 cells/well into 96 well plates containing 150 μl of DMEM/HamsF12 media supplemented with either 20 ng/ml of bFGF (Invitrogen) and 20 ng/ml of EGF (Invitrogen) or 20 ng/ml bFGF and 10 ng/ml of EGF. Cultures were maintained for a total of 6 weeks in a 95% humidified air atmosphere at 37°C and 5% CO_2. The presence of tumorspheres was evaluated at weekly intervals using phase contrast microscopy at 20× magnification. Images were photographed using a Nikon P5000 digital camera.

2.5. Enzyme-Linked Immunosorbent Assay

Supernatant from Granta cells, MS5 cells, Granta/MS5 co-cultures and Granta TIC and non-TIC/MS5 co-cultures were collected and quantified for *interleukin 8* (IL-8) using enzyme-linked immunosorbent assay (ELISA). The Quantikine Immunoassay Kit (R&D Systems, Minneapolis, MN) was utilized and all procedures were followed according to the manufacturer's protocol. The lower limit of sensitivity for the assay is 3.5 pg/ml with a dynamic range between 3.5 pg/ml and 2000 pg/ml. Intra-assay coefficient of variation ranges from 5.4% - 6.5% and inter-assay coefficient of variation from 6.1% to 9.7%. For analyses of IL-8 secretion from Granta and MS5 cells, 2.0×10^6 cells/ml were used. These cultures were maintained for 3 days prior to collection of supernatants. The cells were then re-suspended in fresh media and maintained in culture for another 3 days prior to collection of additional supernatant. For Granta/MS5 co-cultures, 1.0×10^6 MS5 cells were plated and maintained as previously described. Once MS5 cells reached 75% confluency, 1.0×10^6 Granta cells were plated and grown in standard growth media as previously described. The supernatants from Granta/MS5 co-cultures were collected at 1, 3, 7 and 14 day intervals for the assessment of IL-8 levels over time. All supernatant was passed through a 70 μM strainer for removal of residual cell debris. For each analysis, the supernatants from triplicate cultures were evaluated.

2.6. *In-Vivo* Analyses

All procedures on animals were followed in compliance with the UNMC Animal Care and Use Committee. Three-five animals were maintained in a stainless steel cage and were given food and water ad libitum. Granta TIC and non-TIC populations were subcutaneously injected into the hind flanks of 3 - 5 week old female NOD-scid IL2Rgnull (NSG) mice (Jackson Laboratories; Bar Harbor, ME). Dilutions of 10, 100 and 1000 SP and non-SP cells and 10, 100 and 500 $CD133^+/CD44^+$ and $CD133^-/CD44^-$ cells were prepared as described by Quintana *et al* (2008). Additionally, 10, 100 and 1000 $CD133^+/CD44^+$ and $CD133^-/CD44^-$ cells were resuspended at a 1:8 dilution in hyaluronan (Hyaluronex; Lexington, KY). Single SP or non-SP cells were sorted using FACS into 96 well plates and were re-suspended at a 1:4 dilution in Matrigel. When tumors reached 1 - 1.5 cm, animals were necropsied. Tumor volume was assessed using the formula for an ellipsoid: $4/3\ \pi r^1 r^2 r^3$. As a control, Matrigel and vehicle were injected alone into either the right or left shoulders of 2 NSG mice.

2.7. Histolopathology and Flow Cytometry

Murine tissues including the lung, right femur, and kidney and portions of the spleen, small intestine, liver and kidney were fixed in 10% neutral buffered formalin for at least 24 hours and subjected to histopathological analysis using hematoxylin and eosin (H&E) staining (Eppley Cancer Center Histology Core Facility, UNMC). The remaining murine tissues were evaluated for human CD20 expression using flow cytometry. The lung was cut into 5 mm pieces and digested in 1 mg/ml collagenase V (Sigma-Aldrich) and 500 μg/ml elastase (Sigma-Aldrich) for 30 minutes at 37°C. Bone marrow from the right femur was extracted using a 22 gauge syringe. Remaining tissues were subjected to mechanical disruption using a blunt end syringe. Tissues were filtered in 70 μM cell strainers. Between 3.0×10^5 and 1.0×10^6 cells were stained 1:11 with PE-CD20 (BD Biosciences). Flow cytometry assessed CD20 species cross-reactivity in the tissues from a control NSG mouse. H&E staining and SP analyses were performed as previously described.

2.8. Statistical Analyses

All data are presented as the mean ± SEM. Linear regression (Sigma Plot v 9.0; San Jose, CA) produced the line of best fit for CAFC assays. Graphs were made in Sigma Plot v 9.0 or GraphPad Prism v4.02 (GraphPad Software Inc. La Jolla, CA). Student's t test was utilized for all remaining analyses. A P value ≤ 0.05 was considered significant.

3. RESULTS

3.1. SP and $CD133^+/CD44^+$ Cells Are Present in Granta

Initially, we sought to identify whether Granta cells possessed populations of cells, identified through use of Hoescht exclusion, (e.g. the SP) or expression of the hematopoietic stem cell marker CD133 [21] in conjunction with CD44, widely used markers for identification of TICs [14-16,18,24]. The SP phenotype was observed in Granta and was represented at an average of 6.4% ± 1.8% (range: 0% - 35.2%) (**Figure 1(Aa)**). Validation of the SP was confirmed through the incorporation of verapamil, an ABCG2 transport blocker (**Figure 1(Ab)**). Granta cells additionally possessed a small population of $CD133^+/CD44^+$ cells which represented 0.06% ± 0.03% (range: 0% - 0.39%) of the gated population. Examples of the unstained Granta control (**Figure 1(Ac)**) and Granta $CD133^+/CD44^+$ cells (**Figure 1(Ad)**) are shown. Overall, these analyses suggest that Granta possess subpopulations of cells bearing stem cell-like properties and points to the SP as being a more robust marker of putative TICs.

3.2. SP Cells Are Enriched for Cobblestone Area-Forming Cells

The cobblestone area forming cell (CAFC) assay is considered one of the best *in-vitro* techniques for the identification of stem cells [44,45]. The presence of stem and progenitor cells is visualized when a stem or progenitor cell migrates below a stromal cell layer and self-renews to form a colony of cells, which resemble a cobblestone in appearance [44,45]. Utilizing this technique, limiting dilutions of Granta SP and non-SP cells and $CD133^+/CD44^+$ and $CD133^-/CD44^-$ cells were plated onto a semi-confluent monolayer of MS5 cells, chosen for its known role in supporting long term maintenance of HSCs *in-vitro* [45,46] and evaluated at weekly intervals for the presence of cobblestones. At the end of the 5 week analysis, the CAFC frequencies of Granta $CD133^+/CD44^+$ and $CD133^-/CD44^-$ cells were not significantly different: 1/415 and 1/755 cells (P = 0.09) (**Table 1**), respectively. Granta SP cells, however, were enriched for stem cell-like cells, having a CAFC frequency of 1/970 cells while non-SP cells had a CAFC frequency of 1/4350 cells (P = 0.02) (**Table 1**). It is important to note that cell dilutions corresponding to 33,300, 11,100 and 3700 cells/well were not included in SP and non-SP CAFC assays as they yielded non-responsive wells from non-SP cells, resulting in a shifted CAFC curve which could not be evaluated. It is possible that these high cell numbers may have overwhelmed the conditions of the assay. **Figures 1(Ba)** and **1(Bb)** illustrate the presence and absence of cobblestones from Granta SP and non-SP cells, respectively.

Interestingly, 1000 SP cells were observed to form spheres in the tumorsphere assay, a technique utilized to detect self-renewal of both stem cell populations and TICs [47-50]. These spheres were detected as early as 2 weeks in culture (**Figure 1(C)**). Lower limits of SP cells (1, 10 and 100) and all tested dilutions of non-SP cells (1, 10, 100 and 1000) were not observed to form tumorpheres. An example illustrating the absence of spheres and identifiable cells is shown for a culture of 1000 non-SP cells (**Figure 1(C)**). Together, the CAFC and tumorsphere results suggest that Granta SP cells are enriched for self-renewing TICs at a dilution which corresponds to a frequency of ~1000 cells.

3.3. Matrigel Enhances the CAFC Frequencies of SP and Non-SP Cells

Since ECM components have been shown to maintain certain stem cell populations in an undifferentiated state [35,51,52], we hypothesized that the addition of Matrigel would enhance the number of self-renewing TICs and thus the CAFC frequencies of putative SP and $CD133^+/CD44^+$ TICs. Limiting dilutions of Granta SP and non-SP cells (33,300 cells/well to 1 cell/well) and $CD133^+/CD44^+$ and $CD133^-/CD44^-$ cells (407 cells/ well to 1 cell/well) were plated onto MS5 cells and the cultures were overlaid with a final concentration of 275 μg/ml of Matrigel. Interestingly, the addition of Matrigel to Granta SP and non-SP/MS5 co-cultures not only significantly increased the CAFC frequencies of both populations, but resulted in intersecting CAFC frequencies of 1/175 for both SP and non-SP cells (P > 0.05) (**Table 1**) (**Figure 1(D)**). Surprisingly, the addition of Matrigel to $CD133^+/CD44^+$ and $CD133^-/CD44^-$/MS5 co-cultures significantly decreased the CAFC frequencies to 1/4850

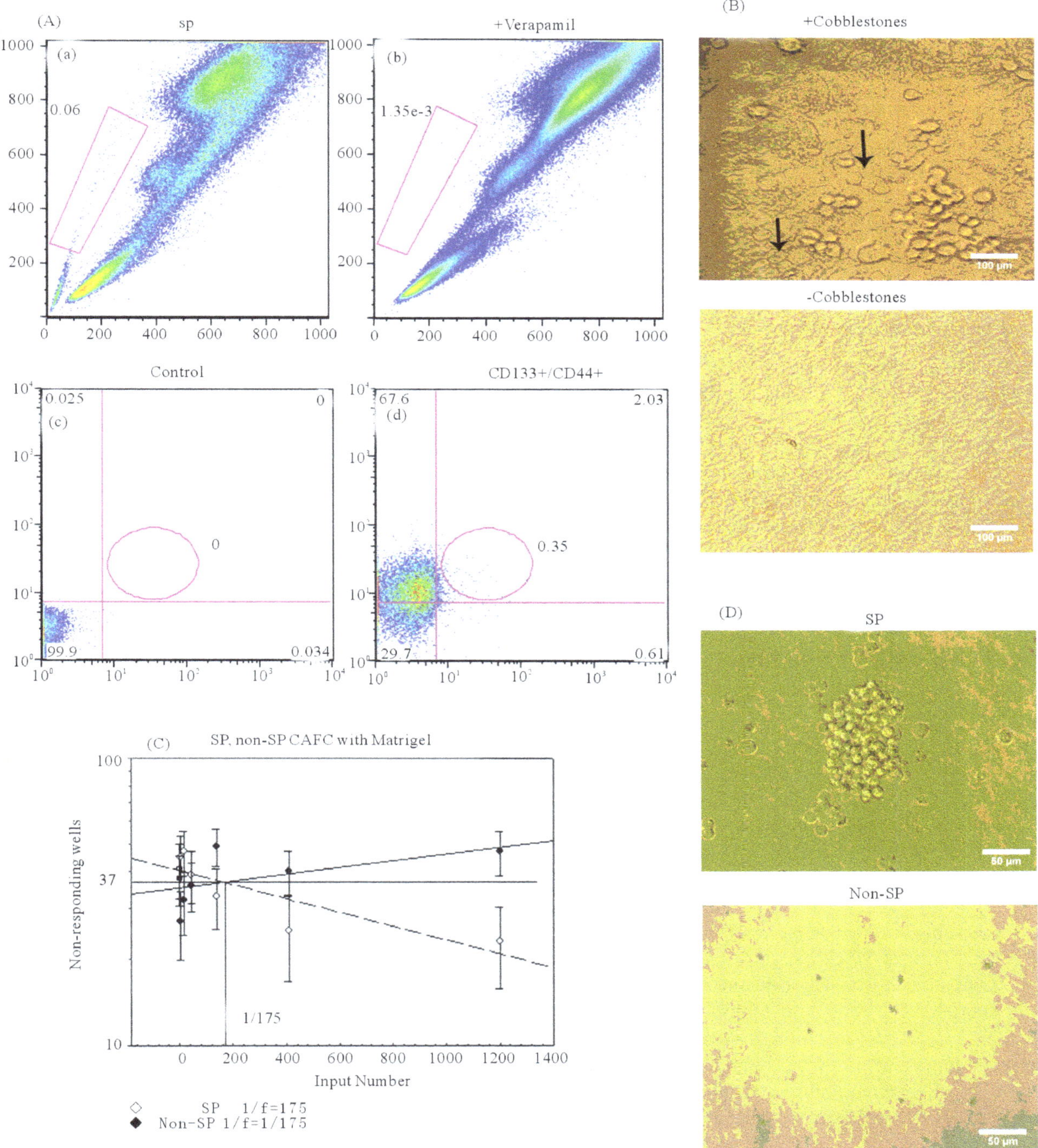

Figure 1. Granta possess populations of cells with stem cell-like properties. (Aa) The SP phenotype was identified in Granta cells and occurred at a frequency of 6.4% ± 1.8% (range: 0% - 35.2%) of the population. (Ab) Verapamil confirmed the presence of SP cells. (Ac) Quadrants for the analysis of CD133/CD44-expressing cells were defined in unstained Granta cells. (Ad) $CD133^+/CD44^+$ cells, indicated by the oval in Q2, were present in Granta cells and occurred at a frequency of 0.06% ± 0.03% (range: 0% - 0.39%). (B) Images illustrating the presence of phase-dark cobblestones (indicated by the black arrows) from a 2 week culture of SP/MS5 cells and absence of cobblestones from non-SP/MS5 cells maintained in culture for 5 weeks. Images were captured at ×100 magnification. (C) The presence of a tumorsphere was observed from 1000 SP cells maintained in culture for 2 weeks. Tumorsphere formation was not observed from 1000 non-SP cells maintained in culture for 6 weeks. Images were captured at ×200 magnification. (D) The CAFC frequencies of Granta SP and non-SP cells overlaid with 275 µg/ml Matrigel is demarcated by the line representing 37% non-responding wells and was determined to be 1/175 cells for both cell populations. 95% confidence intervals are indicated by the error bars. $^*P \leq 0.05$; $^{**}P \leq 0.01$; $^{***}P \leq 0.001$.

Table 1. Granta TIC and non-TIC CAFC frequencies.

Cell Type	Treatment	CAFC Frequency	Student's T-test
CD133$^+$/CD44$^+$	No Treatment Matrigel	1/415 1/4 850	<0.01
CD133$^-$/CD44$^-$	No Treatment Matrigel	1/755 1/2 575	<0.01
SP	No Treatment Matrigel	1/970 1/175	<0.01
Non-SP	No Treatment Matrigel	1/4 350 1/175	<0.01

and 1/2575, respectively, in comparison to co-cultures without Matrigel ($P < 0.01$) (**Table 1**). Together, these data not only demonstrate that Matrigel has opposing effects on the CAFC frequencies of SP and non-SP cells and CD133$^+$/CD44$^+$ and CD133$^-$/CD44$^-$ cells, but additionally demonstrates that micro-environmental components, rather than phenotype differences, may be a more important factor in promoting stem cell-like behaviors of Granta SP and non-SP cells.

3.4. Matrigel Expedites Tumor Formation of Granta SP and Non-SP Cells

We sought to determine whether Matrigel enhanced the tumorigenic properties of Granta SP and CD133$^+$/CD44$^+$ cells, a property reported by others [38-40]. Palpable tumors from Matrigel injections of 10, 100 and 1000 SP and non-SP cells were evident in 100% of tested cases and arose within an average time of 34 ± 0.9 days following cell injection. Examples of tumors derived from the injections of 10 Matrigel-mixed SP and 10 Matrigel-mixed non-SP cells are shown (**Figures 2(Aa)** and **2(Ab)**). Remarkably, a tumor arose from the injection of a single Matrigel-mixed SP cell at 70 days post injection (**Figures 2(Ac)** and **2(B)**). Tumors did not; however, arise from single cell injections of Matrigel-mixed non-SP cells at 160 days post-injection. Overall, significant differences in tumor volumes between Matrigel-mixed SP and non-SP cells were not observed (**Figure 2(C)**). In the absence of Matrigel, tumors arose in two animals injected with 1000 and 100 vehicle-mixed SP cells; however, the tumor volumes were 2.4× and 1.4× less than their counterpart Matrigel-mixed tumors, respectively. Tumors did not develop from vehicle-injected non-SP cells nor did they form from control Matrigel or vehicle injections, demonstrating that these inoculums were not tumorigenic alone. **Figure 2(D)** depicts the frequency of tumor formation in Matrigel and vehicle-mixed SP and non-SP cells. CD133$^+$/CD44$^+$ and CD133$^-$/CD44$^-$ cells were also evaluated for their tumor-forming capabilities. Both cell populations were injected into NSG mice in the presence and absence of Matrigel or hyaluronan, chosen as CD44 preferentially interacts with hyaluronan [22]. **Table 2** provides a summary of findings from Matrigel and vehicle-mixed injections of SP and non-SP cells. Surprisingly, tumors did not arise by 160 days post-injection from Matrigel and hyaluronan-mixed CD133$^+$/CD44$^+$ and CD133$^-$/CD44$^-$ cells (data not shown). Similarly, vehicle-mixed injections of CD133$^+$/CD44$^+$ and CD133$^-$/CD44$^-$ cells did not give rise to tumors at 160 days post-injection. Taken together, these results suggest that phenotypic differences in tumor formation from SP and non-SP cells may be irrelevant in the presence of Matrigel but may be necessary for tumor establishment and growth in the absence of Matrigel. CD133$^+$/CD44$^+$ and CD133$^-$/CD44$^-$ cells are not capable of tumor formation under the tested conditions.

In order to validate that tumors obtained from SP and non-SP cells were from Granta cells, flow cytometry was employed to quantify cell surface CD20. Flow cytometry detected enriched levels of CD20 positive cells from SP and non-SP-derived tumors (**Figures 2(Ea) and (Eb)**). SP and non-SP-derived tumors had an average tumor CD20 expression of 82% ± 6%. Together, these data confirm that tumor specimens were derived from human MCL cells.

3.5. SP Fractions Were Identified in SP and Non-SP Derived Tumors

Flow cytometry was utilized to assess the presence of the SP in Matrigel-mixed SP and non-SP-derived tumors. SP fractions were found in tumors arising from injections of both SP (**Figure 2(Ec)**) and non-SP cells (**Figure 2(Ed)**). The mean SP expression was the same for tumors derived from Matrigel-mixed SP and non-SP cells: 1.1% ± 0.5% and 1.1% ± 0.3%, respectively ($P = 0.4$) and was 1.4% ± 0.7% in vehicle-mixed SP cells ($P > 0.05$: Matrigel-mixed non-SP and SP-derived tumors). Together, these data strongly suggest that the SP phenotype is malleable and may be modulated by microenvironmental factors.

3.6. SP and Non-SP Derived Tumors Cells Are Capable of Spread to Distant Organs

In order to evaluate the metastatic capabilities of SP and non-SP cells, several murine organs including the bone marrow, spleen, lung, small intestine, liver and kidney were harvested and assessed for the presence of tumor cells using H&E staining and flow cytometry. H&E staining did not reveal the presence of distinct tumor nodules in any of the tissues examined (data not shown). Given the limitations of H&E/immunostaining to small regions of tissue sections, we elected to utilize flow cytometry on intact, prepared tissues to investigate whether human CD20 cells, indicative of metastasizing Granta cells, were present in the aforementioned organs. Human CD20-positive cells were detected by flow cytometry in all evaluated tissues, with the greatest level of detection observed in the small intestine **(Figure 3)**, a common metastatic site for non-Hodgkin's lymphomas [53]. Taken together, these results indicate that while identifiable nodular tumors were not detected in potential metastatic sites, human CD20 expression was observed and quantified in murine tissues indicating that Granta cells from SP and non-SP injections most likely migrated to these distant sites.

3.7. IL-8 Levels Are Significantly Elevated in Granta/MS5 Co-Cultures

We examined IL-8 levels, chosen due to its implications in tumor invasion and metastasis [54], in the conditioned media (CM) of Granta and MS5 cells after 3 and 6 days in culture. IL-8 was also evaluated in Granta MS5 co-cultures at several days along the culture period and was further investigated in co-cultures of Granta TIC and non-TIC populations with MS5 cells. IL-8 was found to be secreted at negligible levels from MS5 cells after 3 (**Figure 4(A)**) and 6 days (data not shown) in culture and highly secreted from Granta cells after 3 (**Figure 4(A)**)

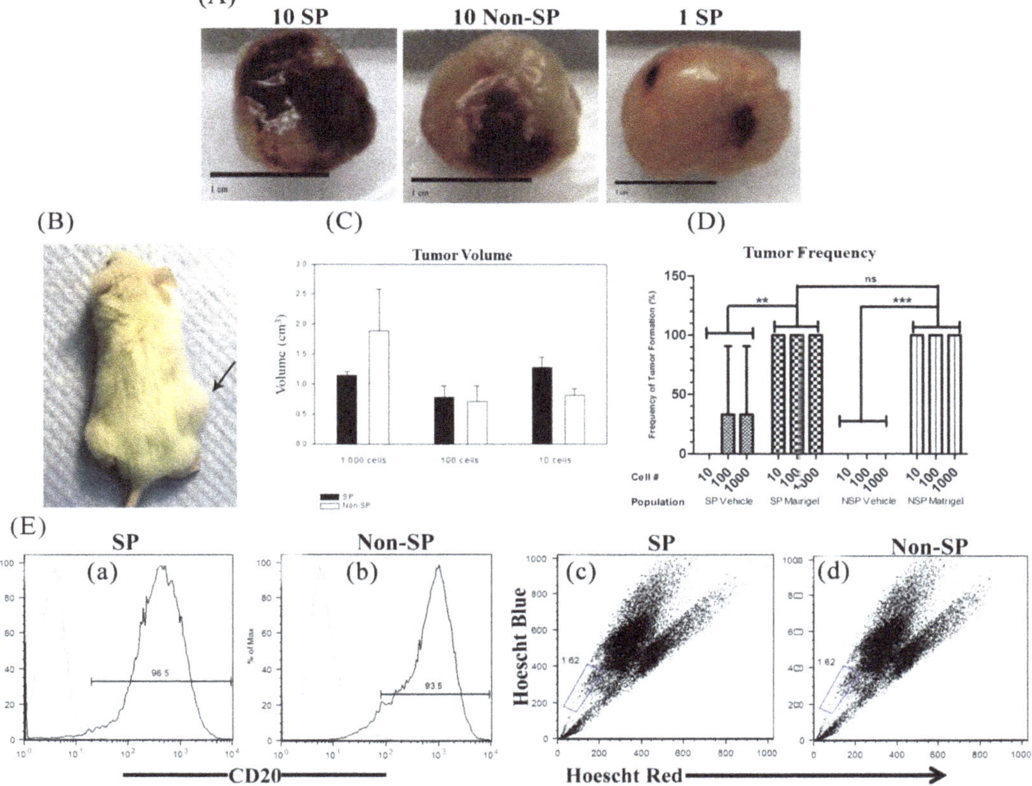

Figure 2. Tumor specimens and characteristics of Matrigel-mixed SP and non-SP cells. (A) Tumor specimens obtained from Matrigel-mixed 10 SP cells, 10 non-SP cells and 1 SP cell. Scale bars represent 1 cm. (B) NSG mouse harboring a tumor from the injection of a single Matrigel-mixed SP cell. (C) Tumor volumes were not statistically significantly different between SP and non-SP-derived tumors at corresponding dilutions. (D) The frequency of tumor formation was the same for all tested dilutions of Matrigel-mixed SP and non-SP cells and occurred 100% of the time. Tumor formation of vehicle-mixed SP cells occurred 33% of the time and did not result from vehicle-mixed non-SP cells. (E) Flow cytometry demonstrated the presence of cell surface CD20 expression ((a) and (b)) and SPs ((c) and (d)) in tumors arising from 10 SP and 10 non-SP cells.

Table 2. Tumor Formation from Granta SP and non-SP cells.

Cells	Inoculum	Tumor Formation (+/−) 1	10	100	1000	Avg Weeks to Tumor Palpability 1	10	100	1000	P value
SP	Vehicle	NA	0/4	1/3	1/3	NA	NT	4.8	4.7	0.003
	Matrigel	1/5	4/4	3/3	3/3	10	5.2 ± 0.4	5 ± 0.3	4.4 ± 0.1	
Non-SP	Vehicle	NA	0/3	0/3	0/3	NA	NT	NT	NT	<0.001
	Matrigel	0/5	4/4	3/3	3/3	NT	5.3 ± 0.2	4.7 ± 0.2	4.3 ± 0.04	

N/A Not applicable; N/T No Tumor; Avg Average.

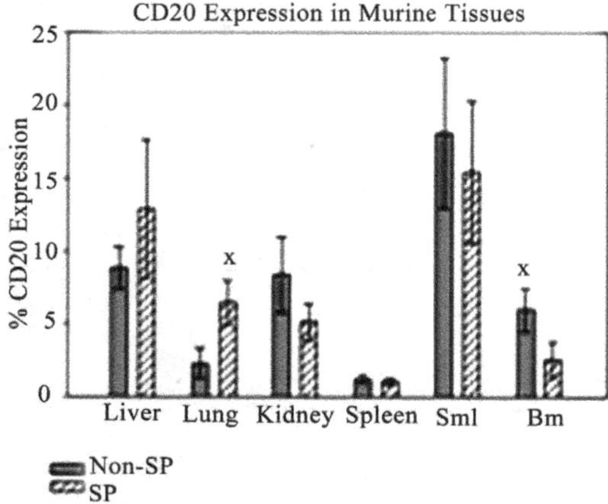

Figure 3. Granta cells spread to distant murine tissues. CD20-positive cells were detected in all murine tissues from SP and non-SP-injected NSG mice. All values are averages and presented as a percentage of the total CD20-positive cells minus control. SMI: Small Intestine. BM: Bone Marrow. $^{X}P \leq 0.05$.

and 6 days (data not shown) in culture. Interestingly, it was noted that the greatest level of IL-8 secretion oc curred in a time dependent manner in Granta/MS5 co-cultures **(Figure 4(B))**. Surprisingly, it was found that IL-8 secretion was significantly higher in SP/MS5 co-cultures than in non-SP/MS5 co-cultures where IL-8 was not detectable **(Figure 4(C))**. Regarding CD133^{+}/ CD44^{+} and CD133^{-}/CD44^{-} cells co-cultured with MS5, IL-8 was not significantly different **(Figure 4(C))**. Together, these studies suggest that MS5 cells alone do not secrete appreciable levels of IL-8, but significantly contribute to IL-8 levels when cultured in direct contact with Granta cells. Moreover, these results further suggest that IL-8 is predominantly secreted from co-cultures of SP/MS5, but not appreciably from co-cultures of MS5 with non-SP, CD133^{+}/CD44^{+} and CD133^{-}/CD44^{-} cells.

4. DISCUSSION

Here, we report that the Granta MCL cell line possesses subpopulations of cells expressing stem cell functions and markers. For the purpose of more closely mimicking the *in-vivo* environment, we evaluated the stem cell-like and tumor-forming capabilities of Granta SP and CD133^{+}/CD44^{+} cells in the presence of micro-environmental components found in Matrigel. While numerous reports have documented the existence of rare sub-populations of TICs in a variety of carcinomas, the majority of these studies have failed to consider the role of the microenvironment in modulating the stem cell-like and tumor-forming properties of such cells. Thus, the question remains as to whether properties associated with TICs are mediated through mechanisms solely related to intrinsic or extrinsic factors, or some combination of both.

Our results demonstrate that when assessed for the presence of stem and progenitor cells, evaluated using the CAFC assay, Granta SP cells were highly enriched for stem cell-like cells. The ability of Granta cell populations to form cobblestones in the CAFC assay is in contrast to observations from Kurtova *et al.* (2009) who reported that Granta cells were incapable of cobblestone formation. It's possible that this discrepancy may have arisen due to the type of fibroblasts used in these assays. For instance, it has been documented that certain murine and human fibroblast cell lines are incapable of supporting the long-term maintenance of human HSCs *in-vitro* [46,55,56]. Since the MS5 cell line has been shown to reliably support the quantification and long term maintenance of HSCs *in-vitro* [45,46], we employed this cell line for analyses of stem and progenitor cell frequencies and believe it to be a valid cell line for this purpose. In this manner, our data not only demonstrates that the SP isolation technique better enriches for cells possessing stem cell-like properties in Granta, but warrants caution in the choice of fibroblast cell lines for the purpose of identifying and/or supporting putative stem cell populations.

Further investigating the *in-vitro* stem cell-like properties of putative Granta TIC cells, we observed that Matrigel had discordant effects on SP and CD133^{+}/ CD44^{+} cells, enhancing and depressing the CAFC frequencies, respectively. Interestingly, Matrigel endowed both SP and non-SP cells with a concordantly enriched

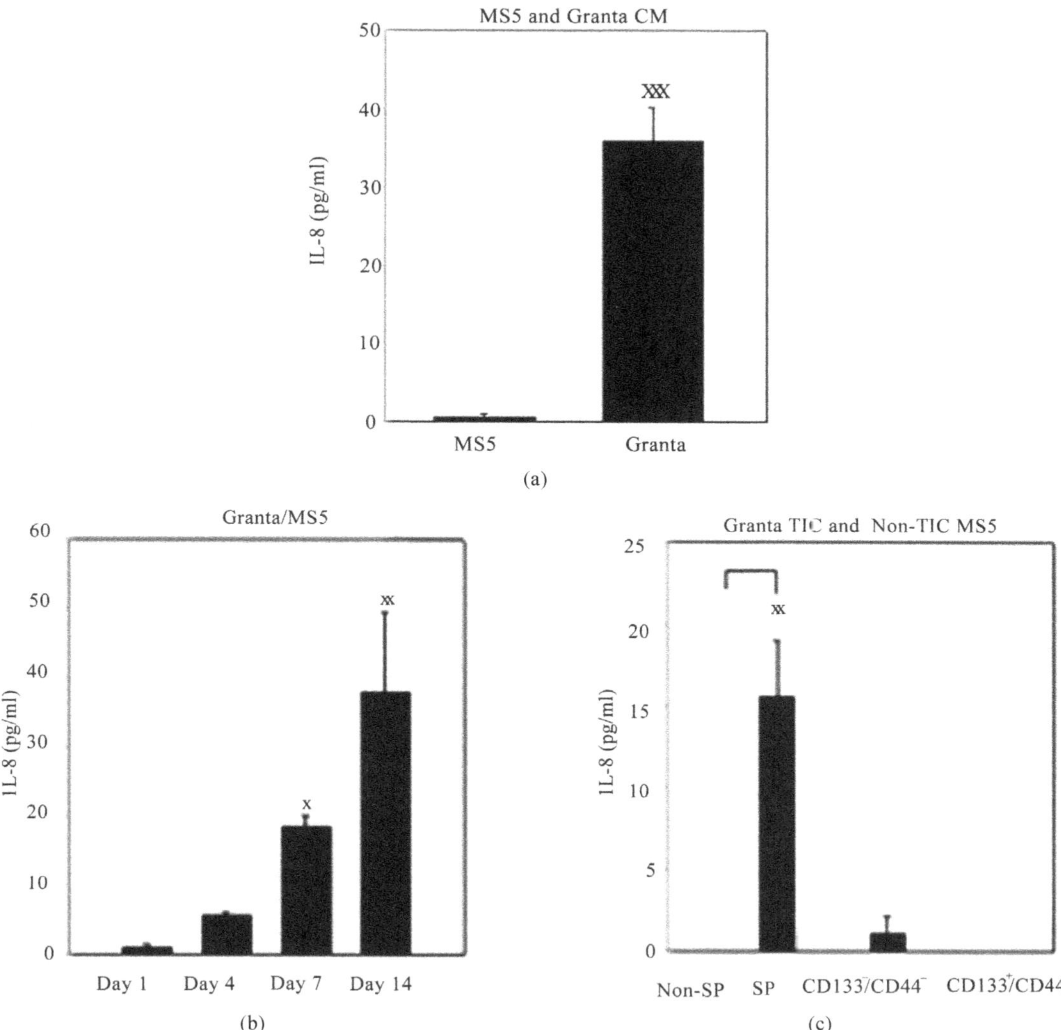

Figure 4. IL-8 secretion was significantly elevated in Granta and co-cultures of Granta and Granta SP with MS5. Secreted IL-8 was significantly elevated in (A) Granta CM (B) Granta/MS5 CM, with increasing IL-8 observed during the culture period. All comparisons were made against baseline (day 1) IL-8 secretion. (C) IL-8 secretion was significantly elevated in SP/MS5 co-cultures and was negligibly detected in non-SP/MS5 co-cultures. Detectable IL-8 was observed from $CD133^-/CD44^-$ /MS5 co-cultures, but was negligibly secreted from $CD133^+/CD44^+$ /MS5 co-cultures . $^{X}P \leq 0.05$; $^{XX}P \leq 0.01$; $^{XXX}P \leq 0.001$.

proportion of cells exhibiting a stem cell phenotype. A similar observation was made by Cao *et al.* [57] who reported that non-SP cells in nasopharyngeal carcinomas could be induced to express the SP phenotype when cultured in the conditioned media of macrophage-like cells, a cell type comprising the microenvironment. Our results suggest that the microenvironment plays an important role in modulating a stem cell-like phenotype of Granta SP and non-SP cells. Matrigel did not, however, enrich for stem cell-like cells in the $CD133^+/CD44^+$ population. It's possible that Matrigel may not have provided the requisite ECM constituents for facilitating a stem cell phenotype. For instance, the main ligand for CD44 is HA [22], a polysaccharide ECM component reported to be enriched in the tumor microenvironment [58]. Since Matrigel does not contain HA, it's possible that the Matrigel niche does not provide the cues necessary to support the expression of a stem cell-like phenotype from $CD133^+/CD44^+$ cells. However, it should be noted that $CD133^+/CD44^+$ may not enrich for a population of MCL TICs as evaluated in the CAFC assay.

Recent reports have documented the tumor-forming capabilities of Matrigel-injected TICs [38-40]. Utilizing similar techniques, we demonstrated that both Matrigel-mixed SP and non-SP cells were tumorigenic in NSG mice at dilutions of 10 or more cells. Indeed, the microenvironment-mediated control of tumorigenesis is a widely acknowledged phenomenon for unselected tumor cells [59,60] and was reported for thyroid [61] and mesenchymal [62] TICs. In the latter studies, Matrigel-mixed SP and non-SP cells were reported to form tumors in immunocompromised mice [61,62]. While these authors did not attribute their observations to a microenvironment-mediated effect, it is likely, given our data, that the ECM factors found in Matrigel is a more important determinant for influencing tumor formation than SP and non-SP cell phenotype differences. In the absence of Matrigel, intrinsic differences may be important as tumor formation was documented in two instances from vehicle-injected SP cells. Together, these observations would suggest that both intrinsic and extrinsic properties may govern tumor-forming capabilities of Granta SP and non-SP cells. A remarkable observation was the finding that a tumor arose from 1 Matrigel-injected SP cell. While tumors arose in 1/5 cases from the injections of single Matrigel-mixed SP cells, our results are consistent with that of Quintana et al [60], who observed a ~20% tumor formation frequency from the injection of single Matrigel-mixed melanoma cells. Regarding the absence of tumors from single cell injections of Matrigel-mixed non-SP cells, we speculate that intrinsic mechanisms may provide a tumorigenic advantage to SP cells. This potentially suggests that interactions and communications between tumor cells may be an important means by which non-SP cells form tumors. In future studies, it will be necessary to address the limiting number of non-SP cells which can reliably form tumors in NSG mice.

The presence of a SP denotes a population of cells capable of self-renewal [27]. We discovered that SP cells were found in tumors derived from Matrigel-mixed SP and non-SP injections. The presence of the SP in Matrigel-mixed non-SP tumors was unexpected and may relate to the transformation ability of Matrigel as previously demonstrated in thyroid cancer cells [61]. This assessment is reasonable when taking into consideration the *in-vitro* results whereby Matrigel significantly enhanced the CAFC frequency of non-SP cells. Together, these data strongly suggest that the SP phenotype is malleable and may be modulated by micro-environmental factors. It will be necessary to determine whether this phenomenon is due to the microenvironment-mediated release of cytokines/chemokines or the acquisition of epigenetic changes facilitating cellular transformation of the target cells.

Metastasis is the greatest determinant of cancer morbidity. Although solid tumor nodules were not detected, diffuse infiltrates of MCL cells were present in all murine tissues examined. While it is unknown as to what caused the discrepancy between the lack of nodular tumor formation in spite of the cellular presence of Granta MCL cells, we hypothesize that cellular to microenvironment interactions likely play a role. In other words, Granta SP and non-SP cells were incapable of forming the appropriate cellular to cellular or non-cellular associations due to host microenvironment-mediated incompatibilities, a postulate set forth by Kelly *et al.* [63]. In this manner, tumor development could not take place despite the presence of MCL cells. It will be important to address whether an orthotopic introduction of a carefully selected human-derived stromal cell line, with Granta SP and non-SP cells may overcome potential species incompatibility constraints.

Neither $CD133^+/CD44^+$ nor $CD133^-/CD44^-$ cells co-mixed with Matrigel or hyaluronan formed tumors. It is possible that either the cell populations themselves and/or the microenvironmental niches were not favorable for growth of these cell populations into tumors. Since hyaluronan principally mediates cellular interactions with CD44 [22], it is puzzling as to why tumors did not develop from $CD133^+/CD44^+$ cells. Given the absence of sequestered growth factors in the hyaluronan matrix, it is possible that hyaluronan in combination with growth factors is necessary for tumor formation from $CD133^+/CD44^+$. In future studies, it will be important to evaluate how a hyaluronan-rich matrix containing growth factors influence tumor development from Granta $CD133^+/CD44^+$ cells.

In conclusion, our results demonstrate that the ECM constituents found in Matrigel are pivotal for stem cell-like and tumor-forming properties of Granta SP and non-SP cells. Additionally, these data point to potential niche specifications regarding the manifestation of tumor formation and stem cell-like properties associated with given subpopulations of tumor cells. Importantly, these data warrant caution in assigning tumor-forming capabilities exclusively to rare TICs.

5. ACKNOWLEDGEMENTS

We gratefully thank Dr. Shantaram Joshi UNMC, Omaha, NE for provision of Granta 519 cells and Dr. John D. Jackson Wake Forest Institute of Regenerative Medicine, Winston Salem, NC for provision of the MS5 cell line. We also thank Dr. Anathbandu Chaudhuri UNMC, Omaha, NE for assistance with animal injections, Valerie Shostrum for assistance with statistical analyses, and Sue Brusnahan UNMC, Omaha, NE and Dr. Sharon Gerecht Johns Hopkins University, Baltimore, MD for critical reading of the manuscript. This work was supported in part by: UNMC Eppley Cancer Center Support Grant P30CA036727; NIA Grant AG024912; Nebraska Tobacco Settlement Biomedical Research Development Fund.

REFERENCES

[1] Campo, E., Raffeld, M. and Jaffe, E.S. (1999) Mantle-cell lymphoma. *Seminars in Hematology*, **36**, 115-127.

[2] Zucca, E., *et al.* (1995) Patterns of survival in mantle cell lymphoma. *Annals of Oncology*, **6**, 257-262.

[3] Pittaluga, S., *et al.* (1996) "Small" B-cell non-Hodgkin's lymphomas with splenomegaly at presentation are either mantle cell lymphoma or marginal zone cell lymphoma. A study based on histology, cytology, immunohistochemistry, and cytogenetic analysis. *American Journal of Surgical Pathology*, **20**, 211-223. doi:10.1097/00000478-199602000-00010

[4] Cohen, P.L., Kurtin, P.J., Donovan, K.A. and Hanson, C.A. (1998) Bone marrow and peripheral blood involvement in mantle cell lymphoma. *British Journal of Haematology*, **101**, 302-310. doi:10.1046/j.1365-2141.1998.00684.x

[5] Marts, B.S., Longo, W.E., Maluf, H. and Vernava 3rd, A.M. (1994) Intermediate lymphocytic lymphoma of the small intestine. Mantle cell lymphoma. *Journal of Clinical Gastroenterology*, **18**, 161-162. doi:10.1097/00004836-199403000-00018

[6] Howard, O.M., *et al.* (2002) Rituximab and CHOP induction therapy for newly diagnosed mantle-cell lymphoma: Molecular complete responses are not predictive of progression-free survival. *Journal of Clinical Oncology*, **20**, 1288-1294. doi:10.1200/JCO.20.5.1288

[7] Nickenig, C., *et al.* (2006) Combined cyclophosphamide, vincristine, doxorubicin, and prednisone (CHOP) improves response rates but not survival and has lower hematologic toxicity compared with combined mitoxantrone, chlorambucil, and prednisone (MCP) in follicular and mantle cell lymphomas: Results of a prospective randomized trial of the German Low-Grade Lymphoma Study Group. *Cancer*, **107**, 1014-1022. doi:10.1002/cncr.22093

[8] Weisenburger, D.D., *et al.* (2000) Mantle cell lymphoma. A clinicopathologic study of 68 cases from the Nebraska Lymphoma Study Group. *American Journal of Hematology*, **64**, 190-196. doi:10.1002/1096-8652(200007)64:3<190::AID-AJH9>3.0.CO;2-B

[9] Dreyling, M., *et al.* (2005) Early consolidation by myeloablative radiochemotherapy followed by autologous stem cell transplantation in first remission significantly prolongs progression-free survival in mantle-cell lymphoma: Results of a prospective randomized trial of the European MCL Network. *Blood*, **105**, 2677-2684. doi:10.1182/blood-2004-10-3883

[10] Freedman, A.S., *et al.* (1998) High-dose chemoradiotherapy and anti-B-cell monoclonal antibody-purged autologous bone marrow transplantation in mantle-cell lymphoma: No evidence for long-term remission. *Journal of Clinical Oncology*, **16**, 13-18.

[11] Ward, R.J. and Dirks, P.B. (2007) Cancer stem cells: At the headwaters of tumor development. *Annual Review of Pathology*, **2**, 175-189. doi:10.1146/annurev.pathol.2.010506.091847

[12] Bonnet, D. and Dick, J.E. (1997) Human acute myeloid leukemia is organized as a hierarchy that originates from a primitive hematopoietic cell. *Nature Medicine*, **3**, 730-737. doi:10.1038/nm0797-730

[13] Al-Hajj, M., Wicha, M.S., Benito-Hernandez, A., Morrison, S.J. and Clarke, M.F. (2003) Prospective identification of tumorigenic breast cancer cells. *Proceedings of the National Academy of Sciences of USA*, **100**, 3983-3988. doi:10.1073/pnas.0530291100

[14] Patrawala, L., *et al.* (2006) Highly purified CD44+ prostate cancer cells from xenograft human tumors are enriched in tumorigenic and metastatic progenitor cells. *Oncogene*, **25**, 1696-1708. doi:10.1038/sj.onc.1209327

[15] Vander Griend, D.J., Karthaus, W.L., Dalrymple, S., Meeker, A., DeMarzo, A.M. and Isaacs, J.T. (2008) The role of CD133 in normal human prostate stem cells and malignant cancer-initiating cells. *Cancer Research*, **68**, 9703-9711. doi:10.1158/0008-5472.CAN-08-3084

[16] Du, L., *et al.* (2008) CD44 is of functional importance for colorectal cancer stem cells. *Clinical Cancer Research*, **14**, 6751-6760. doi:10.1158/1078-0432.CCR-08-1034

[17] Chiba, T., *et al.* (2006) Side population purified from hepatocellular carcinoma cells harbors cancer stem cell-like properties. *Hepatology*, **44**, 240-251. doi:10.1002/hep.21227

[18] Yin, S., *et al.* (2007) CD133 positive hepatocellular carcinoma cells possess high capacity for tumorigenicity. *International Journal of Cancer*, **120**, 1444-1450.

[19] Vega, F., *et al.* (2010) Side population of a murine mantle cell lymphoma model contains tumour-initiating cells responsible for lymphoma maintenance and dissemination. *Journal of Cellular and Molecular Medicine*, **14**, 1532-1545. doi:10.1111/j.1582-4934.2009.00865.x

[20] Chen, Z., *et al.* (2010) Prospective isolation of clonogenic mantle cell lymphoma-initiating cells. *Stem Cell Research*, **5**, 212-225.

[21] Yin, A.H., *et al.* (1997) AC133, a novel marker for human hematopoietic stem and progenitor cells. *Blood*, **90**, 5002-5012.

[22] Aruffo, A., Stamenkovic, I., Melnick, M., Underhill, C.B. and Seed, B. (1990) CD44 is the principal cell surface receptor for hyaluronate. *Cell*, **61**, 1303-1313. doi:10.1016/0092-8674(90)90694-A

[23] Denhardt, D.T., Giachelli, C.M. and Rittling, S.R. (2001) Role of osteopontin in cellular signaling and toxicant injury. *Annual Review of Pharmacology and Toxicology*, **41**, 723-749. doi:10.1146/annurev.pharmtox.41.1.723

[24] Haraguchi, N., *et al.* (2008) CD133+CD44+ population efficiently enriches colon cancer initiating cells. *Annals of Surgical Oncology*, **15**, 2927-2933. doi:10.1245/s10434-008-0074-0

[25] Scharenberg, C.W., Harkey, M.A. and Torok-Storb, B. (2002) The ABCG2 transporter is an efficient Hoechst 33342 efflux pump and is preferentially expressed by immature human hematopoietic progenitors. *Blood*, **99**, 507-512. doi:10.1182/blood.V99.2.507

[26] Goodell, M.A., Brose, K., Paradis, G., Conner, A.S. and Mulligan, R.C. (1996) Isolation and functional properties of murine hematopoietic stem cells that are replicating *in vivo*. *Journal of Experimental Medicine*, **183**, 1797-1806. doi:10.1084/jem.183 4.1797

[27] Mao, Q. and Unadkat, J.D. (2005) Role of the breast cancer resistance protein (ABCG2) in drug transport. *American Association of Pharmaceutical Scientists Journal*, **7**,

E118-E133.

[28] Moore, K.A. and Lemischka, I.R. (2006) Stem cells and their niches. *Science*, **311**, 1880-1885. doi:10.1126/science.1110542

[29] Morrison, S.J. and Spradling, A.C. (2008) Stem cells and niches: Mechanisms that promote stem cell maintenance throughout life. *Cell*, **132**, 598-611. doi:10.1016/j.cell.2008.01.038

[30] Vermeulen, L., *et al.* (2010) Wnt activity defines colon cancer stem cells and is regulated by the microenvironment. *Nature Cell Biology*, **12**, 468-476. doi:10.1038/ncb2048

[31] Calabrese, C., *et al.* (2007) A perivascular niche for brain tumor stem cells. *Cancer Cell*, **11**, 69-82. doi:10.1016/j.ccr.2006.11.020

[32] Calvo, K.R., *et al.* (2008) IL-4 protein expression and basal activation of Erk *in vivo* in follicular lymphoma. *Blood*, **112**, 3818-3826. doi:10.1182/blood-2008-02-138933

[33] Chen, X.D. (2010) Extracellular matrix provides an optimal niche for the maintenance and propagation of mesenchymal stem cells. *Birth Defects Research Part C: Embryo Today*, **90**, 45-54. doi:10.1002/bdrc.20171

[34] Chen, X.D., Dusevich, V., Feng, J.Q., Manolagas, S.C. and Jilka, R.L. (2007) Extracellular matrix made by bone marrow cells facilitates expansion of marrow-derived mesenchymal progenitor cells and prevents their differentiation into osteoblasts. *Journal of Bone Mineral Research*, **22**, 1943-1956. doi:10.1359/jbmr.070725

[35] Kanatsu-Shinohara, M., *et al.* (2005) Long-term culture of mouse male germline stem cells under serum-or feeder-free conditions. *Biology of Reproduction*, **72**, 985-991. doi:10.1095/biolreprod.104.036400

[36] Salasznyk, R.M., Williams, W.A., Boskey, A., Batorsky, A. and Plopper, G.E. (2004) Adhesion to vitronectin and collagen I promotes osteogenic differentiation of human mesenchymal stem cells. *Journal of Biomedicine and Biotechnology*, **2004**, 24-34.

[37] Salasznyk, R.M., Williams, W.A., Boskey, A., Batorsky, A. and Plopper, G.E. (2004) Adhesion to vitronectin and collagen I promotes osteogenic differentiation of human mesenchymal stem cells. *Journal of Biomedicine and Biotechnology*, **1**, 24-34. doi:10.1155/S1110724304306017

[38] Stabenfeldt, S.E., Munglani, G., Garcia, A.J. and LaPlaca, M.C. (2010) Biomimetic microenvironment modulates neural stem cell survival, migration, and differentiation. *Tissue Engineering Part A*, **16**, 3747-3758.

[39] Charafe-Jauffret, E., *et al.* (2009) Breast cancer cell lines contain functional cancer stem cells with metastatic capacity and a distinct molecular signature. *Cancer Research*, **69**, 1302-1313. doi:10.1158/0008-5472.CAN-08-2741

[40] Hansford, L.M., *et al.* (2007) Neuroblastoma cells isolated from bone marrow metastases contain a naturally enriched tumor-initiating cell. *Cancer Research*, **67**, 11234-11243. doi:10.1158/0008-5472.CAN-07-0718

[41] Vassilopoulos, A., Wang, R.H., Petrovas, C., Ambrozak, D., Koup, R. and Deng, C.X. (2008) Identification and characterization of cancer initiating cells from BRCA1 related mammary tumors using markers for normal mammary stem cells. *International Journal of Biological Sciences*, **4**, 133-142. doi:10.7150/ijbs.4.133

[42] Itoh, K., *et al.* (1989) Reproducible establishment of hemopoietic supportive stromal cell lines from murine bone marrow. *Experimental Hematology*, **17**, 145-153.

[43] Weekes, C.D., Kuszynski, C.A. and Sharp, J.G. (2001) VLA-4 mediated adhesion to bone marrow stromal cells confers chemoresistance to adherent lymphoma cells. *Leukemia and Lymphoma*, **40**, 631-645. doi:10.3109/10428190109097661

[44] Taswell, C. (1981) Limiting dilution assays for the determination of immunocompetent cell frequencies. I. Data analysis. *Journal of Immunology*, **126**, 1614-1619.

[45] Ploemacher, R.E., van der Sluijs, J.P., Voerman, J.S. and Brons, N.H. (1989) An *in vitro* limiting-dilution assay of long-term repopulating hematopoietic stem cells in the mouse. *Blood*, **74**, 2755-2763.

[46] Robinson, S.N., Seina, S.M., Gohr, J.C., Kuszynski, C.A. and Sharp, J.G. (2005) Evidence for a qualitative hierarchy within the Hoechst-33342 "side population" (SP) of murine bone marrow cells. *Bone Marrow Transplant*, **35**, 807-818. doi:10.1038/sj.bmt.1704881

[47] Issaad, C., Croisille, L., Katz, A., Vainchenker, W. and Coulombel, L. (1993) A murine stromal cell line allows the proliferation of very primitive human CD34++/CD38- progenitor cells in long-term cultures and semisolid assays. *Blood*, **81**, 2916-2924.

[48] Eramo, A., *et al.* (2008) Identification and expansion of the tumorigenic lung cancer stem cell population. *Cell Death and Differentiation*, **15**, 504-514. doi:10.1038/sj.cdd.4402283

[49] Hermann, P.C., *et al.* (2007) Distinct populations of cancer stem cells determine tumor growth and metastatic activity in human pancreatic cancer. *Cell Stem Cell*, **1**, 313-323. doi:10.1016/j.stem.2007.06.002

[50] Ponti, D., *et al.* (2005) Isolation and *in vitro* propagation of tumorigenic breast cancer cells with stem/progenitor cell properties. *Cancer Research*, **65**, 5506-5511. doi:10.1158/0008-5472.CAN-05-0626

[51] Ricci-Vitiani, L., *et al.* (2007) Identification and expansion of human colon-cancer-initiating cells. *Nature*, **445**, 111-115. doi:10.1038/nature05384

[52] Adams, J.C. and Watt, F.M. (1989) Fibronectin inhibits the terminal differentiation of human keratinocytes. *Nature*, **340**, 307-309. doi:10.1038/340307a0

[53] Xu, C., *et al.* (2001) Feeder-free growth of undifferentiated human embryonic stem cells. *Nature Biotechnology*, **19**, 971-974. doi:10.1038/nbt1001-971

[54] Levine, M.S., Rubesin, S.E., Pantongrag-Brown, L., Buck, J.L. and Herlinger, H. (1997) Non-Hodgkin's lymphoma of the gastrointestinal tract: Radiographic findings. *American Journal of Roentgenology*, **168**, 165-172. doi:10.2214/ajr.168.1.8976941

[55] Waugh, D.J. and Wilson, C. (2008) The interleukin-8 pathway in cancer. *Clinical Cancer Research*, **14**, 6735-6741. doi:10.1158/1078-0432.CCR-07-4843

[56] Kodama, H., *et al.* (1992) *In vitro* proliferation of primitive hemopoietic stem cells supported by stromal cells: Evidence for the presence of a mechanism(s) other than that involving c-kit receptor and its ligand. *Journal of Experimental Medicine*, **176**, 351-361. doi:10.1084/jem.176.2.351

[57] Torok-Storb, B., Iwata, M., Graf, L., Gianotti, J., Horton, H. and Byrne, M.C. (1999) Dissecting the marrow microenvironment. *Annals of the New York Academy of Sciences*, **872**, 164-170. doi:10.1111/j.1749-6632.1999.tb08461.x

[58] Cao, J.X., *et al.* (2010) Pluripotency-associated genes in human nasopharyngeal carcinoma CNE-2 cells are reactivated by a unique epigenetic sub-microenvironment. *BMC Cancer*, **10**, 68. doi:10.1186/1471-2407-10-68

[59] Itano, N., Zhuo, L. and Kimata, K. (2008) Impact of the hyaluronan-rich tumor microenvironment on cancer initiation and progression. *Cancer Science*, **99**, 1720-1725. doi:10.1111/j.1349-7006.2008.00885.x

[60] Mbeunkui, F. and Johann Jr., D.J. (2009) Cancer and the tumor microenvironment: A review of an essential relationship. *Cancer Chemotherapy and Pharmacology*, **63**, 571-582. doi:10.1007/s00280-008-0881-9

[61] Quintana, E., Shackleton, M., Sabel, M.S., Fullen, D.R., Johnson, T.M. and Morrison, S.J. (2008) Efficient tumour formation by single human melanoma cells. *Nature*, **456**, 593-598. doi:10.1038/nature07567

[62] Mitsutake, N., *et al.* (2007) Characterization of side population in thyroid cancer cell lines: Cancer stem-like cells are enriched partly but not exclusively. *Endocrinology*, **148**, 1797-1803. doi:10.1210/en.2006-1553

[63] Wu, C., *et al.* (2007) Side population cells isolated from mesenchymal neoplasms have tumor initiating potential. *Cancer Research*, **67**, 8216-8222. doi:10.1158/0008-5472.CAN-07-0999

[64] Kelly, P.N., Dakic, A., Adams, J.M., Nutt, S.L. and Strasser, A. (2007) Tumor growth need not be driven by rare cancer stem cells. *Science*, **317**, 337. doi:10.1126/science.1142596

5

NSC-induced D-neurons are decreased in striatum of schizophrenia: Possible cause of mesolimbic dopamine hyperactivity

Keiko Ikemoto[1,2]

[1]Department of Neuropsychiatry, Fukushima Medical University, School of Medicine, Fukushima, Japan; ikemoto@fmu.ac.jp
[2]Department of Psychiatry, Iwaki Kyoritsu General Hospital, Iwaki, Japan

ABSTRACT

Neural stem cell (NSC) hypofunction is an etiological hypothesis of schizophrenia. Although dopamine (DA) dysfunction is also a widely accepted hypothesis, molecular background of mesolimbic DA hyperactivity has not yet been well known. Here, the author proposes "D-cell hypothesis", accounting for molecular basis of mesolimbic DA hyperactivity of schizophrenia, by NSC hypofunction and decrease of putative NSC-induced D-cells. The "D-cell" is defined as "non-monoaminergic aromatic L-amino acid decarboxylase (AADC)-containing cell". D-cells produce trace amines, and also take up amine precursors and convert them to amines by decarboxylation. The author reported "dopa-decarboxylating neurons specific to the human striatum", that is, "D-neurons" in the human striatum, and decrease of striatal D-neurons in patients with schizophrenia. Trace amine-associated receptor, type 1 (TAAR1), a subtype of trace amine receptors, having a quite number of ligands such as tyramine, *β*- phenylethylamine (PEA) and methamphetamine, has modulating functions on monoamine neurons. It has been known that reduced binding of ligands to TAAR1 receptors on DA terminal of DA neurons of the midbrain ventral tegmental area (VTA) increased firing frequency of VTA DA neurons. In brains of schizophrenia, NSC hypofunction in the subventricular zone of lateral ventricle may cause decrease of D-neurons in the striatum and nucleus accumbens, and may result in decrease of trace amine signals. Decrease of trace amine signals to TAAR1 on VTA DA neurons may increase firing frequency of VTA DA neurons, and may finally cause mesolimbic DA hyperactivity. Increased stimulation to DA D2 receptors of NSCs might suppress NSC proliferation, and may induce additional mesolimbic DA hyperactivity as well as D-cell decrease. This novel theory, "D-cell hypothesis", possibly explains mesolimbic DA hyperactivity in pathogenesis of schizophrenia.

Keywords: Dopamine; D-Neuron; Ventral Tegmental Area; Schizophrenia; TAAR1

1. INTRODUCTION

Dopamine (DA) dysfunction [1,2], glutamate dysfunction [3,4], or neurodevelopmental deficits [5-8] are widely accepted hypotheses for etiology of schizophrenia. Nevertheless, molecular mechanism of mesolimbic DA hyperactivity [1,2] as DA dysfunction has not yet been well known. In the present review, the author proposes "D-cell hypothesis", for explaining mesolimbic DA hyperactivity of schizophrenia, in which neural stem cell (NSC) dysfunction, and decrease of putative NSC-induced D-cells [9] in the striatum and nucleus accumbens [10] are involved.

1.1. Is "D-Cell" NSC-Like Cell?

The "D-cell" was described, by Jaeger *et al.* [11] in 1983, in the rat central nervous system, and was defined "non-monoaminergic aromatic L-amino acid decarboxylase (AADC)-containing cells" [11]. D-cells produce trace amines [12,13], and may also act as an APUD (amine precursor uptake and decarboxylation) system that takes up amine precursors and converts them to amines by decarboxylation [14]. The localizations of D-cells were specified into 14 groups, from D1 (the spinal cord) to D14 (the bed nucleus of stria terminalis), in caudo-rostral orders of the rat central nervous system, using AADC immunohistochemistry [15,16]. In this usage of classification term, "D" meant decarboxylation. In rodents [14, 17,18], a small number of D-cells were described in the striatum, rostral to D14, and confirmed to be neurons by electro-microscopic observation [14].

The author reported in 1997, "dopa-decarboxylating neurons specific to the human striatum [19-22]", that is, "D-neurons" in the human striatum [21,23] (classified to be D15) [21], and later in 2003, the decrease of D-neurons in the striatum and nucleus accumbens of patients with schizophrenia [10,23]. The decrease of D-neurons must be caused by NSC hypofunction in the subventricular zone of lateral ventricle.

Whereas, it is known that the number of striatal D-neurons increased in parkinsonian model rats with unilateral 6OH-DA lesion in the substantia nigra, and the D-neurons synthesized DA after administration of L-dopa [18].

1.2. Trace Amine-Associated Receptor, Type 1 (TAAR1) Modulates DA Function

Since the cloning of trace amine receptors in 2001 [24,25], enormous efforts have been made for exploring signal transduction of these G-protein coupled receptors located on chromosome focus 6q23.1 [26]. The receptors have been shown to co-localize with dopamine or adrenaline transporters in monoamine neurons, and to modulate the functions of monoamines [27-29].

The trace amine-receptor, type 1 (TAAR1) has been shown to have a quite number of ligands, including tyramine, β-phenylethylamine (PEA), octopamine, and psychostimulants, for example, methamphetamine, 3,4-methylenedioxymethamphetamine (MDMA) and lysergic acid diethylamide (LSD) [24,26,30], and is now a target receptor for exploring novel neuroleptics [31,32].

TAAR1 knockout mice displayed schizophrenia-like behaviors, with a deficit in prepulse inhibition [33]. TAAR1 knockout mice showed greater locomotor response to amphetamine and released more DA (and noradrenaline) in response to amphetamine than wild type mice [33].

It has been clarified that signal increase to TAAR1 receptors on cell membranes of DA neurons in the midbrain ventral tegmental area (VTA) reduces firing frequency of VTA DA neurons [26,31,33].

1.3. D-Cell Hypothesis of Schizophrenia

In **Figure 1**, "D-cell hypothesis", the novel theory for mesolimbic DA hyperactivity in pathogenesis of schizophrenia is outlined. In brains of patients with schizophrenia, NSC hypofunction in the subventricular zone of lateral ventricle [34-36] may induce reduction of D-neurons in the striatum and nucleus accumbens [10], and may result in decrease of trace amines. For example, the ventricular enlargement, noticed in brain imaging studies of schizophrenia, may be caused by NSC hypofunction of the subventricular zone of lateral ventricle [35,36].

The reduction of simulation to TAAR1 on VTA DA neurons may increase firing frequency of VTA DA neurons [31,32], and may cause mesolimbic DA hyperactivity.

DA hyperactivity in the striatum [1,2] might inhibit forebrain NSC proliferation by increasing the stimulation to DA D2 receptors [37], and may lead additional decrease of striatal D-neurons, which may induce additional hyperactivity of mesolimbic DA system.

2. Conclusion

Putative NSC-induced D-cells in the striatum, as trace amine producer, are clue to molecular basis of mesolimbic DA hyperactivity of schizophrenia. Further exploration of signal transduction of D-cells is essential.

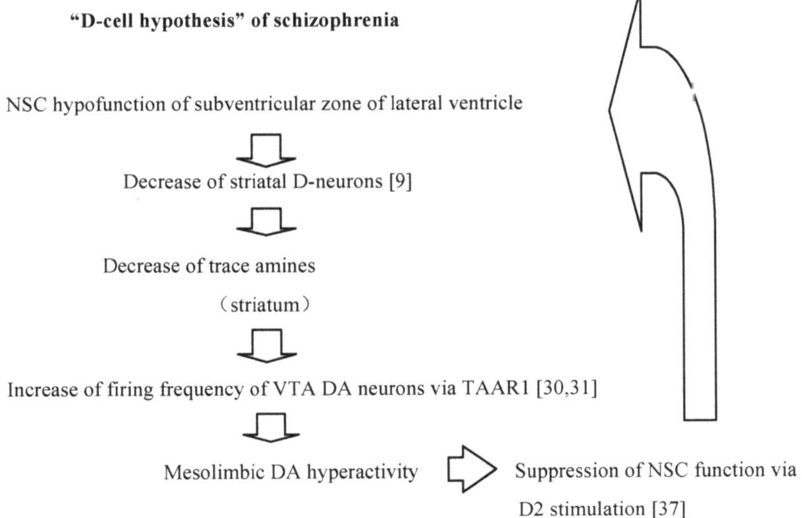

Figure 1. "D-cell hypothesis" of schizophrenia.

3. ACKNOWLEDGEMENTS

The present study was supported by Grant-in-Aid for Scientific Research from Japan Society for the Promotion of Science (JSPS) (C-22591265).

REFERENCES

[1] Hokfelt, T., Ljungdahl, A., Fuxe, K. and Takashima, N. (1974) Dopamine nerve terminals in the rat limbic cortex: Aspects of the dopamine hypothesis of schizophrenia. *Science*, **184**, 177-179. doi:10.1126/science.184.4133.177

[2] Toru, M., Nishikawa, T., Mataga, N. and Takashima, M. (1982) Dopamine metabolism increases in post-mortem schizophrenic basal ganglia. *Journal of Neural Transmission*, **54**, 181-191. doi:10.1007/BF01254928

[3] Watis, L., Chen, S.H., Chua, H.C., Chong, S.A. and Sim, K. (2008) Glutamatergic abnormalities of the thalamus in schizophrenia: A systematic review. *Journal of Neural Transmission*, **115**, 493-511. doi:10.1007/s00702-007-0859-5

[4] Olbrich, H.M., Valerius, G., Rüsch, N., Buchert, M., Thiel, T., Hennig, J., Ebert, D. and Van Elst, L.T. (2008) Frontolimbic glutamate alterations in first episode schizophrenia: Evidence from a magnetic resonance spectroscopy study. *World Journal of Biological Psychiatry*, **9**, 59-63.

[5] Christison, G.W., Casanova, M.F., Weinberger, D.R., Rawlings, R. and Kleinman, J.E. (1989) A quantitative investigation of hippocampal pyramidal cell size, shape, and variability of orientation in schizophrenia. *Archives of General Psychiatry*, **46**, 1027-1032.

[6] Duan, X., Chang, J.H., Ge, S., Faulkner, R.L., Kim, J.Y., Kitabatake, Y., Liu, X.B., Yang, C.H., Jordan, J.D., Ma, D.K., Liu, C.Y., Ganesan, S., Cheng, H.J., Ming, G.L., Lu, B. and Song, H. (2007) Disrupted-in-Schizophrenia 1 regulates integration of newly generated neurons in the adult brain. *Cell*, **130**, 1146-1158. doi:10.1016/j.cell.2007.07.010

[7] Raedler, T.J., Knable, M.B. and Weinberger, D.R. (1998) Schizophrenia as a developmental disorder of the cerebral cortex. *Current Opinion in Neurobiology*, **8**, 157-161. doi:10.1016/S0959-4388(98)80019-6

[8] McGlashan, T.H. and Hoffman, R.E. (2000) Schizophrenia as a disorder of developmentally reduced synaptic connectivity. *Archives of General Psychiatry*, **57**, 637-648.

[9] Ikemoto, K. (2008) Striatal D-neurons: In new viewpoints for neuropsychiatric research using post-mortem brains. *Fukushima Journal of Medical Science*, **54**, 1-3.

[10] Ikemoto, K., Nishimura, A., Oda, T., Nagatsu, I. and Nishi, K. (2003) Number of striatal D-neurons is reduced in autopsy brains of schizophrenics. *Legal Medicine*, **5**, 221-224.doi:10.1016/S1344-6223(02)00117-7

[11] Jaeger, C.B.,Teitelman, G., Joh, T.H., Albert, V.R., Park, D.H. and Reis, D.J. (1983) Some neurons of the rat central nervous system contain aromatic-L-amino-acid decarboxylase but not monoamines. *Science*, **219**, 1233-1235. doi:10.1126/science.6131537

[12] Boulton, A.A. (1974) Amines and theories in psychiatry. *The Lancet*, **304**, 52-53. doi:10.1016/S0140-6736(74)91390-7

[13] Boulton, A.A. and Juorio, A.V. (1979) The tyramines: Are they involved in the psychoses? *Biological psychiatry*, **14**, 413-419.

[14] Komori, K., Fujii, T., Karasawa,N.,Yamada, K., Sakai, M. and Nagatsu, I. (1991) Some neurons of the mouse cortex and caudo-putamen contain aromatic L-amino acid decarboxylase but monoamines. *Acta Histochemica et Cytochemica*, **24**, 571-577. doi:10.1267/ahc.24.571

[15] Jaeger, C.B., Ruggiero, D.A., Albert, V. R., Joh, T.H. and Reis, D.J. (1984) Immunocytochemical localization of aromatic L-amino acid decarboxylase, In: Björklund, A. and Hökfelt, T., Eds., *Handbook of Chemical Neuroanatomy. Vol.* 2: *Classical Transmitters in the CNS, Part I*, Elsevier, Amsterdam, 387-408.

[16] Jaeger, C.B., Ruggiero, D.A., Albert, V.R., Park, D.H., Joh, T.H. and Reis, D.J. (1984) Aromatic L-amino acid decarboxylase in the rat brain: Immunocytochemical localization in neurons of the rat brain stem. *Neuroscience*, **11**, 691-713. doi:10.1016/0306-4522(84)90053-8

[17] Tashiro, Y., Kaneko, T., Sugimoto, T., Nagatsu, I., Kikuchi, H. and Mizuno, N. (1989) Striatal neurons with aromatic L-amino acid decarboxylase-like immunoreactivity in the rat. *Neuroscience Letters*, **100**, 29-34. doi:10.1016/0304-3940(89)90655-1

[18] Mura, A., Linder, J.C., Young, S.J. and Groves, P.M. (2000) Striatal cells containing aromatic L-amino acid decarboxylase: An immunohistochemical comparison with other classes of striatal neurons. *Neuroscience*, **98**, 501-511. doi:10.1016/S0306-4522(00)00154-8

[19] Ikemoto, K., Kitahama, K., Jouvet, A., Arai, R., Nishimura, A., Nishi, K. and Nagatsu, I. (1997) Demonstration of L-dopa decarboxylating neurons specific to human striatum. *Neuroscience Letters*, **232**, 111-114. doi:10.1016/S0304-3940(97)00587-9

[20] Ikemoto, K., Kitahama, K., Jouvet, A., Nishimura, A., Nishi, K., Maeda, T. and Arai, R. (1998) A dopamine-synthesizing cell group demonstrated in the human basal forebrain by dual labeling immunohistochemical technique of tyrosine hydroxylase and aromatic L-amino acid decarboxylase. *Neuroscience Letters*, **243**, 129-132. doi:10.1016/S0304-3940(98)00103-7

[21] Kitahama, K., Ikemoto, K., Jouvet, A., Nagatsu, I., Sakamoto, N. and Pearson, J. (1998) Aromatic L-amino acid decarboxylase and tyrosine hydroxylase immunohistochemistry in the adult human hypothalamus. *Journal of Chemical Neuroanatomy*, **16**, 43-55. doi:10.1016/S0891-0618(98)00060-X

[22] Kitahama, K., Ikemoto, K., Jouvet, A., Araneda, S., Nagatsu, I., Raynaud, B., Nishimura, A., Nishi, K. and Niwa, S. (2009) Aromatic L-amino acid decarboxylase-immunoreactive structures in human midbrain, pons, and medulla. *Journal of Chemical Neuroanatomy*, **38**, 130-140. doi:10.1016/j.jchemneu.2009.06.010

[23] Ikemoto, K. (2004) Significance of human striatal D-neurons: Implications in neuropsychiatric functions. *Progress in Neuro-Psychopharmacology and Biological Psychiatry*, **28**, 429-434. doi:10.1016/j.pnpbp.2003.11.017

[24] Bunzow, J.R., Sonders, M.S., Arttamangkul, S., Harrison, L.M., Zhang, G., Quigley, D.I., Darland, T., Suchland, K.L., Pasumamula, S., Kennedy, J.L., Olson, S.B., Magenis, R.E., Amara, S.G. and Grandy, D.K. (2001) Amphetamine, 3,4-methylenedioxymethamphetamine, lysergic acid diethylamide, and metabolites of the catecholamine neurotransmitters are agonists of a rat trace amine receptor. *Molecular Pharmacology*, **60**, 1181-1188.

[25] Borowsky,.B, Adham,.N, Jones, K.A., Raddatz, R., Artymyshyn, R., Ogozalek, K.L., Durkin, M.M., Lakhlani, P.P., Bonini, J.A., Pathirana, S., Boyle, N., Pu, X., Kouranova, E., Lichtblau, H., Ochoa, F.Y., Branchek, T.A. and Gerald, C. (2001) Trace amines: Identification of a family of mammalian G protein-coupled receptors. *Proceedings of the National Academy of Sciences of USA*, **98**, 8966-8971. doi:10.1073/pnas.151105198

[26] Miller, G.M. (2011) The emerging role of trace amine-associated receptor 1 in the functional regulation of monoamine transporters and dopaminergic activity. *Journal of Neurochemistry*, **116**, 164-176. doi:10.1111/j.1471-4159.2010.07109.x

[27] Xie, Z. and Miller, G.M. (2007) Trace amine-associated receptor 1 is a modulator of the dopamine transporter. *Journal of Pharmacology and Experimental Therapeutics*, **321**, 128-136. doi:10.1124/jpet.106.117382

[28] Xie, Z. and Miller, G.M. (2009) Trace amine-associated receptor 1 as a monoaminergic modulator in brain. *Biochemical Pharmacology*, **78**, 1095-1104. doi:10.1016/j.bcp.2009.05.031

[29] Lindemann, L., Meyer, C.A., Jeanneau, K., Bradaia, A., Ozmen, L., Bluethmann, H., Bettler, B., Wettstein, J.G., Borroni, E., Moreau, J.L. and Hoener, M.C. (2008) Trace amine-associated receptor 1 modulates dopaminergic activity. *Journal of Pharmacology and Experimental Therapeutics*, **324**, 948-956. doi:10.1124/jpet.107.132647

[30] Zucchi, R., Chiellini, G., Scanlan, T.S. and Grandy, D.K. (2006) Trace amine-associated receptors and their ligands. *British Journal of Pharmacology*, **149**, 967-978. doi:10.1038/sj.bjp.0706948

[31] Bradaia, A., Trube, G., Stalder, H., Norcross, R.D., Ozmen, L., Wettstein, J.G., Pinard, A., Buchy, D., Gassmann, M., Hoener, M.C. and Bettler, B. (2009) The selective antagonist EPPTB reveals TAAR1-mediated regulatory mechanisms in dopaminergic neurons of the mesolimbic system. *Proceedings of the National Academy of Sciences of USA*, **106**, 20081-20086. doi:10.1073/pnas.0906522106

[32] Revel, F.G., Moreau, J.L., Gainetdinov, R.R., Bradaia, A., Sotnikova, T.D., Mory, R., Durkin, S., Zbinden, K.G., Norcross, R., Meyer, C.A., Metzler, V., Chaboz, S., Ozmen, L., Trube, G., Pouzet, B., Bettler, B., Caron, M.G., Wettstein, J.G. and Hoener, M.C. (2011) TAAR1 activation modulates monoaminergic neurotransmission, preventing hyperdopaminergic and hypoglutamatergic activity. *Proceedings of the National Academy of Sciences of USA*, **108**, 8485-8490. doi:10.1073/pnas.1103029108

[33] Wolinsky, T.D., Swanson, C.J., Smith, K.E., Zhong, H., Borowsky, B., Seeman, P., Branchek, T. and Gerald, C.P. (2007) The Trace Amine 1 receptor knockout mouse: An animal model with relevance to schizophrenia. *Genes, Brain and Behavior*, **6**, 628-639. doi:10.1111/j.1601-183X.2006.00292.x

[34] Reif, A., Fritzen, S., Finger, M., Strobel, A., Lauer, M., Schmitt, A. and Lesch, K.P. (2006) Neural stem cell proliferation is decreased in schizophrenia, but not in depression. *Molecular Psychiatry*, **11**, 514-522. doi:10.1038/sj.mp.4001791

[35] Degreef, G., Ashtari, M., Bogerts, B., Bilder, R.M., Jody, D.N., Alvir, J.M. and Lieberman, J.A. (1992) Volumes of ventricular system subdivisions measured from magnetic resonance images in first-episode schizophrenic patients. *Archives of General Psychiatry*, **49**, 531-537.

[36] Horga, G., Bernacer, J., Dusi, N., Entis, J., Chu, K., Hazlett, E.A., Haznedar, M.M., Kemether, E., Byne, W. and Buchsbaum, M.S. (2011) Correlations between ventricular enlargement and gray and white matter volumes of cortex, thalamus, striatum, and internal capsule in schizophrenia. *European Archives of Psychiatry and Clinical Neuroscience*, **261**, 467-476. doi:10.1007/s00406-011-0202-x

[37] Kippin, T.E., Kapur, S. and van der Kooy, D. (2005) Dopamine specifically inhibits forebrain neural stem cell-proliferation, suggesting a novel effect of antipsychotic drugs. *The Journal of Neuroscience*, **25**, 5815-5023. doi:10.1523/JNEUROSCI.1120-05.2005

6

Expression of the polycomb group gene *Bmi1* does not affect the prognosis of pediatric acute lymphoblastic leukemia

Teruyuki Kajiume*, Nobutsune Ishikawa, Norioki Ohno, Yasuhiko Sera, Syuhei Karakawa, Masao Kobayashi

Department of Pediatrics, Graduate School of Biomedical Sciences, Hiroshima University, Hiroshima, Japan;
*Corresponding Author: kajiume@hiroshima-u.ac.jp

ABSTRACT

The Polycomb group protein *Bmi1* is a constituent of the Polycomb repressive complex 1, and it is an important molecule for the regulation of the self-renewal of hematopoietic stem cells. In the field of clinical hematology, there are reports that the level of *Bmi1* expression in blast cells is related to the prognosis of acute myeloid leukemia, chronic myeloid leukemia, and myelodysplastic syndrome. We investigated whether the level of *Bmi1* expression in leukemic cells is related to the prognosis and the characteristics of childhood acute lymphoblastic leukemia. In all the leukemic blast cells, *Bmi1* gene expression was lower value than that in normal B cells. There were no correlations between the level of *Bmi1* gene expression in leukemic blast cells and other parameters, including prognosis. Here, we report that the level of *Bmi1* expression in blast cells is not related to the prognosis of pediatric acute lymphoblastic leukemia.

Keywords: Acute Lymphoblastic Leukemia; Leukemic Stem Cell; *Bmi1*; Polycomb

1. INTRODUCTION

Mammalian Polycomb group (PcG) protein complexes can be classified into 2 distinct types, Polycomb repressive complex 1 (PRC1) and PRC2. The PcG protein *Bmi1* is a constituent of PRC1 [1-5]. *Bmi1* is an important molecule for the self-renewal of hematopoietic stem cells (HSCs). The expression of *Bmi1* is generally high in HSCs but decreases after these cells differentiate [6,7]. Some reports in the field of clinical hematology have shown that the expression level of *Bmi1* in blast cells of acute myeloid leukemia (AML), chronic myeloid leukemia (CML), and myelodysplastic syndrome (MDS) can be related to the prognosis of the disease [8-10]. According to these reports, leukemia cells that have a high *Bmi1* expression are correlated with poor prognosis. Cancer stem cells in AML were identified for the first time in 1997. In that study, CD38–/CD34+ cells together with leukemic cells were injected into non-obese diabetic mice with severe combined immunodeficiency disease, and the injected mice developed AML [11]. Subsequently, stem cells of breast cancer, brain tumor, prostate cancer, colon cancer, and pancreatic cancer were successively reported [12-16]. Although there are reports on the stem cells of acute lymphoblastic leukemia, these are fewer than those on other cancers [17,18]. A high expression of *Bmi1*, which has been reported for many cancer stem cells, might be the reason for some cancers becoming chemoresistant [19,20]. We investigated whether *Bmi1* expression is related to the prognosis and cell properties of pediatric acute lymphoblastic leukemia.

2. MATERIALS AND METHODS

2.1. Patients

Because childhood leukemia is usually precursor B leukemia, we limited our investigation to pediatric precursor B acute lymphoblastic leukemia. According to the Declaration of Helsinki, informed consent and permission were obtained from all patients. Leukemic blast cells were collected from patients who had been diagnosed with pediatric precursor B acute lymphoblastic leukemia at Hiroshima university hospital from January 2002 to September 2006. These leukemic blast cells were used for real-time polymerase chain reaction (RT-PCR). Cells were obtained from only those patients in whom the percentage of leukemic cells was higher than 90%, and only CD19+ cells were chosen.

2.2. Flow Cytometric Cell Sorting

The bone marrow-derived cells were labeled with different antibodies to sort each hematopoietic lineage. CD34+/CD38–, CD34+/CD38–/CD10–, CD34+/CD38+/CD10+, CD3+, and CD19+ cells were treated as HSCs, common myeloid progenitors, common lymphoid progenitors, T cells, and B cells, respectively. Dead cells that positively stained with propidium iodide were excluded. The cells were sorted using a FACS Aria system (BD Biosciences, Bedford, MA). Sorted cells with a purity of at least 95% were used for further experimentation.

2.3. Real Time RT-PCR

The TaqMan RT-PCR was used for quantitative gene analysis (TaqMan PCR; Applied Biosystems, Foster City, CA). The sequences of the specific primers were as follows: *Bmi*1, sense primer: 5'-AAA TGC ATC GAA CAA CGA GAA TC-3' and antisense primer: 5'-AAT GAA GTA CCC TCC ACA AAG CA-3'; *GAPDH*, sense primer: 5'-GAA GGT GAA GGT CGG AGT-3' and antisense primer: 5'-CTT TAG GGT AGT GGT AGA AG-3'. The sequences of the 5'-FAM3'-TAMRA labeled probes were as follows: *Bmi*1, 5'-CAG GTG GGG ATT TAG CTC AG-3' and *GAPDH*, 5'-CCG ACT CTT GCC CTT CGA AC-3'. The relative quantification (ΔΔCT method) was used for quantitative analysis.

2.4. Statistical Analysis

The correlation coefficient was analyzed with Pearson product-moment correlation coefficient. Welch's t test was used for analyzed between 2 groups.

3. RESULTS

Firstly, we purified the cell populations of each differentiation stage, including the HSCs from the bone marrow of healthy volunteers and analyzed the expression of the *Bmi*1 gene. The expression of the *Bmi*1 gene is high in HSCs, and decreases when the cells enter the differentiation stage, as shown **Figure 1(a)**. This result is in agreement with a previous report [21]. The inhibition of T-cell differentiation has been reported in *Bmi*1-deficient mice [22]. Therefore, it is thought that *Bmi*1 is essential for T-cell maturation. The expression of the *Bmi*1 gene was high in T cells in moderation. The expression of the *Bmi*1 gene did not increase when B cells underwent differentiation. These results are summarized in the schema (**Figure 1(b)**). The expression of *Bmi*1 in HSCs is 1.0. The expression of the *Bmi*1 gene was lower than HSCs at all hematopoietic stages. In other words, the expression of the *Bmi*1 gene decreased during the differentiation of the hematopoietic cells. In addition, it seems that undifferentiated cells have a high level of *Bmi*1 expression.

Table 1 summarizes the basic data of all participants such as the peripheral blood white blood cell count, cell properties, and age. Unfortunately, 4 patients (Nos. 12 - 14)

Table 1. Summary of the patients' profiles, cell profiles, and the level of *Bmi*1 expression.

case	age	sex	WBC counts in PB at the onset (/mm³)	risk	*Bmi*1/*GAPDH*	positive for [percentage (%)]						hospitalization days	
						CD10	CD19	CD20	CD33	CD34*	CD38		
1	2y8m	M	9400	standard risk	0.241	88.6	88.2	1.8	1.6	86.8	33.5	144	
2	3y1m	M	6900	high risk	0.430	56.2	97.6	25.4	0.3	24.4	99.1	334	
3	6y2m	F	30,910	high risk	0.057	78.4	96.5	22.0	0.9	93.1	76.4	203	
4	0y9m	F	275,400	infant	0.076	89.5	92.7	8.1	0.8	84.2	69.1	436	relapse
5	4y10m	F	5200	standard risk	1.253	91.5	94.1	1.4	56.9	8.9	85.7	166	
6	7y5m	M	9290	high risk	1.683	45.4	79.3	80.7	2.3	0.6	91.5	173	
7	9y2m	M	39,320	high risk	0.127	86.7	89.3	4.3	0.9	61.8	95.8	187	
8	5y5m	F	7920	bcr-abl +	0.040	81.0	84.4	70.8	29.2	59.9	73.8	243	
9	6y0m	F	7600	high risk	0.050	79.6	76.2	21.1	2.6	2.0	98.4	236	
10	1y6m	M	4500	standard risk	0.567	90.9	91.4	62.4	3.1	90.6	82.8	139	
11	8y3m	F	4210	standard risk	1.023	86.6	89.1	18.6	2.7	14.9	91.7	118	
†12	7y3m	F	4900	high risk	0.063	70.7	95.2	4.0	0.4	94.5	98.3	529	relapse
†13	0y1m	F	25,340	infant	0.065	1.5	89.8	2.4	23.1	92.0	99.2	86	
†14	6y9m	F	278,000	bcr-abl +	0.153	91.8	91.4	44.6	0.6	25.2	80.7	364	
†15	1y7m	F	59,770	high risk	0.272	2.0	96.9	3.3	0.4	1.3	91.7	443	

†death case; *$p < 0.05$.

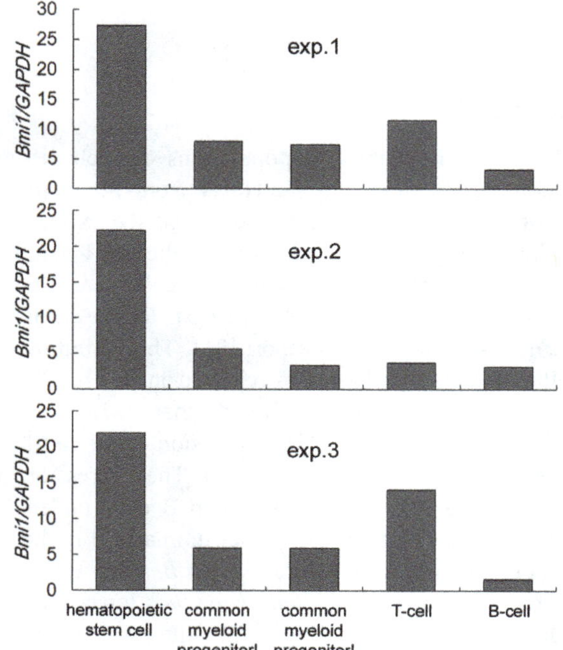

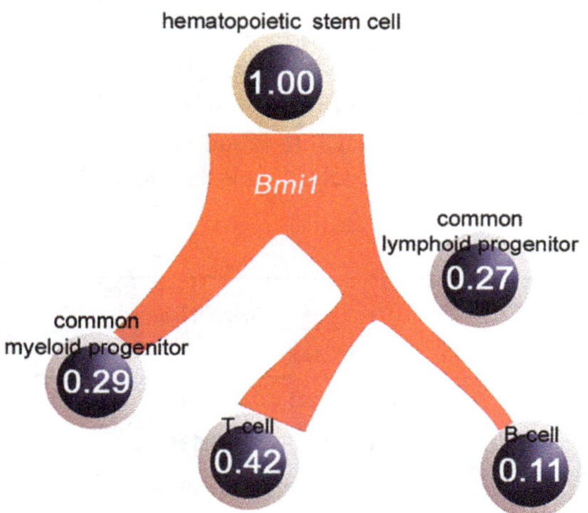

Figure 1. Quantitative analysis of *Bmi*1 gene expression of each hematopoietic cell type. (a) CD34+/CD38–, CD34+/ CD38+/CD10–, CD34+/CD38+/CD10 +, CD3+, and CD19+ cells were treated as HSCs, common myeloid progenitors, common lymphoid progenitors, T cells, and B cells, respectively. The expression of *Bmi*1 increased in immature cells; (b) *Bmi*1 gene expression in each lineage are shown in the schema. The expression of the *Bmi*1 gene decreased during the differentiation of hematopoietic cells.

died in spite of treatment. **Figure 2(a)** compares *Bmi*1 gene expression in the blast cells and B cells (CD19+ cells) from the bone marrow of healthy donors. *Bmi*1 gene expression in all blast cells was low compared to normal B cells. There was no correlation between the prognosis of the patients and the level of *Bmi*1 gene ex-

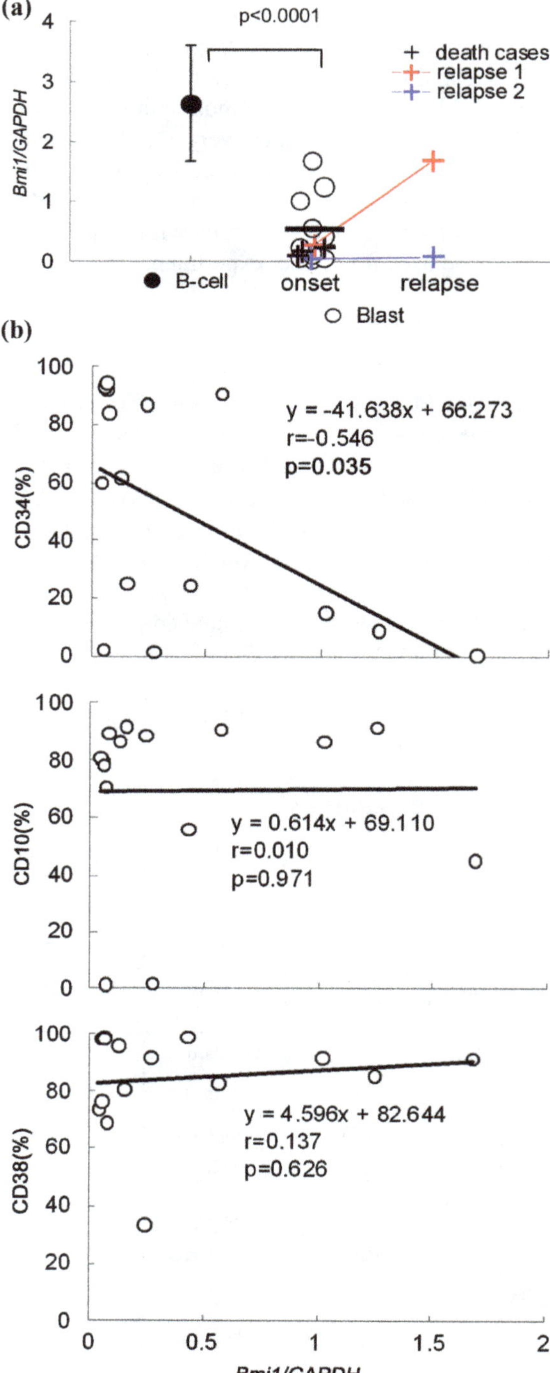

Figure 2. Comparison of the level of *Bmi*1 expression in normal B cells and precursor B cells of acute lymphoblastic leukemia. (a) The level of *Bmi*1 expression is significantly decreased in all leukemic cells as compared to normal B cells. The level of *Bmi*1 expression was not significantly different between recurrent cases and death cases. Error bars indicate standard deviation; (b) There was a correlation between *Bmi*1 gene expression and the cell surface marker CD34. There was no significant difference between other surface markers.

pression. The expression of the *Bmi*1 gene was analyzed using cells from the bone marrow at the time of recurrence in 2 cases (of 4 relapse cases). In one of these 2 cases, *Bmi*1 expression in the blast cells increased from the first onset but did not change in the second case. However, both patients had low expression levels compared to normal B cells. There was a negative correlation between *Bmi*1 gene expression and the cell surface marker CD34 (**Figure 2(b)**). It is known that human HSCs harbor the CD34 antigen. Therefore, we expected that CD34+ cells are undifferentiated cells and express *Bmi*1. However, this result was contrary to our expectation.

4. DISCUSSION

We investigated whether the level of *Bmi*1 gene expression in pediatric precursor B leukemic cells is related to the clinical course, cell profile, and prognosis. There are reports on a relationship between the prognosis of hematopoietic malignancies and *Bmi*1 gene expression. Especially in AML, CML, and MDS, when the expression of the *Bmi*1 gene increased in leukemic blasts, the prognosis was bad [8-10]. Yet, the reason for this is not known. However, the *Bmi*1 protein regulates the p16INK4a protein, which is one of the CDK (cyclin-dependent kinase) inhibitors [23]. In addition, the proliferation of leukemic cells may increase due to *Bmi*1 expression. *Bmi*1 is an essential molecule for the self-renewal of HSCs. It has been reported that the selfrenewal of HSCs reduces remarkably in *Bmi*1-deficient mice [7]. Immature cells such as HSCs have a high expression of *Bmi*1, and *Bmi*1 expression decreases in developed cells during differentiation [21,24]. It has been reported that the expression of the *Bmi*1 gene is high in side population cells such as cancer stem cells in heaptocellular carcinoma [25]. It can be expected that the expression of the *Bmi*1 gene increases in cancer stem cells according to these previous studies. Usually, cancer stem cells are chemoresistant. In addition, it was shown that cancer stem cells are involved in cancer recurrence [26-28]. A high expression of *Bmi*1, which has been reported for many cancer stem cells, might be the reason for some cancers becoming chemoresistant [19,20]. Therefore, there is the possibility that the cancer cells are not exterminated, and the prognosis of the patient worsens. In acute lymphoblastic leukemia, it was reported that CD90+/CD110+ cells in acute lymphoblastic T-cell leukemia, and CD9-overexpressing cells in acute lymphoblastic B-cell leukemia, are cancer stem cells [17,18]. Although these data were collected from in vitro experiments, the existence of cancer stem cells in primary precursor B acute lymphoblastic leukemia cells and pediatric acute lymphoblastic leukemia cells is not clarified yet. In our data, there was the significance of the negative correlation between CD34 and *Bmi*1 expression of blast cells. Generally, it is known that human CD34 positive cells are immature cells. When there are many immature cells, poor prognosis was expected. There were a few reports that CD34 is a prognostic factor in adults with acute myelocytic leukemia [29,30]. However, there were no reports showing the relation between CD34 and prognosis of acute lymphoblastic leukemia. Both CD34 and the expression of *Bmi*1 were not correlated with prognosis in our data. *Bmi*1 expression in pediatric acute lymphoblastic leukemia cells is lower than that in normal B cells. We do not know why the *Bmi*1 expression in pediatric acute lymphoblastic leukemia cells is lower than *Bmi*1 expression in B-cells. Although it is our speculation, pediatric acute lymphoblastic leukemia cells are no longer in immature. Moreover, cancer stem cells in pediatric acute acute lymphoblastic leukemia may be nonexistent.

5. CONCLUSION

We investigated whether the level of *Bmi*1 expression in leukemic cells is related to the prognosis and the characteristics of childhood acute lymphoblastic leukemia. From this result, it will be a very small number even if immature cells like cancer stem cells exist. In addition, there is no correlation between *Bmi*1 expression and the prognosis of pediatric acute lymphoblastic leukemia. Cancer stem cells may not exist in pediatric acute lymphoblastic leukemia. However, the number of people participating in the experiment is not enough in this study. We consider the samples from more patients with leukemia will be necessary to lead certain conclusion.

6. ACKNOWLEDGEMENTS

We are indebted to the pediatric hematologists (Drs. Takashi Sato, M.D., Shinichiro Nishimura, M.D., Hiroshi Kawaguchi, M.D., Kazuhiro Nakamura, M.D., and Mizuka Miki, M.D.) and nurses for providing excellent patient care.

We thank the Analysis Center of Life Science, Hiroshima University, for allowing us to use their facilities.

REFERENCES

[1] Alkema, M.J., Bronk, M., Verhoeven, E., Otte, A., van't Veer, L.J., Berns, A. and van Lohuizen, M. (1997) Identification of *Bmi*1-interacting proteins as constituents of a multimeric mammalian polycomb complex. *Genes & Development*, **11**, 226-240. doi:10.1101/gad.11.2.226

[2] Gunster, M.J., Satijn, D.P., Hamer, K.M., den Blaauwen, J.L., de Bruijn, D., Alkema, M.J., van Lohuizen, M., van Driel, R. and Otte, A.P. (1997) Identification and characterization of interactions between the vertebrate polycomb-group protein *Bmi*1 and human homologs of polyhomeotic. *Molecular and Cellular Biology*, **17**, 2326-2335.

[3] Hashimoto, N., Brock, H.W., Nomura, M., Kyba, M., Hodgson, J., Fujita, Y., Takihara, Y., Shimada, K. and Higashinakagawa, T. (1998) RAE28, *Bmi*1, and M33 are members of heterogeneous multimeric mammalian polycomb group complexes. *Biochemical and Biophysical Research Communications*, **245**, 356-365. doi:10.1006/bbrc.1998.8438

[4] Shao, Z., Raible, F., Mollaaghababa, R., Guyon, J.R., Wu, C.T., Bender, W. and Kingston, R.E. (1999) Stabilization of chromatin structure by PRC1, a polycomb complex. *Cell*, **98**, 37-46. doi:10.1016/S0092-8674(00)80604-2

[5] Francis, N.J., Saurin, A.J., Shao, Z. and Kingston, R.E. (2001) Reconstitution of a functional core polycomb repressive complex. *Molecular Cell*, **8**, 545-556. doi:10.1016/S1097-2765(01)00316-1

[6] Park, I.K., Qian, D., Kiel, M., Becker, M.W., Pihalja, M., Weissman, I.L., Morrison, S.J. and Clarke, M.F. (2003) *Bmi*-1 is required for maintenance of adult self-renewing haematopoietic stem cells. *Nature*, **423**, 302-305.

[7] Lessard, J. and Sauvageau, G. (2003) *Bmi*-1 determines the proliferative capacity of normal and leukaemic stem cells. *Nature*, **423**, 255-260.

[8] Chowdhury, M., Mihara, K., Yasunaga, S., Ohtaki, M., Takihara, Y. and Kimura, A. (2007) Expression of polycomb-group (PcG) protein *Bmi*-1 predicts prognosis in patients with acute myeloid leukemia. *Leukemia*, **21**, 1116-1122. doi:10.1038/sj.leu.2404623

[9] Mohty, M., Yong, A.S., Szydlo, R.M., Apperley, J.F. and Melo, J.V. (2007) The polycomb group *Bmi*1 gene is a molecular marker for predicting prognosis of chronic myeloid leukemia. *Blood*, **110**, 380-383. doi:10.1182/blood-2006-12-065599

[10] Mihara, K., Chowdhury, M., Nakaju, N., Hidani, S., Ihara, A., Hyodo, H., Yasunaga, S., Takihara, Y. and Kimura, A. (2006) *Bmi*-1 is useful as a novel molecular marker for predicting progression of myelodysplastic syndrome and patient prognosis. *Blood*, **107**, 305-308. doi:10.1182/blood-2005-06-2393

[11] Bonnet, D. and Dick, J.E. (1997) Human acute myeloid leukemia is organized as a hierarchy that originates from a primitive hematopoietic cell. *Nature Medicine*, **3**, 730-737. doi:10.1038/nm0797-730

[12] Al-Hajj, M., Wicha, M.S., Benito-Hernandez, A., Morrison, S.J. and Clarke, M.F. (2003) Prospective identification of tumorigenic breast cancer cells. *Proceedings of the National Academy of Sciences of the United States of America*, **100**, 3983-3988. doi: 10.1073/pnas.0530291100

[13] Singh, S.K., Clarke, I.D., Terasaki, M., Bonn, V.E., Hawkins, C., Squire, J. and Dirks, P.B. (2003) Identification of a cancer stem cell in human brain tumors. *Cancer Research*, **63**, 5821-5828.

[14] Xin, L., Lawson, D.A. and Witte, O.N. (2005) The Sca-1 cell surface marker enriches for a prostate-regenerating cell subpopulation that can initiate prostate tumorigenesis. *Proceedings of the National Academy of Sciences of the United States of America*, **102**, 6942-6947. doi:10.1073/pnas.0502320102

[15] Ricci-Vitiani, L., Lombardi, D.G., Pilozzi, E., Biffoni, M., Todaro, M., Peschle, C. and De Maria, R. (2007) Identification and expansion of human colon-cancer-initiating cells. *Nature*, **445**, 111-115.

[16] Li, C., Heidt, D.G., Dalerba, P., Burant, C.F., Zhang, L., Adsay, V., Wicha, M., Clarke, M.F. and Simeone, D.M. (2007) Identification of pancreatic cancer stem cells. *Cancer Research*, **67**, 1030-1037. doi: 10.1158/0008-5472.CAN-06-2030

[17] Yamazaki, H., Nishida, H., Iwata, S., Dang, N.H. and Morimoto, C. (2009) CD90 and CD110 correlate with cancer stem cell potentials in human T-acute lymphoblastic leukemia cells. *Biochemical and Biophysical Research Communications*, **383**, 172-177. doi:10.1016/j.bbrc.2009.03.127

[18] Nishida, H., Yamazaki, H., Yamada, T., Iwata, S., Dang, N.H., Inukai, T., Sugita, K., Ikeda, Y. and Morimoto, C. (2009) CD9 correlates with cancer stem cell potentials in human B-acute lymphoblastic leukemia cells. *Biochemical and Biophysical Research Communications*, **382**, 57-62. doi:10.1016/j.bbrc.2009.02.123

[19] Zhang, S., Balch, C., Chan, M.W., Lai, H.C., Matei, D., Schilder, J.M., Yan, P.S., Huang, T.H. and Nephew, K.P. (2008) Identification and characterization of ovarian cancer-initiating cells from primary human tumors. *Cancer Research*, **68**, 4311-4320. doi:10.1158/0008-5472.CAN-08-0364

[20] Wang, E., Bhattacharyya, S., Szabolcs, A., Rodriguez-Aguayo, C., Jennings, N.B., Lopez-Berestein, G., Mukherjee, P., Sood, A.K. and Bhattacharya, R. (2011) Enhancing chemotherapy response with *Bmi*-1 silencing in ovarian cancer. *PLoS One*, **6**, p. e17918. doi:10.1371/journal.pone.0017918

[21] Lessard, J., Baban, S. and Sauvageau, G. (1998) Stage-specific expression of polycomb group genes in human bone marrow cells. *Blood*, **91**, 1216-1224.

[22] Miyazaki, M., Miyazaki, K., Itoi, M., Katoh, Y., Guo, Y., Kanno, R., Katoh-Fukui, Y., Honda, H., Amagai, T., van Lohuizen, M., Kawamoto, H. and Kanno, M. (2008) Thymocyte proliferation induced by pre-T cell receptor signaling is maintained through polycomb gene product *Bmi*-1-mediated *Cdkn2a* repression. *Immunity*, **28**, 231-245. doi:10.1016/j.immuni.2007.12.013

[23] Jacobs, J.J., Kieboom, K., Marino, S., DePinho, R.A. and van Lohuizen, M. (1999) The oncogene and polycomb-group gene bmi-1 regulates cell proliferation and senescence through the ink4a locus. *Nature*, **397**, 164-168.

[24] Hosen, N., Yamane, T., Muijtjens, M., Pham, K., Clarke, M.F. and Weissman, I.L. (2007) *Bmi*-1-green fluorescent protein-knock-in mice reveal the dynamic regulation of bmi-1 expression in normal and leukemic hematopoietic cells. *Stem Cells*, **25**, 1635-1644. doi:10.1634/stemcells.2006-0229

[25] Chiba, T., Miyagi, S., Saraya, A., Aoki, R., Seki, A., Morita, Y., Yonemitsu, Y., Yokosuka, O., Taniguchi, H., Nakauchi, H. and Iwama, A. (2008) The polycomb gene product *Bmi*1 contributes to the maintenance of tumor-initiating side population cells in hepatocellular carcinoma. *Cancer Research*, **68**, 7742-7749. doi:10.1158/0008-5472.CAN-07-5882

[26] Liu, G., Yuan, X., Zeng, Z., Tunici, P., Ng, H., Abdulkadir,

I.R., Lu, L., Irvin, D., Black, K.L. and Yu, J.S. (2006) Analysis of gene expression and chemoresistance of CD133+ cancer stem cells in glioblastoma. *Molecular Cancer*, **5**, 67-78. doi:10.1186/1476-4598-5-67

[27] Gutova, M., Najbauer, J., Gevorgyan, A., Metz, M.Z., Weng, Y., Shih, C.C. and Aboody, K.S. (2007) Identification of uPAR-positive chemoresistant cells in small cell lung cancer. *PLoS ONE*, **2**, e243. doi:10.1371/journal.pone.0000243

[28] Shafee, N., Smith, C.R., Wei, S., Kim, Y., Mills, G.B., Hortobagyi, G.N., Stanbridge, E.J. and Lee, E.Y. (2008) Cancer stem cells contribute to cisplatin resistance in *Brca1/p*53-mediated mouse mammary tumors. *Cancer Research*, **68**, 3243-3250. doi:10.1158/0008-5472 CAN-07-5480

[29] Geller, R.B., Zahurak, M., Hurwitz, C.A., Burke, P.J., Karp, J.E., Piantadosi, S. and Civin, C.I. (1990) Prognostic importance of immunophenotyping in adults with acute myelocytic leukaemia: The significance of the stem-cell glycoprotein CD34 (My10). *British Journal of Haematology*, **76**, 340-347. doi:10.1111/j.1365-2141.1990.tb06365.x

[30] Myint, H. and Lucie, N.P. (1992) The prognostic significance of the CD34 antigen in acute myeloid leukaemia. *Leukemia & Lymphoma*, **7**, 425-429.

7

Defining umbilical cord blood stem cells

Hamad Ali*, **Fahd Al-Mulla**

Department of Pathology, Human Genetics Unit, Faculty of Medicine, Kuwait University, Kuwait, The State of Kuwait;
*Corresponding Author: hamad.ali@hsc.edu.kw

ABSTRACT

Umbilical cord blood is the blood found in the vessels of the umbilical cord and placenta. It has been shown that this blood contains at least three populations of stem cells, each with unique features and properties. Due to the absence of standardized criteria for characterizing and naming cord blood stem cells, different terms and acronyms have been introduced to describe certain cell populations. Besides the confusion caused by the introduction of these different names, some of the terms used by different groups are inaccurate and misleading when considering the molecular and cellular properties of such cells. Hence, in this review we provide simple and direct descriptions of different populations of stem cells in umbilical cord blood in an attempt to clarify the confusion caused by the existence of multiple names given to certain cord blood stem cells. We also discuss the potential use of umbilical cord blood stem cells as a therapeutic tool for several diseases and disorders in light of ongoing clinical trials.

Keywords: Umbilical Cord Blood; Stem Cell; Embryonic Stem Cell; Adult Stem Cell; Cell Therapy

1. INTRODUCTION

The umbilical cord blood is regarded as the "life line" that supplies the developing fetus with the important nutrition elements and oxygen required for proper fetal development. Beside its role in development, umbilical cord blood has been also involved in therapeutic applications, which was reported for the first time in 1972 by clinicians in the United States to treat a case with lymphoblastic leukemia [1]. In later years, it was used regularly for transplantation in hematology for bone marrow replacement, following either hematological malignancy or bone marrow failure after chemotherapy. Umbilical cord blood use was then restricted to blood-proliferation-based diseases [2,3]. Nevertheless, advances in the production of different tissue groups from umbilical cord blood stem cells, from the three germ layers, has highlighted the additional potential of umbilical cord blood in treatment of other pathological disorders and medical applications including regenerative medicine and tissue engineering [4-6].

Umbilical cord blood contains a highly heterogeneous mixture of cells. This mixture includes hematopoietic cells including erythrocytes and leukocytes. Moreover, umbilical cord blood contains at least three types of stem cells including a population of hematopoietic stem cells (HSCs) and a population of Mesenchymal stem cells (MSCs), which are a multipotent stem cells highly similar to Mesenchymal stem cells (MSCs) of the bone marrow [7,8]. In addition, umbilical cord blood, contains a relatively low concentration of non-hematopoietic multipotent stem cells expressing SSEA-4 protein, a surface marker expressed by embryonic stem cells [9,10], and the transcription factors OCT4, SOX2 and NANOG normally expressed by pluripotent stem cells [10-12]. The potential use of this non-hematopoietic stem cell population in a range of applications underpins the efforts to further characterize and analyze the properties of this unique cell population. Nevertheless, the absence of standardized criteria for characterizing and naming this unique population of cells resulted in the introduction of different names and acronyms for these cells. Such acronyms may have sometimes lead to inaccurate and misleading classification, especially in relation to other types of stem cells. Here, we describe the different types of stem cells that exist in the umbilical cord blood/placenta to ease the misconception and confusion surrounding umbilical cord blood stem cells. Also, we reflect on the advantages of utilizing umbilical cord blood over other sources of stem cells and explore the potential uses of these cells as a therapeutic tool for treating different diseases and disorders.

2. UMBILICAL CORD AND PLACENTA: STRUCTURE, DEVELOPMENT AND FUNCTION

2.1. Umbilical Cord

The umbilical cord is the cord that connects the developing fetus to the placenta. The umbilical cord originates from the same zygote as the fetus. It develops from the yolk sac and allantois by the 5th week of fetal development and replaces the yolk sac as the nutrient supplier for the fetus [13]. The umbilical cord averages 50 - 60 cm in length and about 2 cm in diameter at the end of gestation (**Figure 1**) [14]. It contains three blood vessels, one vein and two arteries, which coil around the vein in a helical configuration [15]. The vein supplies the fetus with nutrient-rich oxygenated blood from the placenta and the arteries takes the nutrient-depleted deoxygenated blood back to the placenta. The three blood vessels are insulated with a gelatinous substance called Wharton's jelly that protects these vessels and prevents their compression [16]. The umbilical cord is connected to the fetus at the abdominal area at the point, which after birth becomes the umbilicus. Once inside the fetus, the vein of the umbilical cord splits into two branches, one joins the hepatic portal vein, which directs blood to the liver and the second allows the majority of blood to bypass the liver and directs it to the fetal heart via the left hepatic vein and inferior vena cava. The umbilical cord arteries branch from the fetal internal iliac artery, which is the main artery in the pelvic area [17].

2.2. Placenta

The placenta is the organ that connects the developing fetus via the umbilical cord to the maternal uterine wall carrying out nutritive, respiratory, and excretory functions [18]. Similar to the umbilical cord, the placenta originate from the same zygote as the fetus. It begins to develop during implantation of the blastocyst into the maternal endometrium and grows throughout pregnancy [19]. Anatomically, the placenta has a dark maroon color and round flat appearance. It averages around 20 cm in diameter and 2.5 cm in thickness at the end of gestation (**Figure 1**).

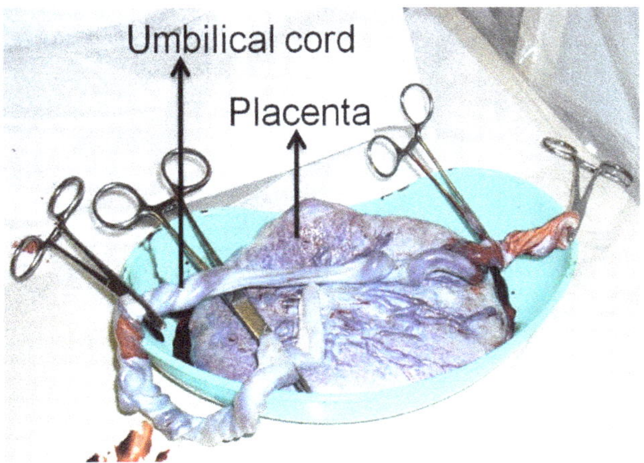

Figure 1. Human placenta and umbilical cord before cord blood collection. Photograph taken minutes after delivery.

The placenta is divided into two portions, the fetal portion and the maternal portion. The fetal portion consists of the chorionic villi, which are villi that merge from the chorion to maximize the contact area with maternal blood. The maternal portion contains the intervillous space, which is the space between the fetal chorionic villi and maternal blood vessels. The delicate walls of the chorionic villi allow the fetal blood to absorb nutrients and oxygen from the maternal blood and discard waste products into it without intermigration of the two blood currents [18,19].

3. UMBILICAL CORD BLOOD CONTAINS DIFFERENT TYPES OF STEM CELLS

The increasing interest in umbilical cord blood emanated from its utilization in hematological applications in the past couple of decades. Previous and current clinical efforts, focused on analyzing and characterizing the constituents of umbilical cord blood. Beside the blood cells, that include erythrocytes, leukocytes and thrombocytes, the umbilical cord blood was found to contain different populations of stem cells, a unique feature not shared with peripheral blood. Scientists and researchers have characterized the following stem cell populations from umbilical cord blood; hematopoietic stem cells (HSCs), multipotent non-hematopoietic stem cells and Mesenchymal stem cells (MSCs) (**Figure 2**).

3.1. Hematopoietic Stem Cells (HSCs)

Haematopoiesis is the process by which blood cells are formed. All blood cellular components are derived from a multipotent stem cell population called hematopoietic stem cells through a series of complex proliferation and differentiation events [20]. Umbilical cord blood has been shown to contain a population of hematopoietic stem cells (HSCs) at different stages of hematopoietic commitment, characterized by their differential expression of hematopoietic antigens CD133, CD34 and CD45 according to a model previously described [21,22]. It has been shown that cord blood hematopoietic stem cells can be selectively induced into specific hematopoietic lineages *in-vitro* including erythroid, megakaryocytic and monocytic lineages [23].

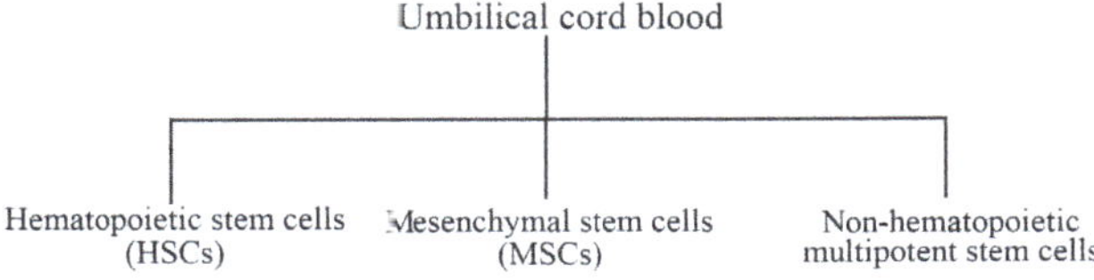

Figure 2. Umbilical cord blood contains at least three populations of stem cells. Each has its unique molecular and cellular properties.

3.2. Mesenchymal Stem Cells (MSCs)

Mesenchymal stem cells (MSCs), are a multipotent stem cell population found originally in the bone marrow [7,8]. These cells have the inherent ability of differentiating into osteogenic, adipogenic and chondrogenic lineages as well as non-mesodermal lineages including neural and hepatic lineages [8,24-26]. MSCs have been also isolated from umbilical cord blood [27-29]. Umbilical cord blood derived MSCs show high morphological and molecular similarities to bone marrow derived MSCs including the lacking of hematopoietic surface antigens CD133, CD34 and CD45 [27,29-31]. Although the isolation of MSCs from umbilical cord blood has been shown to be laborious because of their low number, compared to the bone marrow, cord blood derived MSCs demonstrate higher proliferation capabilities than bone marrow MSCs [29]. Cord blood MSCs have been successfully differentiated *in-vitro* into osteogenic, chondrogenic, neural and hepatic lineages [32-35].

3.3. Multipotent Non-Hematopoietic Stem Cells

A unique population of multipotent non-hematopoietic stem cells has been identified in umbilical cord blood. These stem cells are small in size and exist at low density in cord blood and are negative for the major hematopoietic marker CD45 [9,10,36,37]. This population of cells has been shown to express transcription factors normally expressed by embryonic stem cells including pluripotency key players OCT4, SOX2 and NANOG. In addition, they expressed specific surface markers, which have been used previously to characterize human embryonic stem cell lines. These markers include state-specific embryonic antigens, SSEA-3 and SSEA-4 in addition to tumor rejection antigens TRA1-60 and TRA1-80 [9,10,36, 38,39]. These stem cells have been shown to differentiate into various cell types representing the three germ layers. Many groups have reported successful neural induction of cord blood stem cells representing ectodermal commitment [12,37,40,41], whilst other groups have successfully differentiated cord blood naïve stem cells into endodermic lineages including hepatic and pancreatic cells [5,9], and other groups have reported the successful generation of endothelial cells from cord blood naive stem cells representing the mesodermal lineage [42,43]. Research groups have developed different strategies in attempts to purify cord blood non-hematopoietic stem cells population (**Table 1**). For example, Buzanska *et al.* (2002) developed an immunomagnetic sorting strategy to purify the targeted population. They utilized magnetic beads that can specifically recognize CD34, a surface antigen expressed by hematopoietic stem cells (HSCs), and depleted the CD34-postive cells [44]. The purified CD34-negative cell fraction was reported to express OCT4 and SOX2 [41,45,46]. Forraz *et al.* (2004), utilized the same immunomagnetic depletion strategy used by Buzanska's group but instead of using a single antibody, they used a combination of hematopoietic antibodies including CD45, CD235a, CD38, CD7, CD33, CD56, CD16, CD3, and CD2 in a sequential manner to purify the targeted population, which were reported to make up around 0.1% of the total mononuclear fraction of the cord blood [9,47,48]. Other groups utilized multi-parameter fluorescence-activated cell sorting (FACS) to purify the targeted population. They used a cocktail of antibodies including hematopoietic stem cell markers CD 133, CD34 and the general hematopoietic marker CD45. The CD45-positive cells were eliminated and at the same time the CD133 and CD 34 positive cells were enriched using FACS sorting. Those enriched cells expressed OCT4 and NANOG in addition to surface embryonic marker SSEA-4 [10,49] (**Table 1**).

Table 1. Reported purification and selection methods of umbilical cord blood non-hematopoietic stem cells.

Name of isolated cells	Purification/selection method	Markers expressed	References
Human umbilical cord blood-neural stem cells (HUCB-NSC)	Continuous depletion of CD34 cells (cell line)	OCT4 SOX2	[41,44-46]
Lineage-Negative Stem-Progenitor Cell Population	Immuno-magnetic depletion	TRA-1-60 TRA-1-81 SSEA-4 SSEA-3 OCT4	[9,47-48]
Very small embryonic-like stem cells (VSEL)	FACS sorting	SSEA-4 OCT4 NANOG	[10,49]
Progenitor cord blood cells	CD133 positive selection	NESTIN	[40]
Cord blood derived embryonic-like stem cells (CBE)	Immuno-magnetic depletion	OCT4 SOX2 NANOG	[11]

Due to such marker expression profile, McGuckin *et al.* (2005) named these cells cord blood derived embryonic-like stem cells (CBEs), while Kucia *et al.* (2007) named them very small embryonic-like stem cells (VS ELs). Other groups have also named them cord blood pluripotent stem cells [50,51]. Besides the confusion caused by the introduction of different names and acronyms for these cells (due to the absence of standardized biological/expression or other criteria) the use of terms such as "embryonic-like" and "pluripotent" terms to describe these cells might be inaccurate and misleading. The term "embryonic-like" was given to cells based on their expression of so-called embryonic stem cell markers such as OCT4, the main pluripotency key player in embryonic stem cells [52]. It has been shown that OCT4 has multiple splice variants including OCT4A and OCT4B that differ only in their N terminals whilst having identical C terminals. The splice variants have been shown to have different temporal and spatial expression patterns. Whilst OCT4A was expressed mainly in the nuclei of human embryonic stem cells, OCT4B was detected in many different types of differentiated cells [53,54]. Consequently, McGuckin *et al.* (2005), Kucia *et al.* (2007) and Zhao *et al.* (2006) have all used OCT4 antibodies that were not specific for the OCT4A variant in their studies, and such antibodies have been shown to give positive results on mature hematopoietic cells isolated from adult human peripheral blood [55]. Therefore, drawing conclusions based on such results could be inaccurate. On the other hand, using the term "pluripotent" to describe the differentiation potential of such cells based on the expression profiles of certain markers might not be appropriate even if the cells have been shown to differentiate into some but not all cell types representing the three germ layers. The reason for this is that cord blood stem cells do not form teratomas after transplantation in SCID mice, the current gold standard for determining the pluripotency of human cell lines. Therefore, these stem cells do not satisfy the current criteria for defining them as pluripotent stem cells [56].

Hence to avoid confusion, we suggest naming these cells "non-hematopoietic multipotent stem cells", which defines their differentiation potential and distinguishes them from cord blood hematopoietic stem cells. Such terminology would avoid the inappropriate linking between these cells and embryonic stem cells and better describes their cell biology.

4. WHY UMBILICAL CORD BLOOD STEM CELLS

There has been great debate on the stem cell source of choice for research and clinical applications. Each type of stem cells (embryonic, cord blood, adult) has its advantages and drawbacks when considered for potential clinical applications. Umbilical cord blood offers an alternative source of stem cells with both research and clinical advantages over other sources of stem cells. Moving toward effective clinical applications requires a readily abundant supply of stem cells to provide the needed amounts of stem cells.

With the global birth rate exceeding 140 millions/year, umbilical cord blood can be considered as one of the most abundant sources of stem cells (World health statistics 2011, World Health Organization). In addition, unlike embryonic stem cells, umbilical cord blood stem cells collection is not associated with complicated ethical, religious or political concerns, which makes them more appealing to use in the clinical practice [4,57]. Umbilical cord blood stem cells also show a number of advantages over adult stem cells sources like bone marrow. In addition to the non-invasive collection procedure, umbilical cord blood stem cells show higher proliferating potential and longer telomeres than other adult stem cells [58-60].

Allogenic transplantation with adult HSCs is regarded as a life-saving procedure in the treatment of severe hematological diseases such as hematopoietic malignancies, bone marrow failure syndromes and hereditary immunodeficiency disorders [61]. Yet, this procedure is limited by the availability of suitable HLA-matched donors [62]. Due to the immature HLA status of umbilical cord blood cells, transplantation with cord blood shows better tolerance for HLA-mismatching in comparison with adults HSCs [63]. This unique feature of cord blood allows the safe use of unrelated and HLA-mismatched donor samples when HLA-identical donors are not available, thus providing the clinicians with alternative effective therapeutic options [3,64]. Furthermore, transplantation with HLA-mismatched cord blood samples shows a lower risk of graft-versus-host diseases (GvHD) in comparison with bone marrow transplantation. This is also attributed to the fact that the cells transplanted from umbilical cord blood are more naïve and have lower (HLA) protein expression than adults stem cells including bone marrow stem cells [59,64-66]. In addition, umbilical cord blood transplantation was shown to be associated with a lower risk of infection transmission in comparison with bone marrow transplantation [67]. On the other hand, the low number of stem cells per cord blood unit represents a limitation that is associated with delayed engraftment of these cells into host targeted tissues [62,68]. However, this obstacle has been tackled with the possibility of combining multiple cord blood units in order to increase the final transplanted cell dose resulting in improved engraftment and survival of the transplanted cells [3,61,64,68]. Umbilical cord blood has added advantages over other sources of stem cells. This highlights its potential as the stem cell type of choice for potential treatments of many diseases and disorders for which current form of treatment is inadequate (**Table 2**).

Table 2. Summary of advantages and disadvantages of different stem cell sources.

	Advantages	Disadvantages
Embryonic stem cells	• Pluripotency: can differentiate into any cell type in the body. • Serve as a strong platform for pluripotency, developmental and lineage commitment studies.	• Ethical, religious and political concerns. • Limited number of cells isolated from each embryo. • High chance of transformation into cancer cells (teratomas). • Cells instability *in-vitro* due to lack of proper imprinting patterns.
Umbilical cord blood stem cells	• No ethical, religious or political controversies. • Collection procedure is totally safe and non-invasive • Abundant supply. • Low viral contamination. • Ability to store cord blood units in cord blood banks. • No risk of teratoma formation. • Lower risk of graft-versus-host diseases (GvHD). • Tolerance of HLA-mismatching. • Higher proliferation capacity compared with adult stem cells.	• Limited number of stem cells per single cord blood unit.
Adult stem cells	• No ethical, religious or political controversies. • Effective in generation their tissue of origin. • No risk of teratoma formation. • Established clinical history.	• Often invasive collection procedure. • Limited cell numbers in human body tissues. • Limited differentiation capabilities. • Limited supply. • Limited availability of HLA-match donors.

Table 3. Currently active clinical trials using umbilical cord blood to treat different diseases and conditions.

Targeted disease/condition	**Status**	**Sponsor**	**Clinical Trials.gov Identifier**
Hematologic Neoplasms; Bone Marrow Failure Syndromes	Recruiting participants	University of British Columbia, Canada	NCT00897260
Traumatic Brain Injury	Recruiting participants (phase II)	The University of Texas Health Science Center, Houston, USA	NCT01251003
Hematologic Malignancies	Recruiting participants (phase II)	Fred Hutchinson Cancer Research Center, USA	NCT01175785
Inborn Errors of Metabolism	Recruiting participants (phase I)	Duke University, USA	NCT00692926
Cerebral Palsy	Recruiting participants (phase II)	Duke University, USA	NCT01147653
Leukemia Lymphoma Multiple Myeloma Aplastic Anemia	Recruiting participants (phase II)	Tufts Medical Center, USA	NCT00676806
Spinal cord injuries	Recruiting participants (phase II)	China Spinal Cord Injury Network, China	NCT01046786
Hematologic Malignancies	Recruiting participants (phase II)	Memorial Sloan-Kettering Cancer Center, USA	NCT00739141
Hearing Loss	Recruiting participants (phase I)	Memorial Hermann Healthcare System, USA	NCT01343394
Hypoplastic Left Heart Syndrome	Recruiting participants (phase I)	Duke University, USA	NCT01445041
Type 1 Diabetes	Recruiting participants (phase II)	University of Florida, USA	NCT00873925
Myelodysplastic Syndrome (MDS) Severe Aplastic Anemia (SAA)	Recruiting participants (phase II)	National Heart, Lung, and Blood Institute (NHLBI), USA	NCT00604201

5. THE CLINICAL POTENTIAL OF UMBILICAL CORD BLOOD STEM CELLS

Clinical applications of umbilical cord blood date back to the early 1970s, where it was used to treat lymphoblastic leukemia patients [1]. Since then, it was used regularly in hematology transplantations as a replacement for bone marrow following hematological malignancy or bone marrow failure [2,3]. The discovery of the unique non-hematopoietic multipotent stem cells in cord blood and the ability to differentiate these cells into many different cell types highlighted the potential use of umbilical cord blood as a therapeutic tool for a wider range of diseases and disorders. Umbilical cord blood has already been utilized in a number of clinical trials aimed to treat certain neurological diseases including hypoxic-ischemic encephalopathy and spastic cerebral palsy, several media reports have indicated remarkable improvements in kids treated but official reports are yet to be published. In another currently active trial, umbilical cord blood is being utilized to treat people with spinal cord injuries. Umbilical cord blood is also currently involved in clinical trials treating different hematological conditions, inborn errors of metabolism, diabetes and heart disorders (**Table 3**). Clinical trials are still at its early stages but early indications suggest high potential and hope toward developing effective therapies for the disorders and injuries using umbilical cord blood.

6. CONCLUSIONS

Umbilical cord blood can be viewed as a promising source of stem cells for research and clinical applications. It is ethically sound, its abundant supply, immunological immaturity and high plasticity makes it superior to other sources of stem cells. Umbilical cord blood contains at least three different populations of stem cells including hematopoietic stem cells (HSCs), Mesenchymal stem cells (MSCs) and a unique population of non-hematopoietic multipotent stem cells. Supported by *in-vitro* and preclinical studies, umbilical cord blood has been utilized in many different clinical trials aiming to treat a wide range of diseases and disorders. Although still at early stages, preliminary results from these clinical trials demonstrated high potential and hope toward developing effective therapies for various diseases and disorders for which current mode of therapy is inadequate.

7. ACKNOWLEDGEMENTS

We would like to thank Professor Susan Lindsay and Dr Sajjad Ahmad from Institute of Genetic Medicine in University of Newcastle for their support and help.

REFERENCES

[1] Ende, M. and Ende, N (1972) Hematopoietic transplantation by means of fetal (cord) blood: A new method. *Virginia Medical Monthly* 1918, **99**, 276-280.

[2] Gluckman, E., Broxmeyer, H.A., Auerbach, A.D., Friedman, H.S., Douglas, G.W., Devergie, A., Esperou, H., Thierry, D., Socie, G., Lehn, P., *et al.* (1989) Hematopoietic reconstitution in a patient with Fanconi's anemia by means of umbilical-cord blood from an HLA-identical sibling. *New England Journal of Medicine*, **321**, 1174-1178. doi:10.1056/NEJM198910263211707

[3] Slatter, M.A., Bhattacharya, A., Flood, T.J., Abinun, M., Cant, A.J. and Gennery, A.R. (2006) Use of two unrelated umbilical cord stem cell units in stem cell transplantation for Wiskott-Aldrich syndrome. *Pediatric Blood Cancer*, **47**, 332-334. doi:10.1002/pbc.20450

[4] Watt, S.M. and Contreras, M. (2005) Stem cell medicine: Umbilical cord blood and its stem cell potential. *Seminars in Fetal and Neonatal Medicine*, **10**, 209-220. doi:10.1016/j.siny.2005.02.001

[5] Denner, L., Bodenburg, Y., Zhao, J.G., Howe, M., Cappo, J., Tilton, R.G., Copland, J.A., Forraz, N., McGuckin, C. and Urban, R. (2007) Directed engineering of umbilical cord blood stem cells to produce C-peptide and insulin. *Cell Proliferation*, **40**, 367-380. doi:10.1111/j.1365-2184.2007.00439.x

[6] Ali, H. and Bahbahani, H. (2010) Umbilical cord blood stem cells—Potential therapeutic tool for neural injuries and disorders. *Acta Neurobiologiae Experimentalis*, **70**, 316-324.

[7] Short, B., Brouard, N., Occhiodoro-Scott, T., Ramakrishnan, A. and Simmons, P.J. (2003) Mesenchymal stem cells. *Archives of Medical Research*, **34**, 565-571. doi:10.1016/j.arcmed.2003.09.007

[8] Pittenger, M.F., Mackay, A.M., Beck, S.C., Jaiswal, R.K., Douglas, R., Mosca, J.D., Moorman, M.A., Simonetti, D.W., Craig, S. and Marshak, D.R. (1999) Multilineage potential of adult human mesenchymal stem cells. *Science*, **284**, 143-147. doi:10.1126/science.284.5411.143

[9] McGuckin, C.P., Forraz, N., Baradez, M.O., Navran, S., Zhao, J., Urban, R , Tilton, R. and Denner, L. (2005) Production of stem cells with embryonic characteristics from human umbilical cord blood. *Cell Proliferation*, **38**, 245-255. doi:10.1111/j.1365-2184.2005.00346.x

[10] Kucia, M., Halasa, M., Wysoczynski, M., Baskiewicz-Masiuk, M., Moldenhawer, S., Zuba-Surma, E., Czajka, R., Wojakowski, W., Machalinski, B. and Ratajczak, M.Z. (2007) Morphological and molecular characterization of novel population of CXCR4+ SSEA-4+ Oct-4+ very small embryonic-like cells purified from human cord blood: Preliminary report. *Leukemia*, **21**, 297-303. doi:10.1038/sj.leu.2404470

[11] McGuckin, C., Jurga, M., Ali, H., Strbad, M. and Forraz, N. (2008) Culture of embryonic-like stem cells from human umbilical cord blood and onward differentiation to neural cells *in vitro*. *Nature Protocols*, **3**, 1046-1055. doi:10.1038/nprot.2008.69

[12] Ali, H., Jurga, M., Kurgonaite, K., Forraz, N. and McGuckin, C. (2009) Defined serum-free culturing conditions for neural tissue engineering of human cord blood stem cells. *Acta Neurobiologiae Experimentalis*, **69**, 12-23.

[13] Exalto, N. (1995) Early human nutrition. *European Journal of Obstetrics & Gynecology and Reproductive Biology*, **61**, 3-6. doi:10.1016/0028-2243(95)02146-J

[14] Di Naro, E., Ghezzi, F., Raio, L., Franchi, M. and D'Addario, V. (2001) Umbilical cord morphology and pregnancy outcome. *European Journal of Obstetrics & Gynecology and Reproductive Biology*, **96**, 150-157. doi:10.1016/S0301-2115(00)00470-X

[15] Chaurasia, B.D. and Agarwal, B.M. (1979) Helical structure of the human umbilical cord. *Acta Anatomica*, **103**, 226-230. doi:10.1159/000145013

[16] Ferguson, V.L. and Dodson, R.B. (2009) Bioengineering aspects of the umbilical cord. *European Journal of Obstetrics & Gynecology and Reproductive Biology*, **144**, Suppl. **1**, S108-S113. doi:10.1016/j.ejogrb.2009.02.024

[17] Currarino, G., Stannard, M.W. and Kolni, H. (1991) Umbilical vein draining into the inferior vena cava via the internal iliac vein, bypassing the liver. *Pediatric Radiology*, **21**, 265-266. doi:10.1007/BF02018619

[18] Desforges, M. and Sibley, C.P. (2010) Placental nutrient supply and fetal growth. *International Journal of Developmental Biology*, **54**, 377-390. doi:10.1387/ijdb.082765md

[19] Cross, J.C., Nakano, H., Natale, D.R., Simmons, D.G. and Watson, E.D. (2006) Branching morphogenesis during development of placental villi. *Differentiation*, **74**, 393-401. doi:10.1111/j.1432-0436.2006.00103.x

[20] Muller-Sieburg, C.E., Cho, R.H., Thoman, M., Adkins, B. and Sieburg, H.B. (2002) Deterministic regulation of hematopoietic stem cell self-renewal and differentiation. *Blood*, **100**, 1302-1309.

[21] McGuckin, C.P., Pearce, D., Forraz, N., Tooze, J.A., Watt, S.M. and Pettengell, R. (2003) Multiparametric analysis of immature cell populations in umbilical cord blood and bone marrow. *European Journal of Haematology*, **71**, 341-350. doi:10.1034/j.1600-0609.2003.00153.x

[22] McGuckin, C.P., Basford, C., Hanger, K., Habibollah, S. and Forraz, N. (2007) Cord blood revelations: The importance of being a first born girl, big, on time and to a young mother! *Early Human Development*, **83**, 733-741. doi:10.1016/j.earlhumdev.2007.09.001

[23] Felli, N., Cianetti, L., Pelosi, E., Care, A., Liu, C.G., Calin, G.A., Rossi, S., Peschle, C., Marziali, G. and Giuliani, A. (2010) Hematopoietic differentiation: A coordinated dynamical process towards attractor stable states. *BMC Systems Biology*, **4**, 85. doi:10.1186/1752-0509-4-85

[24] da Silva Meirelles, L., Chagastelles, P.C. and Nardi, N.B. (2006) Mesenchymal stem cells reside in virtually all post-natal organs and tissues. *Journal of Cell Science*, **119**, 2204-2213. doi:10.1242/jcs.02932

[25] Black, I.B. and Woodbury, D. (2001) Adult rat and human bone marrow stromal stem cells differentiate into neurons. *Blood Cells, Molecules & Diseases*, **27**, 632-636. doi:10.1006/bcmd.2001.0423

[26] Krause, D.S., Theise, N.D., Collector, M.I., Henegariu, O., Hwang, S., Gardner, R., Neutzel, S. and Sharkis, S.J. (2001) Multi-organ, multi-lineage engraftment by a single bone marrow-derived stem cell. *Cell*, **105**, 369-377. doi:10.1016/S0092-8674(01)00328-2

[27] Erices, A., Conget, P. and Minguell, J.J. (2000) Mesenchymal progenitor cells in human umbilical cord blood. *British Journal of Haematology*, **109**, 235-242. doi:10.1046/j.1365-2141.2000.01986.x

[28] Kern, S., Eichler, H., Stoeve, J., Kluter, H. and Bieback, K. (2006) Comparative analysis of mesenchymal stem cells from bone marrow, umbilical cord blood, or adipose tissue. *Stem Cells*, **24**, 1294-1301. doi:10.1634/stemcells.2005-0342

[29] Bieback, K., Kern, S., Kluter, H. and Eichler, H. (2004) Critical parameters for the isolation of mesenchymal stem cells from umbilical cord blood. *Stem Cells*, **22**, 625-634. doi:10.1634/stemcells.22-4-625

[30] Lee, O.K., Kuo, T.K., Chen, W.M., Lee, K.D., Hsieh, S.L. and Chen, T.H. (2004) Isolation of multipotent mesenchymal stem cells from umbilical cord blood. *Blood*, **103**, 1669-1675. doi:10.1182/blood-2003-05-1670

[31] Lindner, U., Kramer, J., Rohwedel, J. and Schlenke, P. (2010) Mesenchymal stem or stromal cells: Toward a better understanding of their biology? *Transfusion Medicine and Hemotherapy*, **37**, 75-83. doi:10.1159/000290897

[32] Liu, G., Ye, X., Zhu, Y., Li, Y., Sun, J., Cui, L. and Cao, Y. (2011) Osteogenic differentiation of GFP-labeled human umbilical cord blood derived mesenchymal stem cells after cryopreservation. *Cryobiology*, **63**, 125-128. doi:10.1016/j.cryobiol.2011.05.005

[33] Zhang, X., Hirai, M., Cantero, S., Ciubotariu, R., Dobrila, L., Hirsh, A., Igura, K., Satoh, H., Yokomi, I., Nishimura, T., Yamaguchi, S., Yoshimura, K., Rubinstein, P. and Takahashi, T.A. (2011) Isolation and characterization of mesenchymal stem cells from human umbilical cord blood: reevaluation of critical factors for successful isolation and high ability to proliferate and differentiate to chondrocytes as compared to mesenchymal stem cells from bone marrow and adipose tissue. *Journal of Cellular Biochemistry*, **112**, 1206-1218. doi:10.1002/jcb.23042

[34] Tio, M., Tan, K.H., Lee, W., Wang, T.T. and Udolph, G. (2010) Roles of db-cAMP, IBMX and RA in aspects of neural differentiation of cord blood derived mesenchymal-like stem cells. *PLoS One*, **5**, E9398. doi:10.1371/journal.pone.0009398

[35] Kang, X.Q., Zang, W.J., Bao, L.J., Li, D.L., Song, T.S., Xu, X.L. and Yu, X.J. (2005) Fibroblast growth factor-4 and hepatocyte growth factor induce differentiation of human umbilical cord blood-derived mesenchymal stem cells into hepatocytes. *World Journal of Gastroenterology*, **11**, 7461-7465.

[36] Zhao, Y., Wang, H. and Mazzone, T. (2006) Identification of stem cells from human umbilical cord blood with embryonic and hematopoietic characteristics. *Experimental Cell Research*, **312**, 2454-2464. doi:10.1016/j.yexcr.2006.04.008

[37] Ali, H., Forraz, N., McGuckin, C.P., Jurga, M., Lindsay, S., Ip, B.K., Trevelyan, A., Basford, C., Habibollah, S., Ahmad, S., Clowry, G.J. and Bayatti, N. (2011) *In vitro* modelling of cortical neurogenesis by sequential induction of human umbilical cord blood stem cells. *Stem Cell Review*, **43**, 215-227.

[38] Adewumi, O., Aflatoonian, B., *et al.* (2007) Characterization of human embryonic stem cell lines by the international stem cell initiative. *National Biotechnology*, **25**, 803-816. doi:10.1038/nbt1318

[39] Inamdar, M.S., Venu, P., Srinivas, M.S., Rao, K. and VijayRaghavan, K. (2009) Derivation and characterization of two sibling human embryonic stem cell lines from discarded grade III embryos. *Stem Cells and Development*, **18**, 423-433. doi:10.1089/scd.2008.0131

[40] Zangiacomi, V., Balon, N., Maddens, S., Lapierre, V., Tiberghien, P., Schlichter, R., Versaux-Botteri, C. and Deschaseaux, F. (2008) Cord blood-derived neurons are originated from CD133+/CD34 stem/progenitor cells in a cell-to-cell contact dependent manner. *Stem Cells and Development*, **17**, 1005-1016. doi:10.1089/scd.2007.0248

[41] Habich, A., Jurga, M., Markiewicz, I., Lukomska, B., Bany-Laszewicz, U. and Domanska-Janik, K. (2006) Early appearance of stem/progenitor cells with neural-like characteristics in human cord blood mononuclear fraction cultured *in vitro*. *Experimental Hematology*, **34**, 914-925. doi:10.1016/j.exphem.2006.03.010

[42] Senegaglia, A.C., Barboza, L.A., Dallagiovanna, B., Aita, C.A., Hansen, P., Rebelatto, C.L., Aguiar, A.M., Miyague, N.I., Shigunov, P., Barchiki, F., Correa, A., Olandoski, M., Krieger, M.A. and Brofman, P.R. (2010) Are purified or expanded cord blood-derived CD133+ cells better at improving cardiac function? *Experimental Biology and Medicine*, **235**, 119-129. doi:10.1258/ebm.2009.009194

[43] Ma, N., Ladilov, Y., Kaminski, A., Piechaczek, C., Choi, Y.H., Li, W., Steinhoff, G. and Stamm, C. (2006) Umbilical cord blood cell transplantation for myocardial regeneration. *Transplantation Proceedings*, **38**, 771-773. doi:10.1016/j.transproceed.2006.01.061

[44] Buzanska, L., Machaj, E.K., Zablocka, B., Pojda, Z. and Domanska-Janik, K. (2002) Human cord blood-derived cells attain neuronal and glial features *in vitro*. *Journal of Cell Science*, **115**, 2131-2138.

[45] Buzanska, L., Jurga, M. and Domanska-Janik, K. (2006) Neuronal differentiation of human umbilical cord blood neural stem-like cell line. *Neurodegenerative Diseases*, **3**, 19-26. doi:10.1159/000092088

[46] Buzanska, L., Jurga, M., Stachowiak, E.K., Stachowiak, M.K. and Domanska-Janik, K. (2006) Neural stem-like cell line derived from a nonhematopoietic population of human umbilical cord blood. *Stem Cells and Development*, **15**, 391-406. doi:10.1089/scd.2006.15.391

[47] Forraz, N., Pettengell, R. and McGuckin, C.P. (2004) Characterization of a lineage-negative stem-progenitor cell population optimized for *ex vivo* expansion and enriched for LTC-IC. *Stem Cells*, **22**, 100-108. doi:10.1634/stemcells.22-1-100

[48] McGuckin, C.P., Forraz, N., Allouard, Q. and Pettengell, R. (2004) Umbilical cord blood stem cells can expand hematopoietic and neuroglial progenitors *in vitro*. *Experimental Cell Research*, **295**, 350-359. doi:10.1016/j.yexcr.2003.12.028

[49] Halasa, M., Baskiewicz-Masiuk, M., Dabkowska, E. and Machalinski, B. (2008) An efficient two-step method to purify very small embryonic-like (VSEL) stem cells from umbilical cord blood (UCB). *Folia Histochemica et Cytobiologica*, **46**, 239-243. doi:10.2478/v10042-008-0036-1

[50] Leeb, C., Jurga, M., McGuckin, C., Moriggl, R. and Kenner, L. (2010) Promising new sources for pluripotent stem cells. *Stem Cell Review*, **6**, 15-26. doi:10.1007/s12015-009-9102-0

[51] Harris, D.T. and Rogers, I. (2007) Umbilical cord blood: A unique source of pluripotent stem cells for regenerative medicine. *Current Stem Cell Research & Therapy*, **2**, 301-309. doi:10.2174/157488807782793790

[52] Buitrago, W. and Roop, D.R. (2007) Oct-4: The almighty POUripotent regulator? *Journal of Investigative Dermatology*, **127**, 260-262. doi:10.1038/sj.jid.5700654

[53] Cauffman, G., Liebaers, I., Van Steirteghem, A. and Van de Velde, H. (2006) POU5F1 isoforms show different expression patterns in human embryonic stem cells and preimplantation embryos. *Stem Cells*, **24**, 2685-2691. doi:10.1634/stemcells.2005-0611

[54] Lee, J., Kim, H.K., Rho, J.Y., Han, Y.M. and Kim, J. (2006) The human OCT-4 isoforms differ in their ability to confer self-renewal. *Journal of Biological Chemistry*, **281**, 33554-33565. doi:10.1074/jbc.M603937200

[55] Zangrossi, S., Marabese, M., Broggini, M., Giordano, R., D'Erasmo, M., Montelatici, E., Intini, D., Neri, A., Pesce, M., Rebulla, P. and Lazzari, L. (2007) Oct-4 expression in adult human differentiated cells challenges its role as a pure stem cell marker. *Stem Cells*, **25**, 1675-1680. doi:10.1634/stemcells.2006-0611

[56] Sangeetha, V.M., Kale, V.P. and Limaye, L.S. (2010) Expansion of cord blood CD34 cells in presence of zVADfmk and zLLYfmk improved their *in vitro* functionality and *in vivo* engraftment in NOD/SCID mouse. *PLoS One*, **5**, E12221.

[57] Ballen, K.K., Barker, J.N., Stewart, S.K., Greene, M.F. and Lane, T.A. (2008) Collection and preservation of cord blood for personal use. *Biology of Blood and Marrow Transplantation*, **14**, 356-363. doi:10.1016/j.bbmt.2007.11.005

[58] Pipes, B.L., Tsang, T., Peng, S.X., Fiederlein, R., Graham, M. and Harris, D.T. (2006) Telomere length changes after umbilical cord blood transplant. *Transfusion*, **46**, 1038-1043. doi:10.1111/j.1537-2995.2006.00839.x

[59] Slatter, M.A. and Gennery, A.R. (2006) Umbilical cord stem cell transplantation for primary immunodeficiencies. *Expert Opinion on Biological Therapy*, **6**, 555-565. doi:10.1517/14712598.6.6.555

[60] Kim, D.K., Fujiki, Y., Fukushima, T., Ema, H., Shibuya, A. and Nakauchi, H. (1999) Comparison of hematopoietic activities of human bone marrow and umbilical cord blood CD34 positive and negative cells. *Stem Cells*, **17**, 286-294. doi:10.1002/stem.170286

[61] Brunstein, C.G. and Wagner, J.E. (2006) Cord blood transplantation for adults. *Vox Sanguinis*, **91**, 195-205. doi:10.1111/j.1423-0410.2006.00823.x

[62] Tse, W. and Laughlin, M.J. (2005) Umbilical cord blood transplantation: A new alternative option. *American Society of Hematology Education Program*, 377-383.

[63] Liu, E., Law, H.K. and Lau, Y.L. (2004) Tolerance associated with cord blood transplantation may depend on the state of host dendritic cells. *British Journal of Haematology*, **126**, 517-526. doi:10.1111/j.1365-2141.2004.05061.x

[64] Ringden, O., Okas, M., Uhlin, M., Uzunel, M., Remberger, M. and Mattsson, J. (2008) Unrelated cord blood and mismatched unrelated volunteer donor transplants, two alternatives in patients who lack an HLA-identical donor. *Bone Marrow Transplant*, **42**, 643-648. doi:10.1038/bmt.2008.239

[65] Fasouliotis, S.J. and Schenker, J.G. (2000) Human umbilical cord blood banking and transplantation: A state of the art. *European Journal of Obstetrics & Gynecology and Reproductive Biology*, **90**, 13-25. doi:10.1016/S0301-2115(99)00214-6

[66] Mochizuki, K., Kikuta, A., Ito, M., Akaihata, M., Sano, H., Ohto, H. and Hosoya, M. (2008) Successful unrelated cord blood transplantation for chronic granulomatous disease: A case report and review of the literature. *Pediatric Transplantation*, **13**, 384-389. doi:10.1111/j.1399-3046.2008.00996.x

[67] Behzad-Behbahani, A., Pouransari, R., Tabei, S.Z., Rahiminejad, M.S., Robati, M., Yaghobi, R., Nourani, H., Ramzi, M.M., Farhadi-Andarabi, A., Mojiri, A., Rahsaz, M., Banihashemi, M. and Zare, N. (2005) Risk of viral transmission via bone marrow progenitor cells versus umbilical cord blood hematopoietic stem cells in bone marrow transplantation. *Transplantation Proceedings*, **37**, 3211-3212. doi:10.1016/j.transproceed.2005.07.007

[68] Stanevsky, A., Goldstein, G. and Nagler, A. (2009) Umbilical cord blood transplantation: Pros, cons and beyond. *Blood Reviews*, **23**, 199-204. doi:10.1016/j.blre.2009.02.001

8

Molecular confirmation of CHARGE syndrome from umbilical cord blood stem cells from a deceased newborn and identification of a new mutation in the exon 29 of the *CHD7* gene

Nélida Montano[1*], Andrea Quadrelli[1], Aubrey Milunsky[2], Alicia Vaglio[1], Roberto Quadrelli[1]

[1]Instituto de Genética Médica, Hospital Italiano, Montevideo, Uruguay; *Corresponding Author: rquadr@dedicado.net.uy
[2]Center for Human Genetics, Boston University School of Medicine, Boston, USA

ABSTRACT

CHARGE syndrome (Coloboma of the eye, Heart defects, Atresia of the choanae, Retardation of growth and/or development, Genital and/or urinary abnormalities, and Ear abnormalities) is an autosomal dominant disorder characterized by a specific and a recognizable pattern of anomalies. De novo mutations in the *CHD7* gene are the major cause of CHARGE syndrome. Here, we present a family who sought genetic counseling because of a newborn with dysmorphic features suggesting CHARGE syndrome. The baby died three months later. Afterwards, a molecular genetic testing for sequence analysis of the *CHD7* coding region was performed with DNA extracted from umbilical cord blood stem cells confirming the diagnosis of CHARGE syndrome. Although the diagnosis is first suspected clinically, in the newborn case presented here, we illustrate the importance of the molecular testing to confirm the diagnosis, and to enable precise genetic counseling. Also, even though cord blood has been stored in private banks for more than ten years, there is as yet no routine clinical application of autologous (self-donation) hematopoietic stem cells from cord blood. Now, we illustrate for the first time the usefulness of umbilical cord blood stem cells for diagnosis and genetic counseling in a case that involve a dead propositus.

Keywords: CHARGE Syndrome; *CHD7* Gene; Genetic Counseling; Umbilical Cord Blood Stem Cells

1. INTRODUCTION

CHARGE syndrome is an autosomal dominant disorder with a prevalence of about one in 10,000 [1]. The acronym CHARGE is based on the cardinal features identified when the syndrome was delineated: coloboma, heart malformation, choanal atresia, retardation of growth and/or development, genital anomalies and ear anomalies [2]. The life expectancy of patients with CHARGE syndrome varies widely, with individuals living anywhere from five days to at least 46 years [1,3,4]. Mutations in the *CHD7* gene were identified as causative for CHARGE syndrome in approximately 2/3 of patients with a clinical diagnosis of CHARGE syndrome [5,6]. Of the *CHD7* mutations reported thus far, approximately 72% are nonsense or frameshift, 13% are splice site, and 10% are missense [4]. Recurrent mutations are rare, and clear genotype-phenotype correlations have not been recognized [3,4,7]. *CHD7* is located in 8q12.1; it is 188kb in size, consists of 37 coding exons and one non-coding exon, and codes for a 2997 amino-acid protein. The function of *CHD7* protein is still largely unknown [2]. Pathogeny of the CHARGE remains puzzling: *CHD7* is a regulatory element that potentially affects a large number of development pathways, explaining the pleiotropic nature of its phenotypic spectrum [2]. Originally, the diagnosis of CHARGE syndrome included the identification of four to six cardinal signs, one being either choanal atresia or a coloboma [2]. Afterward, new diagnostic criteria were developed, expanding the original picture to encompass brainstem anomalies and visceral malformations [8] or focusing on the coloboma-choanal atresia-abnormal semicircular canals triad, and giving a formal definition for partial and atypical CHARGE syndromes [2,9]. A combination of coloboma, choanal atresia and abnormal semicircular canals (3C) is highly predictive of the presence of a *CHD7* mutation [2]. Prenatal diagnosis of CHARGE syndrome has been reported at least twice, although more than 200 newborns and infants with CHARGE syndrome have been described [2,10].

Here, we present a family who sought genetic counseling because of a newborn with dysmorphic features suggesting CHARGE syndrome. The baby died three months later. A molecular genetic testing for sequence analysis of the *CHD7* coding region was performed with DNA extracted from umbilical cord blood stem cells. Umbilical cord blood stem cells can be viewed as the stem cells source of choice for clinical and non-clinical research applications [11]. Between other reasons, umbilical cord blood stem cells can be considered as one of the most abundant sources of non-embryonic stem cells, the collection is non-invasive, can be stored and cryopreserved in cord blood banks for later uses and occupy and intermediate age stage between the embryonic stem cells and the adult stem cells, which lead to a higher proliferating potential [11,12]. At this time, we illustrate for the first time the usefulness of umbilical cord blood stem cells for cases that involve a dead propositus.

2. MATERIALS AND METHODS

This case is about a family who sought genetic counseling because of a newborn with dysmorphic features including a square-shaped face with narrow bifrontal diameter, broad nasal bridge, short webbed neck, ocular asimmetry with left palpebral ptosis and ear and hand anomalies. The baby also showed chorioretineal coloboma, choanal atresia, anterior located anus and congenital heart disease. Visual and auditory evoked potentials were defined as pathological. The presenting features suggested the diagnosis of CHARGE syndrome. We recommended a sequence analysis of the *CHD7* coding region but it was not performed at that time. The baby died three months later. Afterwards, the family decided to perform the molecular genetic testing. DNA was extracted from umbilical cord blood stem cells stored in the New England Cryogenic Center (NECC) and the sequence analysis of the *CHD7* coding region was performed in the Center for Human Genetics (Boston University School of Medicine). Analysis of blood samples from patient's parents was also recommended.

Molecular Genetic Testing

DNA from the baby patient was extracted from umbilical cord blood stem cells. Briefly, fluorescence labeled PCR primers in exon flanking regions were used to amplify and sequence coding exons 2 - 38 in the *CHD7* gene in both directions. Exon numbering is based on the NCBI reference NM_017780.2 sequence (2010). This service is performed pursuant to an agreement with Roche Molecular Systems, Inc. This test was developed and its performance characteristics determined by the Center for Human Genetics as required by the CLIA'88 regulations.

DNA from patient's parents was performed on peripheral blood lymphocytes. Briefly, PCR amplification and automated fluorescence sequencing was performed on exon 29 and its intervening sequence and exon 38 and its intervening sequence of the *CHD7* gene.

Also, paternity and maternity testing was performed. Briefly, PCR analysis was used to test the DNA samples for 16 polymorphic markers using the ABI Identifier kit. Amplified DNA fragments were resolved by capillary gel electrophoresis. A paternity index was calculated based on marker frequencies in the population that are published or as derived from our accumulated database (Center for Human Genetics, Boston University School of Medicine).

3. RESULTS

Paternity and maternity was confirmed. DNA samples from the umbilical cord blood stem cells were tested at 16 unlinked DNA marker loci and the baby shares alleles with patient's alleged parents at all 16 tested loci. Analysis of the umbilical cord blood stem cells revealed that the baby was heterozygous for the L1898X alteration in exon 29 of the *CHD7* gene. This alteration has not been previously reported in the literature; however, given that it is a truncating alteration, it likely confirms a diagnosis of CHARGE syndrome. This patient was also found to be heterozygous for the G2914R alteration in exon 38 of the *CHD7*. No additional mutations were found in the remaining 35 exons of *CHD7*. Given the above result, analysis by multiplex ligation-dependant probe amplification (MLPA) to detect whole-exon or whole-gene deletions/duplications in *CHD7* was not performed. These analyses detect approximately 65% of mutations in individuals with clinically diagnosed CHARGE syndrome.

On the other hand, patient's father was found to be negative for the L1898X alteration in exon 29 of the *CHD7* gene, previously identified in this patient's son. Patient's mother was also found to be negative for the L1898X alteration in exon 29 of the *CHD7* gene but heterozygous for the G2914R alteration in exon 38 of the *CHD7* gene. The certainty of the molecular test result exceeds 99%.

Hence, patient's parents were found to be negative for the L1898X mutation, which was interpreted as responsible for the clinical condition of CHARGE syndrome in the newborn. The mutation G2914R, found both in the mother's patient and the child, was considered to be a variant without pathological significance.

4. DISCUSSION

CHARGE syndrome is a clinical diagnosis; the clinical scores have shown their robustness, as almost all patients with *CHD7* mutation are in accord with them

[2]. Although the diagnosis is first suspected clinically, in the newborn case presented here, we illustrate the importance of the molecular testing of the *CHD*7 gene to confirm the diagnosis, and to enable precise genetic counseling. The molecular testing allowed the identification of a new mutation in exon 29 of the *CHD*7 gene from umbilical cord blood stem cells. Published mutation in *CHD*7 are scattered throughout the gene, and do not show preferential domain aggregation nor hot spot; mutations were shown to be dominantly transmitted in some families, and proven recurrence of a mutation in two sibs confirmed the possibility of germinal mosaicism [2]. Most of the mutations are truncating mutations that are likely to result in haploinsufficiency and most of the affected individuals have *de novo* mutations [7]. In the case presented here, the results suggest that the CHARGE syndrome of the newborn correspond to a *de novo* mutation with low risk of recurrence in future pregnancies of the couple. In fact, almost all cases of CHARGE syndrome are sporadic, although a small number of cases of familial CHARGE syndrome and parent-to-child transmission of *CHD*7 mutations have been reported [4]. As a result of the established diagnosis in this case, with low risk of recurrence, the couple decided to undergo a new pregnancy. The pregnancy outcome was an unaffected boy.

Here, we also illustrate for the first time the usefulness of umbilical cord blood stem cells for cases that involve a dead propositus. Privately run cord blood banks store cord blood for donors' own use and keep this for a certain period of time, for a fee that the parents pay to the company. As indicated before, it is possible that the parents regard this service as a sort of "biological life insurance policy" for their children; however, a scientific rationale and an indication for the use of such services are thus far lacking [13]. Allogenic umbilical cord blood stem cells (obtained from healthy donors, rather than from the patient to be treated), have been in routine use worldwide for more than ten years in the treatment of hematopoietic diseases [13,14]. On the other hand, autologous stem cells from cord blood have poor prospects for use in regenerative medicine, because they have to be cryopreserved until use [13]. In fact, there is as yet no routine clinical application of autologous hematopoietic stem cells from cord blood (self-donation of blood), even though cord blood has been stored in private banks for more than ten years [13]. Now, we demonstrate the value of umbilical cord blood stem cells for diagnosis and genetic counseling in a case that involve a dead propositus. This by itself may not be surprising but may encourage storing of cord blood not only for future stem cell-based therapies but to identify significant polymorphisms and mutations that may aid families after death of fetuses or other situations where tissues may not be available.

REFERENCES

[1] Issekutz, K.A., Graham, J.M. Jr., Prasad, C., Smith, I.M. and Blake, K.D. (2005) An epidemiological analysis of CHARGE syndrome: Preliminary results from a Canadian study. *American Journal of Medical Genetics Part A*, **133**, 309-317. doi:10.1002/ajmg.a.30560

[2] Sanlaville, D. and Verloes, A. (2007) CHARGE syndrome: An update. *European Journal of Medical Genetics*, **15**, 389-399.

[3] Jongmans, M.C., Admiraal, R.J., Van Der Donk, K.P., Vissers, L.E., *et al.* (2006) CHARGE syndrome: The phenotypic spectrum of mutations in the *CHD*7 gene. *Journal of Medical Genetics*, **43**, 306-314. doi:10.1136/jmg.2005.036061

[4] Zentner, G.E., Layman W.S., Martin, D.M. and Scacheri, P.C. (2010) Molecular and phenotypic aspects of *CHD*7 mutation in CHARGE syndrome. *American Journal of Medical Genetics Part A*, **152**, 674-686. doi:10.1002/ajmg.a.33323

[5] Vissers, L.E., Van Ravenswaaij, C.M., Admiraal, R., *et al.* (2004) Mutations in a new member of the chromodomain gene family cause CHARGE syndrome. *Nature Genetics*, **36**, 955-957. doi:10.1038/ng1407

[6] Johnson, D.S., Morrison, N., Grant, L., *et al.* (2006) Confirmation of *CHD*7 as a cause of CHARGE association identified by mapping a balanced chromosome translocation in affected monozygotic twins. *Journal of Medical Genetics*, **43**, 280-284. doi:10.1136/jmg.2005.032946

[7] Lalani, S.R., Safiullah, A.M., Fernbach, S.D., Harutyunyan, K.G., *et al.* (2006) Spectrum of *CHD*7 mutations in 110 individuals with CHARGE syndrome and genotype-phenotype correlation. *American Journal of Human Genetics*, **78**, 303-314. doi:10.1086/500273

[8] Blake, K.D., Davenport, S.L., Hall, B.D., *et al.* (1998) CHARGE association: An update and review for the primary pediatrician. *Clinical Pediatrics*, **37**, 159-173. doi:10.1177/000992289803700302

[9] Verloes, A. (2005) Updated diagnostic criteria for CHARGE syndrome: A proposal. *American Journal of Medical Genetics Part A*, **133**, 306-308. doi:10.1002/ajmg.a.30559

[10] Sanlaville, D., Etchevers, H.C., Gonzales, M., Martinovic, J., Clément-Ziza, M., *et al.* (2006) Phenotypic spectrum of CHARGE syndrome in fetuses with *CHD*7 truncating mutations correlates with expression during human development. *Journal of Medical Genetics*, **43**, 211-217. doi:10.1136/jmg.2005.036160

[11] Ali, H. and Bahbahani. H. (2010) Umbilical cord blood stem cells—Potential therapeutic tool for neural injuries and disorders. *Acta Neurobiologiae Experimentalis*, **70**, 316-324.

[12] Watt, S. and Contreras, M. (2005) Stem cell medicine: Umbilical cord blood and its stem cell potential. *Seminars in Fetal and Neonatal Medicine*, **10**, 209-220. doi:10.1016/j.siny.2005.02.001

[13] Reimann, V., Creutzig, U. and Kögler, G. (2009) Stem

cells derived from cord blood in transplantation and regenerative medicine. *Deutsches Aerzteblatt international*, **106**, 831-836.

[14] Verneris, M.R., Brunstein, C.G., Barker, J., Macmillan, M.L., Defor, T., McKenna, D.H., *et al.* (2009) Relapse risk after umbilical cord blood transplantation: enhanced graft versus leukemia effect in recipients of tow units. *Blood*, **114**, 4293-4299. doi:10.1182/blood-2009-05-220525

9

Similar effects of mouse and human *pub* gene on proliferation and embryoid bodies formation in mouse embryonic stem cells *in vitro*

Ekaterina Novosadova, Nella Khaydarova, Ekaterina Manuilova, Elena Arsenyeva, Andrey Lebedev, Vyacheslav Tarantul, Igor Grivennikov

Institute of Molecular Genetics, Russian Academy of Sciences, Moscow, Russia; novek-img@ma l.ru, grivigan@mail.ru

ABSTRACT

Previously we have demonstrated that *pub* gene modulates expression of PU.1 transcription factor and plays an important role in differentiation of embryonic stem cells not only at early stages (during formation of embryoid bodies), but also during differentiation into ectodermal, mesodermal and endodermal derivatives *in vitro*. We have compared the influence of elevated expression of two homological genes *mpub* and *hpub* of mouse and human respectively on early stages of differentiation of murine embryonic stem cells. Overexpression of both genes caused an increase in the number of formed embryoid bodies but did not alter the proliferative activity of transfected embryonic stem cells. It was also observed that expression of *mpub* and *hpub* led to decreased expression of *pu.*1 mRNA.

Keywords: Embryonic Stem Cells; Transfection; Gene Pub; Proliferation

1. INTRODUCTION

Pub belongs to TRIM protein family. This family usually is composed of three zinc-binding domains: RING (R) domain, B-box type 1 (B1) domain and B-box type 2 (B2) domain, followed by coiled-coil (CC) domain [1].

Genes, related to TRIM family are involved in diverse cellular processes, such as growth, differentiation and transcription regulation [2]. For example, the gene coding RFP (RET finger protein) was cloned as transforming gene from human lymphoma cells. *Rfp* gained its transforming activity only if expressed as recombinant fuse protein when its DNA sequence was integrated with fragment coding tyrosine kinase of RET protein [2]. It was shown that RFP protein is present in nuclei and cytosol of cells of wide range of tissues as well as was shown it's interaction with transcriptional regulator (EPC), these facts suggest possible involvement of the abovementioned TRIM family member in processes of cellular and differentiation and proliferation [2].

Another distinguished member of the current family is the PML protein. PML plays an important role in maintenance of genome stability [3,4].

Mutations and structural changes in domains lead to diseases such as familial Mediterranean fever (FMF), Opitz syndrome, dwarfism, as well as malignancies such as promyelocytic leukemia or thyroid carcinoma.

This suggests that TRIM family members play important role in many biological processes [5].

Previously we have shown that human gene *hpub* is excessively expressed in human immunoblast lymphomas [6]. In mouse the high level of mRNA of the homologue *mpub* was observed in spleen, thymus, liver and low level in brain, kidney and skeletal muscle [1]. It was shown that *mpub* binds the master transcription factor PU.1 and is capable to modulate its transcriptional activity [1].

On the basis of this data and considering Pub structure it can be assumed that current protein possesses regulatory fuctions and is able to influence the processes of cellular growth and differentiation [7,8].

Embryonic stem (ES) cells present a unique model for investigation of processes of differentiation into derivatives of three primary germ layers *in vitro* as well as *in vivo*.

In specific cultivation conditions ES cells are capable to go into spontaneous differentiation generating muscular, hematopoietic, neuronal or other derivatives [9,10].

Its also well known that directed differentiation of ES cells can be achieved by addition of different exogenic growth and differentiation factors into the culture media or by the genetic modifications [11,12].

2. MATERIALS AND METHODS

2.1. Cell Cultures

Mouse R1 line ES cells (kindly presented by Alan

Nagy, Mount Sinai Hospital, Toronto, Canada) was isolated from agouti-color (129/Sv × 129/SvJ) F1 line mouse blastocytes. Cell were cultured at 37°C and with 5% CO_2 in α-MEM medium (Sigma, USA) containing 15% fetal bovine serum (FBS) (Gibco, USA), 0.1 mM 2-mercaptethanol, 2 mM L-glutamin, nonessential amino acids (Gibco, USA), nucleosides, vitamins, and antibiotic gentamicin (20 μg/ml). Mitomycin-C (3 μg/ml) treated primary fibroblasts derived from 11 - 12 day mouse embryos were used as feeder layers. Fibroblast cultures were grown in DMEM (Sigma, USA), containing 10% FBS, 2 mM L-glutamine and antibiotic gentamycin (20 μg/ml). When ES cells were cultured in absence of feeder layer recombinant leukemia inhibitory factor (LIF) was added into the culture media (Sigma, USA) to final concentration of 10 ng/ml, to block the spontaneous differentiation of ES cells. Cells were passaged every 72 hours.

2.2. Plasmids Used for ES Cell Transfection

The *pPB* plasmid used in current work was constructed on the base of commercially-available *pcDNA*3 vector (Promega, USA). The recombinant plasmid *pPB* was obtained by cloning full 4450 b.p. cDNA sequence of human *hpub* (Blast 2 database number: gi 15208662) between restriction sites *HindIII* and *NotI*.

The plasmid pub-myc was kindly provided by kindly provided by Hirofumi Nishizumi, (University of Tokyo, 2-11-16 Yayoi, Bunkyo-ku, Tokyo 113-0032, Japan) [2]. The vector contained cDNA sequence of mouse *pub* gene, expressed as fuse protein with myc-epitiope, which allowed further detection of *pub* protein product, using commercial antibodies against myc-epitope. To obtain the control plasmid k-myc, the pub-myc vector was enzymatically digested by specific endonuclease removing the sequence of *pub* between *XhoI* restriction sites and ligating the sticky ends. Plasmid DNA was isolated from transformed *E. coli XL*1 cells Qiagen DNA isolation kit (USA). Plasmid DNA used for transfection was redissolved in sterile water after ethanol precipitation to final concentration of 2 μg/ml.

2.3. Transfection of ES Cells with Unifectin-56

The day before transfection ES cells were seeded on 35 mm Petri dishes covered with gelatin by 5×10^5 per dish with standard culture media. The next day the plasmid DNA was introduced to cells combined with Unifectin-56 (Unifect. The transfection group. Russia) according to producer's protocol. Plasmids k-myc and pub-myc were used for transfection in concentration of 6 mcg per 1 million of cells. For estimation of transfection efficiency the pEGFP-C1 plasmid was used, which contained the enhanced green fluorescent protein gene sequence.

2.4. Isolation of Protein Homogenates from Mammalian Cells

Protein homogenates were isolated from transfected and control cells and EB as previously reported by as [13].

2.5. Protein Electrophoresis in Polyacrylamide Gel

Electrophoretic separation was performed according to Laemmli [14].

2.6. Western Blotting

After electrophoretic separation, proteins were transferred on a Hybond ECL nitrocellulose membrane (Amersham, England) using a Bio-Rad blotting unit at 0.8 mA/cm^2 for 90 min. Polyclonal rabbit antibodies against TRIM 14 (Aviva Systems biology, USA) and mouse antibidies anti-myc (Invitrogen, USA) were used for detection of protein bands on the nitrocellulose membrane. Antibodies against rabbit IgG and mouse IgG conjugated with horseradish peroxidase (IMTEKRussia) were used as secondary antibodies. Complexes were visualized using ECL kit (Amersham, England).

2.7. Test on Pluripotency of Transfected ES Cells

Alkaline phosphatase and SSEA-1 detection was demonstrated as described [15].

2.8. Total RNA Isolation and RT-PCR

Total RNA from ES cells cultivated without the feeder layer in the presence of LIF, EBs was isolated by phenol-chloroform extraction method using a YellowSolve kit (Clonogen, Russia). Reverse transcription was performed using a kit from Silex (Russia) according to the protocol and recommendations of the manufacturer. DNA synthesis was run with 0.5 μg total RNA at 37°C for 1 h in 20 μl of reaction mixture containing 0.05 μg of random hexa-primers and 100 units of moloney murine leukemia virus reverse transcriptase. The reaction was stopped by 10 min incubation at 70°C, the cDNA samples were stored at –20°C.

Polymerase chain reaction (PCR) was run in 25 μl reaction mixture containing Taq-buffer, 1.5 mM mixture of dNTP, 1.25 unit "colored" Taq polymerase (Sintol, Russia), 0.5 μl cDNA sample and 10 pmol of each of the following primers:

For *gapdh*:

5'-TCCATGACAACTTTGGCATTGTGG-3'
5'-GTTGCTGTTGAAGTCGCAGGAGAC-3'
For *pu.*1
5'-CCCGGATGTGCTTCCCTTAT-3'
5'-TCCAAGCCATCAGCTTCTCC-3'
For *mpub*:
5'-CCCATTTGGAAGACGCCG-3'
5'-AGGGTGGCTCAGCTCCG-3'

PCR conditions for the gene *gapdh* were the following: start, 2 min, 95°C, 27 cycles: 95°C, 1 min; 66°C, 45 s; 72°C, 45 s. PCR conditions for the gene *pu.*1 were the following: start, 2 min, 52°C; 35 cycles: 94°C, 30 s; 59°C, 30 s; 72°C, 30 s.

The PCR products were separated in 1.5% agarose gel, visualized using ethidium bromide, and analyzed in BioDocAnalyze system (Biometra, FRG).

Fluorescence intensity was measured for the following products: 375 bp (*gapdh*), 120 bp (*pu.*1), 328 bp (*mpub*) in UV light.

2.9. Evaluation of ES Cells Proliferation

To evaluate cell growth, ES cells were plated on the dishes (d = 35 mm) about 150,000 cells per dish, covered with gelatin, in 2 ml standard medium for stem cells with addition of LIF (10 ng/ml). Cell numbers were estimated on day 3 after plating by direct counting in Goryaev chamber under Olympus CKX41 microscope (Olympus, Japan). Not less than six dishes were counted for each line.

2.10. Induction of ES Cells Differentiation and EB Formation

To induce differentiation with formation of EB, the cells were isolated form the feeder layer fibroblasts: treated with tripsin, centrifuged, and then the suspension was incubated in a Petri dish (d = 60 mm) (Nunc, Denmark) for 15 - 30 min. During this time, the main part of the fibroblasts attached to the bottom of the dish, while stem cells remained in suspension. For EB formation, suspended cells were plated on Petri dish (d = 35 mm) (Nunc, Denmark), about 200,000 cells per dish, or on 96-well U-form plates (Costar, Netherlands), 1000 cells per well and then placed into CO_2-incubator (5% CO_2). The EB were counted on day 3 after formation of the first EB.

2.11. Statistical Analysis

The results were processed with SigmaPlot for Windows and Origin for Windows (Jandel Scientific). The results were presented as mean ± SE. The sets of data were compared using the multiway ANOVA. Difference was considered significant at $p < 0.05$.

3. RESULTS

For obtaining the tranisntly-transfected polyclonal lines of ES cells we have used the pub-myc plasmid, bearing cDNA sequence of murine mpub coexpressed with myc epitope. The above plasmid was kindly provided by our Japanese colleagues [1]. k-myc vector was constructed based on the pub-myc plasmid in which the *pub* sequence was removed by endonuclease digestion and was used as the control.

By transfection of ES cell line R1 we have obtained two polyclonal cultures of ES-pub-myc (carrying transgene) and ES-myc control line. By using RT-PCR we have shown the increase of expression of *mpub* gene both in *mpub* transfected undifferentiated. ES cells (ES-pub-myc) and in embryoid bodies formed by these cells, compared to control line ES-myc (data not shown).

Earlier we have obtained the polyclonal line ES-hpub (carrying human *hpub* gene) and corresponding control line ES-DNA3, as well as embryoid bodies from these lines [16].

Using Western-blot analysis we have shown the presence of protein product hPUB in *hpub* transfected cells and embryoid bodies formed by them (**Figure 1**).

Also the presence of protein product mPub was shown in cell line ES-pub-myc (**Figure 2**).

Next we have estimated the level of endogenous expression of *mpub* in polyclonal lines obtained earlier, carrying the human *hpub* gene. As a consequence of earlier experiments it was shown that in cells carrying human transgenic *hpub* (ES-hpub) as well as in control line the expression of endogenous *mpub* was unaltered (**Figure 3**).

All transfected ES cells expressed cell surface markers specific for undifferentiated ES cells including stage-specific embryonic antigen SSEA-1 and alkaline phosphatase (**Figure 4**).

It was shown previously that *mpub* gene product sup-

Figure 1. Western blotting of hpub-transfected undifferentiated ES cells end EB. 1. ES-hPub; 2. EB-hPub; 3. ES-DNA3 (control); 4. EB-DNA3 (control); 5. The positive control Jurcat cell.

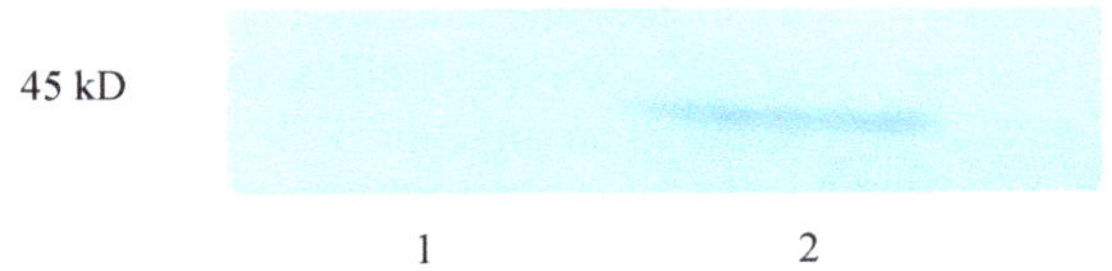

Figure 2. Western blotting of *mpub*-transfected undifferentiated ES cells. 1. ES-myc (control); 2. ES-pub-myc.

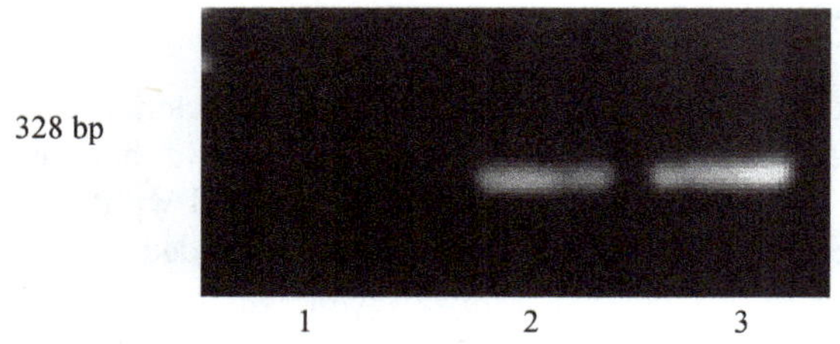

Figure 3. Expression of endogenous *mpub* in undifferentiated ES cells transfected with human *hpub.* 1. Negative control (mixture of RNA for RT-PCR); 2. ES-DNA3 cells; 3. ES-hPub cells.

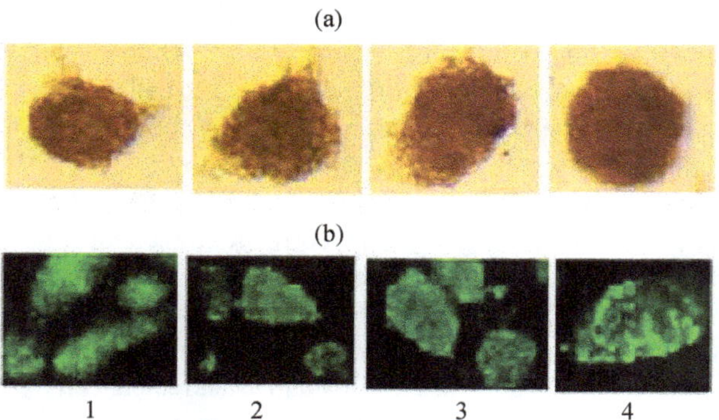

Figure 4. Expression of cell surface markers by transfected MESC. (a) Alkaline phosphatase, (b) SSEA-1. 1. Cells ES-myc (control); 2. Cells ES-pub-myc; 3. Cells ES- DNA3 (control); 4. Cells ES-hpub, ×200.

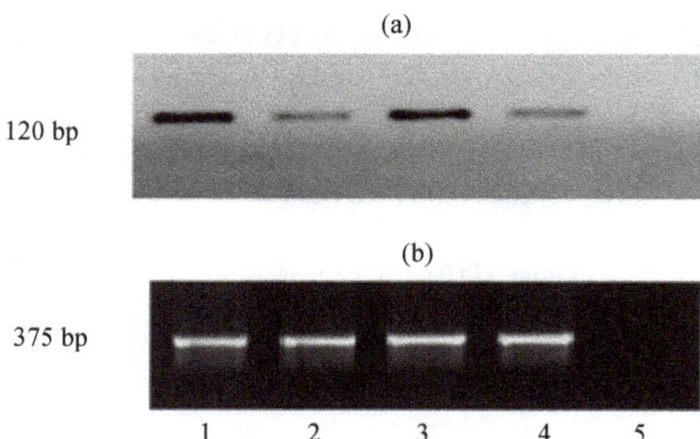

Figure 5. Expression of *pu.*1. (a) and *gapdh* (b) in undifferentiated ES cells transfected with human and mouse genes *pub*. 1. Cells ES-myc (control); 2. Cells ES-pub-myc; 3. Cells ES - DNA3 (control); 4. Cells ES-hpub; 5. Negative control (mixture of RNA for RT-PCR).

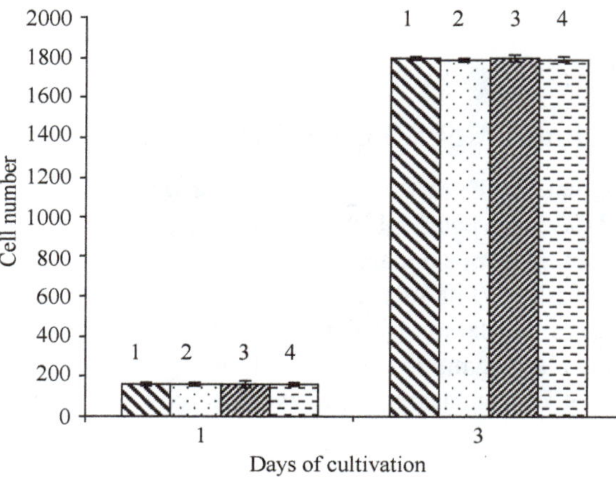

Figure 6. Influence of overexpression of *hpub* and *mpub genes* on proliferative activity of ES cells. 1. ES-DNA3 (control); 2. ES-hPub; 3. ES-myc (control); 4. ES-pub-myc.

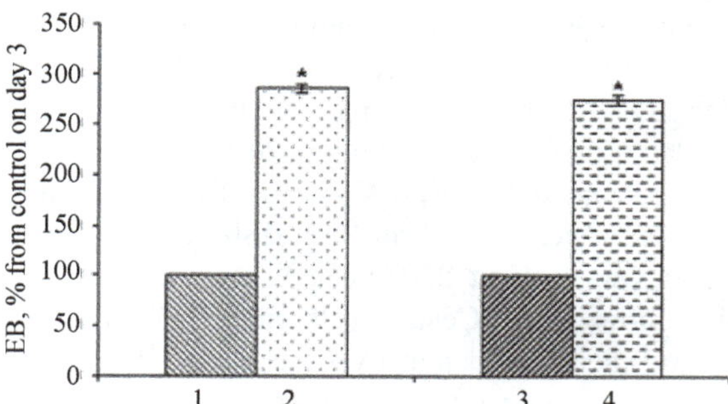

Figure 7. Influence of overexpression of *hpub* and *mpub* genes on EB formation. 1. EB-DNA3 (control); 2. EB-hPub; 3. EB-myc (control); 4. EB-pub-myc. Maximal amount of EBs in control line at 1 and 3 days after the initiation of formation was taken up as 100%. $^*p < 0.05$.

presses the biological activity of transcriptional factor PU.1 [1]. However, the data concerning the possible influence of *mpub* on *pu.*1 expression level are absent in the current literature.

We have examined how the overexpression of *mpub* and *hpub* would influence the expression of endogenous *pu.*1. We have shown that overexpression of either human *hpub* or murine *mpub* caused decrease in expression of endogenous *pu.*1 in cultured transfected ES cells (**Figure 5**).

Comparing the proliferative activity of all four experimental and control lines, no difference was revealed (**Figure 6**).

The above data suggests *mpub* gene product as well as *hpub* do not have considerable influence on proliferaition of undifferentiated ES cells. Next we have compared the time and the number of formed embryoid bodies in cells overexpressing *mpub* and *hpub* and in control lines.

It was shown that the ES-hpub cell line expressing *hpub* gene, as well as in the line ES-pub-myc overexpressing murine *mpub* the embryoid bodies formed approximately 1 day earlier than in control lines (transfected with pcDNA3 and k-myc plasimds resprectively).

Data, presented on **Figure** 7, gives evidence that expression of *mpub* or *hpub* in ES cells substantially influences the early stages of their differentiation, namely the embryoid body formation. After three days after seeding in conditions inducing the formation of EBs their number in ES-hPub and ES-pub-myc cultures was approximately

2.5 times above the number in control cultures.

4. DISCUSSION

It has been established that *pub* gene can modulate the transcriptional activity of PU.1, whisch is the one of the most significant factors controlling hematopoietic differentiation. [1] Recently it was shown, that PU.1 participates in the maintenance of pluripotence of ES cells and demonstrates its effects on earliest stages of differentiation of these cells [17].

The goal of our research is studying the *pub* gene functions. For this purpose we have created earlier the experimental models of murine ES cells overexpressing human *hpub* gene and with decreased expression of endogenous *mpub* of mouse. We have shown significant effect of this gene on various differentiation stages and directions of cellular differentiation, including the EB formation [18].

It is unquestionable that correct transgene function depends not only on its expression stability but also its possible transcriptional and posttranscriptional modifications, such as processing, protein translation regulation to allow the correct further interactions with proteins and other molecules. This is especially actual when heterologous expression systems are used in the experiment. Due to a high homology level of human *hpub* and murine *mpub* genes, we have made an assumption that murine cells transfected with human *hpub* sequence are capable to synthesize the mature biologically active protein Pub.

To check our assumption we have compared the effects of genes *hpub* and *mpub* in populations of transfected ES cells. Comparing the proliferative activity of experimental and control lines no significant difference between these lines were observed. The data on time of EB formation and number of formed embryoid bodies did not reveal any differences in effects of *mpub* and *hpub*.

As we have previously demonstrated [1] *pub* gene product physically interacts with PU.1 transcription factor, which is the one of the most important proteins in regulation of hematopoiesis, inhibiting its activity. We were the first to demonstrate that either *mpub* or *hpub* overexpression led to decrease in expression of *pu.*1 mRNA in mouse ES cells.

In summary, as result of carried experiments we have shown the analogous influence of overexpression of *mpub* and *hpub* genes on proliferation and embryoid body formation in cultured murine ES cells, as well as its negative influence on *pu.*1 expression level.

5. ACKNOWLEDGEMENTS

This study was partially supported by Russian Foundation for Basic Research (Grant N 11-04-01337, 10-04-00656a) and Ministry of education and science of Russian Federation (Grant N 14.740.11.0171).

REFERENCES

[1] Hirose, S., Nishizumi, H. and Sakano, H. (2003) Pub, a novel PU.1 binding protein, regulates the transcriptional activeity of PU.1. *Biochemical and Biophysical Research Communications*, **311**, 351-360. doi:10.1016/j.bbrc.2003.09.212

[2] Shimono, Y., Murakami, H., Hasegawa, Y. and Takahashi, M. (2000) RET finger protein is atranscriptional repressor and interacts with enhancer of polycomb that has dual transcriptional functions. *The Journal of Biological Chemistry*, **275**, 39411-39419. doi:10.1074/jbc.M006585200

[3] Jensen, K., Shiels, C. and Freemont, P. (2001) PML protein isoforms and the RBCC/TRIM motif. *Oncogene*, **20**, 7223-7233. doi:10.1038/sj.onc.1204765

[4] Zhong, S., Hu, P., Ye T., Stan, R., Ellis, N. and Pandolfi, P. (1999) A role for PML and the nuclear body in genomic stability. *Oncogene*, **18**, 7941-7947. doi:10.1038/sj.onc.1203367

[5] Reymond, A., Meroni, G., Fantozzi, A., Merla, G., Cairo, S., Luzi, L., Riganelli, D., Zanaria, E., Messali, S., Cainarca, S., Guffanti, A., Minucci, S., Pelicci, P. and Ballabio, A. (2001) The tripartite motif family identifies cell compartments. *The EMBO Journal*, **20**, 2140-2151. doi:10.1093/emboj/20.9.2140

[6] Nenasheva, V., Maksimov, V., Nikolaev, A. and Tarantul, V. (2001) Comparative analysis of the level of gene transcription in two types of HIV-associated lymphoma. *Mol Gen Mikrobiol Virusol*, **4**, 27-31.

[7] Reddy, B., Etkin, L. and Freemont, P. (1992) A novel zinc finger coiled-coil domain in a family of nuclear proteins. *Trends in Biochemical Sciences*, **17**, 344-345. doi:10.1016/0968-0004(92)90308-V

[8] Borden, K. (1998) RING fingers and B-boxes: Zinc-binding protein-protein interaction domains. *Biochemistry and Cell Biology*, **76**, 351-358. doi:10.1139/o98-021

[9] Doetschman, T., Eistetter, H., Katz, M., Schmidt, W. and Kemler, R. (1985) The *in vitro* development of blastocyst-derived embryonic stem cell lines: Formation of visceral yolk sac, blood islands and myocardium. *Journal of Embryology & Experimental Morphology*, **87**, 27-45.

[10] Hübner, K., Fuhrmann, G., Christenson, L., Kehler, J., Reinbold, R., De La Fuente, R., Wood, J., Strauss, J., Boiani, M. and Schöler, H. (2003) Derivation of oocytes from mouse embryonic stem cells. *Science*, **300**, 1251-1256. doi:10.1126/science.1083452

[11] Wobus, A., Holzhausen, H., Jäkel, P. and Schöneich, J. (1984) Characterization of a pluripotent stem cell line derived from a mouse embryo. *Experimental Cell Research*, **152**, 212-219. doi:10.1016/0014-4827(84)90246-5

[12] Geijsen, N., Horoschak, M., Kim, K., Gribnau, J., Egga, K. and Daley, G. (2004) Derivation of embryonic germ cells and male gametes from embryonic stem cells. *Nature*, **427**, 148-154.

[13] Bobrysheva, I., Grigorenco, A., Novosadova, E., Kal'ina, N., Arsenyeva, E., Grivennikov, I., Tarantul, V. and Ro-

gaev, E. (2003) Effects of human presenilin 1 isoforms on proliferation and survival of rat pheochromocytoma cell line PC12. *Biochemistry*, **68**, 611-617. doi:10.1023/A:1024605523743

[14] Laemmli, U. (1970) Cleavage of structural proteins during the assembly of the head of bacteriophage T4. *Nature*, **227**, 680-685. doi:10.1038/227680a0

[15] Manuilova, E., Arsenyeva, N., Khaidarova, N., Shugurova, I., Tarantul, V. and Grivennikov, I. (2008) Different effects of regulatory genes (tat, nef) of human immunodeficiency virus type 1 (HIV-1) on the proliferation and differentiation of mouse embryonic stem cells *in vitro*. *International Journal of Biomedical Science*, **4**, 29-37.

[16] Novosadova, E., Manuilova, E., Arsenyeva, E., Khaidarova, N., Dolotov, O., Inozemtseva, L., Kozachenkov, K., Tarantul, V. and Grivennikov, I. (2005) Opposite effects increased and decreased expression of the pub gene on the formation embryoid bodies of embryonic stem cells *in vitro*. *Cell Technologies in Biology and Medicine*, **3**, 174-179.

[17] Abujarour, R., Efe, J. and Ding, S. (2010) Genome-wide gain-of-function screen identifies novel regulators of pluripotency. *Stem Cells*, **28**, 1487-1497. doi:10.1002/stem.472

[18] Novosadova, E., Manuilova, E., Arsenyeva, E., Lebedev, A., Khaydarova, N., Tarantul, V. and Grivennikov, I. (2009) Influence of *pub* gene expression on differentiation of mouse embryonic stem cells into derivatives of ecto-, meso-, and endoderm *in vitro*. *Acta Naturae*, **2**, 93-97.

10

Rat adult stem cell differentiation into immature retinal cells

Ma Teresa González-Garza[*]**, Jorge E. Moreno-Cuevas**

Servicio de Terapia Celular, School of Medicine, Tecnológico de Monterrey, Monterrey, México;
[*]Corresponding Author: mtgonzalezgarza@itesm.mx

ABSTRACT

Cell therapy has been proposed as an alternative treatment for retinal diseases. Applications involving stem cells have shown that undifferentiated cells fail to engraft and cannot convert to retinal cells. However, positive results have been reported for retinal precursor cells, suggesting that this approach is the best option. Unfortunately, the source of this cell type is controversial. Predifferentiated adult stem cells may provide an alternative source of cells. The present study proposes a sequential culture media aimed at inducing cells from this source into a preretinal-like lineage. Rat bone marrow stem cells were cultivated in a neuroinduction mix medium for 24 h. The sequence involves immunocytochemistry to detect nestin and tubulin III to demonstrate the cell's neuronal lineage, followed by incubation in retinal-induction mixed medium for 24 h. RT-PCR was performed to detect expression of Brn3b, Pax6, THY1.1, Opn4, and Ath5 genes. Immunocytochemistry results showed increased expression of nestin and tubulin III after 24 h of incubation in the neuroinduction medium. RT-PCR showed slightly increased expression of Pax6, THY1.1, and Opn4 after 48 h of sequential incubation in the neuroinduction and predifferentiation media. Brn3b and Ath5 gene expression increased markedly. These results suggest that mesenchymal stem cells have a high predisposition to differentiate into preretinal-like cells with minimal time in culture. These cells may provide a viable alternative for restoring damaged retinas.

Keywords: Cell Therapy; MSC; Regenerative Medicine; Retinal Diseases; Stem Cells

1. INTRODUCTION

Retinal diseases represent a major source of visual disability worldwide. Glaucoma, the most common cause of retinal injury, is caused by metabolic or genetic diseases [1]. In this condition, ganglion cells are lost as part of the optic nerve degeneration [2]. At present, there are no therapeutic options for functional recovery of the nerve because it is derived from the retinal cell axon [3,4]. Cell therapy is a potential alternative for restoring damaged cells in neurodegenerative diseases [5], including retinopathies. It has been suggested that recovery of ganglion cells and their grown axons might be feasible and, if so, might restore the optic nerve [6-8]. With this target in mind, several groups have focused on the possible engraftment of differentiated or undifferentiated embryonic stem cells (ESCs) into animal models of damaged retinas. The results show that retinal cells derived from human and animal ESCs migrate and engraft into damaged retinas, where the cells differentiate into functional photoreceptors and restore light responses in animals [9-16]. Although ESCs have been suggested as possible repositories of retinal cells, the feasibility of applying these techniques to human clinical protocols are distant because of the ethical and immunological implications.

Current methods of somatic cell reprogramming have developed protocols for generating retinal cell types. These studies have shown that induced pluripotent stem cells (iPSCs) from human fibroblasts can differentiate into retinal progenitor cells [17,18]. Even though these results are promising, these progenitor cells are still slow and inefficient, and some doubts have emerged about their altered genetics and limited viability [18-21].

Adult undifferentiated or differentiated stem cells have also been used for retinal replacement. Among them, Schwann cells have been transplanted intravitreally into an optic nerve transaction model, and the results showed promising retinal ganglion cell (RGC) survival [22]. Adult hippocampal neural progenitor cells also show engraftment, survival capability, and morphological transformation reminiscent of retinal neurons and an extension of processes into the optic nerve [23-26]. Retinal pigment epithelium cells (RPECs) can engraft into and survive in Bruch's membrane [27-32], although in clinical trials in patients with advanced age-related macular degeneration, allogenically transplanted human RPECs have a high rejection rate [33].

Adult stem cell transplantation using cells obtained from the blood or bone marrow and predifferentiated in culture is another promising alternative for retinal regeneration in humans. Preclinical studies with bone marrow cells transplanted into the retina have shown that the inoculated cells produce a high rate of neovascularization, engraft and possibly differentiate into cells of neuronal lineage, and delay retinal degeneration [34-37]. Although one study reported that a degenerated retina cannot itself provide the signals to induce the differentiation of retinal stem cells (RSCs) into photoreceptors [38], the best results were obtained when predifferentiated cells were transplanted; the results were even better than were those with completely differentiated cells [39]. Studies of transplanted retinal precursor cells (RPC) have suggested that the predifferentiation of RSCs is the best option for recovery of a damage retina [38,40].

Several mixed media have been suggested to induce adult stem cell differentiation into neuronal lineage cells or ganglion cells. The formulas of those media include growth factors and chemical compounds involved in neuronal lineage and ganglion differentiation [41-43]. The present study focused on the development of a sequential culture medium aimed at inducing adult stem cells to differentiate into immature neuronal cells and then into immature retinal cells in a minimal time, that would provide an option for the treatment of retinal disease.

2. MATERIALS AND METHODS

2.1. Mesenchymal Cell Isolation and Culture

Mesenchymal stem cells (MSCs) were obtained from adult Wistar male rats, weighing about 220 g. The femurs were washed with Hank's solution to extrude the marrow from the central canal (Gibco, Grand Island, NY, USA) and filtered through a 70 μm cell strainer (BD Falcon, Bedford, MA, USA). After centrifugation, cells were resuspended in Dulbecco's modified Eagle medium (DMEM-F12) containing 20% fetal bovine serum (FBS) and 1% antibiotics (streptomycin-penicillin, Gibco). Cells were seeded in a 100 mm culture dish (Corning Inc., Corning, NY, USA) at 37°C and 5% CO_2 in a humid chamber for 24 h. To remove nonadherent cells, the cells were washed with phosphate-buffered saline (PBS), pH 7.4, and the culture medium was replaced with DMEM-F12 containing 10% FBS and 1% antibiotics. After 10 days, the cells reached 80% confluence and were harvested by incubation with 0.25% trypsin and 1 mM EDTA (Gibco) for 10 min at 37°C. The obtained cells were split 1:3 for the experiments.

2.2. Predifferentiated Medium and Induction Medium

For stem cell induction into neuronal lineage cells, the cells were incubated for 24 h in predifferentiation medium (PM) comprising DMEM-F12 plus 0.1 μM retinoic acid, 1 mM *β*-mercaptoethanol, 10 ng/ml fibroblast growth factor 8 (Sigma, St. Louis, MO, USA), and 2 mM glutamine (Invitrogen, Grand Island, NY, USA). To induce retinal lineage cells, a modification of a previously described protocol was used (17). This induction medium (IM) comprised PM plus 10 ng/ml Insulin Growth Factor -1 (Sigma), 10 ng/ml Dickkopf-1-related protein (Dkk1; R&D Systems, Minneapolis, MN, USA) and 10 ng/ml Noggin (GenWay Biotech, Inc., San Diego, CA, USA). Immunocytochemistry and Reverse transcription polymerase chain reaction RT-PCR analysis was performed after 24 h of incubation in IM.

2.3. Immunocytochemistry

Circular glass cover slips treated with poly-l-lysine (Sigma) were placed into 24-well microplates (Corning, Inc.) for immunocytochemistry, and the cells were cultured at a density of 1×10^5 cells/well for 24 h in PM and then for 24 h in IM. The cells were fixed with 4% paraformaldehyde for 10 min; washed three times with PBS, pH 7.4; and then permeabilized with 0.3% Triton X-100 in PBS for 5 min. Nonspecific antibody reactions were blocked with 5% bovine sera albumin (BSA) in PBS for 1 h. To confirm the neuronal lineage, cells were incubated overnight at 4°C with primary mouse monoclonal antibodies to nestin (1:5000; R&D Systems) and *β*-tubulin III (1:2000; Promega, Madison, WI, USA) diluted in 1% BSA in PBS. To confirm the ganglion lineage, cells were incubated with monoclonal anti-Pax6 (Santa Cruz Biotechnology, Santa Cruz, CA, USA), anti-Thy (1:400; Abcam [MRC OX-7]), and polyclonal anti-Brn3b (1:50; R&D Systems [sc-31989]). The cells were washed three times with PBS and incubated with secondary goat anti-mouse-Fc—fluorescein isothiocyanate (FITC) (Pierce Biotechnology, Thermo Fisher Scientific, Rockford, IL, USA) and donkey anti-goat IgG—FITC (Santa Cruz Biotechnology) for 2 h in the dark. The nuclei were stained with 4',6-diamidino-2-phenylindole (DAPI, Santa Cruz Biotechnology). The cover slips with stained cells were mounted on slides with 90% glycerol in PBS and sealed. The cells were analyzed under a fluorescence microscope (Imager Z1 Zeiss, Jena, Germany). Images were taken using an AxioCam HRm camera system coupled to the microscope.

2.4. RNA Isolation and RT-PCR

MSCs were added to poly-l-lysine-treated six-well microplates (Corning Inc.) at a density of 5×10^5 cells/well and cultured for 2 h and 24 h. Total RNA was isolated from undifferentiated mesenchymal cells, and from cells incubated in PM and IM using a binding silica column kit (GenElute Mammalian Total RNA, Sigma). The amount and quality of RNA were determined on a GeneQuant Pro Spectrophotometer (Amersham Biosciences, ambridge, UK). RT-PCR was performed in a Px2 Thermal Cycler (Thermo Electron Co, Milford, USA) using one-step reactions (Qiagen, Crawley, UK). All primers were obtained from MWG-Biotech, Huntsville, AL, USA, and are described on **Table 1**. The RT-PCR reactions were performed in a final volume of 50 μl with 1 μg of total RNA, according to the Qiagen One-Step RT-PCR protocol. PCR reactions were resolved on 2% agarose gels. The bands were observed under UV light and photographed in a UVP High-performance UV Transilluminator (DigiDoc-IT, Cambridge, UK) and analyzed with the GelAnalyzer program. Rat retinal tissue from two-month-old adult Wistar male rats was used as the positive control.

2.5. Statistics

The statistical differences amongst groups were analyzed using unpaired Student's t-test. Significance was set at a p-value of less than 0.05. Statistical analyses were performed with SPSS software (v. 17.0; SPSS Inc., Chicago, IL). For each variable under study, medians, standard deviations, and ranges were calculated.

3. RESULTS

3.1. Cell Culture and Predifferentiation

Primary culture of stem cells recovered from the rat bone marrow showed characteristic Colony forming units (CFU) formation after 8 days incubation in DMEM-F12 medium (**Figure 1(A)**). After 12 days, the culture reached 80% confluence (**Figure 1(B)**). On passage 4, the cells were incubated in PM medium for 24 h. Light microscopy showed morphological changes from typical fibroblast-like cells to cells with a triangular body and long projections (**Figure 1(C)**), which were longer in cells incubated for 24 h in IM. In the latter incubation, some types of contact, which resembled dendritic contacts, were observed between the cells (**Figure 1(D)**).

3.2. Immunocytochemistry

To probe the possible neuronal lineage, nestin and tubulin III were detected by immunocytochemistry in cells cultured for 24 h in PM. Slight positive expression of tubulin III was observed around the nucleus in cells cultured in the control medium. The expression of tubulin III increased markedly in cells incubated for 24 h in PM, and its distribution was detected throughout the cytoplasm (**Figures 2(A)** and **(B)**). A similar distribution was observed for nestin in cells cultured in the control medium, and the amount of protein increased in cells cultured in PM. Immunocytochemistry also confirmed the morphological modification of the cells from fibroblast-like cells to cells with a triangular body and long projections (**Figures 2(C)** and **(D)**).

To detect the possible predifferentiation to the retinal lineage, after incubation for 24 h in PM and then for 24 h in IM, the cells were stained with antibodies to Thy1.1, Pax6, and Brn3b. Thy1.1 immunodetection showed slight staining around the nucleus of the cells incubated in control medium (**Figure 3(A)**). The staining increased markedly in cells incubated in PM medium for 24 h follow by 24 h in IM. These cells also showed modifications of the cell morphology including the presence of long cytoplasmic projections (**Figure 3(B)**). Immunodetection of Pax6 and Brn3b showed a different distribution. These genes are expressed in the nucleus, therefore we

Table 1. Primers used for RT-PCR gene detection.

gene	sense	antisense
GAPDH	GTGGGGCAGCCCAGAACATC	CCAGGCGGCATGTCAGATCC
Tuj1	TGGCCACCGTCTTCCGTGGG	TCTCCCCCTCCTCCTCGGCA
nestin	CCCCAGGCTGAGGGGATCCAG	GGCATCTCCTACCCCCGGGAC
Ath5	TGCCGCAATGGGGCCAGG	AGCTGGCCATGGGGAAGGAC
Brn3b	CACCATCCGCCCCACCACAG	CTCCGAGGAGGGCCTTGGCT
Thy 1.1	CGAGTCTCGGGCCAGAATCCCA	CAGGAGCAGCAGCAGCCAGG
Pax6	TGTCCAACGGATGTGTGAGT	TTTCCCAAGCAAAGATGGAC
Opn4	CCATAGCATTCACGGTGTTG	TTATTTTCCCGTGCCTTGTC

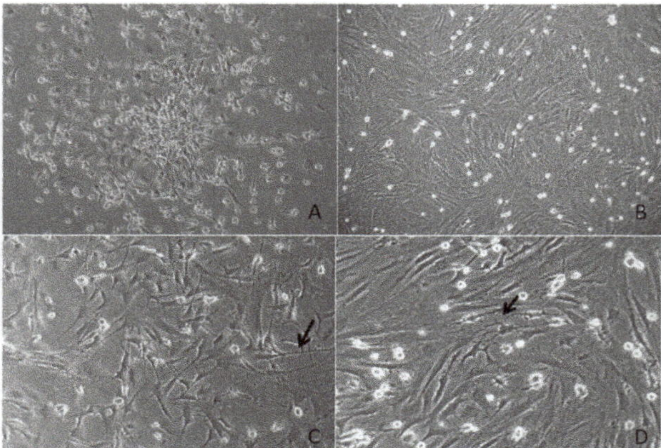

Figure 1. Light microscopy of rat stem cells cultured in control and induction media. (A) Primary culture of stem cells recovered from the rat bone marrow showed characteristic CPU; (B) Confluent culture after 12 days in control medium; (C) Stem cells after 24 h of culture in PM showing triangular bodies with long projections (arrow); (D) Stem cells after 24 h of culture in PM plus 24 h of culture in IM showing cytoplasmic elongation (arrow).

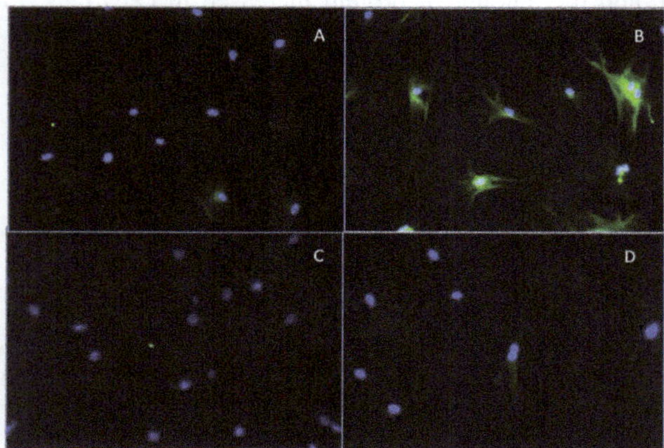

Figure 2. Representative images of immunofluorescent detection of β-tubulin III and nestin in rat stem cells. (A) Positive staining for β-tubulin III was detected around the nucleus (green) in stem cells incubated in control medium; (B) After 24 h of incubation in PM, the distribution was detected throughout the cytoplasm. The nucleus is labeled with 4',6-diamidino-2-phenylindole (DAPI) (blue); (C) Representative images of nestin immunodetection in stem cells cultured in control medium show its detection around the nucleus (green); (D) Immunodetection of nestin in stem cells cultured in PM medium for 24 h showing its distribution throughout the cytoplasm. The nucleus is labeled with DAPI (blue).

did not use DAPI during the immunodetection because nuclear staining could give false information. Immunodetection showed barely detectable staining for these proteins in cells incubated with control medium (**Figures 3(C)** and **(E)**).

However, staining increased markedly after incubation for 24 h in PM plus 24 h with IM (**Figures 3(D)** and **(F)**).

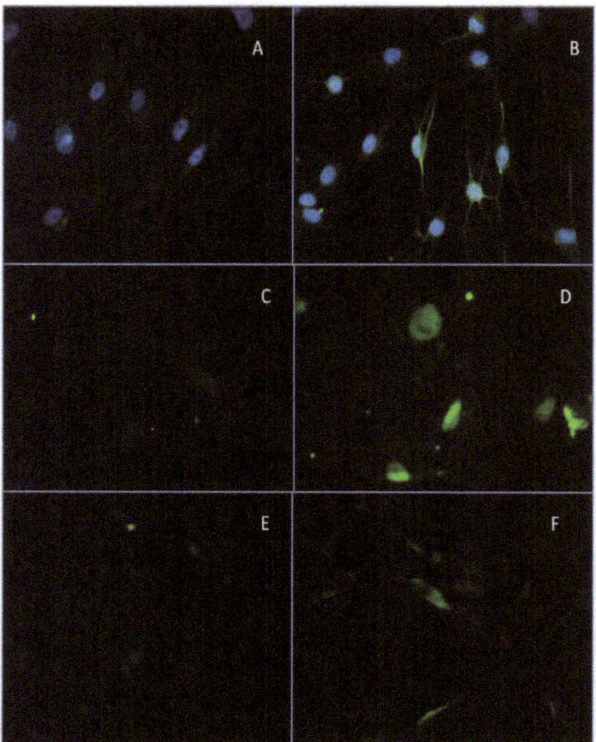

Figure 3. Representative images of Thy1.1 immunodetection. (A) Immunodetection of Thy1.1 in stem cells cultured in control medium; (B) Immunodetection of Thy1.1 in stem cells cultured in PM medium for 24 h and in IM for 24 h; (C) Immunodetection of Brn3b in stem cells cultured in control medium; (D) Positive immunodetection of Brn3b in stem cells cultured in PM for 24 h and in IM medium for 24 h; (E) Immunodetection of Pax6 in stem cells cultured in control medium; (F) Immunodetection of Pax6 gen in stem cells cultured in PM for 24 h and in IM medium for 24 h.

3.3. RT-PCR

Pax6, Opn4, Brn3b, Thy1.1, and Ath5 gene transcription was detected in stem cells cultured in control medium. The expression levels differed between genes. The expression levels were highest for Pax6, Thy1.1, and Opn4; lower for Brn3b, and marginal for Ath5. After culture of stem cells for 24 h in PM followed by 24 h with IM, expression of Brn3b and Ath5 increased by fivefold and threefold, respectively, compared with cells incubated in the control medium. Only minor levels of Pax6, Thy1.1, and Opn4 expression were observed (**Figure 4**).

4. DISCUSSION

The use of adult stem cells to restore retinal cells has been shown to be effective without the need for the cells to go through the path of full differentiation into a retinal cell. There is evidence that cells must be predifferentiated but not differentiated to allow proper retinal integra-

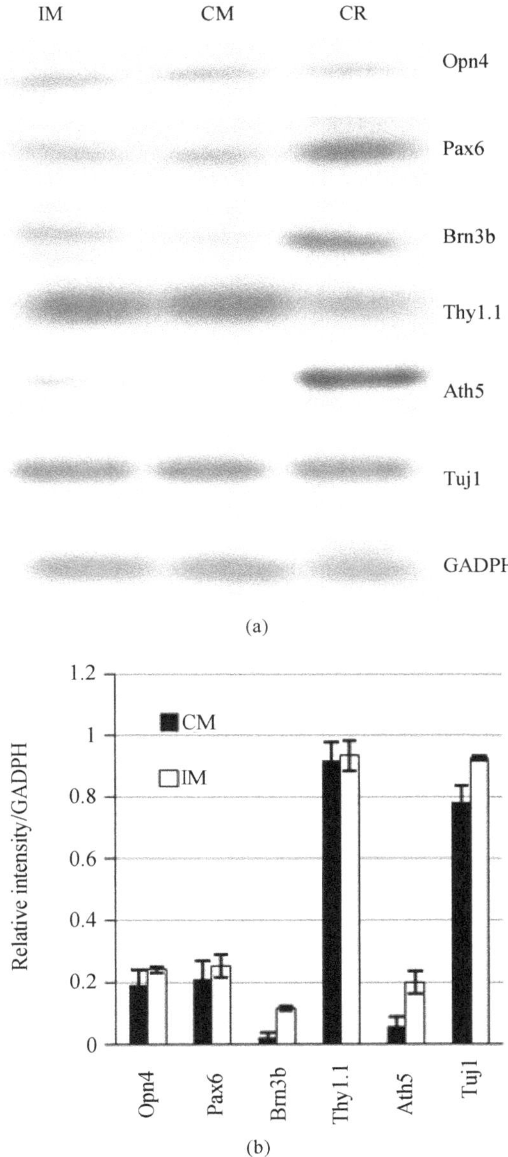

Figure 4. RT-PCR products for Pax6, Brn3b, Opn4, Thy1.1, and Ath5 in mesenchymal stem cells. (a) Image of the results of gel agarose electrophoresis of RT-PCR products from mRNA from cells cultured in DMEM-F12 medium plus 5% BSA (CM), or induction medium (IM). mRNA from rat retina was used as the positive control (CR); (b) Graphic representation of the relative intensity of RT-PCR products of cells cultured in CM or IM.

tion [39]. Thus, it is important to design a medium that will obtain predifferentiated retinal cells. In this study, stem cells were cultured in a PM designed to induce predifferentiation to cells of the neuronal lineage. These cells expressed nestin and tubulin III, confirming their predifferentiation into the neuronal lineage. Nestin is a neuroectodermal marker also expressed in RSCs and in most cells in the RGC layer [44,45]. Tubulin III, also a neuronal marker, is present in both immature and mature neurons. After the differentiation into the neuronal lineage was confirmed, the cells were incubated with IM supplemented with Dkk1, Noggin, and IGF-1. Dkk1 promotes stem cell differentiation into a preretinal stage [46-49], Noggin promotes neurogenesis *in vitro* and inhibits glial cell differentiation [50], and IGF-1 is essential for normal growth and central nervous system development [51]. This combination induces the differentiation of iPSCs and human embryonic cells into derived photoreceptors [10,17].

To support this preretinal linage, the gene expression of Pax6, Brn3b, THY1.1, Opn4, and Ath5 was analyzed. Pax6 plays an important role as a transcription factor in the master regulatory gene needed for the establishment of the retinal field in the forebrain neuroectoderm. This transcription factor is essential for the proliferation and expansion of RSCs *in vitro* [52,53]. In cultured retinal progenitor cells, Pax6 and Brn3b expression has been confirmed as a positive marker during differentiation [54-56]. Brn3b is a transcription factor for POU proteins involved in differentiation of RGCs and is regulated by Ath5 [57]. More importantly, Brn3b promotes RGC differentiation and suppresses non-RGC differentiation [58]. Ath5 over expression increases RGCs [59-61]. In our system, MSCs expressed all the genes tested at baseline. This observation has been reported for other neuronal genes in MSCs, but apparently these are not functionally [40,62]. However, the overexpression of Brn3b and Ath5 detected in the cells incubated in the sequential media suggest that the cells could become functional RGCs.

This is an important finding because of the pluripotency of RSCs and their ability to differentiate into various retinal cell types, including photoreceptors [40,42].

5. CONCLUSION

These findings open the possibility for assessing the potency of these cells and their role in the replacement of cells lost in damaged retinas. These findings also raise the possibility of using autologous transplantation to minimize the risk of immune rejection.

6. ACKNOWLEDGEMENTS

This work was funded partially by endowments from Instituto Tecnologico de Estudios Superiores de Monterrey (cat-134) and the Zambrano-Hellion Foundation. The authors express their appreciation to Rosa Maria de la Rosa and Griselda Bautista for technical assistance.

REFERENCES

[1] Quigley, H.A. and Broman, A.T. (2006) The number of

people with glaucoma worldwide in 2010 and 2020. *British Journal of Ophthalmology*, **90**, 262-267. doi:10.1136/bjo.2005.081224

[2] Morgan, J.E. (2000) Optic nerve head structure in glaucoma: Astrocytes as mediators of axonal damage. *Eye*, **14**, 437-444. doi:10.1038/eye.2000.128

[3] Quigley, H.A., Nickells, R.W., Kerrigan, L.A, Pease, ME, Thibault, D.J. and Zack, D.J. (1995) Retinal ganglion cell death in experimental glaucoma and after axotomy occurs by apoptosis. *Investigative Ophthalmology and Visual Science*, **36**, 774-786.

[4] Soto, I., Pease, M.E., Son, J.L., Shi, X., Quigley, H.A. and Marsh-Armstrong, N. (2011) Retinal ganglion cell loss in a rat ocular hypertension model is sectorial and involves early optic nerve axon loss. *Investigative Ophthalmology and Visual Science*, **52**, 434-441. doi:10.1167/iovs.10-5856

[5] Hess, D.C and Borlongan, C.V. (2008) Stem cells and neurological conditions. *Cell Proliferation*, **41**, 94-114. doi:10.1111/j.1365-2184.2008.00486.x

[6] Daley, G.Q. and Scadden, D.T. (2008) Prospects for stem cell-based therapy. *Cell*, **132**, 544-548. doi:10.1016/j.cell.2008.02.009

[7] Enzmann, V., Yolcu, E., Kaplan, H.J, and Ildstad, S.T. (2009) Stem cells as tools in regenerative therapy for retinal degeneration. *Archives of Ophthalmology*, **127**, 563-571. doi:10.1001/archophthalmol.2009.65

[8] Ballios, B.G. and van der Kooy, D. (2010) Biology and therapeutic potential of adult retinal stem cells. *Canadian Journal of Ophthalmology*, **45**, 342-351.

[9] Adolph, A.R., Zucker, C.L., Ehinger, B. and Bergström, A. (1994) Function and structure in retinal transplants. *Journal of Neural Transplantation and Plasticity*, **5**, 147-161. doi:10.1155/NP.1994.147

[10] Lamba, D.A., Karl, M.O., Ware, C.B. and Reh, T.A. (2006) Efficient generation of retinal progenitor cells from human embryonic stem cells. *Proceedings of the National Academy of Sciences of USA*, **103**, 12769-12774. doi:10.1073/pnas.0601990103

[11] Meyer, J.S., Katz, M.L., Maruniak, J.A. and Kirk, M.D. (2006) Embryonic stem cell-derived neural progenitors incorporate into degenerating retina and enhance survival of host photoreceptors. *Stem Cells*, **24**, 274-283. doi:10.1634/stemcells.2005-0059

[12] Banin, E., Obolensky, A., Idelson, M., Hemo, I., Reinhardtz, E., Pijarsky, E., Ben-Hur, T. and Reubinoff, B. (2006) Retinal incorporation and differentiation of neural precursors derived from human embryonic stem cells. *Stem Cells*, **24**, 246-257. doi:10.1634/stemcells.2005-0009

[13] Lamba, D.A., Gust, J. and Reh, T.A. (2009) Transplantation of human embryonic stem cell-derived photoreceptors restores some visual function in *Crx*-deficient mice. *Cell Stem Cell*, **4**, 73-79. doi:10.1016/j.stem.2008.10.015

[14] Aoki, H., Hara, A., Niwa, M., Yamada, Y. and Kunisada, T. (2009) *In vitro* and *in vivo* differentiation of human embryonic stem cells into retina-like organs and comparison with that from mouse pluripotent epiblast stem cells. *Development Dynamics*, **238**, 2266-2279. doi:10.1002/dvdy.22008

[15] Francis, P.J., Wang, S., Zhang, Y., Brown, A., Hwang, T., McFarland, T.J., Jeffrey, B.G., Lu, B., Wright, L., Appukuttan, B., Wilson, D.J, Stout. J.T., Neuringer, M., Gamm, D.M. and Lund, R.D. (2009) Subretinal transplantation of forebrain progenitor cells in nonhuman primates: Survival and intact retinal function. *Investigative Ophthalmology and Visual Science*, **50**, 3425-3431. doi:10.1167/iovs.08-2908

[16] Wang, S., Girman, S., Lu, B., Bischoff, N., Holmes, T., Shearer, R., Wright, L.S., Svendsen, C.N., Gamm, D.M. and Lund, R.D. (2008) Long-term vision rescue by human neural progenitors in a rat model of photoreceptor degeneration. *Investigative Ophthalmology and Visual Science*, **49**, 3201-3206. doi:10.1167/iovs.08-1831

[17] Lamba, D.A., McUsic, A., Hirata, R.K., Wang, P-R., Russell, D. and Reh, T.A. (2010) Generation, purification and transplantation of photoreceptors derived from human induced pluripotent stem cells. *PLoS ONE*, **5**, e8763. doi:10.1371/journal.pone.0008763

[18] Kokkinaki, M., Sahibzada, N. and Golestaneh, N. (2011) Human induced pluripotent stem-derived retinal pigment epithelium (RPE) cells exhibition transport, membrane potential, polarized VEGF secretion and gene expression pattern similar to native RPE. *Stem Cells*, **29**, 825-835. doi:10.1002/stem.635

[19] Mao, W., Yan, R.T. and Wang, S.Z. (2008) Reprogramming chick RPE progeny cells to differentiate towards retinal neurons by ash1. *Molecular Vision*, **14**, 2309-2320.

[20] Belmonte, J.C., Ellis, J., Hochedlinger, K. and Yamanaka S. (2009) Induced pluripotent stem cells and reprogramming: Seeing the science through the hype. *Nature Reviews Genetics*, **10**, 878-883.

[21] Wang, S.Z., Ma, W., Yan, R.T. and Mao, W. (2010) Generating retinal neurons by reprogramming retinal pigment epithelial cells. *Expert Opinion on Biological Therapy*, **10**, 1227-1239.

[22] Li, S., Hu, B., Tay, D., So, K.F. and Yip, H.K. (2004) Intravitreal transplants of Schwann cells and fibroblasts promote the survival of axotomized retinal ganglion cells in rats. *Brain Research*, **1029**, 56-64. doi:10.1016/j.brainres.2004.09.038

[23] Takahashi, M., Palmer, T.D., Takahashi, J. and Gage, F.H. (1998) Widespread integration and survival of adult-derived neural progenitor cells in the developing optic retina. *Molecular and Cellular Neuroscience*, **12**, 340-348. doi:10.1006/mcne.1998.0721

[24] Nishida, A., Takahashi, M., Tanihara, H., Nakano, I., Takahashi, J.B., Mizoguchi, A., Ide., C. and Honda, Y. (2000) Incorporation and differentiation of hippocampus-derived neural stem cells transplanted in injured adult rat retina. *Investigative Ophthalmology and Visual Science*, **41**, 4268-4274.

[25] Kurimoto, Y., Shibuki, H., Kaneko, Y., Ichikawa, M., Kurokawa, T., Takahashi, M. and Yoshimura, N. (2001) Transplantation of adult rat hippocampus-derived neural stem cells into retina injured by transient ischemia. *Neuroscience Letter*, **306**, 57-60.

doi:10.1016/S0304-3940(01)01857-2

[26] Guo, Y., Saloupis, P., Shaw, S.J. and Rickman, D.W. (2003) Engraftment of adult neural progenitor cells transplanted to rat retina injured by transient ischemia. *Investigative Ophthalmology and Visual Science*, **44**, 3194-3201. doi:10.1167/iovs.02-0875

[27] Sheedlo, H.J., Li, L.X. and Turner, J.E. (1989) Functional and structural characteristics of photoreceptor cells rescued in RPE-cell grafted retinas of RCS dystrophic rats. *Experimental Eye Research*, **48**, 841-854. doi:10.1016/0014-4835(89)90067-5

[28] Sauve, Y., Klassen, H., Whiteley, S.J.O. and Lund R.D. (1998) Visual field loss in RCS rats and the effect of RPE cell transplantation. *Experimental Neurology*, **152**, 243-250. doi:10.1006/exnr.1998.6849

[29] Klassen, H., Whiteley, S.J.O., Young, M.J. and Lund R.D. (2001) Graft location affects functional rescue following RPE cell transplantation in the RCS rat. *Experimental Neurology*, **169**, 114-121. doi:10.1006/exnr.2000.7617

[30] Gouras, P., Lopez, R., Kjeldbye, H., Sullivan, B. and Brittis, M. (1989) Transplantation of retinal epithelium prevents photoreceptor degeneration in the RCS rat. *Progress in Clinical and Biological Research*, **314**, 659-671.

[31] Phillips, S.J., Sadda, S.R., Tso, M.O., Humayan, M.S., de Juan, E. Jr. and Binder, S. (2003) Autologous transplantation of retinal pigment epithelium after mechanical debridement of Bruch's membrane. *Current Eye Research*, **26**, 81-88.

[32] Hu, Y., Zhang, T., Wu, J., Li, Y., Lu, X., Qian, F., Yin, Z. and Ma, Z. (2008) Autologous transplantation of RPE with partial-thickness choroid after mechanical debridement of Bruch membrane in the rabbit. *Investigative Ophthalmology and Visual Science*, **49**, 3185-3192. doi:10.1167/iovs.07-1299

[33] Algvere, P.V., Gouras, P. and Dafgard Kopp, E. (1999) Long-term outcome of RPE allografts in non-immunosuppressed patients with AMD. *European Journal of Ophthalmology*, **9**, 217-230.

[34] Tomita, M., Adachi, Y., Yamada, H., Takahashi, K., Kiuchi, K., Oyaizu, H., Ikebukuro, K., Kaneda, H., Matsumura, M. and Ikehara, S. (2002) Bone marrow-derived stem cells can differentiate into retinal cells in injured rat retina. *Stem Cells*, **20**, 279-283. doi:10.1634/stemcells.20-4-279

[35] Tomita, M., Yamada, H., Adachi, Y., Cui, Y., Yamada, E., Higuchi, A., Minamino, K., Suzuki, Y., Matsumura, M. and kehara, S. (2004) Choroidal neovascularization is provided by bone marrow cells. *Stem Cells*, **22**, 21-26. doi:10.1634/stemcells.22-1-21

[36] Inoue, Y., Iriyama, A., Ueno, S., Takahashi, H., Kondo, M., Tamaki, Y., Araie, M. and Yanagi, Y. (2007) Subretinal transplantation of bone marrow mesenchymal stem cells delays retinal degeneration in the RCS rat model of retinal degeneration. *Experimental Eye Research*, **85**, 234-241. doi:10.1016/j.exer.2007.04.007

[37] Lund, R.D., Wang, S., Lu, B., Girman, S., Holmes, T., Sauvé, Y., Messina, D.J., Harris, I.R., Kihm, A.J., Harmon, A.M., Chin, F.Y., Gosiewska, A. and Mistry, S.K. (2007) Cells isolated from umbilical cord tissue rescue photoreceptors and visual functions in a rodent model of retinal disease. *Stem Cells*, **25**, 602-611. doi:10.1634/stemcells.2006-0308

[38] Canola, K., Angenieux, B., Tekaya, M., Quiambao, A., Naash, M.I., Munier, F.L., Schorderet, D.F. and Arsenijevic, Y. (2007) Retinal stem cells transplanted into models of late stages of retinitis pigmentosa preferentially adopt a glial or a retinal ganglion cell fate. *Investigative Ophthalmology and Visual Science*, **48**, 446-454. doi:10.1167/iovs.06-0190

[39] MacLaren, R.E., Pearson, R.A., MacNeil, A., Douglas, R.H., Salt, T.E., Akimoto, M., Swaroop, A., Sowden, J.C. and Ali, R.R. (2006) Retinal repair by transplantation of photoreceptor precursors. *Nature*, **444**, 203-207.

[40] Coles, B.L., Angénieux, B., Inoue, T., Del Rio-Tsonis, K., Spence, J.R. McInnes, R.R., Arsenijevic, Y. and van der Kooy, D. (2004) Facile isolation and the characterization of human retinal stem cells. *Proceedings of the National Academic of Science of the USA*, **101**, 15772-15777. doi:10.1073/pnas.0401596101

[41] Yang, J., Klassen, H., Pries, M., Wang, W. and Nissen, M.H. (2006) Aqueous humor enhances the proliferation of rat retinal precursor cells in culture, and this effect is partially reproduced by ascorbic acid. *Stem Cells*, **24**, 2766-2775. doi:10.1634/stemcells.2006-0103

[42] Merhi-Soussi, F., Angénieux, B., Canola, K., Kostic, C., Tekaya, M., Hornfeld, D. and Arsenijevic Y. (2006) High yield of cells committed to the photoreceptor fate from expanded mouse retinal stem cells. *Stem Cells*, **24**, 2060-2070. doi:10.1634/stemcells.2005-0311

[43] Mori, T., Kiyono, T., Imabayashi, H., Takeda, Y., Tsuchiya, K., Miyoshi, S., Makino, H., Matsumoto, K., Saito, H., Ogawa, S., Sakamoto, M., Hata, J. and Umezawa, A. (2005) Combination of hTERT and *bmi*-1, E6, or E7 induces prolongation of the life span of bone marrow stromal cells from an elderly donor without affecting their neurogenic potential. *Molecular and Cellular Biology*, **25**, 5183-5195. doi:10.1128/MCB.25.12.5183-5195.2005

[44] Ahmad, I., Tang, L. and Pham, H. (2000) Identification of neural progenitors in the adult mammalian eye. *Biochemical and Biophysical Research Communications*, **270**, 517-521. doi:10.1006/bbrc.2000.2473

[45] Mayer, E.J., Hughes, E.H., Carter, D.A. and Dick, A.D. (2003) Nestin positive cells in adult human retina and in epiretinal membranes. *British Journal of Ophthalmology*, **87**, 1154-1158. doi:10.1136/bjo.87.9.1154

[46] Mukhopadhyay, M., Shtrom, S., Rodriguez-Esteban, C., Chen, L., Tsukui, T., Gomer, L., Dorward, D.W., Glinka, A., Grinberg, A., Huang, S.P., Niehrs, C., Izpisúa Belmonte, J.C. and Westphal, H. (2001) *Dickkopf1* is required for embryonic head induction and limb morphogenesis in the mouse. *Developmental Cell*, **1**, 423-434. doi:10.1016/S1534-5807(01)00041-7

[47] Mukhopadhyay, M., Gorivodsky, M., Shtrom, S., Grinberg, A., Niehrs, C., Morasso, M.I. and Westphal, H. (2006) Dkk2 plays an essential role in the corneal fate of the ocular surface epithelium. *Development*, **133**, 2149-2154. doi:10.1242/dev.02381

[48] Glinka, A., Wu, W., Delius, H., Monaghan, A.P., Blumen-

stock, C. and Niehrs, C. (1998) Dickkopf-1 is a member of a new family of secreted proteins and functions in head induction. *Nature*, **391**, 357-362.

[49] Pera, E.M., Wessely, O., Li, S.Y. and De Robertis, E, M. (2001) Neural and head induction by insulin-like growth factor signals. *Developmental Cell*, **1**, 655-665. doi:10.1016/S1534-5807(01)00069-7

[50] Lim, D.A., Tramontin, A.D., Trevejo, J.M., Herrera, D.G., García-Verdugo, J.M. and Alvarez-Buylla, A. (2000) Noggin antagonizes BMP signaling to create a niche for adult neurogenesis. *Neuron*, **28**, 713-726. doi:10.1016/S0896-6273(00)00148-3

[51] Hollis, E.R. II., Lu, P., Blesch, A. and Tuszynski, M.H. (2009) IGF-I gene delivery promotes corticospinal neuronal survival but not regeneration after adult CNS injury. *Experimental Neurology*, **215**, 53-59. doi:10.1016/j.expneurol.2008.09.014

[52] Xu. S., Sunderland, M.E., Coles, BL, Kam, A., Holowacz, T., Ashery-Padan, R., Marquardt, T., McInnes, R.R, and van der Kooy, D. (2007) The proliferation and expansion of retinal stem cells require functional *pax*6. *Development Biology*, **304**, 713-721. doi:10.1016/j.ydbio.2007.01.021

[53] Zaghloul, N.A. and Moody, S.A. (2007) Alterations of *rx*1 and *pax*6 expression levels at neural plate stages differentially affect the production of retinal cell types and maintenance of retinal stem cell qualities. *Developmental Biology*, **306**, 222-240. doi:10.1016/j.ydbio.2007.03.017

[54] Gu, P., Yang, J., Wang, J., Young, M.J. and Klassen, H. (2009) Sequential changes in the gene expression profile of murine retinal progenitor cells during the induction of differentiation. *Molecular Vision*, **15**, 2111-2122.

[55] Schmitt, S., Aftab, U., Jiang, C., Redenti, S., Klassen, H., Miljan, E., Sinden, J. and Young, M. (2009) Molecular characterization of human retinal progenitor cells. *Investigative Ophthalmology and Visual Science*, **50**, 5901-5908. doi:10.1167/iovs.08-3067

[56] Klassen, H., Kiilgaard, J.F., Zahir, T., Ziaeian, B., Kirov, I., Scherfig, E., Warfvinge, K. and Young, M.J. (2007) Progenitor cells from the porcine neural retina express photoreceptor markers after transplantation to the subretinal space of allorecipients. *Stem Cells*, **25**, 1222-1230. doi:10.1634/stemcells.2006-0541

[57] Klassen, H., Sakaguchi, S., Young, M. (2004) Stem cells and retinal repair. *Progress in Retinal and Eye Research*, **23**, 149-181. doi:10.1016/j.preteyeres.2004.01.002

[58] Qiu, F., Jiang, H., Xiang, M. (2008) A comprehensive negative regulatory program controlled by Brn3b to ensure ganglion cell specification from multipotential retinal precursors. *Journal of Neuroscience*, **28**, 3392-3403. doi:10.1523/JNEUROSCI.0043-08.2008

[59] Liu. W., Mo, Z. and Xiang M. (2001) The *Ath*5 proneural genes function upstream of *Brn*3 POU domain transcripttion factor genes to promote retinal ganglion cell development. *Proceeding of National Academic Science of the USA*. **98**, 1649-1654. doi:10.1073/pnas.98.4.1649

[60] Ma, W., Yan, R.T., Xie, W. and Wang, S.Z. (2004) A role of *ath*5 in inducing *neuro*D and the photoreceptor pathway. *Journal of Neuroscience*, **24**, 7150-7158. doi:10.1523/JNEUROSCI.2266-04.2004

[61] Tondreau, T., Lagneaux, L., Dejeneffe, M., Massy, M., Mortier, C., Delforge, A. and Bron, D. (2004) Bone marrow-derived mesenchymal stem cells already express specific neural proteins before any differentiation. *Differentiation*, **72**, 319-326. doi:10.1111/j.1432-0436.2004.07207003.x

[62] Mareschi, K., Novara, M., Rustichelli, D., Ferrero, I., Guido, D., Carbone, E., Medico, E., Madon, E., Vercelli, A. and Fagioli, F. (2006) Neural differentiation of human mesenchymal stem cells: Evidence of neuronal markers and eag K^+ channel types. *Experimental Hematology*, **34**, 1563-1575. doi:10.1016/j.exphem.2006.06.020

11

Plasmid vector based generation of transgenic mesenchymal stem cells with stable expression of reporter gene in caprine

Manish Kumar[1], Renu Singh[1], Kuldeep Kumar[1], Pranjali Agarwal[1], Puspendra Saswat Mahapatra[1], Abhisek Kumar Saxena[2], Ajay Kumar[3], Subrata Kumar Bhanja[4], Dhruba Malakar[5], Rajendra Singh[6], Bikas C. Das[1], Sadhan Bag[1*]

[1]Division of Physiology and Climatolxcogy, Indian Veterinary Research Institute, Bareilly, India;
[*]Corresponding Author: bag658@gmail.com
[2]Division of Surgery, Indian Veterinary Research Institute, Bareilly, India
[3]Division of Biochemistry, Indian Veterinary Research Institute, Bareilly, India
[4]Central Avian research Institute, Bareilly, India
[5]Animal Biotechnology Center, National Dairy Research Institute, Karnal, India
[6]Division of Pathology, Indian Veterinary Research Institute, Bareilly, India

ABSTRACT

The production of cells capable of expressing gene(s) of interest is important for a variety of applications in biomedicine and biotechnology, including gene therapy and a novel method of stem cell therapy in the various diseases. Achieving high levels of transgene expression for the longer period of time, without adversely affecting cell viability and differentiation capacity of the cells, is crucial. In the present study, we investigated the efficiency of plasmid vector for the production of transgenic cMSCs and examined any functional change of cells after transfection. To do so first we have collected bone marrows from the adult goats and cultured them for isolation of mesenchymal stem cells (cBM-MSCs). These cells were characterized using MSC specific markers including differentiation into osteocytes and adipocytes. Transfection with plasmid vector did not adversely affect cBM-MSCs morphology, viability or differentia-tion potential, and transgene expression levels were unaffected beyond passage 12th. The results indicated that we have been able to generate transgenic caprine MSC (tcBM-MSC) and transfection of cBM-MSCs using plasmid vector resulted in very high and stable transfection efficiency. This finding may have considerable significance in improving the efficacy of MSC-based therapies and their tracking in animal model.

Keywords: Transgenic MSC; Caprine; Plasmid Vector; Characterisation; *In Vitro* Differentiation

1. INTRODUCTION

Mesenchymal stem cells (MSCs) are multipotent, self-renewing cell population isolated from different sources especially from bone marrow and look extremely promising due to their potential to differentiation into cells of different lineages including chondrocytes, osteoblasts and adipocytes [1], their trans-differentiation potentiality to form connective tissue like, muscle, heart, blood vessels and nerves etc. [2-4], their ability to home to sites of injury after systemic delivery [5,6] and their evasion of normal host immune responses [7], easy to isolate from almost all individuals as well as their ability not to form teratomas [8]. These cells are currently being used for transplantation into various diseases viz improvement to myocardial and cerebral function (after cerebral infarction), repair of liver damage [9], bone fracture [10], healing of wound [11,12], repair of damaged ligaments and joint damage [13,14], repair of spinal cord injury [15,16] etc.

So far most of the applications of MSC have been studied in laboratory animal with an aim of their application in human being. However, recently MSC of domestic animals are being studied in-depth and in near future these cells would be used for therapeutics in divergent areas of diseases as well as a vehicle for gene delivery. However, to understand their regenerative potentiality, thorough transplantation studies should be undertaken. But one of the challenges lies in tracking stem cells following *in vivo* transplantation to understand the fate of the transplanted cells.

While there are many ways to label and track cells, but the transgenic MSC expressing green fluorescent protein (GFP) has been found efficient because it can be detected with high sensitivity and specificity, combined with its relative ease of insertion, expression, and detection [17]. Currently many methods are available to produce transgenic cells for the functional studies of genes, drug discovery and gene therapy. But attempts have been made to generate transgenic MSC with reporter gene in different species using viral and non viral based vectors [18] with varying success. In most of the studies it has been reported that plasmid vector is very less efficient [18] and stable transgenic MSC could not be generated. However, comparatively stable transgenic MSC [19] has been generated using viral based transgenesis particularly lentivirus in different species including human beings [20-23].

So far very less attempts have been made to generate stable transgenic MSC in domestic animal [24]. Therefore, in the present study, an attempt was made to transfect bone marrow derived caprine MSC using a plasmid vector with reporter gene so that transgenic stem cells can be generated for their further use in transplantation studies.

2. MATERIALS AND METHODS

All the chemicals used in this study were procured from Sigma, unless indicated. The primary and secondary antibodies used for immunocytochemistry and FACS analysis were purchased from Santa Cruz Biotechnology, USA.

2.1. Isolation and Expansion of cBM-MSCs

The goats of around one year old of either sex were selected for bone marrow collection which were maintained in the Animal Shed of Physiology and Climatology Division, Indian Veterinary Research Institute, Izatnagar, India. The permission for institute ethical committee was taken for collection of bone marrow from caprine. The selected goat was anesthetized using standard protocol. The area of iliac crest (site of collection) on either side was prepared aseptically. The bone marrow aspirate was collected with the help of an 18G bone marrow biopsy needle from the lateral aspect of iliac crest. About 4 - 5 ml bone marrow aspirate was drawn/aspirated. Immediately after collection bone marrow aspirate brought to the laboratory and processed.

The marrow sample was diluted with equal amount of Dulbecco's phosphate buffered saline (DPBS, Invitrogen, #cat. 14190-144) and slowly layered onto 10 ml of Ficol-Hypaque (Sigma, #cat. 1077). The sample was subjected to centrifuge at 2000 rpm for 30 min and the nucleated cells were collected from the interface. The cells were washed with two volumes of DPBS and collected by centrifugation at 2000 rpm for 10 min. The cells were resuspended, counted and plated at 2×10^5 cells/cm^2 in T-25 tissue culture flasks. The cells were maintained in culture medium with antibiotics (mixture of 100 units/ml of penicillin and 100 μg/ml of streptomycin (Gibco #cat. 15140-122) in incubator with atmosphere of 5% CO_2, 95% humidity at 37°C for 48 hours. The culture medium used for cell propagations was DMEM-low glucose (HyClone, #cat. SH30021.01) + 15% serum. After 48 hours of primary culture, the non adherent cells were removed by changing the medium. The medium was changed every third days thereafter. The confluent cells were propagated 1.3 ratios with trypsinisation method.

2.2. Assessment of Cell Viability Using Probes for Membrane Integrity

Approximately 10^6 cBM-MSCs were suspended in 1 ml PBS in 15 ml centrifuge tube and 2 μg propidium iodide (PI) was added. After incubation on ice for 5 min in dark, the cells were analysed on flow cytometer with excitation at 488 nm and emission collected at >550 nm.

2.3. Chromosome Analysis

The chromosome analysis was done using conventional Giemsa staining method. In early growing (48 hr of seeding) cBM-MSCs, culture media was replaced by colcemid (0.05 μg/ml, PAA, #cat. J01-003) containing media & incubated for 15 hrs at 37°C, 5% CO_2 in CO_2 incubator. The cells were trypsinized and treated with 0.56% KCl hypotonic solution for 30 min. After this, cells pellet were treated with 3.1 methanol, acetic acid and slides were prepared using this. The slides were stained with Giemsa stain and observed under microscope at 100× in oil immersion.

2.4. *In Vitro* Differentiation

To induce adipogenic differentiation, normal and transgenic MSCs were cultured to near confluence and the complete media was replaced by adipogenic induction medium consisting of DMEM containing + 10% FBS (Gibco, #cat. 16000-044) and antibiotics + 100 nmol-Dexamethasone (Sigma, #cat. D2915) + 50 mg/ml-indomethacin (Sigma, #cat.17378.) + 10 μg/ml – insulin (Sigma, #cat.I6634). The induction medium was changed every 3 days. At the end of the differentiation period, cells were fixed with 4% paraformaldehyde for 10 min and lipid droplets were stained by Oil Red O (Sigma, #cat.O0625) staining.

To induce osteogenic differentiation, the confluent cBM-MSC were incubated in osteogenic induction medium consisting of DMEM medium containing 10% FBS, antibiotics, 10 nmol Dexamethasone (Sigma #cat. D2915), 10 mmol glycerophosphate (Sigma #cat. G9422), 0.3 mM-L ascorbic acid (Sigma #cat. A4403). The induction medium was changed every 3 days. The bone matrix mineralization was evaluated by Alizarin red S (Sigma #cat. A5533) staining. The induced cells were also examined for alkaline phosphatase activity. For further confirmation of differentiation, RNA was isolated from differentiated cells and cDNA was synthesised from RNA for real time PCR analysis of osteogenic and adipogenic gene expression.

2.5. Alkaline Phosphatase Staining

The cBM-MSCs were *in vitro* differentiated cells were subjected to alkaline phosphatase staining. Cell monolayer was rinsed in DPBS, fixed in 4% paraformaldehyde and then overlaid with AP stain, (Naphthol AS-MX Phosphate (0.5 mg/ml) and Fast Red TR salt (1 mg/ml) (Millipore, USA) mixed in 100 mM Tris-HCl, pH-8.2) for 4 hours at 37°C, rinsed again with DPBS. Stained cells were observed under inverted light microscope (Olympus-1X51S8F3, Japan).

2.6. Immunocytochemistry

Normal as well as transgenic cBM-MSCs, cultured on cover slip in six well plate up to 70% - 80% confluency were fixed using 4% paraformaldehyde in 1X PBS for 20 min and were washed thrice with 1× PBS at room temperature. The cells were incubated in permeabialization solution containing 0.3% Triton X-100 and 4% BSA in PBS 20 min for detection of intracellular markers. The cells were washed thrice with 1× PBS at room temperature. Non specific binding sites were blocked with 10% normal goat serum in PBS for 40 min at room temperature and the cells were washed thrice with 1X PBS. Cells were treated with primary antibodies from Santacruiz viz CD105 (#sc-19793), CD90 (#sc-9162) and CD73 (#sc-25603) (1200 dilution) for each markers for overnight at 4°C and washed thrice with 1× PBS. The cells were then incubated with respective secondary antibodies (1800 dilution) for one hour at room temperature and washed thrice with 1× PBS. The cells were counter stained with DAPI to stain the nucleus. The cells were examined under ZEISS fluorescent microscope. Mesenchymal stem cells were stained simultaneously without addition of primary antibody as control for each antibody.

2.7. FACS Analysis

FACS analysis was performed to investigate the expression of MSCs specific transcriptional markers viz. CD-73 (#sc-25603), CD-105 (#sc-19793) as well as hematopoitic stem cells marker CD-45 (#sc-25590) in cBM-MSCs. Cells were harvested and aliquoted at a density of 1.0×10^6 cells/ml for each staining. The cell suspensions were incubated for 15 min at 4°C (on ice) with 10% normal goat serum in PBS to block nonspecific binding of the primary antibody. After washing the cells were incubated with primary antibodies against CD-73 and CD-105 overnight at a conc. of 2 µg/ml at 4°C. After three DPBS washes, cells were incubated with FITC conjugated anti goat secondary antibody for 2 hr at 4°C in dark. Thereafter, the cells were fixed with 1% PFA for 5 min. Cells were washed thrice and analyzed using a flow cytometer (Becton Dickinson, San Jose, CA, USA) using a negative control processed in similar manner but without primary antibody. The data obtained was analyzed using Cell Quest program and plotted as single parameter histogram.

2.8. *In-Vitro* Transdifferentiation of Mesenchymal Stem Cells into Neurons

The normal and transgenic cBM-MSCs at passage four were induced to become neuronal-like cells under *in vitro* conditions as per given methods [25]. Briefly, subconfluent (approximately 80% - 85% confluent) cultures of cBM-MSCs were maintained in DMEM + 20% FBS. Twenty-four hours prior to neuronal induction, media were replaced with pre-induction media consisting of DMEM + 20% FBS − 1 mM β-mercaptoethanol (BME) (Sigma #cat. M7522). To initiate neuronal differentiation, the preinduction media were removed, and the cells were transferred to neuronal induction media composed of DMEM + 2 - 10 mM BME. Cells were fixed for immunocytochemistry at times ranging from 24 hr to 6 days post-induction. The cells were observed every 12 hr for change in morphology. Differentiated cBM-MSCs were fixed in 4% paraformaldehyde and processed for immunostaining using neuron specific markers. Molecular characterizations of differentiated cells were also done to validate the neuronal differentiations.

2.9. Real Time PCR

For gene expression analysis, different passage of cBM-MSCs and ifferentiated cells were isolated by using Trypsin-EDTA and washed with 1X PBS. The cells were transferred in 2 ml DNAase and RNAse free tube for RNA isolation. The total RNA was isolated using mini RNA kit as per manufacturer's protocol (Zymo Research, Cat No. R1005). The cDNA were synthesized from total RNA using cDNA synthesis kit (Biorad, Cat No. 170 - 8891) as per the manufacturer's instructions.

The gene expression of cBM-MSC and transdiferentiated cells were analysed by Real Time Polymerase Chain Reaction (Biorad) and Evagreen supermix (Biorad, Cat No. 172-5200), as a double stranded DNA-specific fluorescent dye. For real time amplification of genes, primers were designed in beacon software. The reaction mix was prepared in a volume of 10 µl by mixing 3.0 µl nuclease free water, 5.0 µl Evagreen supermix, 0.5 µl of forward and reverse primer each and 1.0 µl of cDNA. The conditions for thermocycling were as follow, initial denaturation at 95˚C for 30 sec followed by 40 cycles (denaturation at 95˚C for 3 sec, annealing for 10 sec at specific temperature for each gene as mentioned in **Table 1**.

2.10. Transfection of cBM-MSCs

A total number of 50,000 cells were plated per well in a 12-well tissue culture plate. After 24 hours of culture, Lipofectamine-2000 mediated (LF2000) (1 mg/mL) (#cat no. 31985-062, Invitrogen) transient transfection was performed according to the protocol given by the supplier (Invitrogen), varying transfection reagent volumes and the amount of DNA (pAcGFP1-C1, Cat No-632470, Clonotech, USA) were carried out in OPTIMEM1 (Gibco), without serum or antibiotics. In one well of 24 well tissue culture dish, first dilution of amplified plasmid DNA (0.8 - 1.6 µg) in 100µl of Opti-MEM®I (Cat. No. 31985, Gibco) was done followed by a gentle mixing. Appropriate amount of lipofectamine was mixed well in 100 µl of Opti-MEM®I medium in another well and incubated for 5 min at room temperature. After the incubation, diluted plasmid DNA and Lipofectamine-2000 was mixed together (total volume now 200 µl) followed by further incubation for 25 - 30 min at room temperature to allow the DNA-Lipofectamine 2000 complexes to form. Before the transfection, culture medium of MSC was changed to serum and antibiotics free DMEM and washed with it (serum and antibiotic free DMEM medium) twice before addition of DNA and Lipofectamine complex. Once the plasmid DNA and lipofectamine complex was ready to use, 800 µl fresh media was added to it and the total content was mixed gently by rocking the plate back and forth. The complex was added on the semi confluent cBM-MSCs and the cells were kept in CO_2 incubator at 37˚C. The cells were observed under microscope and after six hours of transfection, the medium was replaced with fresh one ml DMEM supplemented with serum. Expression of GFP which indicated successful transfection was observed after 24 hr of transfection under fluorescence microscope. After 72 hr of transfection, the previous media was replaced by selection media containing neomycin (G418, sigma) @ 300 µg/ml which was continued at least for two weeks. Subsequently tcBM-MSC were passaged and propagated to increase the cell population and characterized to check for the MSC characteristics as that of the primary MSC culture.

3. RESULTS

3.1. Growth and Culture Characteristics of cBM-MSCs

Bone marrow was harvested from iliac crest of the goats and buffy coat was separated from the bone marrow and cells were plated into 25 mm culture flask at the density of 5×10^5 cells using DMEM culture media (**Figure 1(A)**). Non-adherent cells were carefully removed after 48 hours and fresh medium was replaced. Thereafter, this step was repeated every 24 hours for up to 96 hours of initial culture. Then, the adherent cells (passage 0) were washed with 1× Dulbecco's phosphate-buffer

Table 1. Primers and conditions used for gene specific real time PCR analysis.

S. No	Target Gene	Primer sequence, 5'-3'	Annealing temperature (˚C)	Product (bp)	Reference sequence accession no.
1.	GAPDH	f 5'ggagaaacctgccaagtatg3' r 5'tgagtgtcgctgttgaagtc3'	65	126	DQ152956.1
2.	THY1 (CD90)	f 5'cctcctgctaacagtcttac3' r 5'atccttggtggtgaagttg3'	60	271	BC104530
3.	ENG (CD105)	f 5'agcgatggcatgactctg3' r 5'aggctgtccgtgttgatg3'	65	251	NM_001076397
4.	CD73	f 5'aacacacagtggtgctctcttcc3' r 5'tgttgtcttgggtgtgtgtgcctaga3'	60	401	BC114093.1
5	ADIPSIN	f 5'-caccatcactgagcgaatga-3' R 5'-ttgtggttgccgcagat-3'	60	138	BC102479.1
6	OSTEOCALCIN	f 5'-cttcgtgtccaagcaggag-3' r 5'-tccagcggatctgggtag-3'	60	99	AY661470.1
7	CD34	f 5'-cagcctctacgatgtctc-3' r 5'-gtaataatggaagaagtcaca-3'	60	276	AB021662
8	CD45	f 5'-aaccgctctctcaaccatag-3' r 5'-tcatcttccacgcagtctac-3'	60	288	AJ400864

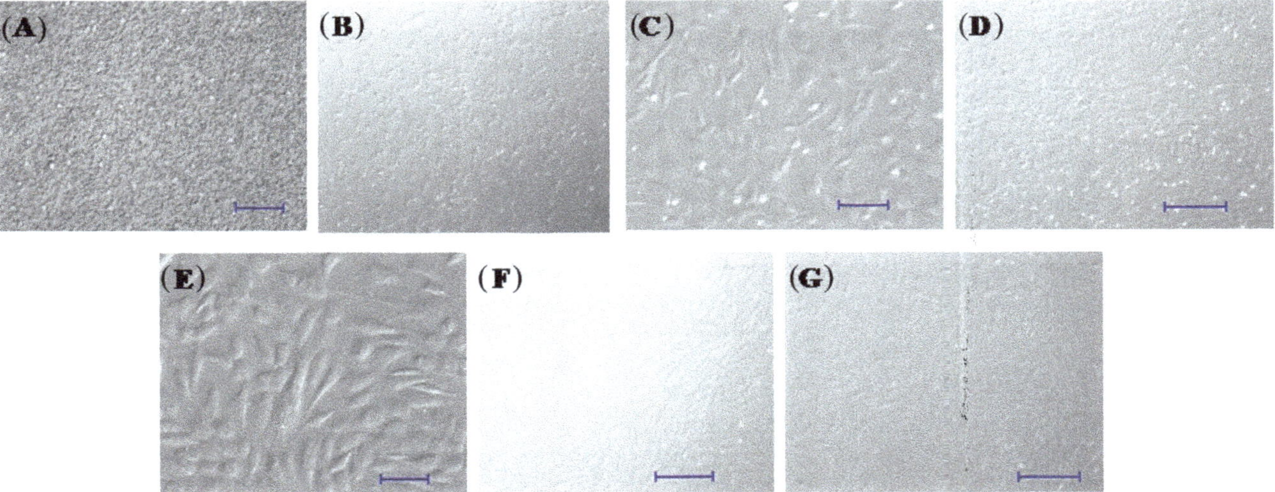

Figure 1. Bone marrow was collected from iliac crest of adult goat and immediately processed for the separation of nucleated cells using density gradient medium by centrifugation method and cells were cultured in DMEM low glucose with FBS and antibiotic. (A) day of culture after centrifugation and proper washing of cells. (B) Cells acquiring the spindle shape on day 6th of culture after frequent change of medium. (C) Day 8th of culture cells are more confluent and showing typical MSC like morphology. (D) On Day 11th cells are approximately 70% - 80% confluent. (E) Cells of passage 5th showing typical spindle shape. (F) Cells of passage 10 and (G) Cells of passage 15th. Scale bar—(A), (C), & (E) 200 μm and (B), (D), (F) & (G) 500 μm.

saline (1X DPBS), and fresh medium was added every 3 - 4 days. The initial adherent cells were observed as triangle or spindle shaped morphology within 5 - 6 days (**Figure 1(B)**). In 7 - 8 days culture became more confluent (**Figure 1(C)**), and reached 80% - 90% of confluence within 10 - 11 days (**Figure 1(D)**). In subsequent passages, cBM-MSCs maintained their characteristic spindle-shape (**Figure 1(E)**), passage 10th (**Figure 1(F)**). The cells were propagated and brought beyond 15th passage (**Figure 1(G)**).

3.2. Characterisation of cBM-MSCs

Analysis of transcript abundance of target genes based real time PCR assay showed that under standard culture conditions, cBM-MSCs were found positive for CD105 and CD90 (**Figure 2(a)**) but negative for haematopoietic cell surface markers like CD45 and CD34 (**Figure 2(b)**). Furthermore, corresponding cell surface marker proteins were successfully localized in passage four cBM-MSCs monolayer via immunocytochemistry such as CD105 (**Figures 3(a)-(c)**), CD90 (**Figures 3(d)-(f)**) and CD73 (**Figures 3(g)-(i)**). Nucleus was counter stained with DAPI.

3.3. FACS Analysis

To verify the cells derived from the caprine bone marrow are mesenchymal stem cells, a panel of antibodies against MSC markers was chosen to evaluate that the cultured cells are MSC. The CD73 and CD105 positive cells were 65.73% (**Figure 4(g)**) and 73.29% (**Figures 4(a)** and **(b)**), respectively and only 0.07% cells were expressed the CD45 which indicated negative for haemopoietic cells (**Figure 4(c)**), these results indicate that the cultured cells were MSC.

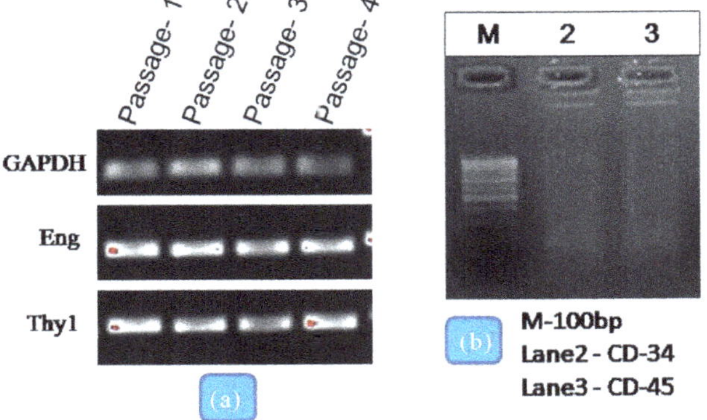

Figure 2. For gene expression analysis, the cultured of different passage were used for checking MSC specific genes by real time PCR. Passage 1 to 4 were used for analysis of Eng (Endoglin) and Thyl and reveled that cells were positive for these markers. Passage fourth cells were also checked for the expression of MSC negative marker CD34 and CD45 and no expression were found in the cultured cells. Gel electrophoresis of PCR amplified products of cBM-MSCs in 2% agarose gel (a) Showing the house keeping and MSCs specific markers Eng and Thy1. (b) Passage four cells were negative for CD34 and CD45.

The cell viability during passaging was checked by FASC analysis after staining by PI stain indicated that around that 92% cells were healthy and 8% cells were dead (**Figure 4(d)**).

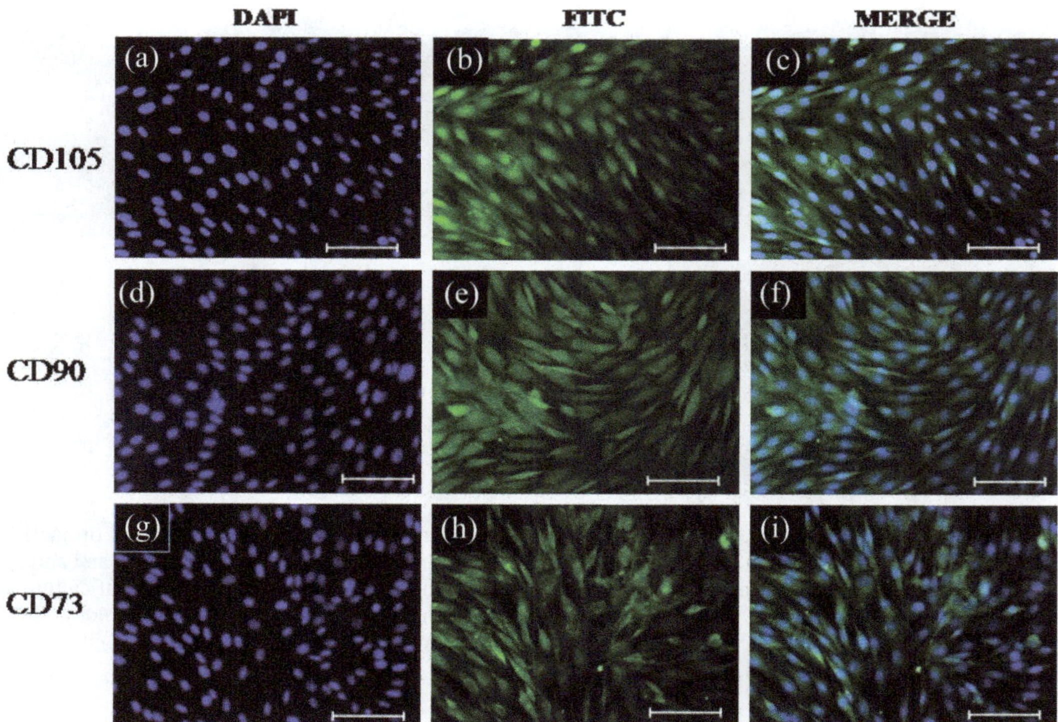

Figure 3. Immunolocalization of surface antigens associated markers in cBM-MSCs monolayer. Cells were stained with primary antibodies directed against CD105 (b), CD90 (e), and CD73 (h), and stained by FITC conjugated secondary antibodies. In alternative panels, (a), (d) & (g) representative fields of DAPI. In next panels (c), (f), (i) is merger photographs of DAPI and FTTC (Scalebar = 100 μm).

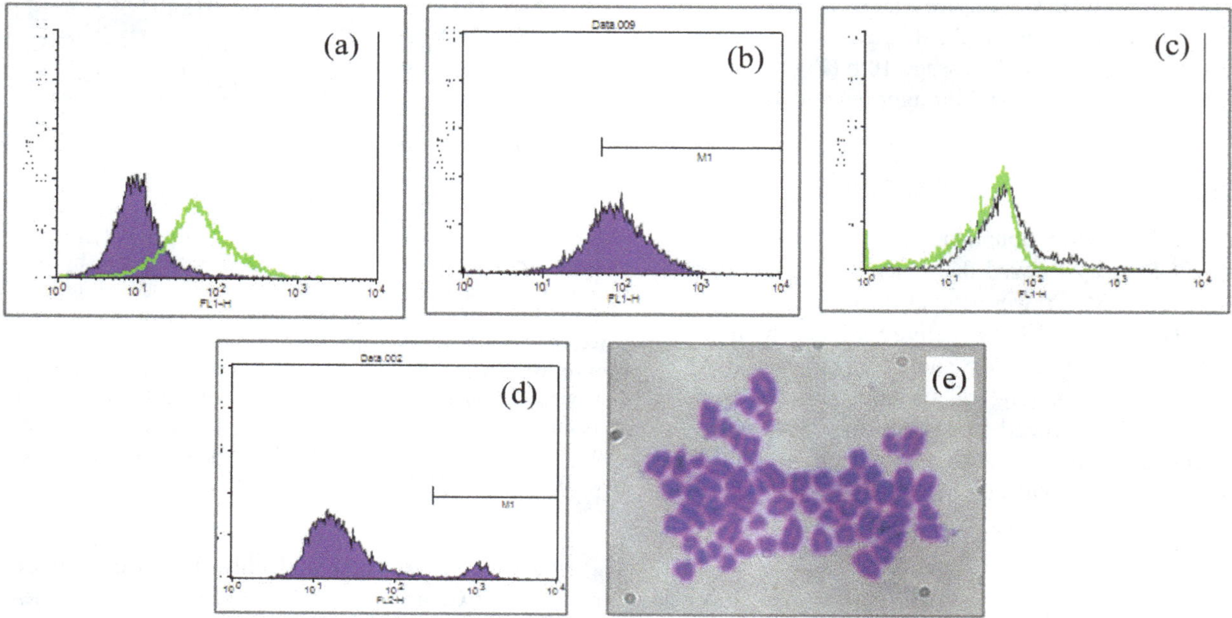

Figure 4. The cultured cBM-MSCs of passage four were used for FACS analysis. MSC specific genes CD73 and CD105 as well as negative marker CD45 were used to ruled out the contamination of other cells. Calibrated histogram representing the number of events in the Y-axis and FTTC-fluorescent intensity (FLH-1) on X-axis. (a) The shadowed histogram indicate 65.73% positive for CD-73. (b) 73.29% for CD-105 and (c) CD-45 showed 0.07%. (d) Passage four cells were used to check the cellular viability and integrity of plasma membrane of cells by FACS analysis after PI staining and 92% cells were live and around 8% cells were found dead. (e) cBM-MSCs showed normal chromosomes during *in vitro* culture.

Chromosome analysis during *in vitro* propagation indicated the normal pattern of caprine chromosomes (**Figure 4(e)**).

3.4. Multi-Differentiation Potential of cBM-MSCs

To induce the adipogenesis, after 21 days of co-culture with specific induction media, small lipid droplets appeared within the cytoplasm of cBM-MSCs. Reddish colored lipid droplets could be demonstrated by Oil Red O staining on 21st day of culture indicative of positive result for primary MSC culture (**Figure 5(a)**). The control were incubated in normal DMEM culture medium for the same period of time at for the treatment and stained with Oil Red O staining, and showed negative for the presence of lipid droplet (**Figure 5(b)**).

To induce the osteogenic differentiation, 70% - 80% confluence cells was replaced by differentiation medium and cultured for 21 days and media was changed periodically. After 7th - 8th day of co-incubation the cellular aggregates were observed in osteogenic differentiation culture plates and gradually increased till the end of the experiment. These aggregates in culture plate were characterized by calcium deposits, which were demonstrated reddish brownish when stained with Alizarin red stain (**Figure 5(c)**) as well as alkaline phosphatase staining (**Figure 5(e)**), control shows no any change after staining (**Figure 5(d)**). Control was negative for Alizarin red stain which indicated the absence of calcium deposit.

Differentiated cBM-MSCs into adipogenic and osteogenic cells were characterized by molecular methods by real time PCR using osteogenic and adipogenic specific markers. Gel picture of PCR products shows positive for both Osteocalcin and Adipsin (**Figure 5(f)**) and negative for control.

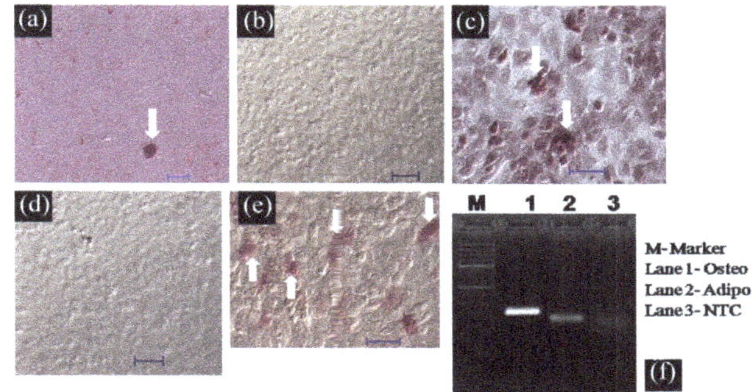

Figure 5. cBM-MSCs were *in vitro* differentiated into osteocytes and adipocytes. (a) Adipogenesis induced lipid droplets observed in red color after specific Oil Red O staining in *in vitro* cultured cBM-MSCs (Scale bar = 200 μm). (b) Control for adipogenic differentiations, absence of lipid droplet. (c) On osteogenic differentiation of cBM-MSCs, brownish colored mineral deposition (arrow) as demonstrated by alizarin red staining (Scale bar = 200 μm). (d) Control showing negative for the same. (e) Alkaline phosphatase positive cells. (f) *In vitro* differentiated cBM-MSCs in adipogenic and osteogenic cells were used for molecular characterization using real time PCR. Gel electrophoresis of PCR amplified products of cBM-MSCs in 2% agarose gel.

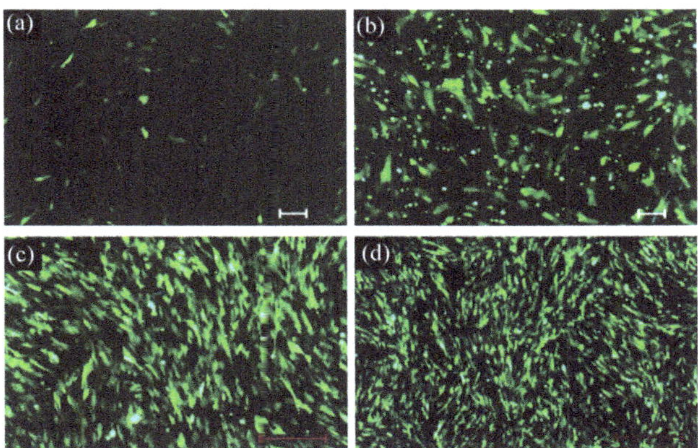

Figure 6. Passage three cBM-MSCs were plated in a 12-well tissue culture plate 24 hrs before the transfection procedure. DNA/Lipofectamine complex was prepared and adherent cells were washed with FBS and antibiotic free media and complex was added. (a) After 12 hrs of transfection, few cells started showing green colour under fluorescent microscope (Olympus, Japan). (b) 24 hrs of transfection more number of cells were showing the green colour. (c) After 72 hrs, large number of cells were expressing the green fluorencence. (d) Green color was stable at 96 hrs indicating continued GFP expression (Scale bar (a) & (b) 200 μm, (c) & (d) 500 μm).

3.5. Generation of Transgenic Mesenchymal Stem Cells and Their Characterization

Once the cBM-MSCs was characterized by molecular method, immunocytochemistry, FACS and *in vitro* differentiation into other mesenchymal lineage like adipocytes and osteocytes and checked for the normal karyotyping, these cells were used for the generation of transgenic cells. After the establishment of primary culture as MSC, early passage cBM-MSCs were transfected by plasmid vector using lipfectamine as a vehicle in 12 wells plate. After 12 hr of transfection, few cells were started showing GFP expression (**Figure 6(a)**) and it was increased in subsequent hours (**Figure 6(b)**), and was stable after 72 hr of transfection (**Figures 6(c)** and **(d)**). More than 67% cells were positive for the GFP expression as observed by FACS analysis (**Figure 7(F)**). After 72 hr, the cells were kept in the selection media containing 300 μg/ml G418, and continued in the selection medium. The cells were further passaged and propagated subsequently to increase the cells populations. At passage 3rd, cells were checked for GFP expression and 97% cells were showing GFP expression under fluorescent microscope. The tcBM-MSCs were successfully propagated beyond 12th passage by sub culturing them with

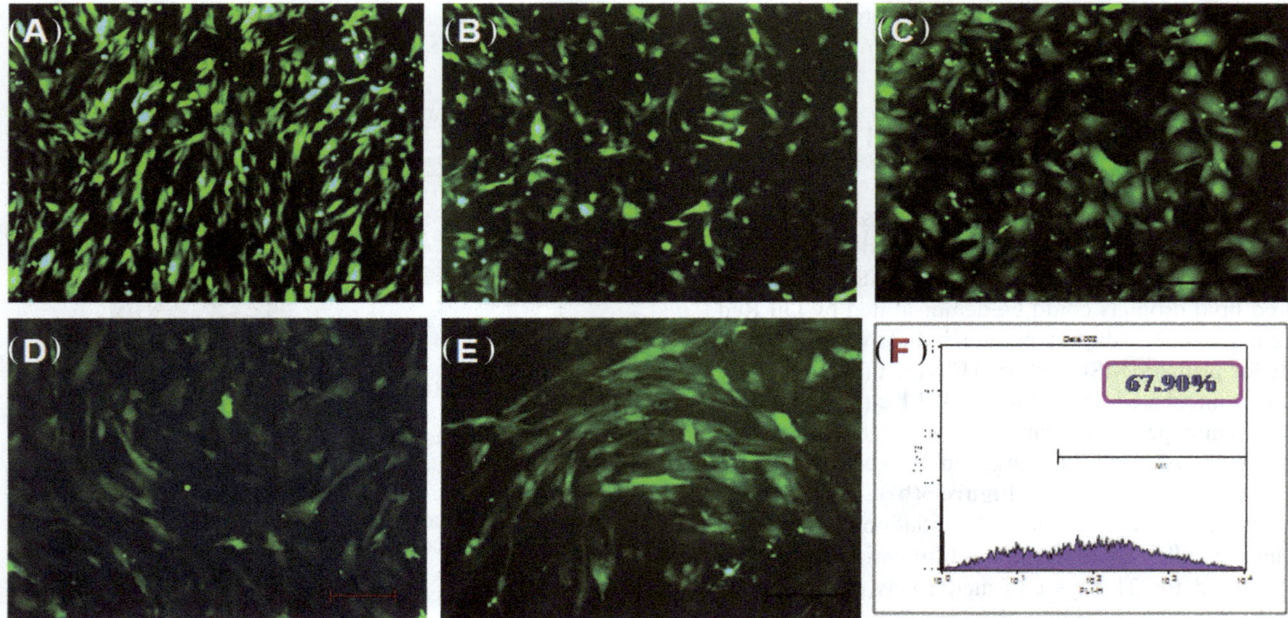

Figure 7. Transgenic cells were passaged and propagated further and reached beyond passage 12th. (A) Passage one cells are showing the green fluorescence. (B) Passage 3rd cells. (C) Passage 5th cells. (D) Passage 8th cells continued showing GFP expression. (E) Passage 10th cells are showing the stable GFP expression. (F) In first passage around 67.9% cells expressing the GFP when checked by FACS. Scale bar 500 μm.

trypsinization and the cells were maintaining the GFP expression during different passage (**Figure 7**). These cells were used for the transplantation studies in rabbit model (data not shown).

To establish that the transfection did not change the MSC characteristics, the tcB-MSCs were further characterized for MSC characteristics. The cell viability of tcB-MSCs checked by FASC analysis indicated that around that 91.45% cells were healthy and 8.55% cells were dead (**Figure 8(a)**). The tcB-MSCs carried normal pattern of caprine chromosomes (**Figure 8(b)**).

3.6. Characterization of tcBM-MSCs

Analysis of transcript abundance of target genes based real time PCR assay showed that under standard culture conditions, transgenic MSCs were found positive for CD73, CD90 and CD105 (**Figure 8(c)**) and negative for haematopoietic cell surface markers like CD45 and CD34 (**Figure 8(d)**). Furthermore, corresponding cell surface marker proteins were also successfully localized in tcBM-MSCs monolayer via immunocytochemistry such as CD73, CD90 and CD90 using alexaflour (**Figure 9**) it showed positive for the above MSC specific markers.

3.7. Multi-Differentiation Potential of tcBM-MSCs

The tcBM-MSCs also successfully differentiated into

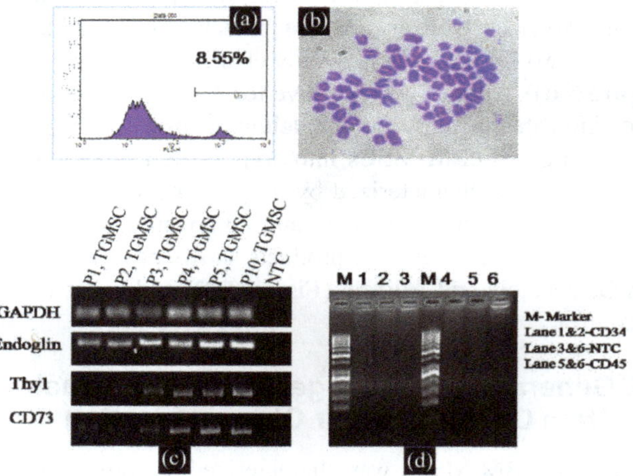

Figure 8. (a) Passage 3rd transgenic cells were used to check the cell viability after PI staining by FACS analysis and around 91.45% cells live and 8.55% cells were dead. (b) Passage 3rd transgenic cells were used for chromosome analysis and found the normal chromosomes. For gene expression analysis, these transgenic cells of different passage were used checked for MSC specific genes by real time PCR. Passage 1 to 5 and 10 were used for analysis of Eng. Thyl and CD73 reveled that cells are positive for the specific said markers, passage 2nd cells were also checked for the expression of MSC negative marker including CD34 and CD45 and no expression were found in the cultured cells. Gel electrophoresis of PCR amplified products of transgenic cBM-MSCs in 2% agarose gel. (c) Showing positive the house keeping and MSCs specific markers endoglin, Thyl and CD73. (d) Passage 2nd cells were negative for CD34 and CD45.

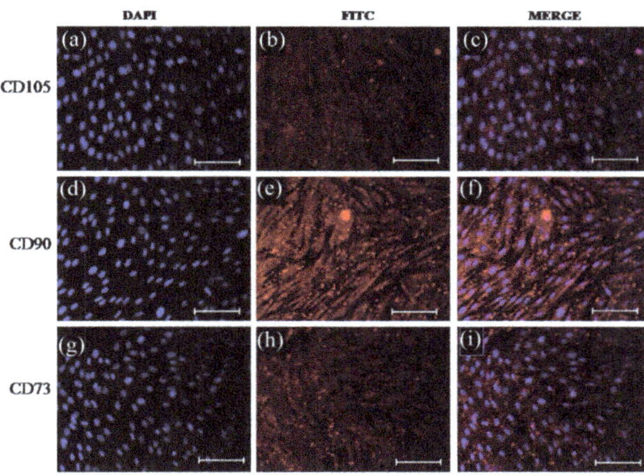

Figure 9. Immunolocalization of surface antigens associated markers in transgenic cBM-MSCs monolayer were done. Cells were stained with primary antibodies directed against CD105 (b), CD90 (e), and CD73 (h), and stained by FITC conjugated secondary antibodies. In alternative panels, (a) (d) and (g) representative fields of DAPI. In next panels (c), (f), (i) is merger photographs of DAPI and FITC (Scalebar = 100 μm).

adipogenic (**Figure 10(a)**) as well as osteogenic cells (**Figure 10(c)**) which was comparable with non transfected MSC cells. Differentiated cBM-MSCs into adipogenic and osteogenic cells were characterized by molecular methods using real time PCR. Gel electrophoresis of PCR products showed positive for Osteocalcin and Adipsin markers (**Figure 10(f)**).

3.8. Transdifferentiation of Transgenic MSC into Neurons

Passage 3rd tcBM-MSCs were used to transdifferentiate into neurons. Initially cells were maintained in sub confluent cultures in serum-containing medium supplemented with 1mM BME for 24 hr for pre-induction. Cells become rounded in structure after 24 hr of pre-induction (**Figure 11(a)**). To effect neuronal differentiation, the previous media were replaced by serum-free medium containing 2 - 8 mM BME. Cells were observed 12 hr of exposure to differentiation media, change in morphology of some of the cBM-MSCs were apparent. Responsive cells progressively assumed neuronal morphological characteristics over the first 24 hr of neuronal induction. Initially, cytoplasm in the flat cBM-MSCs retracted towards the nucleus, forming a contracted multipolar, cell body, protruding membranous, process-like extensions peripherally (**Figure 11(b)**). Over the subsequent hours, cell bodies became increasingly spherical and the cells adopted the morphological features typical of neurons such as refractile cell bodies and long branching processes. Processes continued to elaborate, displaying primary, secondary branches few cells showed tertiary branching also. Even after transdifferentiation of tcBM-MSCs

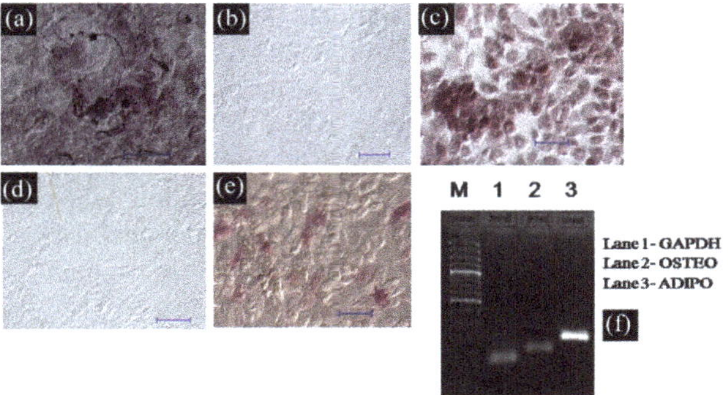

Figure 10. cBM-MSCs were *in vitro* differentiated into osteocytes and adipocytes. (a) Adipogenesis induced lipid droplets observed in res color after specific Oil Red O staining in *in vitro* cultured cBM-MSCs (Scale bar = 200 μm). (b) Control for adipogenic differentiations, absence of lipid droplet. (c) On osteogenic differentiation, brownish colored mineral deposition (arrow) were observed as demonstrated by alizarin red staining (Scale bar = 200 μm). (d) Control showing negative for the alizarin red staining. (e) Alkaline phosphatase positive cells. (f) *In vitro* differentiated cBM-MSCs in adipogenic and osteogenic cells were used for molecular characterization using real time PCR. Gel electrophoresis of PCR amplified products of cBM-MSCs in 2% agarose gel.

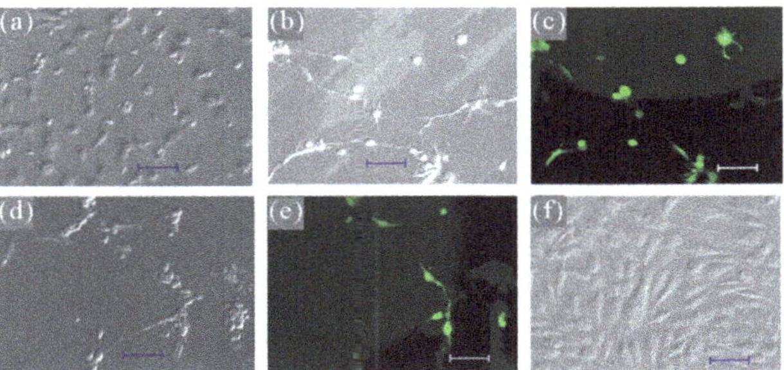

Figure 11. Neuronal differentiation of transgenic cBM-MSCs, passage four cells were used for the transdifferentiation into neurons. (a) After 24 hrs of pre-induction, cytoplasm were retracted toward nucleus and cBM-MSCs became rounded in structure. (b) Cytoplasm retracted towards the nucleus, forming a contracted multipolar, cell body, protruding membranous, process-like extensions peripherally. (c) fluorescent photographs of same field taken under. The neuronal differentiation protocol was initiated once the cells were sub confluent.

expressing the GFP under fluorescent microscope which indicate the stable transfection of the cBM-MSC (**Figures 11(c)** and **(e)**). Control was run simultaneously and no change in morphology of cells was observed (**Figure 11(f)**).

4. DISCUSSION

Mesenchymal stem cells show great promises as a biological therapeutic for a diverse range of unmet medical needs. The reasons for this are many and include, ease of isolation and expansion in culture, multipotency, paracrine effects, immunomodulatory properties, migratory behavior and ethical considerations. Though the bone marrow may be the preferred homing organ for MSCs injected intravenously in the normal untroubled animal [26-28], but this is not the case when inflammation is present in the animal, in this condition MSC appear to preferentially home to the site of inflammation when injected intravenously [29,30]. MSC may demonstrate plasticity beyond their traditional mesodermal lineage, in that they have been induced to generate, *in vitro* at least, into tissues of both ectodermal (neurons) and endodermal (hepatocytes) nature [31,32]. In addition, their ease and reproducibility of isolation, high expansion potential and capacity for useful modification using molecular biological engineering techniques, make them good candidates for the repair and regeneration of a large variety of tissues. They have been shown in preclinical studies to improve many incurable disease including myocardial function, cerebral function, liver damage and joint damage [33-38]. MSC appear to have a major advantage over many other cell types for cellular therapy, in that they are immunologically privileged and in large out bred animals can generally be transplanted across MHC barriers without the need for immunosuppression [39]. This has important implications for the therapeutic application of MSC [40].

The present study was carried out to isolate caprine MSC from bone marrow and generation of transgenic MSC using plasmid based vector for their future use in cell based therapeutics and transgenic animal production. The present study was focused with isolation of MSC from caprine bone marrow and generation of transgenic MSC using plasmid based vector. We had successfully isolated caprine MSC showing typical mesenchymal fibroblastic phenotypes (**Figure 1**) which were similar to the other reports [41,42]. The isolated cBM-MSCs were positive for CD90 and CD105 and negative for CD45 and CD34 (**Figure 3**), suggesting that the established cBM-MSCs were not from hematopoietic lineages [43-46]. We also demonstrated through differentiation studies that cBM-MSCs have the potentials to differentiate into adipogenic and osteogenic cell lineages (**Figures 5(a)** and **(c)**) as was observed by other researcher [47] who reported that murine MSCs can be differentiated into several specialized mesodermal cell types like bone, tendon, cartilage, musle and heart.

The production of cells capable of expressing gene(s) of interest is important for a variety of applications in biomedicine and biotechnology, including gene therapy and a novel method of stem cells therapy in the various diseases. Achieving high levels of transgene expression for the longer period of time, without adversely affecting cell viability and differentiation capacity of the cells, is crucial. Tracking of cells after transplantation into the animal is necessary to check the ability of MSC in regeneration of particular tissue. It will enhance the importance of stem cells therapy in the treatment of incurable disease. A variety of studies using vectors based on oncogenic retroviruses have been attempted to transduce MSCs, but there have been problems due to a number of issues. A major limitation of transduction approaches involving oncogenic retroviral vectors such as Moloney murine leukaemia virus (MoMLV) is a general lack of long-term transgene expression [48,49], possibly due to the inactivation of the retroviral long terminal repeat vectors based on murine stem cell virus appear to be less prone to transcriptional silencing of viral gene expression and, thus, appear to be more promising. Transduction of MSCs with MoMLV and murine stem cell virus-based vectors were shown to be inefficient, as they required drug selection to enrich transduced cells [49,50], multiple rounds of transduction for several days [51-53], or highly concentrated vector stocks [54]. To bypass safety concerns associated with viral vectors and other instrument handling, alternative, non-viral based methods for trans gene delivery were established for MSCs. Unfortunately, traditional transfection methods have shown little success in delivering plasmid DNA into primary MSCs, usually resulting in low transfection efficiencies and high cell mortality.

In the present experiment, the plasmid vector pAc-GFP1-C1 was chosen to transfect the cBM-MSCs and we generated the stable transgenic caprine bone marrow MSCs (tcBM-MSCs). In primary culture of transfected cells around 67% was expressing GFP (**Figure 7(F)**) and after antibiotic selection about 97% cells were showing GFP expression at third passage (**Figure 2**). The tcBM-MSCs were successfully propagated beyond twelfth passage (P12) and the cells showed robust GFP expression throughout the passages. One group of researcher [55] reported that by plasmid, transfected MSC have shown high viabilities (>90%) and recoveries (>52%) while maintaining their multipotency, this might be an advantageous transfection strategy when the goal is to express a therapeutic gene in a safe and transient way.

To verify that the transgenic cells retained typical MSC characters following transfection, the tcBM-MSCs cells were checked for expression of MSC specific genes by different methods and found positive for the expression of MSC specific genes CD73, CD90 and CD105 by imuunostaining as well as RTPCR, and negative for CD45 and CD34. The tcBM-MSCs were also readily differentiated into adipocytes and osteocytes. Present study suggested that the tcBM-MSCs had the similar characteristics and potential as normal MSC. Present results are accordance with the other reports [56] where they have demonstrated that Using Lentiviral vector, they were able to show specific stable suppression of eGFP expression in MSCs and hESCs with no alteration in the ability of the transduced cells to [56].

Presently, the widely used method to transfer genes to MSC is performed through defective viruses, such as adenovirus, lentivirus, and retrovirus [57]. When MSCs are used to compensate or correct a genetic pathology and must express the therapeutic gene for the duration of a patient's life (permanent expression), integrating viruses, such as lentivirus or retrovirus, are preferred because of their well-known capacity for long-term expression. On the contrary, when MSCs are used to treat noninherited diseases and are only required to express the therapeutic gene for a short period of time (transient expression), nonintegrating vectors including adenoviruses and nonviral gene delivery systems are preferred [58]. Recent results from several labs have indicated that HIV-1-based vectors are very efficient at delivering and expressing transgenes into MSCs [21,23,59]. A single round of transduction using unconcentrated HIV-1-based lentiviral vectors led to the efficient transduction of human MSCs and sustained transgene expression for up to at least 5 months [20]. An advantage of lentiviral vectors over vectors based on oncogenic retroviruses is that they are capable of transducing non-dividing cells [60]. One researchor [61] described a method for efficiently transducing murine MSC using lentiviral vectors. In case of adenoviral vectors, transgene delivery by unmodified adenoviral (Ad) vectors appears to be inefficient as far as MSCs are concerned. Some researcher [62] have used Ad vectors to deliver reporter genes into *ex vivo* expanded MPCs. Only 19% of the cells expressed the transgene, possibly due to the absence of the corresponding Coxsackie adenovirus receptor receptor on such cells [63].

Although viral vectors permit efficient transgene delivery, but safety concerns associated with viral transduction have prompted a search for alternative non-viral gene delivery methods [56]. Unfortunately, traditional transfection methods have shown little success in delivering plasmid DNA into primary MSCs, usually resulting in low transfection efficiencies and high cell mortality. Development of a novel, noninvasive transgene delivery protocol, based on the principle of electric field-induced molecular vibration [64]. This promising procedure did not interfere with the normal cellular differentiation activities of human and chick mesenchymal progenitors. In a recent report [65] described liposome-based transfection methods to introduce transgenes and small interfering RNAs (siRNAs) into human MSCs. Transfected MSC maintained their proliferation capacity paired with the ability to differentiate into different mesodermal lineages (bone, cartilage and fat) without loss of transgene expression. Transfection efficiencies ranged from 2% to 35%, resulting from using a Lipid/DNA ratio of 1.25 with a transgene expression of 7 days [56]. Stable transfection of plasmid DNA into rat MSCs by electroporation was successful [66].

To verify that the transgenic cells retained typical MSC characters following transfection the tcBM-MSCs cells were further characterized. The transgenic MSC were expressing MSC specific genes CD73, CD90 and CD105 (**Figure 8(c)**) and were negative for CD45 and CD34 (**Figures 8(d)** and **9(a)-(i)**). Further, these cells also retained the capacity to differentiate into adipocytes, osteoblasts and neuronal cells (**Figures 10(a)** and **(c)**).

5. CONCLUSION

In the present study MSC has been isolated and characterized from bone marrow and a transgenic MSC is generated with stable GFP expression in caprine using plasmid vector. It was also observed that the transgenic MSC retained all the MSC characteristrtics as well as differentiation potentiality including neurons allowing these cells for application in cell therapy with tracking ability. To the best of our knowledge this is the first report in domestic animals to generate transgenic MSCs using non-viral vector.

6. ACKNOWLEDGEMENTS

Authors are thankful to Director, Indian Veterinary Research Institute (IVRI) and NAIP, ICAR for providing necessary financial assistance and support for completing this work.

REFERENCES

[1] Pittenger, M.F., Mackay, A.M., Beck, S.C., Jaiswal, R.K., Douglas, R., Mosca, J.D., Moorman, M.A., Simonetti, D.W., Craig, S. and Marshak, D.R. (1999) Multilineage potential of adult human mesenchymal stem cells. *Science*, **284**, 143-147. http://dx.doi.org/10.1126/science.284.5411.143

[2] Caplan, A.I. (2007) Adult mesenchymal stem cells for tissue engineering versus regenerative medicine. *Journal of Cell Physiology*, **213**, 341-347. http://dx.doi.org/10.1002/jcp.21200

[3] Makino, S., Fukuda, K., Miyoshi, S., Konishi, F., Kodama, H., Pan, J., Sano, M., Takahashi, T., Hori, S., Abe, H., Hata, J., Umezawa, A. and Ogawa, S. (1999) Cardiomyocytes can be generated from marrow stromal cells *in vitro*. *Journal of Clinical Investigation*, **103**, 697-705. http://dx.doi.org/10.1172/JCI5298

[4] Kopen, G.C., Prockop, D.J. and Phinney, D.G. (1999) Marrow stromal cells migrate throughout forebrain and cerebellum, and they differentiate into astrocytes after injection into neonatal mouse brains. *Proceedings of the National Academy of Sciences of the United States of America*, **96**, 10711-10716. http://dx.doi.org/10.1073/pnas.96.19.10711

[5] Barry, F.P. and Murphy, J.M. (2004) Mesenchymal stem cells, clinical applications and biological characterization. *International Journal of Biochemical and Cell Biology*, **36**, 568-584. http://dx.doi.org/10.1016/j.biocel.2003.11.001

[6] Mahmood, A., Lu, D., Lu, M. and Chopp, M. (2003) Treatment of traumatic brain injury in adult rats with intravenous administration of human bone marrow stromal cells. *Neurosurgery*, **53**, 697-702. http://dx.doi.org/10.1227/01.NEU.0000079333.61863.AA

[7] Ryan, J.M., Barry, F., Murphy, J.M. and Mahon, B.P. (2007) Interferon-gamma does not break, but promotes the immunosuppressive capacity of adult human mesenchymal stem cells. *Clinical Experimental Immunology*, **149**, 353-363. http://dx.doi.org/10.1111/j.1365-2249.2007.03422.x

[8] Kumar, S., Chanda, D. and Ponnazhagan, S. (2008) Therapeutic potential of genetically modified mesenchymal stem cells. *Gene Therapy*, **15**, 711-715. http://dx.doi.org/10.1038/gt.2008.35

[9] Orlic, D., Kajstura, J., Chimenti, S., Limana, F., Jakoniuk, I. and Quaini, F. (2001) Mobilized bone marrow cells repair the infarcted heart, improving function and survival. *Proceedings of the National Academy of Sciences of the United States of America*, **98**, 10344. http://dx.doi.org/10.1073/pnas.181177898

[10] Hibi, H., Yamada, Y. and Kagami, H. (2006) Distraction osteogenesis assisted by tissue engineering in an irradiated mandible, a case report. *International Journal of Oral Maxillofac Implants*, **21**, 141.

[11] Yoshikawa, T., Mitsuno, H., Nonaka, I., Sen, Y., Kawanishi, K., Inada, Y., Takakura, Y., Okuchi, K. and Nonomura, A. (2008) Wound therapy by marrow mesenchymal cell transplantation. *Plastic and Reconstructive Surgery*, **121**, 860. http://dx.doi.org/10.1097/01.prs.0000299922.96006.24

[12] Sasaki, M., Abe, R., Fujita, Y., Ando, S., Inokuma, D. and Shimizu, H. (2008) Mesenchymal stem cells are recruited into wounded skin and contribute to wound repair by transdifferentiation into multiple skin cell type. *Journal of Immunology*, **180**, 2581.

[13] Ringden, O., Uzunel, M., Rasmusson, I., Remberger, M., Sundberg, B., Lonnies, H. Marschall, H.U., Dlugosz, A., Szakos, A., Hassan, Z., Omazic, B., Aschan, J., Barkholt, L. and Le Blanc, K. (2006) Mesenchymal stem cells for treatment of therapy-resistant graftversus-host disease. *Transplantation*, **81**, 1390-1397. http://dx.doi.org/10.1097/01.tp.0000214462.63943.14

[14] Amado, L.C., Saliaris, A.P., Schuleri, K.H., St John, M., Xie, J.S., Cattaneo, S., Durand, D.J., Fitton, T., Kuang, J.Q., Stewart, G., Lehrke, S., Baumgartner, W.W., Martin, B.J., Heldman, A.W. and Hare, J.M. (2005) Cardiac repair with intramyocardial injection of allogeneic mesenchymal stem cells after myocardial infarction. *Proceedings of the National Academy of Sciences of the United States of America*, **102**, 11474-11479. http://dx.doi.org/10.1073/pnas.0504388102

[15] McDonald, J.W. and Becker, D. (2003) Spinal cord injury, promising interventions and realistic goals. *American Journal of Physical Medicine & Rehabilitation*, **82**, 38. http://dx.doi.org/10.1097/01.PHM.0000086994.53716.17

[16] Reiss, K., Mentlein, R., Sievers, J. and Hartmann, D. (2002) Stromal cell-derived factor 1 is secreted by meningeal cells and acts as chemotactic factor on neuronal stem cells of the cerebellar external granular layer. *Neuroscience*, **115**, 295. http://dx.doi.org/10.1016/S0306-4522(02)00307-X

[17] Okabe, M., Ikawa, M., Kominami, K., Nakanishi, T. and Nishimune, Y. (1997) "Green mice" as a source of ubiquitous green cells. *FEBS*, **407**, 313. http://dx.doi.org/10.1016/S0014-5793(97)00313-X

[18] McMahon, J.M., Conroy, S., Lyons, M., Greiser, U., O'shea, C., Strappe, P., Howard, L., Murphy, M., Barry, F. and O'brien, T. (2006) Gene transfer into rat mesenchymal stem cells, a comparative study of viral and nonviral vectors. *Stem Cells and Development*, **15**, 87. http://dx.doi.org/10.1089/scd.2006.15.87

[19] McGinley, L., McMahon, J., Strappe, P., Barry, F., Murphy, M., O'Toole, D. and O'Brien1, T. (2011) Lentiviral vector mediated modification of mesenchymal stem cells and enhanced survival in an *in vitro* model of ischaemia. *Stem Cell Research and Therapy*, **12**, 1-18.

[20] Zhang, X.Y., La Russa, V.F., Bao, L., Kolls, J., Schwarzenberger, P. and Reiser, J. (2002) Lentiviral vectors for sustained transgene expression in human bone marrow-derived stromal cells. *Molecular Therapy*, **5**, 555-565. http://dx.doi.org/10.1006/mthe.2002.0585

[21] Totsugawa, T., Kobayashi, N., Okitsu, T., Noguchi, H., Watanabe, T., Matsumura, T., Maruyama, M., Fujiwara, T., Sakaguchi, M. and Tanaka, N. (2002) Lentiviral transfer of the LacZ gene into human endothelial cells and human bone marrow mesenchymal stem cells. *Cell Transplantation*, **11**, 481-488.

[22] Davis, B.M., Humeau, L., Slepushkin, V., Binder, G., Korshalla, L., Ni, Y., Ogunjimi, E.O., Chang, L.F., Lu, X. and Dropulic, B. (2004) ABC transporter inhibitors that are substrates enhance lentiviral vector transduction into primitive haematopoietic progenitor cells. *Blood*, **104**, 364-373. http://dx.doi.org/10.1182/blood-2003-07-2363

[23] Chan, J., O'donoghue, K., de la Fuente, J., Roberts, I.A., Kumar, S., Morgan, E.J. and Fisk, M.N. (2005) Human fetal mesenchymal stem cells as vehicles for gene delivery. *Stem Cells*, **23**, 93-102. http://dx.doi.org/10.1634/stemcells.2004-0138

[24] Kumar, M., Yasotha, T., Singh, R.K., Singh, R., Kumar, K., Ranjan, R., Chetan, D., Das, B.C. and Bag, S. (2013) Generation of transgenic mesenchymal stem cells expressing GFP as reporter gene using no viral vector in caprine. *Indian Journal of Experimental Biology*, **51**, 502-509.

[25] Woodbury, D., Reynolds, K. and Black, I.B. (2002) Adult bone marrow stromal stem cells express germline, ectodermal, endodermal, and mesodermal genes prior to neurogenesis. *Journal of Neuroscience Research*, **96**, 908-917. http://dx.doi.org/10.1002/jnr.10365

[26] Wynn, R.F., Hart, C.A., Corradi-Perini, C., O'Neill, L., Evans, C.A., Wraith, J.E., Fairbairn, L.J. and Bellantuono, I. (2004) A small proportion of mesenchymal stem cells strongly expresses functionally active CXCR4 receptor capable of promoting migration to bone marrow. *Blood*, **104**, 2643-2645. http://dx.doi.org/10.1182/blood-2004-02-0526

[27] Devine, S.M., Bartholomew, A.M., Mahmud, N., Nelson, M., Patil, S., Hardy, W., Sturgeon, C., Hewett, T., Chung,

T., Stock, W., Sher, D., Weissman, S., Ferrer, K., Mosca, J., Deans, R., Moseley, A. and Hoffman, R. (2001) Mesenchymal stem cells are capable of homing to the bone marrow of non-human primates following systemic infusion. *Experimental Hematology*, **29**, 244-255. http://dx.doi.org/10.1016/S0301-472X(00)00635-4

[28] Bensidhoum, M., Chapel, A., Francois, A., Demarquay, C., Mazurier, C., Fouillard, L., Bouchet, S., Bertho, J.M., Gourmelon, P., Aigueperse, J., Charbord, P., Gorin, N.C., Thierry, D. and Lopez, M. (2004) Homing of *in vitro* expanded Stro-1- or Stro-1+ human mesenchymal stem cells into the NOD/SCID mouse and their role in supporting human CD34 cell engraftment. *Blood*, **103**, 3313-3319. http://dx.doi.org/10.1182/blood-2003-04-1121

[29] Chapel, A., Bertho, J.M., Bensidhoum, M., Fouillard, L., Young, R.G., Frick, J., Demarquay, C., Cuvelier, F., Mathieu, E., Trompier, F., Dudoignon, N., Germain, C., Mazurier, C., Aigueperse, J., Borneman, J., Gorin, N.C., Gourmelon, P. and Thierry, D. (2003) Mesenchymal stem cells home to injured tissues when co-infused with hematopoietic cells to treat a radiation-induced multi-organ failure syndrome. *Journal of Gene Medicine*, **5**, 1028-1038. http://dx.doi.org/10.1002/jgm.452

[30] Ortiz, L.A., Gambelli, F., McBride, C., Gaupp, D., Baddoo, M. and Kaminski, N. (2003) Mesenchymal stem cell engraftment in lung is enhanced in response to bleomycin exposure and ameliorates its fibrotic effects. *Proceedings of the National Academy of Sciences of the United States of America*, **100**, 8407-8411. http://dx.doi.org/10.1073/pnas.1432929100

[31] Lee, C.I., Kohn, D.B., Ekert, J.E. and Tarantal, A.F. (2004) Morphological analysis and lentiviral transduction of fetal monkey bone marrow-derived mesenchymal stem cells. *Molecular Therapy*, **9**, 112-123. http://dx.doi.org/10.1016/j.ymthe.2003.09.019

[32] Jiang, Y., Jahagirdar, B.N., Reinhardt, R.L., Schwartz, R.E., Keene, C.D., Ortiz-Gonzalez, X.R., Reyes, M., Lenvik, T., Lund, T., Blackstad, M., Du, J., Aldrich, S., Lisberg, A., Low, W.C., Largaespada, D.A. and Verfaillie, C.M. (2002) Pluripotency of mesenchymal stem cells derived from adult marrow. *Nature*, **418**, 41-49. http://dx.doi.org/10.1038/nature00870

[33] Deans, R.J. and Moseley, A.B. (2000) Mesenchymal stem cells, biology and potential clinical uses. *Experimental Hematology*, **28**, 875-884. http://dx.doi.org/10.1016/S0301-472X(00)00482-3

[34] Itescu, S., Schuster, M.D. and Kocher, A.A. (2003) New directions in strategies using cell therapy for heart disease. *Journal of Molecular Medicine*, **81**, 288-296.

[35] Toma, C., Pittenger, M.F., Cahill, K.S., Byrne, B.J. and Kessler, P.D. (2002) Human mesenchymal stem cells differentiate to a cardiomyocyte phenotype in the adult murine heart. *Circulation*, **105**, 93-98. http://dx.doi.org/10.1161/hc0102.101442

[36] Fang, B., Shi, M., Liao, L., Yang, S., Liu, Y. and Zhao, R.C. (2004) Systemic infusion of FLK1(+) mesenchymal stem cells ameliorate carbon tetrachloride induced liver fibrosis in mice. *Transplantation*, **78**, 83-88. http://dx.doi.org/10.1097/01.TP.0000128326.95294.14

[37] Murphy, J.M., Fink, D.J., Hunziker, E.B. and Barry, F.P. (2003) Stem cell therapy in a caprine model of osteoarthritis. *Arthritis Rheumtment*, **48**, 3464-3474. http://dx.doi.org/10.1002/art.11365

[38] Orlic, D., Kajstura, J., Chimenti, S., Jakoniuk, I., Anderson, S.M., Li, B., Pickel, J., McKay, R., Nadal-Ginard, B., David, M., Bodine, D.M., Leri, A. and Anversa, P. (2001) Bone marrow cells regenerate infarcted myocardium. *Nature*, **410**, 701-705. http://dx.doi.org/10.1038/35070587

[39] Devine, S.M., Cobbs, C., Jennings, M., Bartholomew, A. and Hoffman, R. (2003) Mesenchymal stem cells distribute to a wide range of tissues following systemic infusion into nonhuman primates. *Blood*, **101**, 2999-3001. http://dx.doi.org/10.1182/blood-2002-06-1830

[40] Sordi, V., Malosio, M.L., Marchesi, F., Mercalli, A., Melzi, R., Giordano, T., Belmonte, N., Ferrari, G., Leone, B.E., Bertuzzi, F., Zerbini, G., Allavena, P., Bonifacio, E. and Piemonti, L. (2005) Bone marrow mesenchymal stem cells express a restricted set of functionally active chemo kine receptors capable of promoting migration to pancreatic islets. *Blood*, **106**, 419-427. http://dx.doi.org/10.1182/blood-2004-09-3507

[41] Simmons, P.J. and Torok-Storb, B. (1991) Identification of stromal cell precursors in human bone marrow by a novel monoclonal antbody-STRO-1. *Blood*, **78**, 55-62.

[42] Rosada, C., Justesen, J., Melsvik, D., Ebbesen, P. and Kassem, M. (2003) The human umbilical cord blood, a potential source for osteoblast progenitor cells. *Calcif Tissue International*, **72**, 135-142. http://dx.doi.org/10.1007/s00223-002-2002-9

[43] Haynesworth, S.E., Goshima, J., Goldberg, W.M. and Caplan, A.I. (1992) Characterization of cells with osteogenic potential from human marrow. *Bone*, **13**, 81-88. http://dx.doi.org/10.1016/8756-3282(92)90364-3

[44] Sacchetti, B., Funari, A., Michienzi, S., Di Cesare, S., Piersanti, S., Saggio, I., Tagliafico, E., Ferrari, S., Robey, P.G., Riminucci, M. and Bianco, P. (2007) Self-renewing osteoprogenitors in bone marrow sinusoids can organize a hematopoietic microenvironment. *Cell*, **131**, 324-336. http://dx.doi.org/10.1016/j.cell.2007.08.025

[45] Kassem, M., Kristiansen, M. and Abdallah, B.M. (2004) Mesenchymal stem cells, cell biology and potential use in therapy. *Basic Clinical, Pharmacology and Toxicology*, **95**, 209-214. http://dx.doi.org/10.1111/j.1742-7843.2004.pto950502.x

[46] Krabbe, C., Zimmer, J. and Meyer, M. (2005) Neural transdifferentiation of mesenchymal stem cells—A critical review. *APMIS*, **113**, 831-844. http://dx.doi.org/10.1111/j.1600-0463.2005.apm_3061.x

[47] Woodbury, D., Reynolds, K. and Black, I.B. (2002). Adult bone marrow stromal stem cells express germline, ectodermal, endodermal, and mesodermal genes prior to neurogenesis. *Journal of Neuroscience Research*, **69**, 908-917. http://dx.doi.org/10.1002/jnr.10365

[48] Chuah, M.K., Van Damme, A., Zwinnen, H., Goovaerts, I., Vanslembrouck, V., Collen, D. and VandenDriessche, T. (2000) Long-term persistence of human bone marrow stromal cells transduced with Factor VIII-retroviral vectors and transient production of therapeutic levels of hu-

man Factor VIII in nonmyeloablated immunodeficient mice. *Human Gene Therapy*, **11**, 729-738. http://dx.doi.org/10.1089/10430340050015626

[49] Schwarz, E.J., Alexander, G.M., Prockop, D.J. and Azizi, S.A. (1999) Multipotential marrow stromal cells transduced to produce L-DOPA, engraftment in a rat model of Parkinson's disease. *Human Gene Therapy*, **10**, 2539-2549. http://dx.doi.org/10.1089/10430349950016870

[50] Allay, J.A., Dennis, J.E., Haynesworth, S.E., Majumdar, M.K., Clapp, D.W., Shultz, L.D., Caplan, A.I. and Gerson, S.L. (1997) Lacz and interleukin-3 expression *in vivo* after retroviral transduction of marrow-derived human osteogenic mesenchymal progenitors. *Human Gene Therapy*, **8**, 1417-1427. http://dx.doi.org/10.1089/hum.1997.8.12-1417

[51] Marx, J.C., Allay, J.A., Persons, D.A., Nooner, S.A., Hargrove, P.W., Kelly, P.F., Vanin, E.F. and Horwitz, E.M. (1999) High-efficiency transduction and long-term gene expression with a murine stem cell retroviral vector encoding the green fluorescent protein in human marrow stromal cells. *Human Gene Therapy*, **10**, 1163-1173. http://dx.doi.org/10.1089/10430349950018157

[52] Chianget, G.G., Rubin, H.I., Cherington, V., Wang, T., Sobolewski, J., McGrath, C.A., Gaffney, A., Emami, S., Sarver, N., Levine, P.H., Greenberger, J.S. and Hurwitz, D.R. (1999) Bone marrow stromal cell-mediated gene therapy for hemophilia A, *in vitro* expression of human Factor VIII with high biological activity requires the inclusion of the proteolytic site at amino acid 1648. *Human Gene Therapy*, **10**, 61-76. http://dx.doi.org/10.1089/10430349950019192

[53] Chuah, M.K., Brems, H., Vanslembrouck, V., Collen, D. and Vandendriessche, T. (1998) Bone marrow stromal cells as targets for gene therapy of hemophilia A. *Human Gene Therapy*, **9**, 353-365. http://dx.doi.org/10.1089/hum.1998.9.3-353

[54] Jaalouk, D.E., Eliopoulos, N., Couture, C., Mader, S. and Galipeau, J. (2000) Glucocorticoid-inducible retrovector for regulated transgene expression in genetically engineered bone marrow stromal cells. *Human Gene Therapy*, **11**, 1837-1849. http://dx.doi.org/10.1089/10430340050129468

[55] Madeira, C., Mendes, R.D., Ribeiro, S.C., Boura, J.S., Aires-Barros, M.R., da Silva, C.L., and Cabral, J.M.S. (2010) Nonviral gene delivery to mesenchymal stem cells using cationic liposomes for gene and cell therapy. *Journal of Biomedicine and Biotechnology*, **12**, 1-12. http://dx.doi.org/10.1155/2010/735349

[56] Clements, M.O., Godfrey, A., Crossley, J., Wilson, S.J., Takeuchi, Y. and Boshoff, C. (2006) Lentiviral manipulation of gene expression in human adult and embryonic stem cell. *Tissue Engineering*, **12**, 7-13. http://dx.doi.org/10.1089/ten.2006.12.1741

[57] Zhang, X. and Godbey, W.T. (2006) Viral vectors for gene delivery in tissue engineering. *Advance Drug Delivery Reviews*, **58**, 515-534. http://dx.doi.org/10.1016/j.addr.2006.03.006

[58] Park, S.J. and Na, K. (2012) The transfection efficiency of photo sensitizer-induced gene delivery to human MSCs and internalization rates of eGFP and Runx2 genes. *Biomaterials*, **33**, 6485-6494. http://dx.doi.org/10.1016/j.biomaterials.2012.05.040

[59] Devis, B.M., Humeau, L. and Slepushkin, V. (2004) ABC transporter inhibitors that are substrates enhance lentiviral vector transduction into primitive haematopoietic progenitor cells. *Blood*, **104**, 364-373. http://dx.doi.org/10.1182/blood-2003-07-2363

[60] Reiser, J., Harmison, G., Kluepfel-Stahl, S., Brady, R.O., Karlsson, S. and Schubert, M. (1996) Transduction of nondividing cells using pseudotyped defective high-titer HIV Type 1 particles. *Proceedings of the National Academy of Sciences of the United States of America*, **93**, 15266-15271. http://dx.doi.org/10.1073/pnas.93.26.15266

[61] Anjos-Alfonso, F., Siapati, E.K. and Bonnet, D. (2004) *In vivo* contribution of murine mesenchymal stem cells into multiple cell-types under minimal damage conditions. *Journal of Cell Science*, **117**, 5655-5664. http://dx.doi.org/10.1242/jcs.01488

[62] Conget, P.A. and Minguell, J.J. (2000) Adenoviral-mediated gene transfer into *ex vivo* expanded human bone marrow mesenchymal progenitor cells. *Experimental Hematology*, **28**, 382-390. http://dx.doi.org/10.1016/S0301-472X(00)00134-X

[63] Hung, S.C., Lu, C.Y., Shyue, S.K., Liu, H.C. and Ho, L.L. (2004) Lineage differentiation-associated loss of adenoviral susceptibility and Coxsackie-adenovirus receptor expression in human mesenchymal stem cells. *Stem Cells*, **22**, 1321-1329. http://dx.doi.org/10.1634/stemcells.2003-0176

[64] Song, L., Webb, N.E., Song, Y. and Tuan, R.S. (2006) Identification and functional analysis of candidate genes regulating mesenchymal stem cells self-renewal and multipotency. *Stem Cells*, **24**, 1707-1718. http://dx.doi.org/10.1634/stemcells.2005-0604

[65] Hoelters, J., Ciccarella, M., Drechsel, M., Geissler, C., Gülkan, H., Böcker, W., Schieker, M., Jochum, M. and Neth, P. (2005) Nonviral genetic modification mediates effective transgene expression and functional RNA interference in human mesenchymal stem cells. *Journal of Gene Medicine*, **7**, 718-728. http://dx.doi.org/10.1002/jgm.731

[66] Peister, A., Mellad, J.A., Wang, M., Tucker, H.A. and Prockop, D.J. (2004) Stable transfection of MSCs by electroporation. *Gene Therapy*, **11**, 224-228. http://dx.doi.org/10.1038/sj.gt.3302163

12

Increased osteogenesis with hydroxyapatite constructs combined with serially-passaged bone marrow-derived mesenchymal stem cells

Manabu Akahane[1*], Tomoyuki Ueha[2], Takamasa Shimizu[2], Yusuke Inagaki[2], Akira Kido[2], Tomoaki Imamura[1], Kenji Kawate[3], Yasuhito Tanaka[2]

[1]Department of Public Health, Health Management and Policy, Nara Medical University School of Medicine, Nara, Japan;
[*]Corresponding Author: makahane@naramed-u.ac.jp
[2]Department of Orthopedic Surgery, Nara Medical University, Nara, Japan
[3]Department of Artificial Joint and Regenerative Medicine, Nara Medical University, Nara, Japan

ABSTRACT

We have previously reported on both the osteogenic potential of hydroxyapatite (HA) combined with bone marrow-derived mesenchymal stem cells (BMSCs) and a method involving osteogenic matrix cell sheet transplantation of BMSCs. In the present study, we assessed the osteogenic potential of serially-passaged BMSCs, both *in vitro* and *in vivo*. We also assessed whether an additional cell-loading technique can regain the osteogenic potential of the constructs combined with serially-passaged BMSCs. The present study revealed that passage (P) 1 cells cultured in osteogenic-induced medium showed strong positive staining for alkaline phosphatase (ALP) and Alizarin Red S, whereas P3 cells showed faint staining for ALP, with no Alizarin Red S staining. Staining of P1, P2 and P3 cells were progressively weaker, indicating that the osteogenic potential of the serially-passaged rat BMSCs is lost after P3 *in vitro*. The *in vivo* study showed that little bone formation was observed in the HA constructs seeded with P3 cells, 4 weeks after subcutaneous implantation. However, P3 cell/HA constructs which had increased cell-loading showed abundant bone formation within the pores of the HA construct. ALP and osteocalcin mRNA expression in these constructs was significantly higher than that of constructs with regular cell-seeding. The present study indicates that the osteogenic potential of the constructs with serially-passaged BMSCs is increased by additional cell-loading. This method can be applied to cases requiring hard tissue reconstruction, where BMSCs require serial expansion of cells.

Keywords: Osteogenesis; Mesenchymal Stem Cells; Serial Passaging; Hydroxyapatite; Tissue Engineering; Bone Reconstruction

1. INTRODUCTION

Bone marrow contains a population of undifferentiated cells known as mesenchymal stem cells (MSCs) [1,2]. Bone marrow-derived MSCs (BMSCs) have the potential for self-renewal and differentiation into several cell types after culture expansion *in vitro* and *in vivo*, including osteoblastic, chondrocytic, adipocytic and neuronal cells [3-7]. Differentiation into osteoblastic lineage cells after subculture in osteogenic-induced media, containing dexamethasone (Dex), ascorbic acid phosphate and β-glycerophosphate (β-GP), has been shown for rat and human BMSCs [8-11]. The osteogenic phenotypic markers, alkaline phosphatase (ALP) and osteocalcin (OC), can be detected by days 10 - 12 in passage 1 (P1)-cultured cells, including mineralization [12]. The combination of BMSCs with a scaffolding material, such as hydroxyapatite (HA), can promote the formation of new bone tissue *in vivo* after subcutaneous transplantation with freshly isolated bone marrow cells [13] or culture-expanded BMSCs (HA/BMSCs construct) [2,14-17], Recently, we reported a new cell transplantation technique in which BMSCs were cultured in culture medium containing Dex and ascorbic acid phosphate and transplanted as cell sheets [18]. These cell sheets can be combined with HA, in which they resulted in abundant bone formation compared with conventional techniques [17].

Clinical applications of tissue engineered BMSCs have been attempted in a number of therapies, including the treatment of osteonecrosis [19-21]. In these approaches, BMSCs are obtained from the patients, following which they generally need to be expanded by serial passaging *in vitro* as the number of cells generated in primary culture is limited. However, the osteogenic potential of BMSCs might be lost by serial passaging *in vitro*, resulting in decreased osteogenesis after subcutaneous transplantation [8]. Therefore, it is important to determine whether HA constructs combined with serially-passaged BMSCs maintain sufficient osteogenic potential after *in vivo* transplantation. In the present study, we used BMSCs obtained from rat bone marrow and assessed the osteogenic potential of serially-passaged BMSCs, both *in vitro* and *in vivo*. We also assessed whether an additional cell-loading technique, where cells are cultured in osteoblastic cell sheet preparation medium can regain the osteogenic potential of the constructs combined with serially-passaged BMSCs.

2. MATERIALS AND METHODS

2.1. Bone Marrow Cell Preparation and Cell Culture

Approval from the animal experimental review board of Nara Medical University was obtained before beginning the experiments. Institutional guidelines for the care and use of laboratory animals have been observed. We previously reported the method of bone marrow cell preparation [11,18]. Briefly, bone marrow cells were obtained from the femur shafts of 7-week-old male Fischer 344 rats. Both ends of the femur were removed from the epiphysis and the marrow was flushed out using 10 ml of standard culture medium which was expelled from a syringe containing a 20-gauge needle. Standard culture medium consisted of minimal essential medium (MEM; Nacalai Tesque, Kyoto, Japan) containing 15% fetal bovine serum (FBS, JRH Bioscience Inc., KS, USA) and antibiotics (100 U/ml penicillin and 100 µg/ml streptomycin, Nacalai Tesque).

The obtained cells were collected in two T-75 flasks (Falcon, BD, NJ, USA) containing 15 ml of standard culture medium. These cells were known as passage 0 (P0). Cell culture was maintained in a humidified atmosphere of 95% air with 5% CO_2 at 37°C. After reaching confluency, cells were released from the culture substratum using trypsin/EDTA (Gibco, Invitrogen, CA, USA). The released cells were seeded at density of 1×10^4 cells/cm^2 for subculture in T75 flasks (Falcon) for serial passaging to obtain passage 3 (P3) cells. Each passage of cells (P1, P2 and P3) were used for the following experiments.

2.2. ALP and Alizarin Red S Staining

To evaluate the osteogenic potential of serially-passaged cells *in vitro*, P1, P2 and P3 cells were seeded in 6-well plates at density of 1×10^4 cells/cm^2 and cultured with or without osteogenic-induced media containing Dex (10 nM), ascorbic acid phosphate (82 µg/mL) and β-GP (10 mM) for 14 days. Each well was stained with Naphtol-AS-MX phosphate sodium salt (Sigma) and Fast Red Violet B (Nacalai Tesque) for ALP staining. 10 mg of each reagent was dissolved in 20 ml of AMP buffer (1.0 mM $MgCl_2$, 10 mM p-nitrophenyl phosphate in 0.056 M 2-amino-2-methyl-propanol). Cells were incubated with 2 ml of the substrate solution at room temperature for ~2 minutes and rinsed with dH_2O. Alizarin Red S (0.5%) was also used to evaluate calcium deposition, following which cells were rinsed with dH_2O [12,18]. Each experiment contained 3 replicates and was performed in duplicate.

2.3. ALP Activity, Calcium and DNA Concentration *in Vitro*

Cells cultured in 12-well culture plates were used to measure ALP activity, as previously reported [12]. Briefly, P1, P2 and P3 cells, seeded in 12-well plates at a density of 1×10^4 cells/cm^2 and cultured for 14 days with or without osteogenic-induced media containing Dex, ascorbic acid phosphate and β-GP, were scraped into 1 ml of 0.05 M sodium phosphate buffer, 2 mM EDTA and 2 M NaCl, following which they were homogenized and sonicated. To measure the ALP activity of cultured cells, 0.1 ml of the sonicated cell suspension was added to 0.5 ml of 0.2% Nonidet P-40 containing 1 mM $MgCl_2$ and centrifuged at 13,000 rpm for 10 minutes at 4°C. The supernatant was assayed for ALP activity using *p*-nitrophenylphosphate as a substrate. An aliquot (10 µl) of the supernatant was added to 1 ml of 50 mM *p*-nitrophenylphosphate containing 1 mM $MgCl_2$ and the mixture was incubated for 30 minutes at 37°C. Subsequently, 2 ml of 0.2 N NaOH was added to stop the enzymatic reaction and the absorption at 410 nm was measured by spectrophotometry. ALP activity was represented as *p*-nitrophenol release (µmol) after 30 minutes of incubation at 37°C.

Calcium was extracted from the sediment of Nonidet P-40 extract with 500 µl of 20% formic acid for 24 hours at 4°C. An aliquot of the formic acid extract was diluted with strontium solution. Calcium concentration was determined using an atomic absorption spectrometer (AA-610 S; Shimadzu Co., Kyoto, Japan). The sonicated cell suspension was also used for DNA content measurement by fluorescence emission at 458 nm in the presence of 0.5 µg/ml Hoechst 33,258 (Wako Pure Chemical), with calf thymus DNA as the standard (Wako Pure Chemical). Each group comprised of 4 wells. The experiment was performed in duplicate.

2.4. Preparation of HA Constructs Seeded with P3 Cells

We have previously reported the preparation of HA constructs combined with BMSCs (BMSC/HA construct) [12,17]. Briefly, after release from the substratum, P3 cells were centrifuged and resuspended at a density of 1×10^6 cells/ml in standard medium. Air was removed from the HA, which were previously soaked in cell suspension, by vacuum prior to making the constructs. Then, the HA disks were soaked in the cell suspension for 2 hours in a CO_2 incubator at 37°C to create the P3 cell/HA constructs. After soaking in the cell suspension, the construct was transferred into a 12-well plate (Falcon) in 1 mL of osteogenic-induced medium, consisting of standard medium, 82 μg/mL ascorbic acid phosphate (Wako Pure Chemical Industrials, Kyoto, Japan) and 10 nM Dex (Sigma, St. Louis, MO, USA) for further subculture. After 14 days of subculture, the cultured P3 cell/HA constructs were transplanted into a subcutaneous site of syngenic rats for the control group of the *in vivo* experiments.

Porous HA ceramics (50% average void volume, 5 mm in diameter and 2 mm thickness) were used in this study (Cellyard HA scaffold, Pentax Co., Tokyo, Japan). The solid and porous components of the microstructure are interconnected.

2.5. Additional Cell-Loading of the P3 Cell/HA Constructs

We previously reported that BMSCs cultured in standard medium containing Dex and ascorbic acid phosphate resulted in the formation of cell sheets [10,18]. In the present study, additional P3 cells for loading were also prepared in cell sheet culture medium. Briefly, P3 cells were seeded at a density of 1×10^4 cells/cm^2 in 3.5 cm and 10 cm dishes (Falcon) and cultured in standard medium containing Dex (10 nM) and ascorbic acid phosphate (82 μg/mL) (cell sheet preparation medium) until confluent. We used a mechanical retrieval technique for the preparation of additional P3 cells for cell loading of the constructs. The cells were rinsed twice with phosphate-buffered saline (PBS; Gibco) and lifted as sheet structure using a cell-scraper. As P3 cells formed incomeplete cell sheets compared with P1 cells, they were loaded onto P3 cell/HA constructs by a short centrifugation at 900 rpm for 2 min (Kubota 5100, Kubota Corp., Tokyo, Japan). Subsequently, the constructs were transplanted into a subcutaneous site as the additional-loading group. Because we used a number of different cell densities for the additional loading of the constructs, we placed them into two subgroups, according to whether they were cultured in 3.5 cm or 10 cm dishes.

Thus, there were three groups in the *in vivo* study: the P3 cell/HA construct without additional loading (control group), the P3 cell/HA construct cultured in a 3.5 cm dish of P3 cells (small loading group) and the P3 cell/HA construct cultured in a 10 cm dish of P3 cells (large loading group). Each group contained seven HA disks in two recipient rats (three or four disks per rat), which were implanted at subcutaneous sites on their backs. Three disks were used for histology and four for real-time PCR analysis. The experiment was performed in duplicate.

2.6. Sample Harvest and Histological Analysis

Implanted disks were harvested 4 weeks after implantation. HA disks for analysis by real-time PCR were frozen until RNA isolation. Disks for histological evaluation were fixed in 10% buffered formalin after trimming off the excess rat tissue around the HA disc. The HA disks fixed in formalin were decalcified in K-CX solution (Falma Co., Tokyo, Japan) and embedded in paraffin. They were cut parallel down the centre of specimens to the round surface of the HA discs and stained with hematoxylin and eosin (H-E).

2.7. RNA Isolation and Real-Time Quantitative PCR

We measured the gene expression levels of ALP and OC to confirm osteogenesis in the harvested disks. RNA was isolated from four disks from each group using an Isogen RNA extraction kit (Nippon Gene Co. Ltd., Toyama, Japan). Briefly, each sample was placed in Isogen solution containing matrix beads and disrupted with a FastPrep FP24 Cell Disrupter (Qbiogene, Inc., Carlsbad, CA, USA) [12,17]. Subsequently, the remaining steps of RNA isolation were performed according to the manufacturer's instructions. To measure mRNA expression levels, we conducted real-time quantitative PCR (Applied Biosystems StepOnePlus; Applied Biosystems, Norwalk, CT, USA), using primers for ALP, OC and glyceraldehyde-3-phosphate dehydrogenase (GAPDH, internal standard) for rat cDNAs as previously described [22]. Target ALP and OC mRNA levels were compared after correcting to GAPDH mRNA levels as an internal standard, to adjust for differences in the efficiency of reverse transcription between samples. ALP (Rn00564931 m1), OC (Rn 01455285 g1) and GAPDH (Rn99999916 s1) primer and probe sets were purchased from Applied Biosystems (Foster City, CA, USA). Thermal cycle conditions were 20 sec at 95°C for activation of TaqMan Fast Universal PCR Master Mix, followed by 40 cycles of 1 sec at 95°C for denaturing and 20 sec at 60°C for annealing and extension. This experiment was performed in duplicate.

2.8. Statistics

Statistical significant was determined by one-way ANOVA post-hoc multiple comparisons using Tukey's test. A *p* value of 0.05 was considered statistically significant.

3. RESULTS

3.1. Osteogenic Potential of Serial Passaged Cells *in Vitro*

Figure 1 shows ALP (**Figure 1(a)**) and Alizarin Red S staining (**Figure 1(b)**) of BMSCs that were cultured with or without osteogenic-induced medium at P1, P2 and P3. P1 cells cultured with osteogenic-induced medium showed strong positive staining for ALP and Alizarin Red S, whereas P3 cells showed faint staining for ALP and no Alizarin Red S staining. ALP staining in P2 cells seems weaker than in P1 cells and the size of mineralized nodule in P2 cells appears smaller than P1 cells. Progressively weaker staining was seen in P1, P2 and P3 cells, indicating that osteogenic potential of serially-passaged BMSCs is lost by P3. P1, P2 and P3 cells cultured without osteogenic-induced medium were negative for ALP and Alizarin Red S staining.

Figure 2 shows ALP activity and calcium deposition, which were standardized to DNA content in each group. The activity of P2 cells cultured in osteogenic-induced medium were significantly lower than that of the positive control, indicating that passaging of cells decreases the osteoblastic phenotype of cultured cells (**Figure 2(a)**). There was a significant difference in calcium deposition between the positive control and P2 cells, indicating loss of mineralization ability with increasing passage (**Figure 2(b)**).

3.2. Bone Ormation of P3-Cell/HA Constructs after Implantation

Figure 3 shows representative histological sections of the harvested HA constructs 4 weeks after implantation. Little bone formation occurred in the pores of the control group (the P3 cell/HA constructs: **Figure 3(a)**) and the small loading group (P3 cell/HA constructs with 3.5 cm dish P3 cell-loading: **Figure 3(b)**). In contrast, abundant bone formation, including with osteoblasts and osteocytes, was observed in the large loading group (P3 cell/HA constructs with 10 cm dish P3 cell-loading: **Figure 3(c)**).

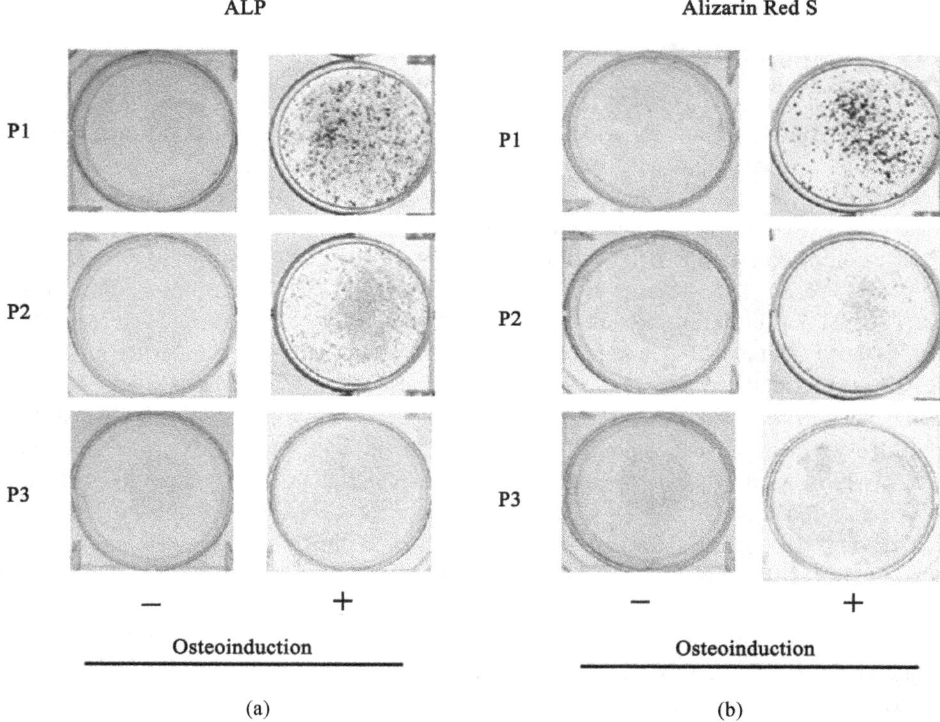

Figure 1. ALP (a) and Alizarin Red S staining (b). P1, P2 and P3 cells were cultured in 6-well plates for 14 days. Positive staining for ALP and Alizarin Red S was observed in P1 cells cultured with osteogenic-induced medium. Progressively weaker staining was seen in P1, P2 and P3 cells cultured with osteogenic-induced medium. By contrast, P1, P2 and P3 cells cultured without osteogenic-induced medium were negative for ALP and Alizarin Red S staining.

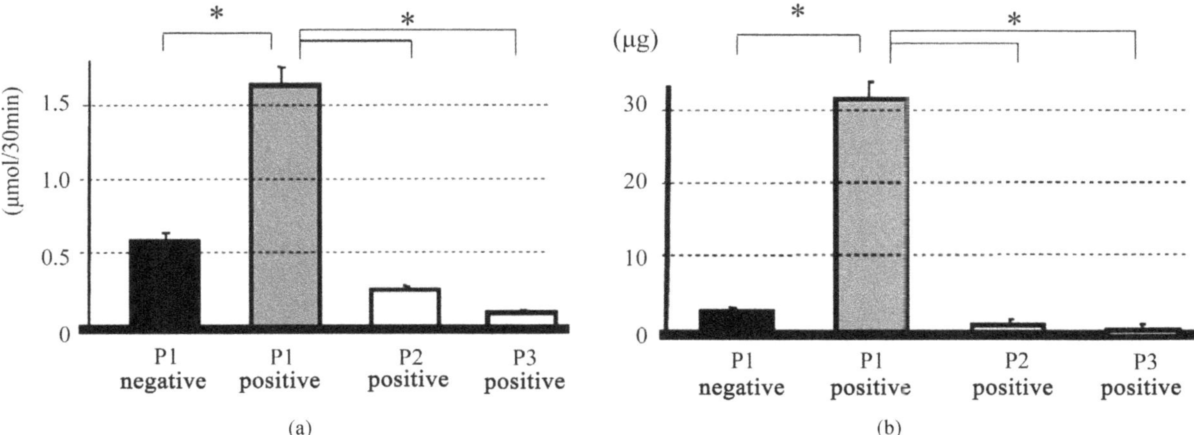

Figure 2. ALP activity (a) and calcium deposition (b), standardized to DNA content. P1 and P2 represent the passage of cells. Positive and negative indicate cells cultured with or without osteogenic-induced medium, respectively. Asterisk indicates $p < 0.05$.

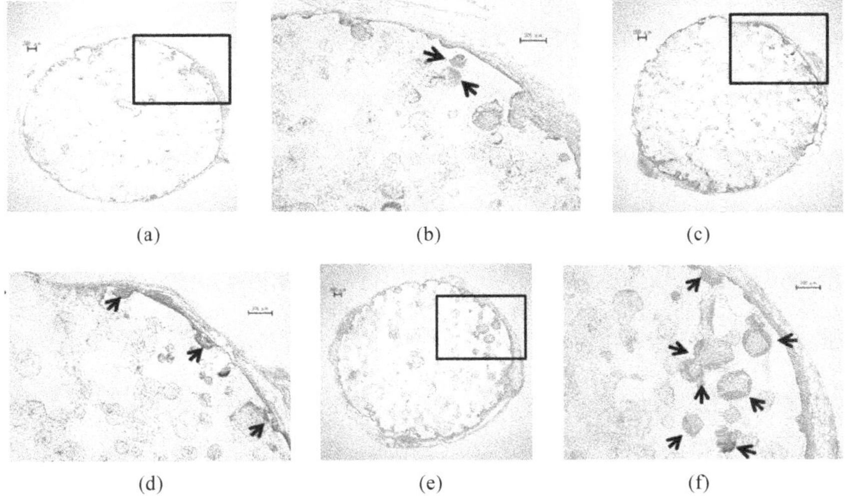

Figure 3. Representative histological sections of the harvested HA constructs 4 weeks after implantation. Little bone formation was observed in the pore of the control group (the P3 cell/HA construct: **Figures 3(a)** and **(b)**) and small cell-loading group (the P3 cell/HA construct with 3.5 cm dish cell-loading: **Figures 3(c)** and **(d)**) In contrast, abundant bone formation together with osteoblasts and osteocytes was seen in large cell-loading group (the P3 cell/HA construct with 10 cm dish cell-loading: **Figures 3(e)** and **(f)**). Arrows indicate bone tissue. Bar = 200 μm.

Figure 4 shows ALP and OC mRNA expression levels evaluated by real-time PCR. The ALP expression in the large loading group was significantly higher than in the control and small loading groups (**Figure 4(a)**). OC expression levels were similar to ALP levels (**Figure 4(b)**).

4. DISCUSSION

The present study shows that serial passaging of BMSCs decreases the osteogenic potential *in vitro*. Consequently, little bone formation was seen in the pore of the construct when P3 cells were combined with HA disk (P3 cell/HA construct) and implanted into a subcutaneous site. However, when additional P3 cells were loaded into the P3 cell/HA construct and implanted, obvious bone formation was seen, indicating that the osteogenic potential of the construct is regained by additional loading of cells cultured in medium with Dex and ascorbic acid. We assume that the additional cell-loading, using the cell sheet culture method with short centrifugation, is more effective at loading cells into the construct than the conventional cell suspension method. Cell suspensions of high cell density can be easily prepared, however, it is difficult to achieve high loading of cells into ceramics. In the present study, we prepared P3 cells using a 3.5 cm

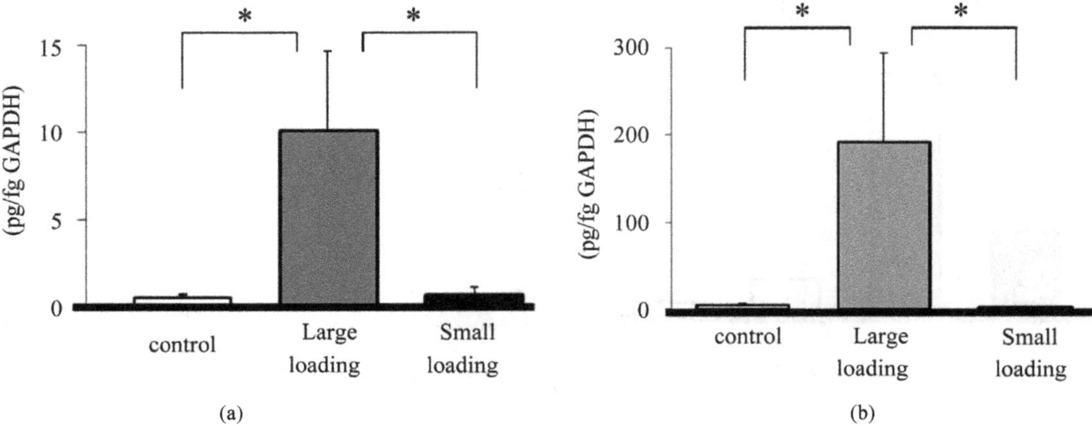

Figure 4. Real-time PCR of ALP and OC mRNA expression. OC expression in the large loading group was significantly higher than those in the control and small loading groups (**Figure 4(a)**). The tendency of ALP expression (**Figure 4(b)**) was similar to OC expression. Control: control group, Large loading: large cell-loading group, Small loading: small cell-loading group. Asterisk indicates $p < 0.05$.

and 10 cm culture dishes. The culture area of 10 cm dish is approximately 5 times larger than the 3.5 cm dish. Consequently, the cell density is also 5 times more in a 10 cm dish. The construct with the 3.5 cm dish P3 cell-loading showed smaller bone formation 4 weeks after implantation compared with the 10 cm dish P3 cell-loading constructs, indicating that the loaded cell number could be an important factor to form bone tissue in the construct combined with serially-passaged cells.

Seeded cells may contain a combination of differentiated and undifferentiated cells after passaging. Differentiated cells have a limited capacity for proliferation [23,24] and as the cells proliferating from the seeded cells are undifferentiated cells, there is a decrease in the percentage of osteogenic cells in the culture [8,25]. Bone marrow cells are a mixed population of cells, including BMSCs, fibroblasts and endothelial cells. After serial passaging, the population of cultured cells changes. Therefore, we assume that percentage of osteogenic cells might decrease during cell culture and result in less ALP activity and mineralization by P2 and P3 passages.

Kumar *et al.* [26] have reported a method for the preparation of cell sheet/HA constructs using a thermosensitive polymer to fabricate the cell sheet. In their report, they showed rapid and complete cellularization to HA by wrapping it with a cell sheet fabricated from a human osteosarcoma cell line. Thus, we think that it is possible to load a lot of cells onto the construct by using the wrapping method with P1 cell sheets. The purpose of the present study was to evaluate the osteogenic potential of serially-passaged cells. We used P3 cells to assess the osteogenic potential of P3 cell/HA constructs. At P3, cell culture with the cell sheet preparation method formed incomplete sheet like fragments. Therefore, we used centrifugation to load the incomplete cell sheet onto the constructs as an additional cell-loading technique. Because little bone formation was seen in the harvested construct with 3.5 cm dish cell-loading, the amount of bone formation could depend on the loading cell number on the HA. The decreased number of osteogenic cells could be compensated by the additional cell-loading from a 10 cm culture dish.

Recently, tissue engineering has been applied clinically [19,20], with some of the technology using cell culture. Bone marrow cells, including BMSCs, can be obtained from patients by needle aspiration and thus the invasiveness is much less compared with harvesting the patient's bone. Therefore, bone marrow cells containing BMSCs are considered a good candidate for tissue-engineered bone. In general, BMSCs need to be expanded by serial passaging to obtain enough cells for their clinical application in tissue engineering. However, the osteogenic potential of cultured BMSCs would be lost after serial passaging. Brugge *et al.* [8] reported that ALP activity and calcium content in cultured cells were not detected at P3 *in vitro*. They also reported that to maintain the osteogenic potential of cells during subcultures requires the addition of Dex to the culture medium as an osteoblastic differentiation factor. However, BMSCs lose their osteogenic potential after several passages even when Dex was added continuously. They concluded that the serial passaging of BMSCs results in the loss of osteogenic potential. A limitation of their report was that it only contained experimental results of an *in vitro* study. Therefore, we decided to examine the osteogenic potential of serially-passaged BMSCs and whether they can differentiate into osteoblasts and subsequently promote bone formation after *in vivo* transplantation. We evaluated the osteogenic potential of P1-P3 cells in this study as lower-passage BMSCs are generally used in clinical applications for tissue-engineered bone reconstruction.

There are a number of limitations of the study that should be acknowledged. First is the use of rat BMSCs in the present study. For the clinical application of this technique, human BMSCs should be used to determine whether our cell-loading method can restore the oseteogenic potential of HA constructs combined with serially-passaged cells. Second, the culture technique for the preparation of cell sheets formed incomplete sheets at P3. Therefore, further improvement of cell sheet preparation for serially-passaged cells is needed. A complete cell sheet created by serial passaging could load large amounts of cells onto the constructs without centrifugation and resulted in increased bone formation. Third, we used only HA in the present study. Other ceramics, such as β-tricalcium phosphate (β-TCP), are also commonly used clinically [27-29]. Therefore, other types of ceramics should be tested to confirm our results.

5. CONCLUSION

The present study indicated that osteogenic potential of BMSCs decreases by serial passaging. However, bone formation could be regained using the additional cell-loading technique. Owing to its usage of serially-passaged cells, this method could be applied in cases of hard tissue reconstruction, which requires the serial passaging of BMSCs to obtain a suitable number of cells. This technique, along with the cell suspension method, can be used to prepare cell-loaded constructs from ceramics, such as HA and β-TCP.

6. ACKNOWLEDGEMENTS

We thank Ms M. Yoshimura and Ms M. Matsumura (Nara Medical University School of Medicine, Japan) for their technical assistance. This study was supported by Takeda Science Foundation.

REFERENCES

[1] Owen, M. (1988) Marrow stromal stem cells. *Journal of Cell Science*, **10**, 63-76.

[2] Ohgushi, H. and Caplan, A.I. (1999) Stem cell technology and bioceramics: From cell to gene engineering. *Journal of Biomedical Materials Research*, **48**, 913-927. doi:10.1002/(SICI)1097-4636(1999)48:6<913::AID-JBM22>3.0.CO;2-0

[3] Ohgushi, H., Yoshikawa, T., Nakajima, H., Tamai, S., Dohi, Y. and Okunaga, K. (1999) Al_2O_3 doped apatite-wollastonite containing glass ceramic provokes osteogenic differentiation of marrow stromal stem cells. *Journal of Biomedical Materials Research*, **44**, 381-388. doi:10.1002/(SICI)1097-4636(19990315)44:4<381::AID-JBM3>3.0.CO;2-E

[4] Sonal, R., Jackson, J.D., Brusnahan, S.K., O'Kane, B. J. and Sharp, J.G. (2012) Characterization of a mesenchymal stem cell line that differentiates to bone and provides niches supporting mouse and human hematopoietic stem cells. *Stem Cell Discovery*, **2**, 5-14. doi:10.4236/scd.2012.21002

[5] Brazelton, T.R., Rossi, F.M., Keshet, G.I. and Blau, H.M. (2000) From marrow to brain: Expression of neuronal phenotypes in adult mice. *Science*, **290**, 1775-1779. doi:10.1126/science.290.5497.1775

[6] Jiang, Y., Jahagirdar, B.N., Reinhardt, R.L., Schwartz, R.E., Keene, C.D., Ortiz-Gonzalez, X.R., Reyes, M., Lenvik, T., Lund, T., Blackstad, M., Du, J., Aldrich, S., Lisberg, A., Low, W.C., Largaespada, D.A. and Verfaillie, C.M. (2002) Pluripotency of mesenchymal stem cells derived from adult marrow. *Nature*, **418**, 41-49. doi:10.1038/nature00870

[7] Krause, D.S. (2002) Plasticity of marrow-derived stem cells. *Gene Therapy*, **9**, 754-758. doi:10.1038/sj.gt.3301760

[8] Ter Brugge, P.J. and Jansen, J.A. (2002) *In vitro* osteogenic differentiation of rat bone marrow cells subcultured with and without dexamethasone. *Tissue Engineering*, **8**, 321-331. doi:10.1089/107632702753725076

[9] Matsushima, A., Kotobuki, N., Tadokoro, M., Kawate, K., Yajima, H., Takakura, Y. and Ohgushi, H. (2009) *In vivo* osteogenic capability of human mesenchymal cells cultured on hydroxyapatite and on beta-tricalcium phosphate. *Artificial Organs*, **33**, 474-481. doi:10.1111/j.1525-1594.2009.00749.x

[10] Akahane, M., Shigematsu, H., Tadokoro, M., Ueha, T., Matsumoto, T., Tohma, Y., Kido, A., Imamura, T. and Tanaka, Y. (2010) Scaffold-free cell sheet injection results in bone formation. *Journal of Tissue Engineering and Regenerative Medicine*, **4**, 404-411. doi:10.1002/term.259

[11] Nakamura, A., Akahane, M., Shigematsu, H., Tadokoro, M., Morita, Y., Ohgushi, H., Dohi, Y., Imamura, T. and Tanaka, Y. (2010) Cell sheet transplantation of cultured mesenchymal stem cells enhances bone formation in a rat nonunion model. *Bone*, **46**, 418-424. doi:10.1016/j.bone.2009.08.048

[12] Nakamura, A., Dohi, Y., Akahane, M., Ohgushi, H., Nakajima, H., Funaoka, H. and Takakura, Y. (2009) Osteocalcin secretion as an early marker of *in vitro* osteogenic differentiation of rat mesenchymal stem cells. *Tissue Engineering Part C: Methods*, **15**, 169-180. doi:10.1089/ten.tec.2007.0334

[13] Akahane, M., Ohgushi, H., Yoshikawa, T., Sempuku, T., Tamai, S., Tabata, S. and Dohi, Y. (1999) Osteogenic phenotype expression of allogeneic rat marrow cells in porous hydroxyapatite ceramics. *Journal of Bone and Mineral Research*, **14**, 561-568. doi:10.1359/jbmr.1999.14.4.561

[14] Bianco, P. and Robey, P.G. (2001) Stem cells in tissue engineering. *Nature*, **414**, 118-121. doi:10.1038/35102181

[15] Dong, J., Kojima, H., Uemura, T., Kikuchi, M., Tateishi, T. and Tanaka, J. (2001) *In vivo* evaluation of a novel porous hydroxyapatite to sustain osteogenesis of transplanted bone marrow-derived osteoblastic cells. *Journal of Biomedical Materials Research*, **57**, 208-216.

doi:10.1002/1097-4636(200111)57:2<208::AID-JBM1160>3.0.CO;2-N

[16] Petite, H., Viateau, V., Bensaid, W., Meunier, A., de Pollak, C., Bourguignon, M., Oudina, K., Sedel, L. and Guillemin, G. (2000) Tissue-engineered bone regeneration. *Nature Biotechnology*, **18**, 959-963. doi:10.1038/79449

[17] Shigematsu, H., Akahane, M., Dohi, Y., Nakamura, A., Ohgushi, H., Imamura, T. and Tanaka, Y. (2010) Osteogenic potential and histological characteristics of mesenchymal stem cell sheet/hydroxyapatite constructs. *The Open Tissue Engineering and Regenerative Medicine Journal*, **2**, 63-70. doi:10.2174/1875043500902010063

[18] Akahane, M., Nakamura, A., Ohgushi, H., Shigematsu, H., Dohi, Y. and Takakura, Y. (2008) Osteogenic matrix sheet-cell transplantation using osteoblastic cell sheet resulted in bone formation without scaffold at an ectopic site. *Journal of Tissue Engineering and Regenerative Medicine*, **2**, 196-201. doi:10.1002/term.81

[19] Wakitani, S., Imoto, K., Yamamoto, T., Saito, M., Murata, N. and Yoneda, M. (2002) Human autologous culture expanded bone marrow mesenchymal cell transplantation for repair of cartilage defects in osteoarthritic knees. *Osteoarthritis and Cartilage*, **10**, 199-206. doi:10.1053/joca.2001.0504

[20] Ohgushi, H., Kotobuki, N., Funaoka, H., Machida, H., Hirose, M., Tanaka, Y. and Takakura, Y. (2005) Tissue engineered ceramic artificial joint—*Ex vivo* osteogenic differentiation of patient mesenchymal cells on total ankle joints for treatment of osteoarthritis. *Biomaterials*, **26**, 4654-4661. doi:10.1016/j.biomaterials.2004.11.055

[21] Kawate, K., Yajima, H., Ohgushi, H., Kotobuki, N., Sugimoto, K., Ohmura, T., Kobata, Y., Shigematsu, K., Kawamura, K., Tamai, K. and Takakura, Y. (2006) Tissue-engineered approach for the treatment of steroid-induced osteonecrosis of the femoral head: Transplantation of autologous mesenchymal stem cells cultured with beta-tricalcium phosphate ceramics and free vascularized fibula. *Artifical Organs*, **30**, 960-962. doi:10.1111/j.1525-1594.2006.00333.x

[22] Akahane, M.T.U., Shimizu, T., Shigematsu, H., Kido, A., Omokawa, S., Kawate, K., Imamura, T. and Y. Tanaka. (2010) Cell Sheet Injection as a technique of osteogenic supply. *International Journal of Stem Cells*, **3**, 138-143.

[23] McCulloch, C.A., Strugurescu, M., Hughes, F., Melcher, A.H. and Aubin, J.E. (1991) Osteogenic progenitor cells in rat bone marrow stromal populations exhibit self-renewal in culture. *Blood*, **77**, 1906-1911.

[24] Aubin, J.E. (1998) Advances in the osteoblast lineage. *Biochemistry and Cell Biology*, **76**, 899-910. doi:10.1139/o99-005

[25] Kadiyala, S., Young, R.G., Thiede, M.A. and Bruder, S.P. (1997) Culture expanded canine mesenchymal stem cells possess osteochondrogenic potential *in vivo* and *in vitro*. *Cell Transplantation*, **6**, 125-134. doi:10.1016/S0963-6897(96)00279-5

[26] Anil, K.P.R., Varma, H.K. and Kumary, T.V. (2005) Rapid and complete cellularization of hydroxyapatite for bone tissue engineering. *Acta Biomaterialia*, **1**, 545-552. doi:10.1016/j.actbio.2005.05.002

[27] Ogose, A., Hotta, T., Hatano, H., Kawashima, H., Tokunaga, K., Endo, N. and Umezu, H. (2002) Histological examination of beta-tricalcium phosphate graft in human femur. *Journal of Biomedical Materials Research*, **63**, 601-604. doi:10.1002/jbm.10380

[28] Yamamoto, T., Onga, T., Marui, T. and Mizuno, K. (2000) Use of hydroxyapatite to fill cavities after excision of benign bone tumours. Clinical results. *Journal of Bone & Joint Surgery*, *British Volume*, **82**, 1117-1120. doi:10.1302/0301-620X.82B8.11194

[29] Schindler, O.S., Cannon, S.R., Briggs, T.W. and Blunn, G.W. (2008) Composite ceramic bone graft substitute in the treatment of locally aggressive benign bone tumours. *Journal of Orthopaedic Surgery* (*Hong Kong*), **16**, 66-74.

13

Human dental pulp stem cells differentiate into neural precursors but not into mature functional neurons

Riikka Aanismaa[1*], Jenna Hautala[1], Annukka Vuorinen[2,3], Susanna Miettinen[2], Susanna Narkilahti[1]

[1]Neuro Group, Institute of Biomedical Technology, University of Tampere, Tampere, Finland;
[*]Corresponding Author: riikka.aanismaa@uta.fi
[2]Adult Stem Cell Group, Institute of Biomedical Technology, University of Tampere, Tampere, Finland
[3]Finnish Student Health Service, Tampere, Finland

ABSTRACT

Large numbers of neuronal cells are needed for regenerative medicine to treat patients suffering from central nervous system diseases and deficits such as Parkinson's disease and spinal cord injury. One suggestion has been the utilization of human dental pulp stem cells (hDPSCs) for production of neuronal cells which would offer a patient-specific cell source for these treatments. Neuronal differentiation of hDPSCs has been described previously. Here, we tested the differentiation of DPSCs into neuronal cells with previously reported protocol and characterized the cells according to their morphology, gene and protein expressions and most importantly according to their spontaneous electrical functionality with microelectrode array platform (MEA). Our results showed that even though hDPSC-derived neural progenitor stage cells could be produced, these cells did not mature further into functional neuronal cells. Thus, utilization of DPSCs as a cell source for producing grafts to treat neurological deficits requires more efforts before being optimal.

Keywords: Dental Pulp Stem Cell; Neural; Differentiation; Neural Networks

1. INTRODUCTION

Human stem cells have been intensively studied due to the possibility to use them for regenerative purposes for neurological diseases such as Parkinson's disease, spinal cord injury, and stroke [1]. Both human pluripotent stem cells, *i.e.* human embryonic [2] and human induced pluripotent [3,4] stem cells, as well as human fetal stem cells [5] have been shown to improve the functional recovery after the disease manifestations in both experimental animals [6] and clinical experiments [7]. The source of cells, however, should be thoroughly considered and assessed due to possible harmful side effects and tissue rejections. Indeed, the most optimal case would be harvesting the stem cells from patient's own body before culturing and differentiating them further and finally transplanting these cells back to the same patient. Stem cells can be obtained from various sources in the human body such as bone marrow and adipose tissue [8,9]. Further, these stem cells have been successfully used in treating leukaemia [10] or bone deficits [11]. The neural differentiation potential of human mesenchymal stem cells is not, however, extensively and reliably shown [8].

One interesting adult stem cell population is the human dental pulp stem cells (hDPSCs). These cells have been shown to be able to differentiate along several pathways, including mesenchymal and neural cells [12,13]. Thus, if they could be differentiated into neural cells in large quantities in vitro, they would offer a promising patient-specific cell population for transplantation therapies. So far, neural differentiation of hDPSCs has been reported [14-18]. HDPSC-derived neural cells have been characterized with gene and protein expression analysis but the most important aspect, the spontaneous electrical activity of the produced neural cells, has not been studied. Currently, it is noted that neuronal cells derived from any of the available stem cell sources should be able to form spontaneous action potentials and further spontaneously active functional neuronal networks. Indeed, it has been shown with human embryonic stem cells [19] and human cord blood stem cells [20] and should also be shown with hDPSCs. Patch clamp analysis has been reported from hDPSC-derived neuronal cells showing typical voltage-activated sodium and potassium currents [16,21] but no actual action potentials have been shown. The neuronal activity properties can also be investigated at network level using microelectrode array (MEA) platform [22].

Here, we performed neural differentiation of hDPSCs with previously published method [16] and characterized the cells using qPCR, immunocytochemistry, and MEA setup. Human embryonic stem cell (hESC)-derived neuronal cells were used as a positive control.

2. MATERIALS AND METHODS

2.1. Isolation and Culture of Human Dental Pulp Stem Cells

Normal impact third molars were collected from young adults (n = 4) (21 - 25 years of age) with their informed consent at Finnish Student Health Service, Tampere, Finland. Three of the pulps were from male and one (pulp 1) from a female patient. The donors did not smoke nor had diabetes or asthma. Two pulps (from maxilla and mandible) from one patient were pooled. The pulp tissue was separated from the crown and the root and placed on 2 ml of DMEM/F12 (Gibco Invitrogen, Carlsbad, CA, USA) supplemented with 10% fetal bovine serum (FBS, Invitrogen), 1% antibiotic-antimycotic (Gentaur, Belgium), and 1% GlutaMax (Invitrogen). Tissue was digested with 3 mg/ml collagenase type I and 4 mg/ml dispase for 1 hour at 37°C, centrifuged, and resuspended with medium described above. Cell suspensions were filtered with 100 μm cell strainer and cells were seeded in 6-well plates (Nunc, Thermo Fisher Scientific, Rochester, NY, USA). Subconfluent cultures were passaged using trypsin in phosphate buffered saline (PBS). Cells were transferred to T-25 cell culture flasks when wells were confluent. Cells were cultured 3 - 6 weeks after isolation to increase the number of cells for the experiments.

2.2. Neural Differentiation

Neural differentiation was conducted with protocol published previously [16]. Briefly, dental pulp stem cells (DPSCs) at passage 2 were seeded at 20,000 cells/cm^2 in 10 μg/ml mouse laminin (Sigma-Aldrich, St Louis, MO, USA)-coated 24- and 48-well plates (Nunc) and 20,000 cells/well in 0.1% polyethyleneimine (PEI) and 20 μg/ml mouse laminin-coated 6-well MEA-plates (MultiChannel Systems, Reutlingen, Germany). The used differentiation protocol consisted of three stages. Epigenetic reprogramming was induced for 48 h with DMEM/F12 supplemented with 10 μM 5-azacytidine (Sigma-Aldrich), 2.5% FBS (Invitrogen), and 10 ng/ml bFGF (R&D Systems, Minneapolis, MN, USA) starting 24 h after cell seeding. Next, neural induction was conducted with DMEM/F12 supplemented with 250 μM IBMX, 50 μM forskolin, 200 nM TPA, 1% ITS (all from Sigma-Aldrich), 1 mM dbcAMP, 10 ng/ml bFGF, 10 ng/ml NGF, and 30 ng/ml NT-3 (all from R&D Systems) for 3 days. Cells were washed with PBS before neural maturation with Neurobasal medium (Gibco Invitrogen) supplemented with 1 mM dbcAMP (Sigma-Aldrich), 1% N2, 1% B27 without vitamin A (both from Gibco Invitrogen), and 30 ng/ml NT-3 for 7 days. All solutions were freshly prepared prior to use. Control cells were maintained in control medium (DMEM/F12 supplemented with 2.5% FBS and 1% penicillin/streptomycin) which was changed as differentiation mediums.

2.3. Quantitative RT-PCR

RNA samples from DPSCs was collected at three time points, at time 0 (before cell plating), after 3 days of neural induction, and after 7 days of neural maturation. Similar samples were also collected from control cells. Total RNA was isolated using NucleoSpin® RNA XS kit (Macherey-Nagel, Germany) according to manufacturer's instructions. Next, 50 ng of total RNA per sample was used for cDNA synthesis using random primers (High Capacity cDNA Reverse Transcription Kit, Applied Biosystems) in a reaction volume of 20 μl. Next, quantitative real-time PCR was performed with Taqman® gene expression assays (Applied Biosystems) with 3 μl cDNA according to manufacturer's instructions in a reaction volume of 15 μl for *Musashi* for neural progenitor cells (Hs01045984_m1), *light neurofilament* for neuronal cells (*NF*68, Hs00196245_m1), *glial fibrillary acid protein* for astrocytes (*GFAP*, Hs00909236_m1), *brain lipid-binding protein* for radial glial cells (*BLBP*, Hs00361426_m1), and *Olig*2 for oligodendrocytes (Hs00377820_m1). GAPDH was used as the internal control (4352934E). Quantitative real-time PCR was performed using the following conditions: 50°C for 2 min, 95°C for 10 min, and 40 cycles of 95°C for 15 s and 60°C for 1 min with ABI 7300. All samples were analyzed as technical triplicates (variation required less than 0.5 CT) and no-template control was used. The data was analyzed with a 7300 System SDS Software (Applied Biosystems). Relative quantification was calculated using $2^{-\Delta\Delta CT}$-method [23]. Gained data was normalized to the expression of GAPDH. The data is presented as mean fold change compared to start point.

2.4. Immunocytochemistry

Samples for immunocytochemistry were collected after neural induction and neural maturation stages. Differentiating DPSCs were fixed with 4% PFA in PBS for 20 min in room temperature (RT). Blocking was conducted with 10% normal donkey serum (NDS), 0.1% TritonX-100, and 1% bovine serum albumin (BSA) in

PBS for 45 min at RT. Cells were washed once with 1% NDS, 0.1% TritonX-100, and 1% BSA in PBS and incubated with primary antibodies diluted to the same solution at 4˚C overnight. Antibodies used were mouse anti-nestin (1:100, Chemicon, Temecula, CA, USA) for neural progenitor cells, mouse anti-β-tubulin$_3$ (1:1200, Sigma-Aldrich) and rabbit anti-microtubule associated protein 2 (MAP-2, 1:600, Chemicon) for neuronal cells, sheep anti-GFAP (1:600, R&D Systems) for astrocytes, and mouse anti-GalC (1:200, Chemicon) for oligodendrocytes. All solutions for GalC stainings were made without TritonX-100. After washing three times with 1% BSA in PBS cells were incubated for 1 hour with Alexa Fluor-488 and/or -568 conjugated with anti-mouse, anti-rabbit, and anti-sheep antibodies (1:400, Molecular Probes/ Invitrogen, Carlsbad, CA, USA). After washing with PBS and phosphate buffer the cells were mounted with Vectashield containing DAPI (4',6-diamidino-2-phenylindole) (Vector Laboratories Inc., Burlingame, CA, USA). Stained cells were imaged with a phase contrast microscope with fluorescence optics (Olympus IX51, Olympus, Finland) and Olympus DP30BW camera. Images were edited with Adobe Photoshop CS2.

2.5. Microelectrode Arrays

HDPSCs were also cultured on planar microelectrode array (MEA) 6-well plates (6 × 9 electrode layout, electrode diameter 30 μm, inter-electrode distance 200 μm, MultiChannel Systems, Reutlingen, Germany) during neural differentiation (n = 8 wells/differentiating cells/pulp and n = 4 wells/control cells/pulp) as previously described for hESC-derived neurons [8]. Measurements were performed 1 - 2 times/week. Measurements were performed with MEA 1060-Inv-BC-amplifier with integrated TPC Temperature controller adjusted to +37˚C and data was recorded with MC_Rack software (all from Multichannel systems). Prior to measurements, MEA plates were sealed with PDMS discs in laminar hood to keep the cultures sterile for repeated measurements. After executing the differentiation protocol, the cells were maintained on MEA plates for additional 1 - 2 weeks to prolong the measurement period to 4 weeks.

2.6. Positive Control

As a positive control we used hESC-derived neuronal cells differentiated with previously published protocol [24]. Briefly, the cells were fixed and stained as described above after 8 weeks of differentiation as neurospheres and then 3 days on mouse laminin-coated 24-wells. 8 weeks old neurospheres were also plated on PEI and mouse laminin-coated MEA-plates and measured 1 - 2 times/week for 4 weeks.

3. RESULTS

3.1. Isolation and Culture of hDPSCs

The culture time before actual neural differentiation experiment varied from 3 to 6 weeks depending on the cell number after isolation. Morphology of dental pulp stem cells in general varied from spindle-shaped fibroblasts to flat cells as previously shown [25].

3.2. Morphology of hDPSCs during Neural Differentiation

After seeding the cells mostly resembled fibroblasts. There were no differences in the morphology after the epigenetic reprogramming. The control cells had, however, proliferated notably more efficiently. After initiating the neural induction stage, the morphology of the cells of three hDPSC lines over went a change; the cells became more round-shaped and some processes were developed. During the following three days the morphology changed further. Many processes could be detected in the cell populations as well as branched cells with round soma resembling astrocytes, neuronal cells, or oligodendrocytes. Differences between hDPSC lines could be observed. **Figure 1(a)** represents the induction stages of all 4 hDPSC lines. In induction stage, according to morphology, pulp 2 derived populations resembled mostly neuronal cells. Pulp 4 was clearly different from the others as no clear neuronal morphologies were detected. The neuronal cell morphologies were detected only during neural induction stage. In the neural maturation stage the cell morphology changed again more into fibroblast-like as the number of processes decreased, as represented in **Figure 1(b)** with pulps 1 and 2.

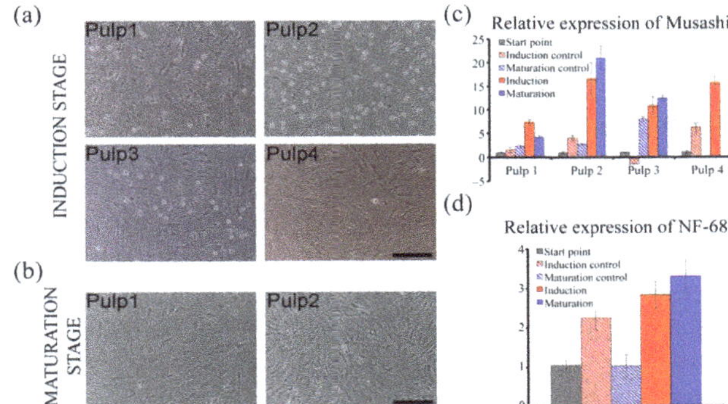

Figure 1. Morphology and gene expression of differentiating DPSC lines. At induction stage: (a) Cells resembling neuronal cells could be detected among pulp 1, 2, and 3 cells but pulp 4 did not seem to be differentiating towards neuronal phenotypes. At maturation stage; (b) The cells of any of the DPSC lines did not seem neuronal whereas more fibroblast-like cells. Increasing *Musashi* expression; (c) Could be detected with all DPSC lines during neural differentiation protocol whereas *NF*-68 expression; (d) Could be detected only with pulp 2 cells. Scale in A and B 100 μm.

3.3. Quantitative RT-PCR

The neural progenitor cell marker Musashi was detectable already in non-differentiated cells and the expression increased with all 4 hDPSC lines during differentiation experiment (**Figure 1(c)**). With three hDPSC lines (pulps 2, 3, and 4) the increment in expression of *Musashi* was at least 10-fold. In line with hDPSC line morphologies during differentiation experiment, the expression of *NF*68 was not detected in any of the DPSC lines expect with pulp 2. In this hDPSC line *NF*68 was expressed already before the differentiation protocol was started and a 3-fold increase in expression could be detected at the maturation stage (**Figure 1(d)**). The expression of *GFAP*, *Olig*2, or *BLBP* was not detected in any of the hDPSC lines at any timepoints.

3.4. Neuronal Cells Were Not Detected with Immunostaining

Variation between hDPSC lines was also detected in protein expression. Neural precursor marker nestin could be detected in cultures after maturation stage with all the studied pulps. Also, control cultures were positive for nestin but the morphology of the cells was different (**Figure 2(a)**). Neuronal marker β-tubulin$_3$ was detected only with pulp 2 after maturation stage but the morphology did not resemble that of neurons (**Figure 2(a)**). MAP-2 staining was negative in all the cultures. Oligodendrocyte marker GalC stained cells after neural induction and maturation stages in pulp 2 as well as in control cultures (**Figure 2(a)**). GFAP-positive astrocytes were not detected among any of the differentiated DPSC lines nor control cultures. As a positive control for immunostaining we used hESC-derived neuronal cells which stained positive for both β-tubulin$_3$ and MAP-2 (**Figure 2(c)**).

3.5. Functional Neuronal Networks Could Not Be Detected

Neuronal network signaling was not detected during 4 weeks follow-up on MEA among hDPSC-derived control or differentiated cultures (**Figure 2(b)**). Neuronal cells derived from hESCs as a positive control formed functional neuronal networks after 2 weeks of culturing on MEA dishes which could be detected as spikes (**Figure 2(c)**).

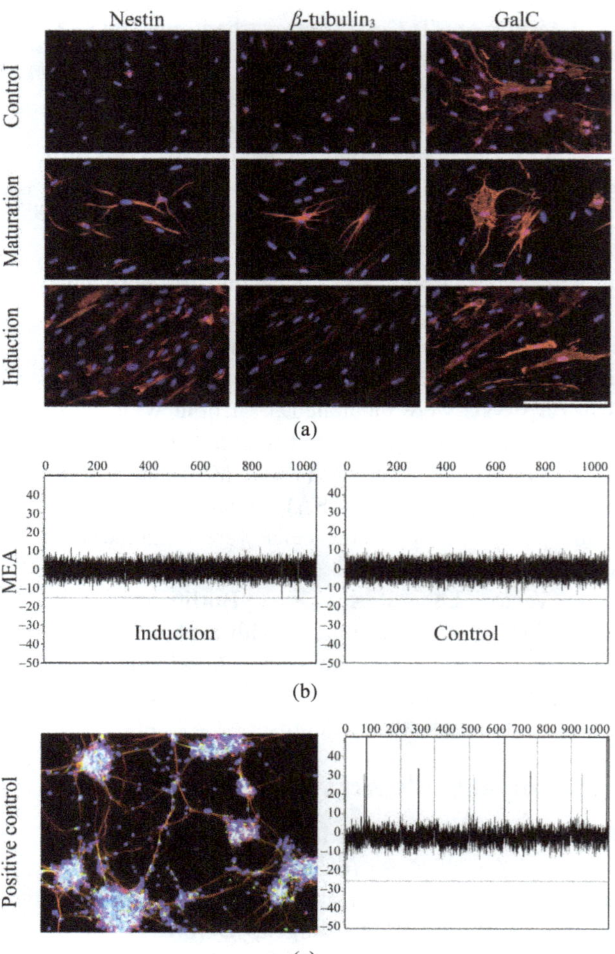

Figure 2. (a) Immunostaining of pulp 2-derived cells during neural differentiation. At neural induction stage no cells stained positive for nestin or β-tubulin$_3$ but some cells stained positive with GalC. At maturation stage some cells stained positive with nestin, β-tubulin$_3$ and GalC. Positive staining could also be detected in control (undifferentiated) cells. Scale 100 µm; (b) No signals could be detected with MEA thus functional neuronal networks were not forming in differentiated or control hDPSCs; (c) HESC-derived neuronal cells were used as a positive control. These cells stained positive with neuronal markers MAP-2 (green) and β-tubulin$_3$ (red) and action potentials could be detected in MEA platform.

4. DISCUSSION

In the present study we differentiated hDPSCs towards neural phenotype with a previously described protocol [16]. We show that, despite of detecting neural gene expression within the differentiating DPSC lines, protein expression of neural or neuronal markers could not reliably be observed and the cells did not form electrically active functional neuronal networks.

The efficient neural differentiation of hDPSCs could be clinically relevant due to opening up possibilities to produce patient-specific cells for treating many neurological deficits. Indeed, some groups have already published the production of neural cells from hDPSCs [14-18,26]. The pulp stem cells hold multipotent nature [27] hence neural differentiation should, in principle, be attainable. The solid production of neuronal cells, however, relies on the cells' electrophysiological properties:

capability of forming spontaneous action potentials and further functional neuronal networks. This aspect remains unanswered in previously published articles.

In this study, the DPSCs did not resemble neural cells morphologically prior to differentiation but neuronal phenotypes could be detected at neural induction phase with 3 hDPSC lines, one (pulp 2) being particularly promising. We could detect increasing expression of *Musashi* in all hDPSC lines during the neural differentiation protocol using quantitative RT-PCR. *Musashi*, however, was also expressed in DPSCs prior to the onset of the differentiation and thus the validity of *Musashi* as a neural precursor marker is somewhat questionable. One major challenge, indeed, is the basal expression of neural genes in undifferentiated hDPSCs. For example, a few of previous studies have shown that expression of another neural progenitor marker *nestin* is negative but the expression of *medium sized neurofilament* is clearly detectable [14,16] while another study discusses expression of *nestin* and *GFAP* in ex vivo-expanded hDPSCs [28]. In contrasts, we could not detect *GFAP* expression at all. Here, *NF*-68 was considered as an important gene to study due to its unequivocal presence in neuronal cells. Indeed, increment in *NF*-68 expression was detected with pulp 2 indicating the presence of neuronal cells. With other pulps, however, expression of this gene was not detected. We studied 4 pulps separately whereas other groups have pooled the pulps collected from several adults [15-18]. To our opinion, the pulp-to-pulp variation should be taken into consideration when collecting cells from human patients.

In immunostaining we could detect nestin positive cells in all pulps after the neural maturation stage which goes hand-in-hand with the *musashi* expression. β-tubulin$_3$ could be detected only with pulp 2 after maturation but the morphology of the positive cells was not typical to neuronal cells. We have been differentiating human pluripotent stem cells to neural lineages routinely [24,29] and are familiar with accurate neural and neuronal morphologies and valid staining with neural, neuronal, and glial markers [24]. To support the lack of neuronal cells we could not detect positive MAP-2 staining with any of the hDPSC lines studied. No GFAP-positive astrocytes were detected either. Interestingly, a few cells from pulp 2 stained positive for oligodendrocytic marker GalC whereas gene expression for *Olig*2 was absent. Whether GalC stains other cell populations in addition to oligodendrocytes remains as an open question as the morphology of the cells was not typical to oligodendrocytes [8,16]. Other published studies do not describe staining with oligodendrocytical markers [14,16,26]. On the other hand, very recent publication shows *in vivo* differentiation of hDPSC to oligodendrocytes after transplantation in to spinal cord lesion [30] which suggests that hDPSCs have potential to differentiate into this particular neural lineage.

None of the differentiated cultures formed spontaneously active neuronal networks. Previous studies have reported the presence of voltage-activated sodium and potassium currents with patch clamp technique [14,16,21] but no evidence of spontaneous action potentials have been shown. Neuron is considered as a neuron by its capability to form action potentials, thus it is the key aspect to show. Further, single action potential forming cells should be able to form electrically active neuronal networks. We used MEA to detect the neuronal network forming properties of differentiating hDPSCs and could not detect any activity within these cultures. Thus, even though neural progenitor gene expression was detected, expression of neuronal proteins and proper neuronal functionality remained undetected. This indicates that neural progenitor stage cells could be produced but they were not maturing further into neuronal cells. The protocol used here has been previously published reporting neuronal cell differentiation from hDPSCs, but the proper functionality was not shown in that study either [16]. Thus, even though Kiraly and co-workers supplemented their maturation medium with B27 containing vitamin-A [16] whereas our B27 supplement did not contain vitamin-A it is highly unlikely that vitamin-A had effects on the end phenotype of the cells. The pulp-to-pulp variation between the patients is another aspect that should be more thoroughly considered when investigating neural differentiation of hDPSCs.

In this study we show that production of functional neuronal cells from dental pulp stem cells is not as straightforward as suggested in previous studies. Even though neural progenitor cells could be produced as indicated by gene expression, their further maturation into functional neuronal cells was unsuccessful. In our study and in previously published articles the amount of detected neuronal cells has not been great and no one has been able to prove the neuronal functionality. For clinical trials the amount of cells needed is millions (ReNeuron www.reneuron.com, StemCells Inc. www.stemcellsinc.com) and thus it seems that for the time-being the most optimal way for large scale production of human neuronal cells remains with the utilization of human pluripotent stem cells.

5. ACKNOWLEDGEMENTS

Use the personnel of IBT Stem cell unit is acknowledged for the support in stem cell research. The study was funded by TEKES Stem-In-Clin project.

REFERENCES

[1] Lindvall, O. and Kokaia, Z. (2010) Stem cells in human

neurodegenerative disorders: Time for clinical translation? *The Journal of Clinical Investigation*, **120**, 29-40. doi:10.1172/JCI40543

[2] Thomson, J.A., Itskovitz-Eldor, J., Shapiro, S.S., Waknitz, M.A., Swiergiel, J.J., Marshall, V.S. and Jones, J.M. (1998) Embryonic stem cell lines derived from human blastocysts. *Science*, **282**, 1145-1147. doi:10.1126/science.282.5391.1145

[3] Takahashi, K., Okita, K., Nakagawa, M. and Yamanaka, S. (2007) Induction of pluripotent stem cells from fibroblast cultures. *Nature Protocols*, **2**, 3081-3089. doi:10.1038/nprot.2007.418

[4] Yu, J., Vodyanik, M.A., Smuga-Otto, K., Antosiewicz-Bourget, J., Frane, J.L., Tian, S., Nie, J., Jonsdottir, G.A., Ruotti, V., Stewart, R., Slukvin, I.I. and Thomson, J.A. (2007) Induced pluripotent stem cell lines derived from human somatic cells. *Science*, **318**, 1917-1920.

[5] Buc-Caron, M.H. (1995) Neuroepithelial progenitor cells explanted from human fetal brain proliferate and differentiate *in vitro*. *Neurobiology of Disease*, **2**, 37-47. doi:10.1006/nbdi.1995.0004

[6] Daadi, M.M., Maag, A.L. and Steinberg, G.K. (2008) Adherent self-renewable human embryonic stem cell-derived neural stem cell line: Functional engraftment in experimental stroke model. *PLoS ONE*, **3**, e1644.

[7] Schwarz, S.C. and Schwarz, J. (2010) Translation of stem cell therapy for neurological diseases. *Translational Research*, **156**, 155-160. doi:10.1016/j.trsl.2010.07.002

[8] Joyce, N., Annett, G., Wirthlin, L., Olson, S., Bauer, G. and Nolta, J.A. (2010) Mesenchymal stem cells for the treatment of neurodegenerative disease. *Regenerative Medicine*, **5**, 933-946. doi:10.2217/rme.10.72

[9] Gimble, J.M., Katz, A.J. and Bunnell, B.A. (2007) Adipose-derived stem cells for regenerative medicine. *Circulation Research*, **100**, 1249-1260. doi:10.1161/01.RES.0000265074.83288.09

[10] Brignier, A.C. and Gewirtz, A.M. (2010) Embryonic and adult stem cell therapy. *The Journal of Allergy and Clinical Immunology*, **125**, S336-S344. doi:10.1016/j.jaci.2009.09.032

[11] Mesimäki, K., Lindroos, B., Törnwall, J., Mauno, J., Lindqvist, C., Kontio, R., Miettinen, S. and Suuronen, R. (2009) Novel maxillary reconstruction with ectopic bone formation by GMP adipose stem cells. *International Journal of Oral and Maxillofacial Surgery*, **38**, 201-209. doi:10.1016/j.ijom.2009.01.001

[12] D'Aquino, R., Graziano, A., Sampaolesi, M., Laino, G., Pirozzi, G., De Rosa, A. and Papaccio, G. (2007) Human postnatal dental pulp cells co-differentiate into osteoblasts and endotheliocytes: A pivotal synergy leading to adult bone tissue formation. *Cell Death and Differentiation*, **14**, 1162-1171. doi:10.1038/sj.cdd.4402121

[13] Nosrat, I.V., Smith, C.A., Mullally, P., Olson, L. and Nosrat, C.A. (2004) Dental pulp cells provide neurotrophic support for dopaminergic neurons and differentiate into neurons *in vitro*; implications for tissue engineering and repair in the nervous system. *European Journal of Neuroscience*, **19**, 2388-2398. doi:10.1111/j.0953-816X.2004.03314.x

[14] Arthur, A., Rychkov, G., Shi, S., Koblar, S.A. and Gronthos, S. (2008) Adult human dental pulp stem cells differentiate toward functionally active neurons under appropriate environmental cues. *Stem Cells*, **26**, 1787-1795. doi:10.1634/stemcells.2007-0979

[15] Ryu, J.S., Ko, K., Lee, J.W., Park, S.B., Byun, S.J., Jeong, E.J., Ko, K. and Choo, Y.K. (2009) Gangliosides are involved in neural differentiation of human dental pulp-derived stem cells. *Biochemical and Biophysical Research Communications*, **387**, 266-271. doi:10.1016/j.bbrc.2009.07.005

[16] Kiraly, M., Porcsalmy, B., Pataki, A., Kadar, K., Jelitai, M., Molnar, B., Hermann, P., Gera, I., Grimm, W.D., Ganss, B., Zsembery, A. and Varga, G. (2009) Simultaneous PKC and cAMP activation induces differentiation of human dental pulp stem cells into functionally active neurons. *Neurochemistry International*, **55**, 323-332. doi:10.1016/j.neuint.2009.03.017

[17] Karaöz, E., Demircan, P.C., Saglam, O., Aksoy, A., Kaymaz, F. and Duruksu, G. (2011) Human dental pulp stem cells demonstrate better neural and epithelial stem cell properties than bone marrow-derived mesenchymal stem cells. *Histochemistry and Cell Biology*, **136**, 455-473. doi:10.1007/s00418-011-0858-3

[18] Nourbakhsh, N., Soleimani, M., Taghipour, Z., Karbalaie, K., Mousavi, S.B., Talebi, A., Nadali, F., Tanhaei, S., Kiyani, G.A., Nematollahi, M., Rabiei, F., Mardani, M., Bahramiyan, H., Torabinejad, M., Nasr-Esfahani, M.H. and Baharvand, H. (2011) Induced *in vitro* differentiation of neural-like cells from human exfoliated deciduous teeth-derived stem cells. *The International Journal of Developmental Biology*, **55**, 189-195. doi:10.1387/ijdb.103090nn

[19] Heikkilä, T.J., Ylä-Outinen, L., Tanskanen, J.M., Lappalainen, R.S., Skottman, H., Suuronen, R., Mikkonen, J.E., Hyttinen, J.A. and Narkilahti, S. (2009) Human embryonic stem cell-derived neuronal cells form spontaneously active neuronal networks *in vitro*. *Experimental Neurology*, **218**, 109-116. doi:10.1016/j.expneurol.2009.04.011

[20] Buzanska, L., Habich, A., Jurga, M., Sypecka, J. and Domanska-Janik, K. (2005) Human cord blood-derived neural stem cell line: Possible implementation in studying neurotoxicity. *Toxicology in Vitro*, **19**, 991-999. doi:10.1016/j.tiv.2005.06.036

[21] Király, M., Kádár, K., Horváthy, D.B., Nardai, P., Rácz, G.Z., Lacza, Z., Varga, G. and Gerber, G. (2011) Integration of neuronally predifferentiated human dental pulp stem cells into rat brain *in vivo*. *Neurochemistry International*, **59**, 371-381. doi:10.1016/j.neuint.2011.01.006

[22] Pine, J. (1980) Recording action potentials from cultured neurons with extracellular microcircuit electrodes. *Journal of Neuroscience Methods*, **2**, 19-31. doi:10.1016/0165-0270(80)90042-4

[23] Livak, K.J. and Schmittgen, T.D. (2001) Analysis of relative gene expression data using real-time quantitative PCR and the $2^{-\Delta\Delta CT}$ method. *Methods*, **4**, 402-408. doi:10.1006/meth.2001.1262

[24] Lappalainen, R.S., Salomaki, M., Yla-Outinen, L., Heikkila, T.J., Hyttinen, J.A., Pihlajamaki, H., Suuronen, R., Skottman, H. and Narkilahti, S. (2010) Similarly derived

and cultured hESC lines show variation in their developmental potential towards neuronal cells in long-term culture. *Regenerative Medicine*, **5**, 749-762. doi:10.2217/rme.10.58

[25] Khanna-Jain, R., Vuorinen, A., Sandor, G.K., Suuronen, R. and Miettinen, S. (2010) Vitamin D_3 metabolites induce osteogenic differentiation in human dental pulp and human dental follicle cells. *The Journal of Steroid Biochemistry and Molecular Biology*, **122**, 133-141. doi:10.1016/j.jsbmb.2010.08.001

[26] Takeyasu, M., Nozaki, T. and Daito, M. (2006) Differentiation of dental pulp stem cells into a neural lineage. *Pediatric Dental Journal*, **16**, 154-162.

[27] Lindroos, B., Maenpaa, K., Ylikomi, T., Oja, H., Suuronen, R. and Miettinen, S. (2008) Characterisation of human dental stem cells and buccal mucosa fibroblasts. *Biochemical and Biophysical Research Communication*, **368**, 329-335. doi:10.1016/j.bbrc.2008.01.081

[28] Nesti, C., Pardini, C., Barachini, S., D'Alessandro, D., Siciliano, G., Murri, L., Petrini, M. and Vaglini, F. (2011) Human dental pulp stem cells protect mouse dopaminergic neurons against MPP^+ or rotenone. *Brain Research*, **1369**, 94-102. doi:10.1016/j.brainres.2010.09.042

[29] Sundberg, M., Skottman, H., Suuronen, R. and Narkilahti, S. (2010) Production and isolation of $NG2^+$ oligodendrocyte precursors from human embryonic stem cells in defined serum-free medium. *Stem Cell Research*, **5**, 91-103. doi:10.1016/j.scr.2010.04.005

[30] Sakai, K., Yamamoto, A., Matsubara, K., Nakamura, S., Naruse, M., Yamagata, M., Sakamoto, K., Tauchi, R., Wakao, N., Imagama, S., Hibi, H., Kadomatsu, K., Ishiguro, N. and Ueda, M. (2012) Human dental pulp-derived stem cells promote locomotor recovery after complete transection of the rat spinal cord by multiple neuro-regenerative mechanisms. *Journal of Clinical Investigation*, **122**, 80-90.

14

Glioblastoma cancer stem cells: Basis for a functional hypothesis

Davide Schiffer[1*], Marta Mellai[1], Laura Annovazzi[1], Angela Piazzi[1,2], Oriana Monzeglio[1], Valentina Caldera[1]

[1]Neuro-Bio-Oncology Center, Policlinico di Monza Foundation (Vercelli)/Consorzio di Neuroscienze, University of Pavia, Pavia Italy; [*]Corresponding Author: davide.schiffer@unito.it
[2]Department of Medical Sciences, University of Piemonte Orientale, Novara, Italy

ABSTRACT

GBM Cancer stem cells (CSCs) are responsible for growth, recurrence and resistance to chemo- and radio-therapy. They are supposed to originate from the transformation of Neural stem cells (NSC) of the Sub-ventricular zone (SVZ) or Sub-granular zone (SGZ) of hippocampus. Alternatively, they can be the expression of a functional status of competence or dedifferentiated cells of the tumor re-acquiring stemness properties. The origin of gliomas has been put in relation with the primitive neuroepithelial cells of the SVZ or NSC or progenitors, as showed by the development of experimental tumors in rats by transplacental ethylnitrosourea administration. The demonstration of CSCs in GBM is based on Neurosphere (NS) and Adherent cell (AC) development in culture. NS share the same genetic alterations with primary tumors and express stemness antigens, whereas AC show differentiation antigens. NS are generated by the most malignant areas of GBM. CSCs are considered at the top of a hierarchy of tumor cells of which the most immature are Nestin^{+}/CD133^{-} cells or established on the basis of EGFR amplification or delta-EGFR. NS in serum conditions differentiate and give origin to AC, the real nature of which is still a matter of discussion. Cells in culture could be simply *in vitro* entities depending on culture methodology. CSCs in GBM could be tumor cells at the end of a dedifferentiation process re-acquiring stemness properties, in an opposite way to what is realized in normal cytogenesis, where stemness is lost progressively with cell differentiation. This interpretation could fit with the origin of the two GBM types, primary and secondary. In primary GBM the tumor originates directly from stem cells or progenitors from SVZ with an accelerated transformation, whereas secondary GBM originates by transformation from astrocytomas arisen through a slow transformation from migrating stem cells and progenitors.

Keywords: Glioblastoma; Stemness; Origin

1. INTRODUCTION

In the last decade a tremendous amount of contributions has been dedicated to the problem of Cancer stem cells (CSCs). In Glioblastoma (GBM) they have been repeatedly demonstrated, interpreted and discussed in relation with the methodology of culture and the starting conceptual viewpoint of the authors. Depending on their attitude as specialists of the field, pathologists/neuro-pathologists, neurobiologists or researchers simply using *in vitro* culture CSCs for resolving neuro-oncological problems, different opinions have been put forward going from CSCs as a special cell type to CSCs as a functional state or a sheer product of the culture. We wanted in this study to discuss the nature of CSCs on the basis of our experience of neuropathologists/neuro-oncologists based on the daily practice with CSCs in the context of diagnosis, genesis and prognosis of gliomas.

2. NERVOUS CYTOGENESIS AND CANCER STEM CELLS

As in other malignancies, in gliomas, Cancer stem cells (CSCs) represent a subset of rare tumor cells capable of self-renewal, tumorigenicity, differentiation and tumor regeneration [1-3] and at the top of a hierarchy of tumor cells [4]. They are supposed to originate from the transformation of Neural stem cells (NSCs), but also from restricted progenitors or more differentiated cells, capable of restoring self-renewal [5-7]. Their source has been identified in the germinal matrices, Sub-ventricular zone (SVZ) or Sub-granular zone (SGZ) of the hippocampus. At variance, they may represent a functional status [8] or dedifferentiated tumor cells which re-acquire stem cell-like properties [2,9,10]. As a matter of fact, gliomas have been produced from dedifferentiated astrocytes [11,12]. Even thought different from the Tumor initiating cells (TICs), identified in the early stages of the tumor, with less mutations and not yet showing the full characteristics of CSCs [13], the two terms are often used inter-changeably [14] also for Glioblastoma multiforme (GBM) [15,16].

CSCs are generally considered as the real target of tumor therapies and from the neuropathologic view point, they are considered in the context of brain function and pathology and under the influence of microenvironments [17].

In the Central nervous system (CNS), NSCs and progenitors occur from the embryo to the adult. Primitive neuroepithelial cells reside in the germinative matrix and give origin to basal progenitors and radial glia, which are found in the telencephalon and generate neurons. In the adult, NSCs are found in the SVZ of the hemispheres, in niches with specific microenvironments [18], composed of A, B and C cells (neuroblasts, quiescent NSCs and transit-amplifying cells, respectively), surrounded by ependymal cells. They are in contact with vessels and send an apical process toward the ventricle, for the stemness maintenance [19]. One of the function of the niche is exactly that to preserve stemness of NSCs [20]. In the mouse, ependymal cells may exist expressing CD133/CD24 and capable of generating neurons, astrocytes and oligodendrocytes [21].

Some cells of GBM show markers of neural progenytors/stem cells, so that its CSCs are considered as deriveing from multipotent NSCs and responsible for growth, recurrence and resistance to therapies, as in other malignnancies. To the first evidence that NSCs of the SVZ are involved in gliomagenesis [22,23], many studies pointed out the glioma origin from aberrant NSCs [2,24-28] and this was confirmed by experiments on animal models [29].

The origin of gliomas from the primitive neuroepithelial cells was demonstrated years ago by the experimenttal production of brain tumors in the rat with nitrosourea derivatives [30]. Ethylnitrosourea (ENU) was administered to the mother rat at the 17th day of gestation and Methylnitrosourea (MNU) to the adult rat [31]. In the first case tumors developed in the offspring migrating from the germinative matrices, proliferating and differentiating. The tumors appeared in the future hemispheres after some cell generations [22,23]. The latency period between the first hit, at the 17th day of gestation, and the first tumor development, was roughly two months and it corresponded in man to the period from i.u. life to the fourth or fifth decade of e.u. life when astrocytomas appear. Tumors by MNU developed from the SVZ or from the SGZ of the hippocampus.

3. THE NATURE OF CSCS AND THE NICHES

GBMs are heterogeneous tumors with undifferentiated and differentiated glia cells and a genetic resemblance with NSCs, beside genetic alterations of the tumor transformation. The demonstration of CSCs in GBM is given by the formation of Neurospheres (NS) in culture media containing growth factors, sharing genetic properties with the primary tumor and antigenic properties with NSCs [32,33]. Adherent cells (AC) develop in serum-containing media which do not show the genetic properties of the tumor and express differentiation antigens [33-35].

The expression by CSCs of the surface glycoprotein CD133, is discussed as representative of stemness and conditioning tumorigenesis [28,36]. The differentiation between + and − cells, based on cell sorting, which is not exempt from impurity problems, is a problem [16]. However, it could be of marginal interest in comparison with other aspects, for example, the Phosphatase and tensin homolog (PTEN) status which correlates with NS growth. $CD133^+$ and $CD133^-$ cells form distinct self-renewing populations, hierarchically organized with $CD133^-$/ $Nestin^+$ as the most immature cells. Cells expressing a range of markers could contribute to the aggressive growth of individual tumors [16]. A CSC hierarchy has been recognized also on the basis of amplified Epidermal growth factor receptor (EGFR) or delta-EGFR [37].

In the SVZ of the mouse, $CD133^+$/$CD24^+$ ependymal cells [21] form a second NSC population composed of and there is a high degree of plasticity in the of exchange between ependymal cells and astrocytes [38]. However, the stage-specific embryonic antigen-1 (SSEA1/CD15) [39] is not expressed in ependymal cells, but it can be positive in ependymoma-derived NS and ependymomas [38]. Among the many regulatory factors of CSCs and NSCs, B lymphoma Mo-MLV insertion region 1 homolog (BMI1) regulates p16 and p19 [40] and is largely expressed in gliomas [41] where it supports invasiveness.

Niches represent a crucial point in the relationship between GBM and its CSCs. To the SVZ [42] and SGZ of hippocampus [43] as niches for NSCs, the white matter could be added as well [44]. Stem cells and quiescent cells are regulated through a balance between proliferation and anti-proliferation signals [45] from which genetic events free cells for tumorigenesis [46]. There is a co-regulation between NSCs and vessels [19,20] and the same happens between microvasculature, cell proliferation and aggressiveness in GBM tumoral niches where stem cells through Vascular endothelial growth factor

(VEGF) support angiogenesis which in turn maintains stem cell survival [47,48], and hypoxia is crucial for both phenomena [49,50]. Proliferating tumor cells are supported by the activation of Hypoxia-inducible factor 1 (HIF-1) which regulates VEGF and platelet-derived growth factor B (PDGF-B) [51,52]. Subsets of Vascular endothelial (VE)-cadherin-positive ($CD144^+$) cells showing CSCs features are capable to start *de novo* vascularisation by differentiating into endothelial cells [53,54].

Stem cells in the adult can be attracted from gliomas [55,56], likely by inflammatory mediators secreted in the damaged CNS from tumor cells, for example, C-X-C chemokine receptor type 4 (CXCR4) [57,58]. Migrating transformed stem cells can be attracted by hypoxia in a neo-niche with its specialized microenvironment [59] or they may contribute to the tumor mass.

Resistance to radio- and chemo-therapy is a feature of CSCs and it is one of the factors responsible for the failure of local control of GBM. Resistance to radio-therapy could be ascribed to the activation of the DNA damage response machinery that increases survival [46]. Inhibition of Checkpoint 1/Checkpoint 2 kinases (Chk1/Chk2) and Poly (ADP-ribose) polymerase 1 (PARP1) make the cells more vulnerable to radiation [60,61]. After irradiation, $CD133^+$ cells accumulate in the irradiated areas [62] through the role played by BMI1 [63].

4. OUR EXPERIENCE ON CSCS AND ON THEIR IDENTIFICATION

In our collection of 21 GBM cell lines, NS developed in growth factor containing media and AC in serum condition in 10 and in 13 cases respectively. NS showed the same genetic alterations and stemness antigens, such as CD133, Musashi.1, Nestin, SOX2 and REST [33] as primary tumors whereas AC expressed differentiation antigens, such as GFAP, Galacto-cerebroside (GalC) and *β*-III Tubulin [33] (**Figure 1**, **Tables 1** and **2**). With the addition of serum to the medium, NS differentiated showing the same antigens as AC. In one case both cell types developed and in another case NS could be obtained from AC by the addition of factors. Our results corresponded, more or less, to previous ones [34,35]: In growth factor containing media NS grew and behaved like NSCs, with clonogenicity and tumorigenicity and with a gene expression profile similar to that of primary tumors; in serum containing media adherent cells developed with no resemblance either to NSCs or primary tumors. They were clearly differentiated.

Microarray studies showed a new categorization of GBM with three subtypes: A Proneural type (PN) with genes of normal brain and neurogenesis and a better prognosis; A Proliferation type (Prolif) with genes of cell proliferation and of poor prognosis and a mesenchymal type (Mes) with genes of angiogenesis activation and poor prognosis [64]. In culture, cell clusters were identified corresponding to the NS and AC showing neurodevelopmental genes and extra-cellular matrix related genes and high and low tumorigenicity, respectively. GBM would be composed by the two phenotypes [34]. Serum cells, even if regaining tumorigenicity in later passages, underwent significant genomic alterations, genetically and biologically different from primary tumors.

NS appear to be the true CSCs and the relevant stem cell property goes lost when they are put in serum conditions; it is restored with the addition of growth factors, but it is very unlikely that they could have preserved the stem cell properties [35]. There are intermediate behaveiours between NS and AC [34]. One wonders, therefore, whether AC are endowed with a partial stemness and what they really are. Monolayer systems of culture, *i.e.* plating NSCs on ornithine, laminin or fibronectin and making them grow flat and adherent with all the features of NS, give different views on CSCs summarized by the sentence "going round or going flat" [65,66]. It would be impossible to compare each other the results of both procedures also taking into account that it is not excluded that NSCs could be nothing else than "physiological players" or *in vitro* entities [67], in line with the repeatedly emphasized concept that culture methodology can influence the expression of CSCs [66,68]. Also in our culture conditions, a hierarchy of CSCs can exist, based not only on molecular features, but also on growth rate, clonogenicity and tumorigenicity, *i.e.* concerning stemness and aggressiveness or differentiation.

Table 1. Stemness and differentiation antigens in glioblastomas and cell lines.

Antigens	Primary tumors	Neurospheres	Adherent cells
CD133	+	++	–
Musashi.1	+	+	–
Nestin	++	++	–
SOX2	++	++	–
GFAP	+/–	–	+
GalC	–	–	+
β-III Tubulin	–	–	+

Table 2. Molecular genetics in glioblastomas and cell lines.

	EGFR amplification	PTEN mutations	TP53 mutations
Primary tumors	+	+	±
Neurospheres	+	+	±
Adherent cells	–	±	–

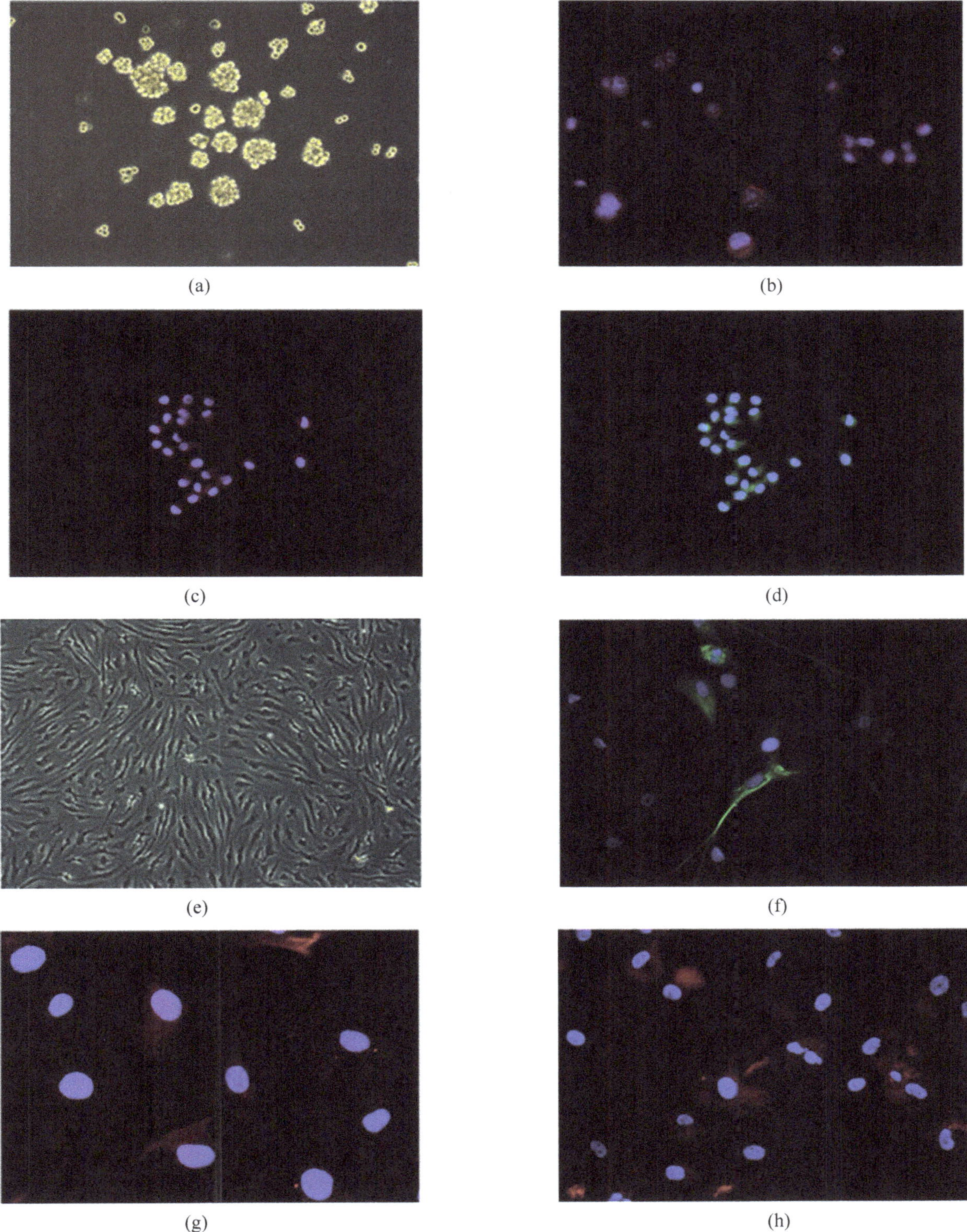

Figure 1. (a) Neurospheres in DMEM/F-12 medium with growth factors (10× magnification); (b) Nestin expression in cytoplasms. Nuclei are counterstained with DAPI (40× magnification); (c) Id. CD133 (20× magnification); (d) Id. Musashi.1 (20× magnification); (e) Adherent cells in DMEM with serum (10× magnification); (f) GFAP expression in cytoplasms. Nuclei are counterstained with DAPI (20× magnification); (g) Id. GalC (20× magnification); (h) Id. β-III Tubulin (20× magnification). Observations were made on a Zeiss Axioskop fluorescence microscope equipped with an AxioCam5MR5c and coupled to an Imaging system (AxioVision Release 4.5, Zeiss).

5. CSCS AND THE TUMOR PHENOTYPE

In our cell line series a correlation was found between NS generation in culture and the phenotype of primary tumors. This was characterized by the highest degree of malignancy with high cell density, high small vessel density, the highest proliferation index and the occurrence of necroses and of perivascular cuffings of tumor cells, expressing much more Nestin than GFAP, and other stemness antigens [33]. It could correspond to the intra-tumoral niches with hypoxic regions where CSCs are promoted or maintained [69-71]. The perivascular location of CSCs is in line with the close relationship among endothelial cells, Nestin and $CD133^+$ cells, with the enhancement of their self-renewal by endothelial cells and the support of CSCs to the vasculature development [46]. This inter-relation might be read in an dynamic perspective, *i.e.* in a functional way, as if stemness may be transient and reversible and niche-dependent [72].

In general, quantitative differences in stemness properties, clonogenicity, tumorigenicity exist between NS and AC and within each category, corresponding to a kind of hierarchy of CSCs [16,37]. Stemness could be distributed in a spectrum covering all the tumor cells with a *crescendo* from quiescent highly differentiated cells, where it is nil, to those in which it reaches the highest degree of expression. As a matter of fact, either NS or AC grow in culture with different rates [2,33] and the capacity to generate NS in culture conditions is not uniform for the different areas of GBM [24,33,73]. Areas increasingly different from the most malignant phenotype seem to progressively generate less NS or AC until to zero. Immature cells expressing Nestin, likely to be CSCs, have been found lining central necroses inside proliferating areas, where HIF-1 is highly expressed [73]; these sites may roughly correspond to those of the tumor where usually the highly malignant phenotype occurs. Practically, all the cells of a tumor are hierarchically distributed with respect to the capacity to produce NS in culture conditions or AC in serum condition. Obviously this does not resolve the question whether stem cells, at the top of the hierarchy represent a cell type or a functional status [66].

6. SIGNIFICANCE OF THE STEM CELL STATUS AND THE ORIGIN OF GBM

Of course, there are genetic determinants of stem cell identity and in the first row there is BMI1 which is believed to represent an oncogenic addition which distinguishes CSCs from NSCs [74,75]. Other pathways are Notch, Hedgehog, Bone morphogenetic protein (BMP), SRY (sex determining region Y)-box 2 (SOX2), Signal transducer and activator of transcription 3 (STAT3) [76-78] and c-MYC [79]. The regulatory factors can be activated or disactivated in the different contexts. In the conception that CSCs are the product of tumor cell dedifferentiation which follows mutation accumulation in the course of malignant transformation [2,8,9], the re-acquisition of stemness properties by the cells could be linked to the activation of the before mentioned pathways. At this point, the two GBM subtypes must be discussed as for their different origin.

Secondary GBM (sGBM) develops from a previous astrocytoma, whereas primary GBM (pGBM) is a *de novo* tumor. They differ as for the genetic configuration, age, and growth speed [80], but not for location and phenotype; at the most they can differ for the spreading modalities [9]. It is not known how *de novo* tumors arise, whereas it is believed that secondary ones originate through anaplasia, *i.e.* through dedifferentiation of tumor cells which follows mutation accumulation [81]. Generally, it is known that GBMs originate either from NSCs or from astrocytes [11] and this could correspond to the distinction between pGBMs and sGBMs. Obviously, it is likely that the two GBM subtypes must originate *ab initio* from the same CSCs. The development of GBM in the emisphere, far away from the SVZ, could be in contrast with its origin from NSCs of the same region, but his can be got over if we refer to the concept of asymmetric division and of migration of progenitors [82]. A path has been traced from mitotically active precursors to the developed tumors [12], which recognizes in transiently dividing progenitors and in somatic stem cells the elements where mutations accumulate; they express also EGFR, present in normal progenitors of SVZ [83]. These cells are the possible source of pGBMs, whereas for sGBMs it is mandatory to refer to a previous astrocytoma.

The two GBM types differ for the expression of mutated Isocitrate dehydrogenase 1-2 (IDH1-2), occurring in sGBM, anaplastic and diffuse astrocytomas and oligodendrogliomas and not in pGBM [84,85]. The mutual exclusion of IDH mutations with EGFR amplification and its association with 1p-19q co-deletion, TP53 mutations and younger age [86-90] are relevant to the timing of IDH mutations, which must be placed between precursors and progenitors. All this means that sGBM originate from tumor cells which have already reached the site of tumor development and the stage of precursors, whereas pGBM originate from cells which transform by mutation accumulation during migration and before reaching the stage of progenitors; they reach the site of development already possessing the genetic equipment of malignancy and keeping or re-acquiring again, at the same time, the features of stem cells. This is something similar to the concept of "maturation arrest" [91] of cells that accumulate mutations and transform before reaching the full maturity or differentiation.

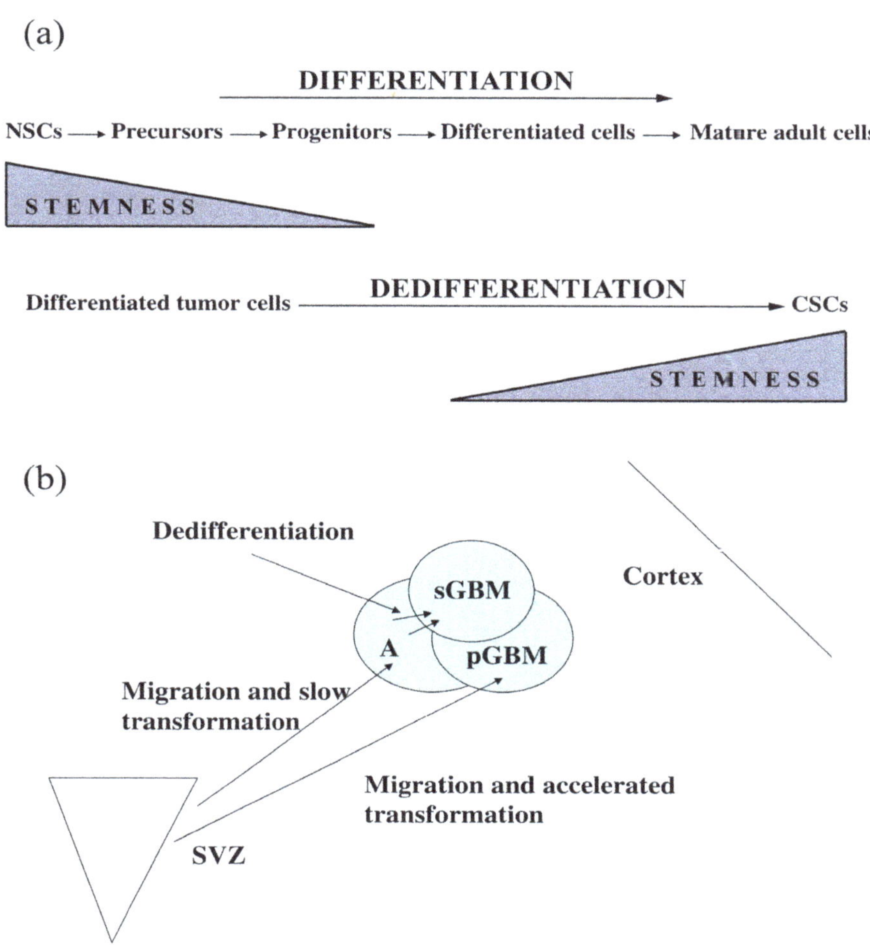

Figure 2. (a) Stemness in differentiation and dedifferentiation; (b) Origin of pGBM and sGBM.

The stemness properties would be acquired in sGBM by dedifferentiation and in pGBM by their preservation (**Figure 2(a)**). The process would be substantially the same, but more rapid and accelerated in pGBM, as already pointed out [17] (**Figure 2(b)**). Stemness would be a condition which is progressively lost during the normal nervous cytogenesis and progressively acquired during dedifferentiation in tumors. In sGBM to obtain NS in culture conditions would be more difficult, because few cells with dedifferentiation reach the stage of stemness, whereas in pGBM it is easier, because most cells already possess it. Stemness would be in this way more a transient status than a fixed feature of a given cell type. The microenvironmental influences are very important in modifying the stemness status, even conceiving GBM in a neo-darwinistic interpretation [17,92].

REFERENCES

[1] Ignatova, T.N., Kukekov, V.G., Laywell, E.D., Suslov, O.N., Vrionis, F.D. and Steindler, D.A. (2002) Human cortical glial tumors contain neural stem-like cells expressing astroglial and neuronal markers *in vitro*. *Glia*, **39**, 193-206. doi:10.1002/glia.10094

[2] Galli, R., Binda, E., Orfanelli, U., Cipelletti, B., Gritti, A., De Vitis, S., Fiocco, R., Foroni, C., Dimeco, F. and Vescovi, A. (2004) Isolation and characterization of tumorigenic, stem-like neural precursors from human glioblastoma. *Cancer Research*, **64**, 7011-7021. doi:10.1158/0008-5472.CAN-04-1364

[3] Yuan, X., Curtin, J., Xiong, Y., Liu, G., Waschsmann-Hogiu, S., Farkas, D.L., Black, K.L. and Yu, J.S. (2004) Isolation of cancer stem cells from adult glioblastoma multiforme. *Oncogene*, **23**, 9392-9400. doi:10.1038/sj.onc.1208311

[4] Visvader, J.E. and Lindeman, G.J. (2008) Cancer stem cells in solid tumours: Accumulating evidence and unresolved questions. *Nature Reviews Cancer*, **8**, 755-768. doi:10.1038/nrc2499

[5] Sanai, N., Alvarez-Buylla, A. and Berger, M.S. (2005) Neural stem cells and the origin of gliomas. *New England Journal of Medicine*, **353**, 811-822. doi:10.1056/NEJMra043666

[6] Liu, Z., Hu, X. Cai, J., Liu, B., Peng, X., Wegner, M. and

Qiu, M. (2007) Induction of oligodendrocyte differentiation by Olig2 and Sox10: Evidence for reciprocal interactions and dosage-dependent mechanisms. *Developmental Biology*, **302**, 683-693. doi:10.1016/j.ydbio.2006.10.007

[7] Stiles, C.D. and Rowitch, D.F. (2008) Glioma stem cells: A midterm exam. *Neuron*, **58**, 832-846. doi:10.1016/j.neuron.2008.05.031

[8] Vescovi, A.L., Galli, R. and Reynolds, B.A. (2006) Brain tumour stem cells. *Nature Reviews Cancer*, **6**, 425-436. doi:10.1038/nrc1889

[9] Uchida, K., Mukai, M., Okano, H. and Kawase, T. (2004) Possible oncogenicity of subventricular zone neural stem cells: Case report. *Neurosurgery*, **55**, 977-978. doi:10.1227/01.NEU.0000137891.99542.43

[10] Schiffer, D., Manazza, A. and Tamagno, I. (2006) Nestin expression in neuroepithelial tumors. *Neuroscience Letters*, **400**, 80-85. doi:10.1016/j.neulet.2006.02.034

[11] Dai, C., Celestino, J.C., Okada, Y., Louis, D.N., Fuller, G.N. and Holland, E.C. (2001) PDGF autocrine stimulation dedifferentiates cultured astrocytes and induces oligodendrogliomas and oligoastrocytomas from neural progenitors and astrocytes *in vivo*. *Genes & Development*, **15**, 1913-1925. doi:10.1016/S1535-6108(02)00046-6

[12] Bachoo, R.M., Maher, E.A., Ligon, K.L., Sharpless, N.E., Chan, S.S., You, M.J., Tang, Y., DeFrances, J., Stover, E., Weissleder, R., Rowitch, D.H., Louis, D.N. and DePinho, R.A. (2002) Epidermal growth factor receptor and Ink4a/Arf: Convergent mechanisms governing terminal differentiation and transformation along the neural stem cell to astrocyte axis. *Cancer Cell*, **1**, 269-277. doi:10.1016/S1535-6108(02)00046-6

[13] Kelly, P.N., Dakic, A., Adams, J.M., Nutt, S.L. and Strasser, A. (2007) Tumor growth need not be driven by rare cancer stem cells. *Science*, **317**, 337. doi:10.1126/science.1142596

[14] Hadjipanayis, C.G. and Van Meir, E.G. (2009) Tumor initiating cells in malignant gliomas: Biology and implications for therapy. *Journal of Molecular Medicine*, **87**, 363-374. doi:10.1007/s00109-009-0440-9

[15] Beier, D., Hau, P., Proescholdt, M., Lohmeier, A., Wischhusen, J., Oefner, P.J., Aigner, L., Brawanski, A. and Bogdahn, U. and Beier, C.P. (2007) CD133(+) and CD133(−) glioblastoma-derived cancer stem cells show differential growth characteristics and molecular profiles. *Cancer Research*, **67**, 4010-4015. doi:10.1158/0008-5472.CAN-06-4180

[16] Chen, R., Nishimura, M.C., Bumbaca, S.M., Kharbanda, S., Forrest, W.F., Kasman, I.M., Greve, J.M., Soriano, R.H., Gilmour, L.L., Rivers, C.S., Modrusan, Z., Nacu, S., Guerrero, S., Edgar, K.A., Wallin, J.J., Lamszus, K., Westphal, M., Heim, S., James, C.D., VandenBerg, S.R., Costello, J.F., Moorefield, S., Cowdrey, C.J., Prados, M. and Phillips, H.S. (2010) A hierarchy of selfrenewing tumor-initiating cell types in glioblastoma. *Cancer Cell*, **17**, 362-375. doi:10.1016/j.ccr.2009.12.049

[17] McLendon, R.E. and Rich, J.N. (2011) Glioblastoma stem cells: A neuropathologist's view. *Journal of Oncology*, **2011**, Article ID: 397195. doi:10.1155/2011/397195

[18] Veeravagu, A., Bababeygy, S.R., Kalani, M.Y., Hou, L.C. and Tse, V. (2008) The cancer stem cell-vascular niche complex in brain tumor formation. *Stem Cells and Development*, **17**, 859-867. doi:10.1089/scd.2008.0047

[19] Mirzadeh, Z., Merkle, F.T., Soriano-Navarro, M., Garcia-Verdugo, J.M. and Alvarez-Buylla, A. (2008) Neural stem cells confer unique pinwheel architecture to the ventricular surface in neurogenic regions of the adult brain. *Cell Stem Cell*, **3**, 265-278. doi:10.1016/j.stem.2008.07.004

[20] Shen, Q., Wang, Y., Kokovay, E., Lin, G., Chuang, S.M., Goderie, S.K., Roysam, B. and Temple, S. (2008) Adult SVZ stem cells lie in a vascular niche: A quantitative analysis of niche cell-cell interactions. *Cell Stem Cell*, **3**, 289-300. doi:10.1016/j.stem.2008.07.026

[21] Coskun, V., Wu, H., Blanchi, B., Tsao, S., Kim, K., Zhao, J., Biancotti, J.C., Hutnick, L., Krueger, R.C. Jr., Fan, G., de Vellis, J. and Sun, Y.E. (2008) $CD133^+$ neural stem cells in the ependyma of mammalian postnatal forebrain. *Proceedings of the National Academy of Sciences of the United States of America*, **105**, 1026-1031. doi:10.1073/pnas.0710000105

[22] Holland, E.C., Celestino, J., Dai, C., Schaefer, L., Sawaya, R.E. and Fuller, G.N. (2000) Combined activation of Ras and Akt in neural progenitors induces glioblastoma formation in mice. *Nature Genetics*, **25**, 55-57. doi:10.1038/75596

[23] Holland, E.C. (2001) Gliomagenesis: Genetic alterations and mouse models. *Nature Reviews Genetics*, **2,** 120-129. doi:10.1038/35052535

[24] Hemmati, H.D., Nakano, I., Lazareff, J.A., Masterman-Smith, M., Geschwind, D.H., Bronner-Fraser, M. and Kornblum, H.I. (2003) Cancerous stem cells can arise from pediatric brain tumors. *Proceedings of the National Academy of Sciences of the United States of America*, **100**, 15178-15183. doi:10.1073/pnas.2036535100

[25] Piccirillo, S.G., Combi, R., Cajola, L., Patrizi, A., Redaelli, S., Bentivegna, A., Baronchelli, S., Maira, G., Pollo, B., Mangiola, A., DiMeco, F., Dalprà, L. and Vescovi, A.L. (2009) Distinct pools of cancer stem-like cells coexist within human glioblastomas and display different tumorigenicity and independent genomic evolution. *Oncogene*, **28**, 1807-1811. doi:10.1038/onc.2009.27

[26] Singh, S.K., Hawkins, C., Clarke, I.D., Squire, J.A., Bayani, J., Hide, T., Henkelman, R.M., Cusimano, M.D. and Dirks, P.B. (2004) Identification of human brain tumour initiating cells. *Nature*, **18432**, 396-401. doi:10.1038/nature03128

[27] Yi, L., Zhou, Z.H., Ping, Y.F., Chen, J.H., Yao, X.H., Feng, H., Lu, J.Y., Wang, J.M. and Bian, X.W. (2007) Isolation and characterization of stem cell-like precursor cells from primary human anaplastic oligoastrocytoma. *Modern Pathology*, **20**, 1061-1068. doi:10.1038/modpathol.3800942

[28] Alcantara Llaguno, S., Chen, J., Kwon, C.H., Jackson, E.L., Li, Y., Burns, D.K., Alvarez-Buylla, A. and Parada, L.F. (2009) Malignant astrocytomas originate from neural stem/progenitor cells in a somatic tumor suppressor mouse model. *Cancer Cell*, **15**, 45-56. doi:10.1016/j.ccr.2008.12.006

[29] Facchino, S., Abdouh, M. and Bernier, G. (2011) Brain

cancer stem cells: Current status on glioblastoma multiforme. *Cancer*, **3**, 1777-1797. doi:10.3390/cancers3021777

[30] Schiffer, D. (1997) Brain tumors. Biology, pathology and clinical references. Springer, Berlin, Heidelberg, New York.

[31] Schiffer, D., Cavalla, P., Dutto, A. and Borsotti, L. (1997) Cell proliferation and invasion in malignant gliomas. *Anticancer Research*, **17**, 61-69.

[32] Schiffer, D., Annovazzi, L., Caldera, V. and Mellai M. (2010) On the origin and growth of gliomas. *Anticancer Research*, **30**, 1977-1998.

[33] Caldera, V., Mellai, M., Annovazzi, L., Piazzi, A., Lanotte, M., Cassoni, P. and Schiffer, D. (2011) Antigenic and genotypic similarity between primary glioblastomas and their derived neurospheres. *Journal of Oncology*, **2011**, Article ID 314962. doi:10.1155/2011/314962

[34] Günther, H.S., Schmidt, N.O., Phillips, H.S., Kemming, D., Kharbanda, S., Soriano, R., Modrusan, Z., Meissner, H., Westphal, M. and Lamszus, K. (2008) Glioblastoma-derived stem cell-enriched cultures form distinct subgroups according to molecular and phenotypic criteria. *Oncogene*, **27**, 2897-2909. doi:10.1038/sj.onc.1210949

[35] Lee, J., Kotliarova, S., Kotliarov, Y., Li, A., Su, Q., Donin, N.M., Pastorino, S., Purow, B.W., Christopher, N., Zhang, W., Park, J.K. and Fine, H.A. (2006) Tumor stem cells derived from glioblastomas cultured in bFGF and EGF more closelymirror the phenotype and genotype of primary tumors than do serum-cultured cell lines. *Cancer Cell*, **9**, 391-403. doi:10.1016/j.ccr.2006.03.030

[36] Campos, B. and Herold-Mende, C.C. (2011) Insight into the complex regulation of CD133 in glioma. *International Journal of Cancer*, **128**, 501-510. doi:10.1002/ijc.25687

[37] Mazzoleni, S., Politi, L.S., Pala, M., Cominelli, M., Franzin, A., Sergi, L., Falini, A., De Palma, M., Bulfone, A., Poliani, P.L. and Galli, R. (2010) Epidermal growth factor receptor expression identifies functionally and molecularly distinct tumor-initiating cells in human glioblastoma multiforme and is required for gliomagenesis. *Cancer Research*, **70**, 7500-7513. doi:10.1158/0008-5472.CAN-10-2353

[38] Nomura, T., Goritz, C., Catchpole, T., Henkemeyer, M. and Frisen, J. (2010) EphB signaling controls lineage plasticity of adult neural stem cell niche cells. *Cell Stem Cell*, **7**, 730-743. doi:10.1016/j.stem.2010.11.009

[39] Son, M.J., Woolard, K., Nam, D.H., Lee, J. and Fine, H.A. (2009) SSEA-1 is an enrichment marker for tumor-initiating cells in human glioblastoma. *Cell Stem Cell*, **4**, 440-452. doi:10.1016/j.stem.2009.03.003

[40] Cui, H., Ma, J., Ding, J., Li, T., Alam, G. and Ding, H.F. (2006) Bmi-1 regulates the differentiation and clonogenic self-renewal of I-type neuroblastoma cells in a concentration-dependent manner. *The Journal of Biological Chemistry*, **281**, 34696-34704. doi:10.1074/jbc.M604009200

[41] Hayry, V., Tynninen, O., Haapasalo, H.K., Wolfer, J., Paulus, W., Hasselblatt, M., Sariola, H., Paetau, A., Sarna, S., Niemela, M., Wartiovaara, K. and Nupponen, N.N. (2008) Stem cell protein BMI-1 is an independent marker for poor prognosis in oligodendroglial tumours. *Neuropathology and Applied Neurobiology*, **34**, 555-563. doi:10.1111/j.1365-2990.2008.00949.x

[42] Sanai, N., Tramontin, A.D., Quiñones-Hinojosa, A., Barbaro, N.M., Gupta, N., Kunwar, S., Lawton, M.T., McDermott, M.W., Parsa, A.T., Manuel-García Verdugo, J., Berger, M.S. and Alvarez-Buylla, A. (2004) Unique astrocyte ribbon in adult human brain contains neural stem cells but lacks chain migration. *Nature*, **427**, 740-744. doi:10.1038/nature02301

[43] Eriksson, P.S., Perfilieva, E., Björk-Eriksson, T., Alborn, A.M., Nordborg, C., Peterson, D.A. and Gage, F.H. (1998) Neurogenesis in the adult human hippocampus. *Nature Medicine*, **4**, 1313-1317. doi:10.1038/3305

[44] Nunes, M.C., Roy, N.S., Keyoung, H.M., Goodman, R.R., McKhann, G. 2nd, Jiang, L., Kang, J., Nedergaard, M. and Goldman, S.A. (2003) Identification and isolation of multipotential neural progenitor cells from the subcortical white matter of the adult human brain. *Nature Medicine*, **9**, 439-447. doi:10.1038/nm837

[45] He, X.C., Zhang, J. and Li, L. (2005) Cellular and molecular regulation of hematopoietic and intestinal stem cell behavior. *Annals of the New York Academy of Sciences*, **1049**, 28-38. doi 10.1196/annals.1334.005

[46] Li, L. and Neaves, W.B. (2006) Normal stem cells and cancer stem cells: The niche matters. *Cancer Research*, **66**, 4553-4557. doi:10.1158/0008-5472.CAN-05-3986

[47] Bao, S., Wu, O., McLendon, R.E., Hao, Y., Shi, Q., Hjelmeland, A.B., Dewhirst, M.W., Bigner, D.D. and Rich J.N. (2006) Glioma stem cells promote radioresistance by preferential activation of the DNA damage response. *Nature*, **444**, 756-760. doi:10.1038/nature05236

[48] Folkins, C., Shaked, Y., Man, S., Tang, T., Lee, C.R., Zhu, Z., Hoffman, R.M. and Kerbel, R.S. (2009) Glioma tumor stem-like cells promote tumor angiogenesis and vasculogenesis via vascular endothelial growth factor and stromal-derived factor 1. *Cancer Research*, **69**, 7243-7251. doi:10.1158/0008-5472.CAN-09-0167

[49] Jensen, R.L., Ragel, B.T., Whang, K. and Gillespie, D. (2006) Inhibition of hypoxia inducible factor-1alpha (HIF-1alpha) decreases vascular endothelial growth factor (VEGF) secretion and tumor growth in malignant gliomas. *Journal of Neuro-Oncology*, **78**, 233-247. doi:10.1007/s11060-005-9103-z

[50] Bar, E.E., Lin, A., Mahairaki, V., Matsui, W. and Eberhart, C.G. (2010) Hypoxia increases the expression of stem-cell markers and promotes clonogenicity in glioblastoma neurospheres. *American Journal of Pathology*, **177**, 1491-1502. doi:10.2353/ajpath.2010.091021

[51] Kourembanas, S., Hannan, R.L. and Faller, D.V. (1990) Oxygen tension regulates the expression of the platelet-derived growth factor-B chain gene in human endothelial cells. *The Journal of Clinical Investigation*, **86**, 670-674. doi:10.1172/JCI114759

[52] Namiki, A., Brogi, E., Kearney, M., Kim, E.A., Wu, T., Couffinhal, T., Varticovski, L. and Isner, J.M. (1995) Hypoxia induces vascular endothelial growth factor in cultured human endothelial cells. *The Journal of Biological Chemistry*, **270**, 31189-31195.

doi:10.1074/jbc.270.52.31189

[53] Wang, R., Chadalavada, K., Wilshire, J., Kowalik, U., Hovinga, K.E., Geber, A., Fligelman, B., Leversha, M., Brennan, C. and Tabar, V. (2010) Glioblastoma stem-like cells give rise to tumour endothelium. *Nature*, **468**, 829-833. doi:10.1038/nature09624

[54] Ricci-Vitiani, L., Pallini, R., Biffoni, M., Todaro, M., Invernici, G., Cenci, T., Maira, G., Parati, E.A., Stassi, G., Larocca, L.M. and De Maria, R. (2010) Tumour vascularization via endothelial differentiation of glioblastoma stem-like cells. *Nature*, **468**, 824-828. doi:10.1038/nature09557

[55] Aboody, K.S., Brown, A., Rainov, N.G., Bower, K.A., Liu, S., Yang, W., Small, J.E., Herrlinger, U., Ourednik, V., Black, P.M., Breakefield, X.O. and Snyder, E.Y. (2000) Neural stem cells display extensive tropism for pathology in adult brain: Evidence from intracranial gliomas. *Proceedings of the National Academy of Sciences of the United States of America*, **97**, 12846-12851. doi:10.1073/pnas.97.23.12846

[56] Glass, R., Synowitz, M., Kronenberg, G., Walzlein, J.H., Markovic, D.S., Wang, L.P., Gast, D., Kiwit, J., Kempermann, G. and Kettenmann, H. (2005) Glioblastoma-induced attraction of endogeneous neural precursor cells is associated with improved survival. *The Journal of Neuroscience*, **25**, 2637-2646. doi:10.1523/JNEUROSCI.5118-04.2005

[57] Ehtesham, M., Yuan, X., Kabos, P., Chung, N.H., Liu, G., Akasaki, Y., Black, K.L. and Yu, J.S. (2004) Glioma tropic neural stem cells consist of astrocytic precursors and their migratory capacity is mediated by CXCR4. *Neoplasia*, **6**, 287-293. doi:10.1593/neo.03427

[58] Oh, M.C. and Lim, D.A. (2009) Novel treatment strategies for malignant gliomas using neural stem cells. *Neurotherapeutics*, **6**, 458-463. doi:10.1016/j.nurt.2009.05.003

[59] Diabira, S. and Morandi, X. (2008) Gliomagenesis and neural stem cells: Key role of hypoxia and concept of tumor "neo-niche". *Medical Hypotheses*, **70**, 96-104. doi:10.1016/j.mehy.2007.04.024

[60] Russo, A.L., Kwon, H.C., Burgan, W.E., Carter, D., Beam, K., Weizheng, X., Zhang, J., Slusher, B.S., Chakravarti, A., Tofilon, P.J. and Camphausen, K. (2009) *In vitro* and *in vivo* radiosensitization of glioblastoma cells by the poly (ADP-ribose) polymerase inhibitor E7016. *Clinical Cancer* Research, **15**, 607-612. doi:10.1158/1078-0432.CCR-08-2079

[61] Chalmers, A.J. (2010) Overcoming resistance of glioblastoma to conventional cytotoxic therapies by the addition of PARP inhibitors. *Anticancer Agents in Medicinal Chemistry*, **10**, 520-533.

[62] Tamura, K., Aoyagi, M., Wakimoto, H., Ando, N., Nariai, T., Yamamoto, M. and Ohno, K. (2010) Accumulation of CD133-positive glioma cells after high-dose irradiation by Gamma Knife surgery plus external beam radiation. *Journal of Neurosurgery*, **113**, 310-318. doi:10.3171/2010.2.JNS091607

[63] Facchino, S., Abdouh, M., Chatoo, W. and Bernier, G. (2010) BMI1 confers radioresistance to normal and cancerous neural stem cells through recruitment of the DNA damage response machinery. *The Journal of Neuroscience*, **30**, 10096-10111. doi:10.1523/JNEUROSCI.1634-10.2010

[64] Phillips, H.S., Kharbanda, S., Chen, R., Forrest, W.F., Soriano, R.H., Wu, T.D., Misra, A., Nigro, J.M., Colman, H., Soroceanu, L., Williams, P.M., Modrusan, Z., Feuerstein, B.G. and Aldape, K. (2006) Molecular subclasses of high-grade glioma predict prognosis, delineate a pattern of disease progression, and resemble stages in neurogenesis. *Cancer Cell*, **9**, 157-173. doi:10.1016/j.ccr.2006.02.019

[65] Pollard, M., Yoshikawa, K., Clarke, I.D., Danovi, D., Stricker, S., Russell, R., Bayani, J., Head, R., Lee, M., Bernstein, M., Squire, J.A., Smith, A. and Dirks, P. (2009) Glioma stem cell lines expanded in adherent culture have tumor-specific phenotypes and are suitable for chemical and genetic screens. *Cell Stem Cell*, **4**, 568-580. doi:10.1016/j.stem.2009.03.014

[66] Reynolds, B.A. and Vescovi, A.L. (2009) Brain cancer stem cells: Think twice before going flat. *Cell Stem Cell*, **5**, 466-467. doi:10.1016/j.stem.2009.10.017

[67] Conti, L. and Cattaneo, E. (2010) Neural stem cell systems: Physiological players or *in vitro* entities? *Nature Reviews Neuroscience*, **11**, 176-187. doi:10.1038/nrn2938

[68] Natsume, A., Kinjo, S., Yuki, K., Kato, T., Ohno, M., Motomura, K., Iwami, K. and Wakabayashi, T. (2011) Glioma-initiating cells and molecular pathology: Implications for therapy. *Brain Tumor Pathology*, **28**, 1-12. doi:10.1007/s10014-010-0011-3

[69] Calabrese, C., Poppleton, H., Kocak, M., Hogg, T.L., Fuller, C., Hamner, B., Oh, E.Y., Gaber, M.W., Finklestein, D., Allen, M., Frank, A., Bayazitov, I.T., Zakharenko, S.S., Gajjar, A., Davidoff, A. and Gilbertson, R.J. (2007) A perivascular niche for brain tumor stem cells. *Cancer Cell*, **11**, 69-82. doi:10.1016/j.ccr.2006.11.020

[70] Kaur, B., Khwaja, F.W., Severson, E.A., Matheny, S.L., Brat, D.J. and Van Meir, E.G. (2005) Hypoxia and the hypoxia-inducible-factor pathway in glioma growth and angiogenesis. *Neuro-Oncology*, **7**, 134-153. doi:10.1215/S1152851704001115

[71] Keith, B. and Simon, M.C. (2007) Hypoxia-inducible factors, stem cells, and cancer. *Cell*, **129**, 465-472. doi:10.1016/j.cell.2007.04.019

[72] Zipori, D. (2004) The nature of stem cells: State rather than entity. *Nature Reviews Genetics*, **5**, 873-878. doi:10.1038/nrg1475

[73] Persano, L., Rampazzo, E., Della Puppa, A., Pistollato, F. and Basso, G. (2011) The three-layer concentric model of glioblastoma: Cancer stem cells, microenvironmental regulation, and therapeutic implications. *Scientific World Journal*, **11**, 1829-1841. doi:10.1100/2011/736480

[74] Felsher, D.W. (2008) Oncogene addiction versus oncogene amnesia: Perhaps more than just a bad habit? *Cancer Research*, **68**, 3081-3086. doi:10.1158/0008-5472.CAN-07-5832

[75] Sharma, S.V. and Settleman, J. (2010) Exploiting the balance between life and death: Targeted cancer therapy and "oncogenic shock". *Biochemical Pharmacology*, **80**,

666-673. doi:10.1016/j.bcp.2010.03.001

[76] Kanamori, M., Kawaguchi, T., Nigro, J.M., Feuerstein, B.G., Berger, M.S., Miele, L. and Pieper, R.O. (2007) Contribution of Notch signaling activation to human glioblastoma multiforme. *Journal of Neurosurgery*, **106**, 417-427. doi:10.3171/jns.2007.106.3.417

[77] Annovazzi, L., Mellai, M., Caldera, V., Valente, G. and Schiffer, D. (2011) SOX2 expression and amplification in gliomas and glioma cell lines. *Cancer Genomics and Proteomics*, **8**, 139-147.

[78] Sherry, M.M., Reeves, A., Wu, J.K. and Cochran, B.H. (2009) STAT3 is required for proliferation and maintenance of multipotency in glioblastoma stem cells. *Stem Cells*, **27**, 2383-2392. doi:10.1002/stem.185

[79] Kim, J., Woo, A.J., Chu, J., Snow, J.W., Fujiwara, Y., Kim, C.G., Cantor, A.B. and Orkin, S.H. (2010) A Myc network accounts for similarities between embryonic stem and cancer cell transcription programs. *Cell*, **143**, 313-324. doi:10.1016/j.cell.2010.09.010

[80] Kleihues, P. and Ohgaki, H. (1999) Primary and secondary glioblastomas: From concept to clinical diagnosis. *Neuro Oncology*, **1**, 44-51.

[81] Louis, D.N., Ohgaki, H., Wiestler, O.D. and Cavenee, W.K. (2007) WHO classification of tumors of the central nervous system, 4th Edition, IARC, Lyon.

[82] Berger, F., Gay, E., Pelletier, L., Tropel, P. and Wion, D. (2004) Development of gliomas: Potential role of asymmetrical cell division of neural stem cells. *The Lancet Oncology*, **5**, 511-514. doi:10.1016/S1470-2045(04)01531-1

[83] Doetsch, F., Petreanu, L., Caille, I., Garcia-Verdugo, J.M. and Alvarez-Buylla, A. (2002) EGF converts transit-amplifying neurogenic precursors in the adult brain into multipotent stem cells. *Neuron*, **36**, 1021-1034. doi:10.1016/S0896-6273(02)01133-9

[84] Balss, J., Meyer, J., Mueller, W., Korshunov, A., Hartmann, C. and von Deimling, A. (2008) Analysis of the IDH1 codon 132 mutation in brain tumors. *Acta Neuropathologica*, **116**, 597-602. doi:10.1007/s00401-008-0455-2

[85] Hartmann, C., Meyer, J., Balss, J., Capper, D., Mueller, W., Christians, A., Felsberg, J., Wolter, M., Mawrin, C., Wick, W., Weller, M., Herold-Mende, C., Unterberg, A., Jeuken, J.W., Wesseling, P., Reifenberger, G. and von Deimling, A. (2009) Type and frequency of IDH1 and IDH2 mutations are related to astrocytic and oligodendroglial differentiation and age: A study of 1010 diffuse gliomas. *Acta Neuropathologica*, **118**, 469-474. doi:10.1007/s00401-009-0561-9

[86] Sanson, M., Marie, Y., Paris, S., Idbaih, A., Laffaire, J., Ducray, F., El Hallani, S., Boisselier, B., Mokhtari, K., Hoang-Xuan, K. and Delattre J.Y. (2009) Isocitrate dehydrogenase 1 codon 132 mutation is an important prognostic biomarker in gliomas. *Journal of Clinical Oncology*, **27**, 4150-4154. doi:10.1200/JCO.2009.21.9832

[87] Yan, H., Parsons, D.W., Jin, G., McLendon, R., Rasheed, B.A., Yuan, W., Kos, I., Batinic-Haberle, I., Jones, S., Riggins, G.J., Friedman, H., Friedman, A., Reardon, D., Herndon, J., Kinzler, K.W., Velculescu, V.E., Vogelstein, B. and Bigner, D.D. (2009) IDH1 and IDH2 mutations in gliomas. *The New England Journal of Medicine*, **360**, 765-773. doi:10.1056/NEJMoa0808710

[88] Van den Bent, M.J., Dubbink, H.J., Marie, Y., Brandes, A.A., Taphoorn, M.J., Wesseling, P., Frenay, M., Tijssen, C.C., Lacombe, D., Idbaih, A., van Marion, R., Kros, J.M., Dinjens, W.N., Gorlia, T. and Sanson, M. (2010) IDH1 and IDH2 mutations are prognostic but not predicttive for outcome in anaplastic oligodendroglial tumors: A report of the European Organization for Research and Treatment of Cancer Brain Tumor Group. *Clinical Cancer Research*, **16**, 1597-1604. doi:10.1158/1078-0432.CCR-09-2902

[89] Labussiere, M., Sanson, M., Idbaih, A. and Delattre, J.Y. (2010) IDH1 gene mutations: A new paradigm in glioma prognosis and therapy? *Oncologist*, **15**, 196-199. doi:10.1634/theoncologist.2009-0218

[90] Mellai, M., Piazzi, A., Caldera, V., Monzeglio, O., Cassoni, P., Valente, G. and Schiffer, D. (2011) IDH1 and IDH2 mutations, immunohistochemistry and associations in a series of brain tumors. *Journal of Neuro-Oncology*, **105**, 345-357. doi:10.1007/s11060-011-0596-3

[91] Cairncross, J.G. (1987) The biology of astrocytoma: Lessons learned from chronic myelogenous leukemia: Hypothesis. *Journal of Neuro-Oncology*, **5**, 99-104. doi:10.1007/BF02571297

[92] Vineis, P. (2006) Misuse of genetic data in environmental epidemiology. *Annals of the New York Academy of Sciences*, **1076**, 163-167. doi:10.1196/annals.1371.060

15

Enrichment of CD9$^+$ spermatogonial stem cells from goat (*Capra aegagrus hircus*) testis using magnetic microbeads

Gautam Kaul[1,2*], Shashi Kumar[1], Sunita Kumari[1]

[1]Biochemistry Department, National Dairy Research Institute, Karnal, India; [*]Corresponding Author: gkndri@gmail.com
[2]King Edward Memorial Hospital, University of Western Australia, Perth, Australia

ABSTRACT

The well documented source for adult multipotent stem cells is spermatogonial stem cells (SSCs) of mammalian testis. It is foundation of spermatogenesis in the testis throughout adult life by balancing self-renewal and differentiation. SSCs isolation from mammalian testis is difficult because of their scarcity and the lack of well characterized cell surface markers. Thus, the isolation of SSCs is of great interest for exploration of spermatogonial physiology and therapeutic approaches for fertility preservation. CD9 is a surface marker expressed in mouse and rat male germline stem cells. In this study, CD9 positive SSCs were successfully isolated from the goat testis using enzymatic digestion followed by three step purification: Differential plating, percoll discontinuous density gradient followed by magnetic activated cell sorting (MACS). Percoll discontinuous density gradient showed significant differences in the percentage of CD9$^+$ SSCs across individual fraction. The fraction 36% and 40% gave the highest percentage of CD9$^+$ SSCs *i.e.* 82% ± 1.2% and 9.2% ± 1.3% respectively. Magnetic activated cell sorting of CD9$^+$ cells in the magnetic fraction of goat testes was in the range of 15% - 18% which is upto threefolds. CD9$^+$ SSCs were further recovered with appreciable efficiency after immunomagnetic isolation by using various bead: cells ratio in which 4:1 ratio gave the highest yield of 69.06 × 10^5 with 18% of CD9$^+$ SSCs. Magnetic activated cell sorting using anti-CD9 antibodies provides an efficient and fast approach as compared to conventional approaches such as differential plating and percoll discontinuous density gradient for enrichment strategy for spermatogonial stem cells from goat testes for undertaking research on basic and applied reproductive biology.

Keywords: SSC; MACS; Testis; CD9$^+$

1. INTRODUCTION

A great excitement and expectation in today's biomedical world is the study of stem cells, owning to their ability to exist in an undifferentiated state and transforming into differing tissue types, depending on what the cells ambient are. In recent years, interest in spermatogonial stem cells (SSCs) have grown due to development of new research tools, which allow the isolation and culture of these cells. SSCs originate from the primordial germ cells (PGCs) that have ability to self-renew and differentiate into committed progenitors, thus maintaining spermatogenesis by unipotent stem cell system throughout adult life for sustained male fertility. The SSCs reside in stem cell niches located on the basement membrane of seminiferous tubules and among the basal portions of sertoli cells [1-3]. SSCs are very unique among other adult stem cells because they can transmit the parental genetic information to subsequent generation. The ability to study SSCs biology has been difficult because of their rarity in the testes and very limited availability of unique phenotypic markers. Several surface protein markers are commonly found on stem cells such as ITGA6 (also known as α6-integrin), ITGB1 (also known as β1-integrin) [4] and CD9 [5]. These markers may facilitate interactions between stem cells and their cognate niches [6]. CD9 is a type III membrane protein having four transmembrane domain and involved in many cellular process such as cell adhesion, migration, proliferation and fusion [7-11]. Flow cytometry and immunohistochemical technique revealed the expression of CD9 on mouse and rat testis cells. These cells were selected with the help of anti-CD9 antibody which resulted in an enrichment of spermatogonial stem cells from intact testis cells by 5 to 7 folds [5]. Success of SSC boilogy study depends on successful obtaining of enough amounts of these cells. The availability of isolation and culture technique will undoubtedly pave the way for innovative research into stem cell biology, leading to further breakthrough in the understanding of spermatogonial physiology and development of powerful tools. Recently magnetic micro beads connected with these markers have been used to enrich SSCs, as the method employed is rapid and effective. These techniques can facilitate the harvesting, culture, cryopreservation or transfection of SSC to preserve the male germ potential and to colonize in the testes of recipient [12,13]. These stem cells can provide a lifetime gamete production in the testis of recipient throughout adult life by balancing self-renewal and differentiation. This can be used as an invaluable tool in modifying the male germ line to generate transgenic animals, to restore male fertility for infertile man and for generation of pluripotent stem cells to differentiate into various cell lineages. Therefore, this present study was designed to enrich and sort goat spermatogonial stem cells (SSCs) by immunomagnetic microbeads, as a first step towards the manipulation and their further studies.

2. MATERIALS AND METHODS

2.1. Collection of Goat Spermatogonial Cell

Testis of normal and healthy goat (5 - 8 month) was collected from slaughter house maintained at karnal, Haryana India. Immediately after slaughter, testis was washed in PBS solution supplemented with 100 IU/ml Penicillin and 100 µg/ml streptomycin. Testis was stored in ice cold PBS and transported to the laboratory. The testis was again washed in sterile PBS containing antibiotic and dissection was done aseptically under laminar airflow hood. Spermatogonial cells (Donor cell) were collected from seminiferous tubule of the testis.

2.2. Donor Cell Preparation

Donor spermatogonial cell from goat testis was collected by following the protocol of Honaramooz *et al.*, 2002 with some minor modifications [14]. In brief, the tunica albuginea and visible connective tissue of testis were aseptically removed. The exposed seminiferous tubules were sequentially digested. First digestion was done by incubating tissue at 30°C in 2 mg/ml Collagenase type IV (Sigma chemical Co., USA, #D5758) in Dulbecco's minimum essential medium (DMEM) for 30 min with intermittent agitation. Further tissues were digested with 1 mg/ml Hyaluronidase (Sigma Chemical Co., USA, #D5758) for 20 min at 37°C followed by rinsing tissue two times in Ca^{2+} free Dulbecco's phosphate buffer saline (DPBS). The tissues were further digested with trypsin at the concentration of 2.5 mg/ml in DPBS. Finally the cells were treated with 7 mg/ml DNaseI (Sigma chemical Co., USA, #D5758) followed by addition of 10% fetal bovine serum (FBS) to terminate enzyme digestion. The resulting cell suspension was filtered subsequently through two nylon mesh with pore size 80 µm and 40 µm, sequentially. The filtrate was centrifuged at 500 ×g for 15 min at 16°C. The pellet so obtained was resuspended in small volume of DMEM. Cell viability was assessed using 0.2% trypan blue in DMEM.

2.3. Identification of SSC

In the cell suspension, SSCs were identified on the basis of their morphology in phase-contrast microscopy. SSCs are large cells with typical spherical shape and a large nucleus/cytoplasm ratio.

2.4. Enrichment of Spermatogonial Cell

The enrichment of spermatogonial cell was done to eliminate contaminating somatic cells (myoid and sertoli cells) from cell suspension. Enrichment was done by incubating the above cell suspension in DMEM containing 10% FBS for overnight at 37°C, 5% CO_2 and 85% relative humidity. During the incubation the sertoli cell and myoid cell were attached to the wall of culture plate due to its anchorage dependency. On the other hand the spermatogonial cells remain in suspension which was removed carefully using pipette. The collected cell suspension was washed in DMEM and viability assessment was done.

2.5. Enrichment of Spermatogonial Stem Cell by Discontinuous Density Gradient

The spermatogonial stem cells were enriched from above cell suspension by following the method of van Pelt *et al.*, 1996; Morena *et al.*, 1996 using discontinuous percoll gradient technique [15,16]. In brief, percoll was first sterilized by autoclaving and used for preparation of iso-osmotic percoll suspension. Iso-osmotic percoll was prepared by mixing 0.6% BSA, 45 µg/ml DNase in 82.2% percoll in DMEM. A discontinuous density gradient (28%, 30%, 32%, 36%, 40%, 50% and 65%) of percoll was prepared by diluting iso-osmotic percoll in diluting medium with final densities of 1.0513, 1.054, 1.056, 1.058, 1.061, 1.077 and 1.095 respectively. The gradient was made in 15 ml graduated tube by adding 1 ml each of percoll solution with different density in a sequence that highest density percoll solution comes in bottom and that of lowest in the top of the tube. The cell suspension containing 0.6% BSA, 45 µg DNase in DMEM was layered on the top of the above gradient and centrifuged at 800 ×g for 30 min at 18°C. The cells were found in the interface between the different density percoll solution were collected and marked as fraction 1 - 8 from top to bottom.

2.6. Enrichment of SSC(s) with Magnetic Beads

Spermatogonial stem cells from above fractionated cells were done by using antibody coated magnetic beads [17]. In this method, cluster of differentiation-9 (CD-9) surface protein was used as marker of spermatogonial stem cell [5]. The paramagnetic beads (Calbiochem) were labelled with anti-CD9 antibody (Miltenyi Biotech) using following the protocol of Cristea *et al.*, 2005 [18]. For magnetic sorting of SSC, percoll fractionated cell suspension (1 - 8) was split to two aliquot. One aliquot was mixed with anti-CD9-labelled magnetic bead in a ration of 1:6 bead per target cell and incubated for 1 hr at 38°C. Another aliquot was used as control. The sorting was done by passing this cell suspension in the steel wool column under magnetic field. For this, the steel wool column was washed in PBS. The non-specific binding sites in the steel wool column were blocked by incubating column in 5% BSA in PBS for 60 min. The column was then flushed with ice-cold PBS containing 1% BSA. Loaded cells were applied to the column under magnetic field. The column was then rinsed three times by 500 µl of PBS containing 1% BSA, under magnetic field. $CD9^+$ cells carry magnetic bead remain in the matrix of the column as long as it is maintained in the magnetic field. The $CD9^+$ cells were finally eluted by removing magnetic field and by rinsing column with PBS with 1% BSA, the collected fraction was designate as sorted fraction. Mature spermatozoa was prepared by same way and used as negative control. The entire sorted fraction obtained after magnetic sorting were analysed in phase contrast microscope under 200× magnification. The number of unsorted, sorted and depleted cells was also counted.

2.7. Immunocharacterisation of SSC

For immunocharacterisation, the sorted fraction was centrifuged at 500 ×g for 15 min. The pellet containing cells were immunostained with anti-CD9 antibody conjugated with phycoerythrin for 1 hr at room temperature [19]. After incubation the cells were rinsed first in PBS with 1% BSA, then PBS only and finally PBS with 1% BSA. The slides were then analysed in a fluorescent microscope under blue filter at 400× magnifications.

2.8. Statistical Analysis

The results are presented as means ± SEM and statistical analysis was performed. Differences were considered significant when the P-value was < 0.05.

3. RESULTS

3.1. Cytological Analysis of Spermatogonial Stem Cell

The phase-contrast microscopy was used to identify spermatogonial stem cells in all the fraction on the basis of SSCs morphology. The unsorted fraction consisted of a heterogeneous single-cell fraction. The magnetic fraction (sorted fraction) consisted of relatively homogenous population of cells (**Figure 1**). whereas the depleted fraction was very much similar to that of the unsorted cell fraction.

3.2. Enrichment of SSCs by Differential Plating

Enzymatic digestion of testicular tissue was done with collagenase in combination with trypsin and hyaluronidase. Sequential enzymatic digestion of the decapsulated testis resulted in a single-cell suspension. After filtration of the cell suspension final cell concentration was found in the range of 5 - 8 × 10^6 cells/g testicular tissue and a mean of 85.5 × 10^6 cells were isolated from a single testis. The cell suspension was checked for $CD9^+$ spermatogonial stem cells and found to be 5.8 ± 1.09 percent. Enrichment of cells by differential plating resulted significant ($P < 0.05$) increase in $CD9^+$ cells (6.9 ± 1.2, **Figure 2**). Viability of the cells were observed using trypan blue and found to be 73 ± 5.1 percent.

3.3. Enrichment of Spermatogonial Stem Cell by Percoll Discontinuous Density Gradient

Second phase of enrichment of spermatogonial stem cells was done by using a gradient of percoll ranges from

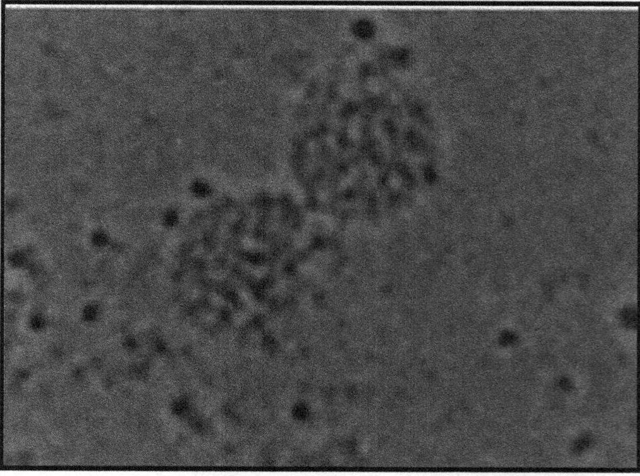

Figure 1. Phase-contrast micrograph showing a homogeneous cell population aggregated with magnetic beads forming large to small clusters in the magnetically sorted faction.

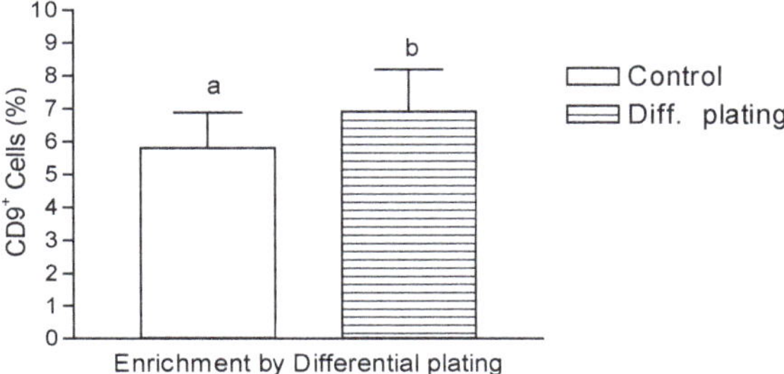

Figure 2. Enrichment of spermatogonia by differential plating method. Number of $CD9^+$ cells slightly enhanced by differenttial plating then the control. Values reported are the mean ± SEM.

28% to 65%. For enrichment gradients were made, cells from differential plating was applied on top and centrifuged. At 28% enrichment of SSC was found to be minimum (0.8 ± 0.22) among all gradient. With increase in percentage of percoll in gradient, the number of $CD9^+$ cells increased significantly upto 36% percoll and decreased gradually upto 65% (**Figure 3**). Enrichment of $CD9^+$ cells were found to be significantly ($P < 0.05$) higher in 36% and 40% percoll compared to other density gradient. Statistically non significant ($P > 0.05$) increase in $CD9^+$ cells were recorded at 40% (9.2 ± 1.30) compared to 36% (8.2 ± 1.2). The results indicate that significant differences in the percentage of $CD9^+$ SSCs population in individual fraction (**Figure 3**). Viability of cells in all the fractions were observed and found to be almost similar (70 ± 3.1).

3.4. Enrichment of Specific Fraction of Percoll Discontinuous Density Gradient by Immunomagnetic Beads

Cell suspension of 36% and 40% fraction were further enriched by immunomagnetic beads tagged with anti-CD9 antibody, showing significantly higher percentage of $CD9^+$ cells in sorted fraction (36%: 17.05 ± 0.5; 40%: 18.2 ± 1.2) compared to unsorted (36%: 8.2 ± 1.2; 40%: 9.2 ± 1.1) and depleted fraction (36%: 4.5 ± 1.02; 40%: 4.4 ± 1.08) in both 36% and 40% percoll gradient. Percentage of $CD9^+$ cells in sorted fraction was statistically non significant ($P > 0.05$) in both 36% and 40% percoll gradient (**Figure 4**). Viability of cells in all the fractions were observed and found to be almost similar (68 ± 5.1).

3.5. Effect of Bead:Cell Ratio on Cell Recovery

Although SSCs represent only 4% of the cells in the testis, these were recovered with appreciable efficiency and purity using a target beads:cell ratio of 4:1 (**Figure 5**). Total number of cells isolated at 4:1 ratio of bead: cells were 69.06 × 10^5 with 18% of $CD9^+$ cells. If a lower number of beads, 2:1, were used, the recovery of the total cell isolated were 41.43 × 10^5 that contain 14% of $CD9^+$ SSCs. When the bead:cell ratio was increased to 6:1, a total of 70.68 × 10^5 cells were isolated but the percentage of $CD9^+$ spermatogonial stem cells recovery was not increased rather its percentage decreased to 8%, as more non target cells were trapped in cell-bead aggregates.

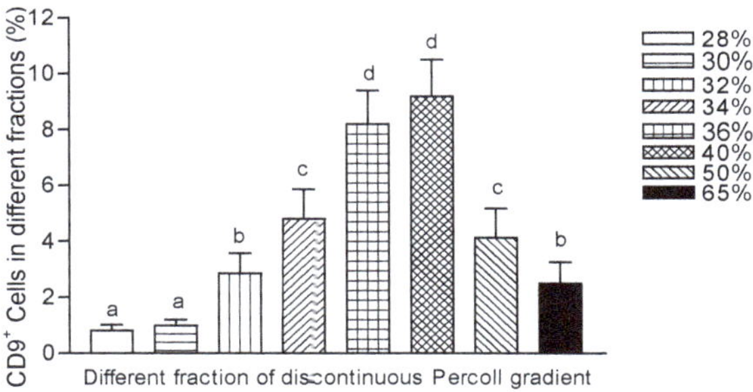

Figure 3. Number of $CD9^+$ cells in different fractions of percoll discontinuous density gradient. The 36% and 40% fraction of the gradient contained the highest percentage of SSCs. Fraction 28% and 30% of the gradient contained the lowest percentage of SSCs. Values reported are the mean ± SEM. Mean showing different letters are significantly different at ($P < 0.05$).

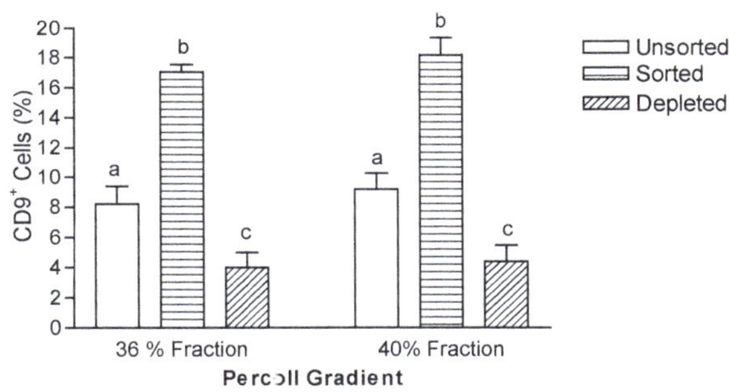

Figure 4. Magnetic sorting of specific fraction of percoll gradient (36% and 40%). Sorted fractions contain more number of $CD9^+$ SSCs in comparison to unsorted fraction. Values are Mean ± SEM of three experiments. Mean showing different letters are significantly different at ($P < 0.05$).

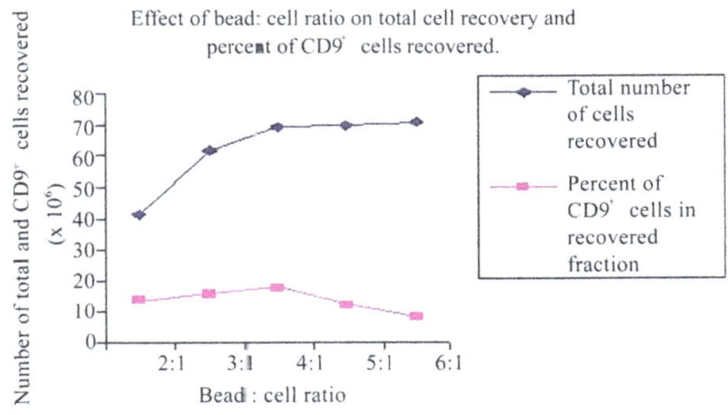

Figure 5. Spermatogonial stem cells were isolated at various bead:cell ratios. The optimal ratio was 4:1 at which the yield of SSCs was highest.

3.6. Immunological Characterization of the Isolated Cell Fractions

The live cells in unsorted, sorted and depleted fractions were characterized using antibody directed against CD9 surface protein by immuno microscopy which revealed that the unsorted fraction contained 5.8% ± 0.66% $CD9^+$ cells. The sorted fraction contained 18.2% ± 1.2% $CD9^+$ cells, indicating three fold enrichment from unsorted fraction (**Figure 6**). The depleted fraction had no significant ($P > 0.05$) depletion of $CD9^+$ cells as compared to the unsorted fraction.

4. DISCUSSION

The isolation of undifferentiated SSCs from mammalian testicular tissue will expand the knowledge of male fertility and aid in developing technologies to enhance reproductive efficiency along with further exploration of SSC characteristics and mechanisms involved in cell fate decisions between self-renewal and differentiation. The conventional techniques that were used in recent years for spermatogonial cell enrichment was either elutriation [20] or velocity sedimentation in a BSA gradient at unit gravity [21,22]. Out of the large population of differentiating germ cells within seminiferous tubules, only a small population of spermatogonia resides at the basement membrane of the adult and fully active seminiferous tubule. The isolation of this small spermatogonial population is technically challenging because of their small number, so magnetic beads are specifically useful for their isolation including stem cells from various tissues [23-25] and organ such as bone marrow, muscle and liver [26-28]. Many molecular markers have been used to identify and study undifferentiated spermatogonia and gonocytes such as promyelocytic leukemia zinc finger protein (PLZF) in rodents, non human primates and pigs [29-32], ubiquitin carboxyl esterase L1 (UCHL1) in the bull [33] and boar [32,34,35], VASA in many species including bulls [36], boars [37], primates [31] & mice [38], CD9 in mouse and rat [5]. The sorting efficiency of intact cells mainly rely on the availability of specific or particular surface markers on the membrane of stem cells. CD9 acts as a surface marker on the spermatogonial stem cells as several literatures reveals its presence [4,5]. Zou *et al.* reported enrichment of female germline stem cells using short-type pituitary gland and brain-cadherin (Stpb-c), CD9 and interferon inducible transmembrane protein 3 (Iftm3, Fragilis) [39]. However, spermatogonial stem cells can be enriched by selection with an antibody against CD9 of these cell surface molecules. Magnetic cell separation has been described as a successful tool for enrichment of SSCs [40,41].

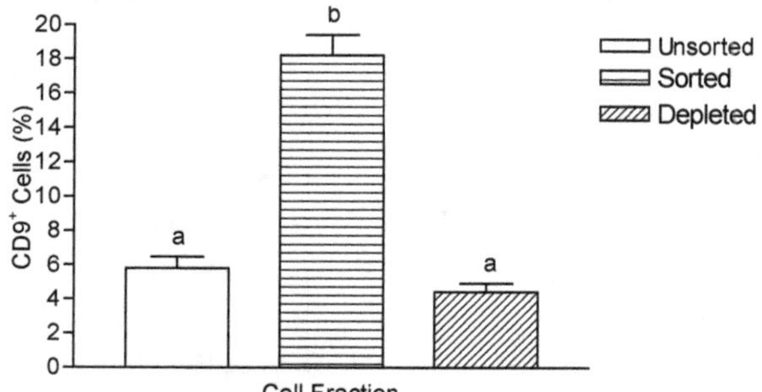

Figure 6. Bar chart of the number of $CD9^+$ cells in the cell fractions obtained after magnetic separation using anti-CD9 antibody conjugated magnetic beads. Cells were isolated from goat testis. The results are shown as mean ± SEM. The unsorted fraction and depleted fraction consisted of low $CD9^+$ cells. The sorted fraction showed high level of $CD9^+$ cells.

In the Present study, we sought to isolate enriched spermatogonial stem cell from goat testis. Our results clearly demonstrated that three step purification viz differential plating, percoll discontinuous density gradient followed by magnetic activated cell sorting (MACS) not only decontaminated mature spermatids, spermatozoa and other somatic cell but also substantially enriched the pool of proliferative SSCs from the enzymatic digested heterogeneous testicular cell population. Spermatogonial stem cells were enriched by conventional method of differential plating leading to 7% purification of $CD9^+$ cells by eliminating the somatic cells (myoid and sertoli cells). This is in correlation with PLZF-positive cells of ovine testis study [42]. Thus, suggesting that efficiency of isolation and/or enrichment of cells appears to depend on the maturity of the testis, as at maturity $CD9^+$ cells seem to be abundant [42]. Further an enrichment of SSCs by using discontinuous percoll gradients were performed and showed maximum enrichment at 36% and 40% fraction which was 8% and 9% respectively. Our result is very much consistent with other enrichment studies such as Polychromatin erythroblasts (PCE) from rat bone marrow [43] and Cardiomyocytes derived from human embryonic stem cells [44] in which percentage of PCE and cardiomyocytes were highest at (1.040/1.058 = 36%) and (40.5%/58.5% and within 58.5%) percoll fraction respectively. The maximum enriched percoll fraction namely 36% and 40% fraction were further enriched by immunomagnetic beads, showing significantly ($P < 0.05$) high SSCs enrichment in sorted fraction as compared to unsorted and depleted fraction. Thus, giving an overall enrichment upto 15% - 18% which is in correlation with other study in which spermatogonial cells were enriched upto 25% - 54% when normal testes from Djungarian hamsters, mice and marmoset monkeys were used [45]. The magnetic separation of these two fractions (36% and 40%) of percoll gradient did not show much more enrichment of $CD9^+$ SSCs in comparison to magnetic separation after enzymatic digestion, which indicates that the efficiency of recovery is independent of the number of SSCs in the starting material but was dependent on the ratio of magnetic beads to SSCs. Hence, SSCs were recovered with appreciable efficiency and purity using a target bead cell ratio of 4:1. If a lower number of beads, 2:1, was used, the recovery decreased significantly. When the bead:cell ratio was increased to 6:1, the $CD9^+$ SSCs recovery was not increased, but more non target cells were trapped in cell-bead aggregates. This is consistent with rat mast cell isolation studies where the optimal bead:cell ratio was 3:1 which gave the highest yield and purity of mast cell [19]. We therefore calculated and characterized the unsorted, sorted and depleted fractions indicating that the $CD9^+$ cells were enriched upto three fold as compared to the presorted fraction and the depleted fraction is widely identical to the unsorted fraction because it contains approximately 98% of all the isolated cells and approximately 90% of the $CD9^+$ cells that were present in the unsorted total cell suspension. This is in correlation with enrichment studies of GFRα1 + spermatogonia from adult primate testes where monkey and human testicular cells enriched GFRα1 + cells were threefold and fivefold respectively [46]. Although the procedure to isolate and to enrich SSCs takes about 5 - 6 hr, the viability of the cells is still high ranging between 65% - 70%. This makes these cells suitable for analysis of mRNA expression and protein synthesis and can also be used for culture, preservation and transplantation.

In this study it has been shown that spermatogonial stem cells were enriched upto 15% - 18% when testes from goats were used. The efficiency of separation is probably determined by the binding affinity of the antibody. Magnetic cell sorting is specifically useful for separation of a few cells from a larger number of unwanted cells in the cell preparation [47-49]. Magnetic cell sorting allows the separation of rare target cells with frequencies down to 1 in 1×10^8. These methodological features render this approach appropriate for the isolation of spermatogonia from mature testes. The availability of isolation and enrichment technique would help in studying underlying molecular mechanisms that regulate germ cell development, mitotic proliferation and differentiation of stem cells, meiosis and their regulation in a vertebrate. Additionally, these tools could provide a novel avenue for genetic modification of the male germline and subsequent generation of transgenic livestock with favourable traits such as disease resistance and production of meat or milk containing components beneficial for human consumption. This method will enable the preparation of enriched spermatogonial suspensions for exploration of physiology, reproductive medicine and therapeutic approaches for fertility preservation.

5. ACKNOWLEDGEMENTS

The authors are grateful to Indian Council of Agricultural Research for providing funds for this piece of work.

REFERENCES

[1] Creemers, L.B., den Ouden, K., van Pelt, A.M.M. and de Rooij, D.G. (2002) Maintenance of adult mouse type A spermatogonia *in vitro*: Influence of serum and growth factors and comparison with prepubertal spermatogonial cell culture. *Reproduction*, **124**, 791-799. doi:10.1530/rep.0.1240791

[2] Creemers, L.B., Meng, X., den Ouden, K., van Pelt, A.M.M., Izadyar, F., Santoro, M., Sariola, H. and de Rooij, D.G. (2002) Transplantation of germ cells from glial cell line-derived neurotrophic factor-overexpressing mice to host testes depleted of endogenous spermatogenesis by fractionated irradiation. *Biology of Reproduction*, **66**, 1579-1584. doi:10.1095/biolreprod66.6.1579

[3] Nagano, M., Ryu, B., Brinster, C.J., Avarbock, M.R. and Brinster, R.L. (2003) Maintenance of mouse male germ line stem cell *in vitro*. *Biology of Reproduction*, **68**, 2207-2214. doi:10.1095/biolreprod.102.014050

[4] Shinohara, T., Avarbock, M.R. and Brinster, R.L. (1999) beta1- and alpha-6-integrin are surface markers on mouse spermatogonial stem cells. *Proceedings of the National Academy of Sciences of the United States of America*, **96**, 5504-5509. doi:10.1073/pnas.96.10.5504

[5] Kanatsu-Shinohara, M., Toyokuni, S. and Shinohara, T. (2004) CD9 is a surface marker on mouse and rat germ line stem cells. *Biology of Reproduction*, **70**, 70-75. doi:10.1095/biolreprod.103.020867

[6] Oka, M., Tagoku, K., Russell, T.L., Nakano, Y., Hamazaki, T., Meyer, E.M., Yokota, T. and Terada, N. (2002) CD9 is associated with leukemia inhibitory factor-mediated maintenance of embryonic stem cells. *Molecular Biology of the Cell*, **13**, 1274-1281. doi:10.1091/mbc.02-01-0600

[7] Ikeyama, S., Koyama, M., Yamaoko, M., Sasada, R. and Miyake, M. (1993) Suppression of cell motility and metastasis by transfection with human motility-related protein (MRP/CD9) DNA. *The Journal of Experimental Medicine*, **177**, 1231-1237. doi:10.1084/jem.177.5.1231

[8] Masellis-Smith, A. and Shaw, A.R. (1994) CD9-regulated adhesion: Anti-CD9 monoclonal antibody induces pre-B cell adhesion to bone marrow fibroblasts through *de novo* recognition of fibronectin. *Journal of Immunology*, **152**, 2768-2777.

[9] Hadjiargyrou, M. and Patterson, P.H. (1995) An anti-CD9 monoclonal antibody promotes adhesion and induces proliferation of Schwann cells *in vitro*. *The Journal of Neuroscience*, **15**, 574-583.

[10] Maecker, H.T., Todd, S.C. and Levy, S. (1997) The tetraspanin superfamily: Molecular facilitators. *Federation of American Societies for Experimental Biology*, **11**, 428-442.

[11] Tachibana, I. and Hemler, M.E. (1999) Role of transmembrane 4 superfamily (TM4SF) proteins CD9 and CD81 in muscle cell fusion and myotube maintenance. *The Journal of Cell Biology*, **146**, 893-904. doi:10.1083/jcb.146.4.893

[12] Avarbock, M., Brinster, C. and Brinster, R. (1996) Re-

constitution of spermatogenesis from frozen spermatogonial stem cells. *Nature Medicine*, **2**, 693-696. doi:10.1038/nm0696-693

[13] Nagano, M. and Brinster, R.L. (1998) Spermatogonial transplantation and reconstitution of donor cell spermatogenesis in recipient mice. *Acta Pathologica Microbiologica et Immunologica Scandinavica*, **106**, 47-57. doi:10.1111/j.1699-0463.1998.tb01318.x

[14] Honaramooz, A., Megee, S. and Dobrinski, I. (2002) Germ cell transplantation in pig. *Biology of Reproduction*, **66**, 21-28. doi:10.1095/biolreprod66.1.21

[15] van Pelt, A., Morena, A., van Dissel-Emiliani, F., Boitani, C., Gaemers, I., de Rooij, D. and Stefanini, M. (1996) Isolation of the synchronized A spermatogonia from adult vitamin A: Deficient rat testes. *Biology of Reproduction*, **55**, 439-444. doi:10.1095/biolreprod55.2.439

[16] Morena, A., Boitani, C., Pesce, M., Felici, M. and Stefanini, M. (1996) Isolation of highly purified type A spermatogonia from prepubertal rat testis. *Journal of Andrology*, **17**, 708-717.

[17] Miltenyi, S., Muller, W., Weichel, W. and Radbruch, A. (1990) High gradient magnetic cell separation with MACS. *Cytometry*, **11**, 231-238. doi:10.1002/cyto.990110203

[18] Cristea, I.M., Williams, R., Chait, B.T. and Rout, M.P. (2005) Fluorescent proteins as proteomic probes. *Molecular and Cellular Proteomics*, **4**, 1933-1941. doi:10.1074/mcp.M500227-MCP200

[19] Jamur, M.C., Grodzki, A.C.G., Moreno, A.N., Swaim, W.D., Siraganian, R.P. and Oliver, C. (1997) Immunomagnetic isolation of rat bone marrow-derived and peritoneal mast cells. *The Journal of Histochemistry and Cytochemistry*, **45**, 1715-1722. doi:10.1177/002215549704501215

[20] Bucci, L.R., Brock, W.A., Johnson, T.S. and Meistrich, M.L. (1986) Isolation and biochemical studies of enriched populations of spermatogonia and early primary spermatocytes from rat testes. *Biology of Reproduction*, **34**, 195-206. doi:10.1095/biolreprod34.1.195

[21] Bellve, A.R., Cavicchia, J.C., Millette, C.F., O'Brien, D.A., Bhatnagar, Y.M. and Dym, M. (1977) Spermatogenic cells of the prepuberal mouse: Isolation and morphological characterization. *The Journal of Cell Biology*, **74**, 68-85. doi:10.1083/jcb.74.1.68

[22] Dym, M., Jia, M., Dirami, G., Price, J.M., Rabin, S.J., Mocchetti, I. and Ravindranath, N. (1995) Expression of c-kit receptor and its autophosphorylation in immature rat type A: Spermatogonia. *Biology of Reproduction*, **52**, 8-19. doi:10.1095/biolreprod52.1.8

[23] Cammareri, P., Lombardo, Y., Francipane, M.G., Bonventre, S., Todaro, M. and Stassi, G. (2008) Isolation and culture of colon cancer stem cells. *Methods in Cell Biology*, **86**, 311-324. doi:10.1016/S0091-679X(08)00014-9

[24] Liu, X.L., Yuan, J.Y., Zhang, J.W., Zhang, X.H. and Wang, R.X. (2007) Differential gene expression in human hematopoietic stem cells specified toward erythroid, megakaryocytic, and granulocytic lineage. *Journal of Leukocyte Biology*, **82**, 986-1002. doi:10.1189/jlb.0107014

[25] Zhang, J., Duan, X., Zhang, H., Deng, Z., Zhou, Z., Wen, N., Smith, A.J., Zhao, W. and Jin, Y. (2006) Isolation of neural crest-derived stem cells from rat embryonic mandibular processes. *Biology of the Cell*, **98**, 567-575. doi:10.1042/BC20060012

[26] Gangopadhyay, N.N., Shen, H., Landreneau, R., Luketich, J.D. and Schuchert, M.J. (2004) Isolation and tracking of a rare lymphoid progenitor cell which facilitates bone marrow transplantation in mice. *Journal of Immunological Methods*, **292**, 73-81. doi:10.1016/j.jim.2004.06.015

[27] Le Grand, F., Auda-Boucher, G., Levitsky, D., Rouaud, T., Fontaine-Perus, J. and Gardahaut, M.F. (2004) Endothelial cells within embryonic skeletal muscles: A potential source of myogenic progenitors. *Experimental Cell Research*, **301**, 232-241. doi:10.1016/j.yexcr.2004.07.028

[28] Qin, A.L., Zhou, X.Q., Zhang, W., Yu, H. and Xie, Q. (2004) Characterization and enrichment of hepatic progenitor cells in adult rat liver. *World Journal of Gastroenterology*, **10**, 1480-1486.

[29] Buaas, F.W., Kirsh, A.L., Sharma, M., McLean, D.J., Morris, J.L., Griswold, M.D., de Rooij, D.G. and Braun, R.E. (2004) PLZF is required in adult male germ cells for stem cell self-renewal. *Nature Genetics*, **36**, 647-652. doi:10.1038/ng1366

[30] Costoya, J.A., Hobbs, R.M., Barna, M., Cattoretti, G., Manova, K., Sukhwani, M., Orwig, K.E., Wolgemuth, D.J. and Pandolfi, P.P. (2004) Essential role of PLZF inmaintenance of spermatogonial stem cells. *Nature Genetics*, **36**, 551-553. doi:10.1038/ng1367

[31] Hermann, B.P., Sukhwani, M., Lin, C.C., Sheng, Y., Tomko, J., Rodriguez, M., Shuttleworth, J.J., McFarland, D., Hobbs, R.M., Pandolfi, P.P., Schatten, G.P. and Orwig, K.E. (2007) Characterization, cryopreservation, and ablation of spermatogonial stem cells in adult rhesus macaques. *Stem Cells*, **25**, 2330-2338. doi:10.1634/stemcells.2007-0143

[32] Luo, J., Megee, S. and Dobrinski, I. (2009) Asymmetric distribution of UCH-L1 in spermatogonia is associated with maintenance and differentiation of spermatogonial stem cells. *Journal of Cellular Physiology*, **220**, 460-468. doi:10.1002/jcp.21789

[33] Herrid, M., Davey, R.J. and Hill, J.R. (2007) Characterization of germ cells from pre-pubertal bull calves in preparation for germ cell transplantation. *Cell and Tissue Research*, **330**, 321-329. doi:10.1007/s00441-007-0445-z

[34] Frankenhuis, M.T., Kramer, M.F. and de Rooij, D.G. (1982) Spermatogenesis in the boar. *The Veterinary Quarterly*, **4**, 57-61. doi:10.1080/01652176.1982.9693840

[35] Luo, J., Megee, S., Rathi, R. and Dobrinski, I. (2006) Protein gene product 9.5 is a spermatogonia-specific marker in the pig testis: Application to enrichment and culture of porcine spermatogonia. *Molecular Reproduction and Development*, **73**, 1531-1540. doi:10.1002/mrd.20529

[36] Bartholomew, R.A. and Parks, J.E. (2007) Identification, localization, and sequencing of fetal bovine vasa homolog. *Animal Reproduction Science*, **101**, 241-251. doi:10.1016/j.anireprosci.2006.09.017

[37] Lee, G.S., Kim, H.S., Lee, S.H., Kang, M.S., Kim, D.Y.,

Lee, C.K., Kang, S.K., Lee, B.C. and Hwang, W.S. (2005) Characterization of pig vasa homolog gene and specific expression in germ cell lineage. *Molecular Reproduction and Development*, **72**, 320-328. doi:10.1002/mrd.20320

[38] Toyooka, Y., Tsuenekawa, N., Takahashi, Y., Matsui, Y., Satoh, M. and Noce, T. (2000) Expression and intercellular localization of mouse vasa-homologue protein during germ cell development. *Mechanisms of Development*, **93**, 139-149. doi:10.1016/S0925-4773(00)00283-5

[39] Zou, K., Hou, L., Sun, K., Xie, W. and Wu, J. (2011) Improved efficiency of female germline stem cell purification using fragilis-based magnetic bead sorting. *Stem Cells and Development*, **20**, 2197-2204.

[40] Hofmann, M.C., Braydich-Stolle, L. and Dym, M. (2005) Isolation of male germ-line stem cells; influence of GDNF. *Developmental Biology*, **279**, 114-124. doi:10.1016/j.ydbio.2004.12.006

[41] Kubota, H., Avarbock, M.R. and Brinster, R.L. (2004) Culture conditions and single growth factors affect fate determination of mouse spermatogonial stem cells. *Biology of Reproduction*, **71**, 722-731. doi:10.1095/biolreprod.104.029207

[42] Borjigin, U., Davey, R., Hutton, K. and Herrid, M. (2010) Expression of promyelocytic leukaemia zinc-finger in ovine testis and its application in evaluating the enrichment efficiency of differential plating. *Reproduction Fertility and Development*, **22**, 733-742. doi:10.1071/RD09237

[43] Asano, H., Deguchi, Y., Kawamura, S. and Inaba, M. (2011) A simple method for enrichment of polychromatic erythroblasts from rat bone marrow, and their proliferation and maturation *in vitro*. *The Journal of Toxicological Sciences*, **435**, 435-444. doi:10.2131/jts.36.435

[44] Xu, C., Police, S., Rao, N. and Carpenter M.K. (2002) Characterization & enrichment of cardiomyocytes derived from human embryonic stem cells. *Circulation Research*, **91**, 501-508. doi:10.1161/01.RES.0000035254.80718.91

[45] von Schonfeldt, V., Krishnamurthy, H., Foppiani, L. and Schlatt, S. (1999) Magnetic cell sorting is a fast & effective method of enriching viable spermatogonia from djungarian hamster, mouse, and marmoset monkey testes. *Biology of Reproduction*, **61**, 582-589. doi:10.1095/biolreprod61.3.582

[46] Gassei, K., Ehmcke, J., Dhir, R. and Schlatt, S. (2010) Magnetic activated cell sorting allows isolation of spermatogonia from adult primate testes and reveals distinct GFRα1-positive subpopulations in men. *Journal of Medical Primatology*, **39**, 83-91. doi:10.1111/j.1600-0684.2009.00397.x

[47] Semple, J.W., Allen, D., Chang, W., Castaldi, P. and Freedman, J. (1993) Rapid separation of $CD4^+$ and $CD19^+$ lymphocyte populations from human peripheral blood by a magnetic activated cell sorter (MACS). *Cytometry*, **14**, 955-960. doi:10.1002/cyto.990140816

[48] Büsch, J., Huber, P., Pflüger, E., Miltenyi, S., Holtz, J. and Radbruch, A. (1994) Enrichment of fetal cells from maternal blood by high gradient magnetic cell sorting (double MACS) for PCR-based genetic analysis. *Prenatal Diagnosis*, **14**, 1129-1140. doi:10.1002/pd.1970141206

[49] Schmitz, B., Radbruch, A., Kümmel, T., Wickenhauser, C., Korb, H., Hansmann, M.L., Thiele, J. and Fischer, R. (1994) Magnetic activated cell sorting (MACS)—A new immunomagnetic method for megakaryocytic cell isolation: Comparison of different separation techniques. *European Journal of Haematology*, **52**, 267-275. doi:10.1111/j.1600-0609.1994.tb00095.x

16

Human adipose tissue-derived stem cells in breast reconstruction following surgery for cancer: A controversial issue

Maria Giovanna Scioli[1], Valerio Cervelli[2], Pietro Gentile[2], Alessandra Bielli[1], Roberto Bellini[1], Augusto Orlandi[1*]

[1]Anatomic Pathology, Department of Biomedicine and Prevention, Tor Vergata University, Rome, Italy;
[*]Corresponding Author: orlandi@uniroma2.it
[2]Plastic Surgery, Department of Biomedicine and Prevention, Tor Vergata University, Rome, Italy

ABSTRACT

Breast cancer is the most common cancer in women. Patients, in particular young women, after surgical removal of the tumor have a poorer quality of life and psychological problems. Plastic surgery procedures for breast reconstruction, including autologous fat grafting, concur to reduce cosmetic and psychological problems. The maintenance of the transplanted fat is partially due to the presence of resident adipose derived-stem cells (ASCs). The latter can be isolated by digestion and centrifugation from the stromal vascular fraction (SVF) of subcutaneous adipose tissue. Intraoperatory SVF/ASC enrichment has been proposed to stabilize and optimalize autologous fat engraftment for breast reconstructive surgery after mastectomy, but the safety of these procedures is still uncertain. Although the literature offers contrasting opinions concerning the effects of ASCs on cancer growth according to the tumor type, at the present time ASC implementation for regenerative medicine therapies should be carefully considered in patients previously treated for breast cancer. At the present, reconstructive therapy utilizing ASC-enriched fat grafting should be postponed until there is no evidence of active disease.

Keywords: Human Adipose-Derived Stem Cells; Breast Cancer; Breast Reconstruction; Fat Grafting

1. INTRODUCTION

Breast cancer is the most common cancer in women. Patients, in particular young women, after surgical removal of the tumor have a poorer quality of life and psychological problems. The use of lumpectomy and adjuvant radiation as surgical approach has contributed to ameliorate cosmetic and functional outcomes. In addition, ameliorated plastic surgery procedures for breast reconstruction, including autologous fat grafting [1], concur to reduce cosmetic and psychological problems. The maintenance of the transplanted fat is partially due to the presence of adipose derived-stem cells (ASCs). The latter can be isolated from the stromal vascular fraction (SVF) after digestion and centrifugation of residual subcutaneous adipose tissue [2]. ASCs maintain the expression of stem cell markers *in vitro* (**Figure 1**). Preliminary reports describe the increased efficacy of autologous fat grafting when associated to SVF enrichment for regenerative surgery purposes [3]. ASCs represent a good model to address questions concerning specific differentiation strategies. ASCs are readily responsive to platelet-derived growth factors and insulin [4,5]. The plasticity of human ASCs offers a stimulating potential in regenerative medicine and surgery [6]. However, a critical review of the literature reveals considerable uncertainty. In particular, the differentiation of ASCs into cell lineages apart from adipocytes has not been conclusively demonstrated in many studies due to the use of rather simplistic approaches, nonspecific histological confirmation, or a small number of specific markers. ASCs have been proposed to stabilize autologous fat grafts for regenerative therapy, but their safety is unknown in the setting of reconstructive surgery after mastectomy. Nevertheless, the full clinical potential of ASCs awaits much deeper investigation. In this sense, it must be clearly evaluated if enrichment with SVF of autologous engrafted fat tissue could be considered a safe pro-

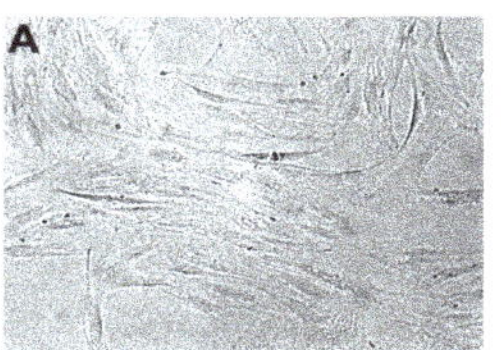

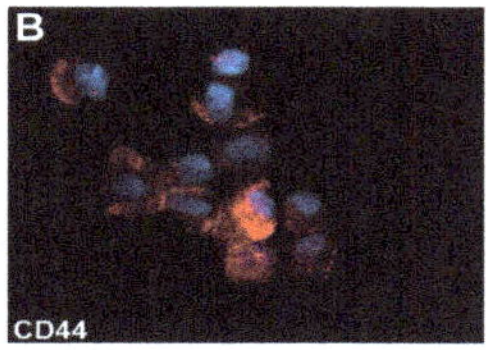

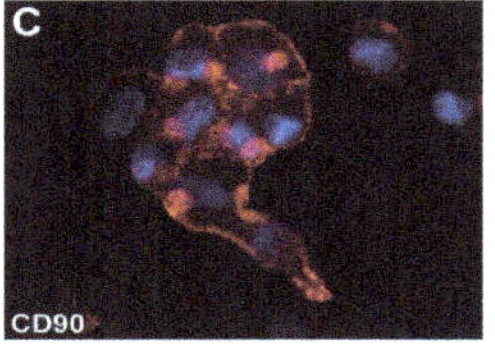

Figure 1. (A) Phase contrast micrograph of ASCs cultured in the presence of 10% FBS. Original magnification 200×. (B)-(C) Immunofluorescent staining for CD44 and CD90 stromal stem cell markers of cultured ASCs. Original magnification, (A): 200×; (B): 600×.

cedure for all patients undergoing breast reconstruction following traditional surgery or new combined therapies for small breast cancers [7].

2. ADIPOSE DERIVED STEM CELLS AND BREAST RECONSTRUCTION

Whilst there has been no direct evidence linking fat grafting in the breast to an increased risk of cancer progression, recent scientific attention has turned to whether the transfer of ASCs-containing SVF could favour an increased risk of breast cancer development or recurrence [6]. The first evidence of interplay between adipose tissue and cancer cells was reported by Manabe *et al.* [8]; they demonstrated that rat mature adipocytes and preadipocytes stimulated proliferation of oestrogen receptor positive breast cancer cell lines in 3D collagen matrices [8]. Successive studies confirmed that ASCs increased proliferation and invasive potential of breast cancer cells [9,10]. Human ASCs co-cultured with MCF7 breast cancer cells secreted transforming growth factor-β1 and regulated the establishment of extracellular matrix [11]. These findings suggest that ASCs may promote cancer diffusion by stimulating the extracellular matrix assembly process. As concerning the role of ASCs in non-breast cancer progression, data are contradictory. Findings similar to those obtained with breast cancer cells were documented with osteosarcoma cells with or without murine mesenchymal stem cells [12]. Opposite conclusions have been made for prostate cancer. ASCs were found to be nontumorigenic and capable to variably reduce tumor growth and prostate tumor establishment in two prostate cancer xenograft models *in vivo*, as well using a soft agar assay *in vitro* [13]. Recent studies indicate that soluble factors from breast cancer cells inhibit adipogenic differentiation while increase proliferation, pro-angiogenic factor secretion, and myofibroblastic differentiation of ASCs [14]. Extracellular matrix deposition increased stiffness and, in turn, facilitated changes in ASC behaviour [14]. The potential concern of autologous fat transfer is that enrichment with ASCs may contribute to stromal support for cancer cells and to deliver locally inflammatory cytokines and/or growth factors, thus facilitating potential residual cancer cell survival and growth. Recent data suggest that a small subpopulation of cancer stem cells is responsible for tumor dedifferentiation, metastasis and chemotherapy resistance. Moreover, malignant cells can reprogram and de-differentiate, so acquiring a stemness phenotype. Inflammatory signals, such as TGF-β, TNF-α, and NF-κB, induce the expression of specific molecules. Transglutaminase 2, is an extracellular matrix molecule that plays a relevant role in TGF-β-driven osteocartilagineous tissue remodeling [15]. Transglutaminase 2 has been recently recognized to drive the ovarian tumor cell phenotypic conversion sustaining the epithelial-mesenchymal transition and stemness appearance [16]. A potentially less stable population of engrafted mesenchymal stem cells likely contribute to inflammatory/growth factor-driven residual breast cancer growth, so representing an undetermined or too high potential risk compared to the aesthetic advantage [17]. Nevertheless, in an interesting study, Zimmerlin *et al.* [18] tested tumorigenesis of tumor cells from metastatic pleural effusion from breast cancer patients in ASC co-cultures. The Authors provided convincing evidence that ASCs enhanced the growth of active, but not resting tumor cells and concluded that reconstructive therapy utilizing ASC-augmented whole fat should be postponed until there is no evidence of active disease [18].

3. CONCLUSION

Current scientific evidence suggests that ASC implementation for regenerative medicine therapies should be carefully considered in patients previously treated for breast cancer. Reconstructive therapy utilizing SVF/ASC-enriched fat grafting should be postponed until there is convincing clinical and anamnestic evidence of absence of active disease.

4. ACKNOWLEDGEMENTS

We thank Ms S. Cappelli for technical assistance. This work was partially supported by a 2012 grant from Transplantation Agency of Lazio, Rome, Italy.

REFERENCES

[1] Missana, M.C., Laurent, I., Barreau, L. and Balleyguier,

C. (2007) Autologous fat transfer in reconstructive breast surgery: Indications, technique and results. *European Journal of Surgical Oncology*, **33**, 685-690. doi:10.1080/02841850112734684б

[2] Mitchell, J.B., McIntosh, K., Zvonic, S., Garrett, S., Floyd, Z.E., Kloster, A., Di Halvorsen, Y., Storms, R.W., Goh, B., Kilroy, G., Wu, X. and Gimble, J.M. (2006) Immunophenotype of human adipose-derived cells: Temporal changes in stromal-associated and stem cell-associated markers. *Stem Cells*, **24**, 376-385. doi:10.1634/stemcells.2005-0234

[3] Cervelli, V., Gentile, P., De Angelis, B., Calabrese, C., Di Stefani, A., Scioli, M.G., Curcio, B.C., Felici, M. and Orlandi, A. (2011) Application of enhanced stromal vascular fraction and fat grafting mixed with PRP in post-traumatic lower extremity ulcers. *Stem Cell Research*, **6**, 103-111. doi:10.1016/j.scr.2010.11.003

[4] Cervelli, V., Scioli, M.G., Gentile, P., Doldo, E., Bonanno, E., Spagnoli, L.G. and Orlandi, A. (2012) Platelet-rich plasma greatly potentiates insulin-induced adipogenic differentiation of human adipose-derived stem cells through a serine/threonine kinase Akt-dependent mechanism and promotes clinical fat graft maintenance. *Stem Cells Translational Medicine*, **1**, 206-220. doi:10.5966/sctm.2011-0052

[5] Gentile, P., Orlandi, A., Scioli, M.G., Di Pasquali, C., Bocchini, I., Curcio, C.B., Floris, M., Fiaschetti, V., Floris, R. and Cervelli, V. (2012) Comparative translational study: The combined use of enhanced stromal vascular fraction and platelet-rich plasma improves fat grafting maintenance in breast reconstruction. *Stem Cells Translational Medicine*, **1**, 341-351. doi:10.5966/sctm.2011-0065

[6] Locke, M., Feisst, V. and Dunbar, P.R. (2011) Concise review: Human adipose-derived stem cells: Separating promise from clinical need. *Stem Cells*, **29**, 404-411. doi:10.1002/stem.593

[7] Manenti, G., Bolacchi, F., Perretta, T., Cossu, E., Pistolese, C.A., Buonomo, O.C., Bonanno, E., Orlandi, A. and Simonetti, G. (2009) Small breast cancers: *In vivo* percutaneous US-guided radiofrequency ablation with dedicated cool-tip radiofrequency system. *Radiology*, **251**, 339-346. doi:10.1148/radiol.2512080905

[8] Manabe, Y., Toda, S., Miyazaki, K. and Sugihara, H. (2003) Mature adipocytes, but not preadipocytes, promote the growth of breast carcinoma cells in collagen gel matrix culture through cancer stromal cell interactions. *The Journal of Pathology*, **201**, 221-228. doi:10.1002/path.1430

[9] Iyengar, P., Combs, T.P., Shah, S.J., *et al.* (2003) Adipocyte-secreted factors synergistically promote mammary tumorigenesis through induction of anti-apoptotic transcriptional programs and protooncogene stabilization. *Oncogene*, **22**, 6408-6423. doi:10.1038/sj.onc.1206737

[10] Xu, Q., Wang, L, Li, H., Han, Q., Li, J., Qu, X., Huang, S. and Zhao R.C. (2012) Mesenchymal stem cells play a potential role in regulating the establishment and maintenance of epithelial-mesenchymal transition in MCF7 human breast cancer cells by paracrine and induced autocrine TGF-β. *International Journal of Oncology*, **41**, 959-968. doi:10.3892/ijo.2012.1541

[11] Yu, J.M., Jun, E.S., Bae, Y.C. and Jung, J.S. (2008) Mesenchymal stem cells derived from human adipose tissues favor tumor cell growth in vivo. *Stem Cells and Development*, **17**, 463-473. doi:10.1089/scd.2007.0181

[12] Perrot, P., Rousseau, J., Bouffaut, A.L., Rédini, F., Cassagnau, E., Deschaseaux, F., Heymann, M.F., Heymann, D., Duteille, F., Trichet, V. and Gouin, F. (2010) Safety concern between autologous fat graft, mesenchymal stem cell and osteosarcoma recurrence. *PLoS One*, **5**, Article ID: e10999. doi:10.1371/journal.pone.0010999

[13] Zolochevska, O., Yu, G., Gimble, J.M. and Figueiredo, M.L. (2012) Pigment epithelial-derived factor and melanoma differentiation associated gene-7 cytokine gene therapies delivered by adipose-derived stromal/mesenchymal stem cells are effective in reducing prostate cancer cell growth. *Stem Cells*, **21**, 1112-1123. doi:10.1089/scd.2011.0247

[14] Chandler, E.M., Seo, B.R., Califano, J.P., Andresen Eguiluz, R.C., Lee, J.S., Yoon, C.J., Tims, D.T., Wang, J.X., Cheng, L., Mohanan, S., Buckley, M.R., Cohen, I., Nikitin, A.Y., Williams, R.M., Gourdon, D., Reinhart-King, C.A. and Fischbach, C. (2012) Implanted adipose progenitor cells as physicochemical regulators of breast cancer. *Proceedings of the National Academy of Sciences of USA*, **109**, 9786-9791. doi:10.1073/pnas.1121160109

[15] Orlandi, A., Oliva, F., Taurisano, G., Candi, E., Di Lascio, A., Melino, G., Spagnoli, L.G. and Tarantino, U. (2009) Transglutaminase-2 differently regulates cartilage destruction and osteophyte formation in a surgical model of osteoarthritis. *Amino Acids*, **36**, 755-763. doi:10.1007/s00726-008-0129-3

[16] Cao, L., Shao, M., Schilder, J., Guise, T., Mohammad, K.S. and Matei, D. (2012) Tissue transglutaminase links TGF-β, epithelial to mesenchymal transition and a stem cell phenotype in ovarian cancer. *Oncogene*, **31**, 2521-2534. doi:10.1038/onc.2011.429

[17] Pearl, P.R., Leedham, S.J. and Pacifico, M.D. (2012) The safety of autologous fat transfer in breast cancer: Lessons from stem cell biology. *Journal of Plastic, Reconstructive & Aesthetic Surgery*, **65**, 283-288. doi:10.1016/j.bjps.2011.07.017

[18] Zimmerlin, L., Donnenberg, A.D., Rubin, J.P., Basse, P., Landreneau, R.J. and Donnenberg, V.S. (2011) Regenerative therapy and cancer: *In vitro* and *in vivo* studies of the interaction between adipose-derived stem cells and breast cancer cells from clinical isolates. *Tissue Engineering Part A*, **17**, 93-106. doi:10.1089/ten.tea.2010.0248

17

The curative effect of the associated cell transplantation on the rabbit myocardial infarction

Zhicheng Fang[1*], Chang'e Zhou[2], Xiang Zheng[1], Boyi Liu[1], Li Chen[1], Chunfeng Shen[1], Pei Liu[1], Yunfei Huang[1]

[1]Department of Intensive Care Unit, Taihe Hospital, Hubei Medicine University, Shiyan, China;
[*]Corresponding Author: 13593751009@139.com
[2]Department of Nephrology, Taihe Hospital, Hubei Medicine University, Shiyan, China

ABSTRACT

Inducing Mesenchymal stem cells to differentiate into cardiomyocycte-like cells and endothelial progenitor cells orientedly and evaluating the curative effect of the associated cell transplantation on the rabbit myocardial infarction (MI). Methods: Mesenchymal stem cells (MSCs) were isolated from the bone marrow of 24 rabbits and cultured in special cell culture medium containing 5-azacytidine (5-AZA), endothelial cell growth supplements (ECGS), vascular endothelial growth factor (VEGF) and basic fibroblast growth factor (BFGF) respectively. The cell transplantation was performed 2 weeks after MI. Rabbits were divided into control group, cardiomyocytes-like cell group, endothelial progenitor cell group and combination group. We used the echocardiography to measure the heart function 2 to 4 weeks after MI, TTC to measure the area of the infarction, flow cytometry to estimate the cell apoptosis. Results: After induced, MSCs were differentiated orientedly into cardiomyocycte-like cells (CLCs) and endothelial progenitor cells (EPCs). CLCs became greater and had a "stick" or "ball" shape. Transmisson electron microscopy showed that the cells had oval nuclei positioned in the central part and well organized myofilaments, atrial granules and mitochomdrion. RT-PCR showed the expression of the atrial natriuretic polypeptide, phospholamban and myosin heavy chain in CLCs. EPCs formed confluent one-celled layer which showed a cobblestone shape by phase-contrast microscope. The expression of CD133 in EPCs was much at first and then descended gradually. Compared with the control group, cell transplantation could improve the heart function, reduce the size of MI, decrease the left ventricular end systole diameter and end diastolic diameter, suppressed cell apoptosis. The curative effect of cell transplantation was better in the associated-cell group than in the single-cell transplantation group (LVEF: 32.49% ± 1.29% vs 53.22% ± 2.13% vs 56.91% ± 2.04% vs 62.61% ± 2.37%, *P* < 0.05; LVESD: 1.23 ± 0.02 vs 0.98 ± 0.04 vs 0.98 ± 0.12 vs 1.11 ± 0.03, *P* < 0.05; LVEDD: 1.53 ± 0.13 vs 1.24 ± 0.02 vs 1.21 ± 0.09 vs 1.01 ± 0.01, *P* < 0.05; the area of infarction: 35.17% ± 0.98% vs 28.61% ± 1.24% vs 29.73% ± 2.11% vs 22.82% ± 3.12%, *P* < 0.05; apotosis: 8.6% ± 0.94% vs 6.94% ± 0.59% vs 6.4% ± 0.27% vs 4.63% ± 0.74%, *P* < 0.05). Conclusions: This study showed that MSCs can differentiate into CLCs and EPCs in the given conditions and the associated cell transplantation is better than the single cell transplantation to treat MI.

Keywords: Mesenchymal Stem Cell; Cardiomyocycte-Like Cell; Endothelial Progenitor Cell; Cell Transplantation

1. INTRODUCTION

The prognosis of the myocardial infarction (MI) has been improved greatly by medication and intervention therapy, but there are still many problems to be resolved. Nowadays, lots of studies show that cell transplantation has positive effect on treating MI. Cardiomyocytes-like cells and endothelial progenitor cells are the two main kinds of cells used for transplantation. Because the former is used for myocardial regeneration and the latter for myocardial ischemia, if we transplanted only one kind of cell, the therapeutic effect is limited. In this study, we explore whether the associated cells transplantation is superior to the single cell transplantation [1,2].

2. METHODS

2.1. Experimental Animals and Cell Transplantation

Ten Japanese big-ear rabbits, including both male and female, weighing 2 - 2.5 kg, were anesthetized with 10% urethane. Additional smaller doses were given as needed to maintain deep anesthesia. Under controlled ventilation, a thoracotomy through a left parasternal incision was performed, the pericardium was incised and the anterior wall of the left ventricle was exposed. The left anterior descending (LAD) coronary artery of the animals was identified and carefully separated, then ligated downstream 2 mm from where the first diagonal artery branches out. After successfully producing an anterior MI, which was confirmed by elevation of the ST segment by more than 0.2 mV in leads I, II and aVL, the rabbits were randomized into four groups, the control group (Cont group), the cardiomyocycte-like cell group (CLC group), the endothelial progenitor cell group (EPC group) and the combination group (Comb group). All the rabbits underwent another thoracotomy after 2 weeks of MI. We identified the necrotic muscle which was pale and had less motion, and then injected 100 μL cell suspensions into six random points at the edge of the necrosis. The Cont group was given saline instead of cell suspension. The cell suspension contained 5×10^7 cells of CLCs, EPCs, or both of them, which had been marked by Brdu before cell transplantation. The total number of cells injected into per rabbit was 3×10^8. Postoperatively, each rabbit received penicillin and gentamicin intramuscularly daily for 7 days, and were treated kindly.

2.2. Mesenchymal Stem Cells (MSCs) Isolation

Bone marrow (4 - 5 mL) was extracted from ilium, moved into Percoll lysis, and centrifuged (1500 rpm, 20 min). The white homogenate with mononuclear cells was moved into another centrifuge tube, washed with DMEM culture medium and centrifuged twice (2000 rpm, 5 min). After that, the cell precipitation (5 mL) was reserved, cultured in the high- and low-sugar DMEM culture medium and blowed evenly. Then the cells were inoculated into culture dish (2×10^6 cells per dish) and ventilated with 5% CO_2 at 37˚C. After 3 - 4 days, the suspended cells were discarded. 5-azacytidine (5-AZA), endothelial cell growth supplements (ECGS), vascular endothelial growth factor (VEGF) and basic fibroblast growth factor (BFGF) were added into the dishes respectively, so as to induce MSCs into CLCs and EPCs. Change the culture medium every 2 or 3 days and observe the cells every day.

2.3. Cardiomyocycte-Like Cells (CLCs) Detection

After adding 5-AZA, we used the phase-contrast microscope to observe the changes of the cell shape every day and used the electron microscope to observe the ultrastructure of CLCs. We also used RT-PCR to analyze the expression of β-myosin heavy main (β-MHC), phospholamban (PHO) and atrial natriuretic polypeptide (ANP) quantificationally.

2.4. Endothelial Progenitor Cells (EPCs) Detection

After adding ECGS, VEGF and BFGF, we used the phase-contrast microscope to observe the changes of the cell shape every day and used the flow cytometry to detect the expression of CD133 every week. The cells were reserved after digested with 0.25% trypsin and discarded the suspension. Mix the cells with 1 mL PBS, filter them by nylon web and centrifuge it at 1000 rpm for 5 min. Then reserve the precipitation and add 20 μL CD133 FITD into it. Finally, we used the flow cytometry to demonstrate the expression rate of CD133 which was showed by the number of the fluorescent cells per 1000 cells.

2.5. Evaluating the Heart Function and Ventricle Remodeling

Echocardiography was performed to assess viable myocardium via parasternal long-axis and short-axis views by a veteran doctor. We measured the left ventricular end systole diameter (LVESD), the left ventricular end diastolic diameter (LVEDD), the left ventricular posterior wall hypertrophy (LVPWH), the fractional shortening (FS), the stork volume (SV) and the left ventricular ejection fraction (LVEF).

2.6. Evaluating the Area of MI and the Apoptosis

After 4 weeks of cell transplantation, we executed the rabbits and took out of the hearts. We cut down the left ventricle and put it into the refrigerator at −80˚C for 3 - 5 min. Then we incised the left ventricle into 2 mm wide slices along the axis from apex to base. The slices were put into the 2% TTC solution and dyed for 30 min at 37˚C. Using the image analysis system to measure the area of the infarction and calculate the area rate in each slice. Repeating 3 times and calcutating the average as the area of MI. 3 plots (5 × 5 mm) were cut from the infarction, washed with the saline and cut into small pieces. digest with 0.25% trypsin and discard the suspension. Mix the left cell precipitation with 1mL PBS, filter and centrifuge (1000 rpm, 5 min). Then reserve the cell precipitation again. We added DNA-PrepTM LPR into it and placed it for 1 min, then added DNA-PrepTM Stain and placed it for 15 - 20 min avoiding the light. We measured the content of the hypodiploid DNA in the total DNA as the apoptosis, repeating 3 times and calculating the average.

3. STATISTICAL ANALYSIS

Continuous variables are presented as mean ± SD. Statistical comparisons among the four groups were made by ANOVA and q test. Statistical computing was performed by use of SPSS (Version 10.0, SPSS Inc.); for all tests, a probability level of $P < 0.05$ was considered significant.

4. RESULTS

4.1. The Morphous of Cardiomyocycte-Like Cells (CLCs) and Endothelial Progenitor Cells (EPCs)

MSCs became bigger after induced by 5-AZA and showed the shape of "short stick" or "pearl" (**Figures 1(a)** and **(b)**). After 2 weeks, the cells syncretized and fusiformly arrayed with directionality. After culturing 3 weeks, the conjunctions among the cells were abundant and the myotube structure appeared, but spontaneous beats were not found. MSCs, induced by ECGS *et al.*, proliferated rapidly after a short period of retention. Within 1 - 2 days, the cells became fusiform and cluster. After 16 - 18 days, the cells were nearly syncretized completedly and showed the shape of cobblestone shope or slabstone (**Figure 2(a)**).

4.2. The Indentification of CLCs and EPCs *in Vitro*

Observed by transmission electron microscope, CLCs had one orbicular-ovate nuclear locating in the center and contained lots of mitochondria. ANPs were at the surrounding of the nuclear with high electron density and its diameter was 200 - 300 μm. The myofilament arrayed lengthways with directionality. But the sarcomere and the intercalated disk could not be discovered (**Figures 1(c)-(e)**). After induced by 5-AZA for 4 - 5 weeks, MSCs expressed the specific protein of ANP, PHO, β-MHC (**Figure 1(f)**). β-MHC was expressed much, while the ANPs were little and showed 3 bonds. In the EPCs group, the rate of CD133 expression was 28.8% ± 3%, 17.6% ± 0.9%, 11.9% ± 0.4% and 7.8% ± 1.3% respectively after the first, second, third and forth week and there was significant difference among these rates (**Table 1**).

4.3. The Area of the MI and the Apoptosis

TTC dying showed the infarction in the Cont group included the the epicardial (Epi) layer, midmyocardial layer and the endocardial (Endo) layer in the anterior wall of left ventricle. However, the infarction in the other 3 groups was limited in or under the the Epi layer (**Figure 3**). The area of MI was smaller in the cell transplantation groups than in the Cont group and was smallest in the associated cell transplantation group. There was no difference between the CLCs group and the EPCs group (**Figure 3**).

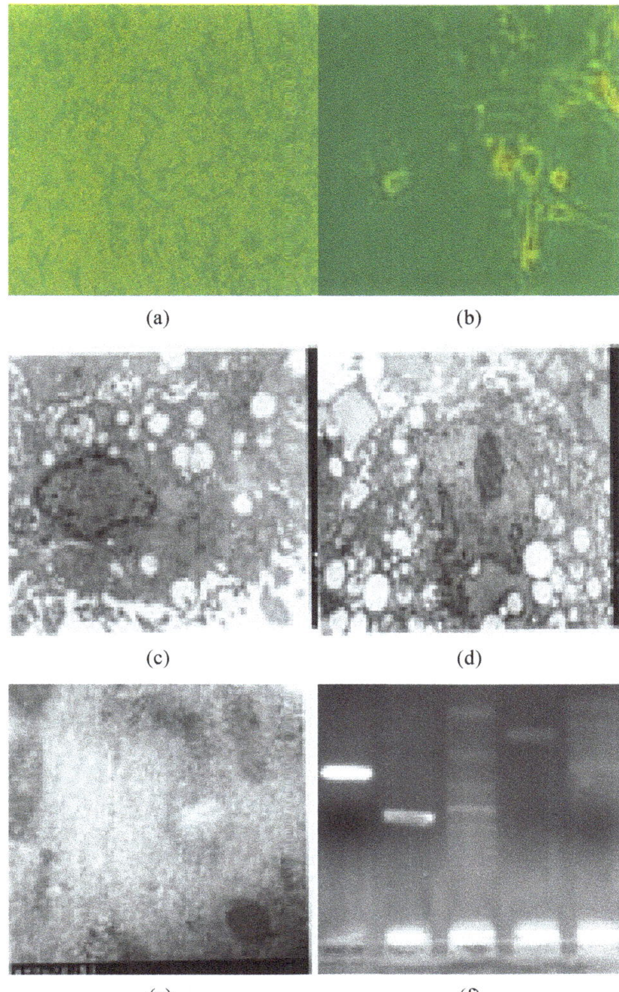

Figure 1. MSCs were induced and differentiated into CLCs by 5-AZA. (a) After 3 days, there were a few of fusiform-shape cells through phase-contrast microscope (×100); (b) After 1 week, there were short stick-like or pearl-like cells through phase-contrast microscope (×100); (c) After 2 weeks, the fusiform-shape cells arrayed with directionality through phase-contrast microscope (×100); (d) After 4 - 5 weeks, the cell showed one orbicular-ovate nuclear locating in the center by transmission electron microscope (×8000); (e) The myofilament arrayed orderly by transmission electron microscope (×8000); (f) The results of RT-PCR. From the left to the right is β-actin, MHC (510000Da), Ladder, PHO (25000Da), ANP (6000Da).

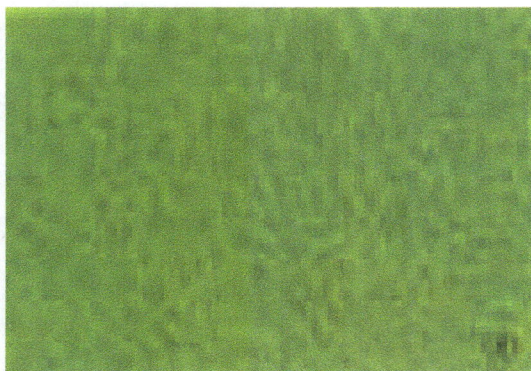

Figure 2. EPCs appeared the typical shape of cobblestone shope or slabstone.

Table 1. The rate of CD133 expression in EPCs at different time.

Time	First week	Second week	Third week	Forth week
CD133 (%)	28.8 ± 3	17.6 ± 0.9※	11.9 ± 0.4※	7.8 ± 1.3※

※$P < 0.05$, compared with each group.

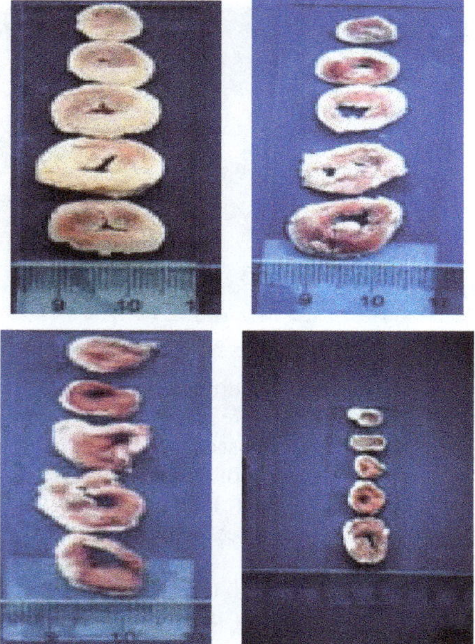

Figure 3. The results of TTC dying.

The pale region showed the infarction. The area of MI from the left to the right is 35.17% ± 0.98% in the cont group, 28.61% ± 1.24%in the CLCs group, 29.73% ± 2.11% in the EPCs group and 22.82% ± 3.12% in the combination group respectively.

5. DISCUSSION

It is important to regenerate myocardial cells and repair the necrotic tissues after MI. And it needs the following conditions to perform these: 1) the capillary web and the big vessels to transport the oxygen and the nutrition; 2) the myocardial cells to proliferate. So it is necessary for the infarcted myocardium to possess the vascular endothelial cells and reproducible myocardial cells. There are myocardial cells in the heart itself and these cells can differentiate into the mature cells to replace the necrotic cells. But the number of these cells is small, what is more, their function decreases gradually with aging, so they can not improve the heart function sufficiently [3]. There have been lots of studies to testify the characters of mesenchymal stem cells (MSCs). It is believed that MSCs can be induced and differentiate into all kinds of mesenchymal tissues, including cardiomyocycte-like cells (CLCs) and endothelial progenitor cells (EPCs), which can regenerate the myocardial cells and the vessels.

5.1. Oriented Differentiatinon of the MSCs

After induced by 5-AZA, MSCs became bigger and appeared obvious myofilament and sarcotubule-like constitution between the cells after 1 week through the phase-contrast microscope. After 10 days, MSCs appeared "short stick" or "pearl" shape and arrayed fusiformly with directionality. Transmission electron microscope showed that the CLCs have one nuclear in the center. They were not binucleate or polynucleate cells and the muscle fibers do not branch. We can distinguish the CLCs from the skeletal muscle cells by these characters [4]. Transmission electron microscope also showed ANPs with the diameter of 200 - 300 μm. ANPs locate at the surrounding of the nuclear. They are special ultrastructures of CLCs [4]. Makino [5] studied the short stick-like or pearl-like cells and found that these cells had sarcomere, intercalated disk and the ultrastructure which could beat spontaneously. So he considered these as the characters of CLCs. However, our study did not find these ultrastructures. The possible reasons are: 1) the cells in Makino's experiment were immortal cells and they are superior to MSCs, as far as the regeneration and the ability of differentiation were concerned; 2) CLCs are not the mature myocardial cells, but the transitional cells [6,7]; 3) the culture medium are different too. The fitting internal environment is important to the cells' maturation.

RT-PCR showed that ANPs, PHO, β-MHC were expressed in CLCs. ANPs is the main component of atrium particle. It has 3 kinds of functional constitutent: α, β, γ, which are not same in the molecular weight and the number of amino acid. So we found 3 bands after electrophoresis. β-MHC is the main component of Myosin. PHO is sarcoplasmic reticulum binding polypeptide and it can activate the calcium pump to increase absorption and storage of the calcium, which leads the myocardium to relaxation. PHO and β-MHC are the special proteins of relaxation and contraction. They take part in the performance of the beat, so they are the markers of the ventricular cells.

The above results indicate that MSCs, after induced, have not only the morphous of CLCs but also the special proteins of contraction and relaxation. They are the molecular foundation of the heart function.

Our former experiments had showed that MSCs could be induced and differentiated into EPCs. EPCs appeared like cobblestone shope or slabstone. They can phagocytize the acetylated low density lipoprotein (LDL). Immunohistochemistry showed there were vWF and te lomerase in EPCs. vWF could become the vessels *in vitro* [8,9]. Recent studies proved that the endothelial precursor cells expressed CD133, CD34 and KDR highly; however, CD133 was expressed only in the endothelial ancestral cell, but not in the endothelial cells (ECs). It is generally believed that CD133 was expressed little by little when EPCs differentiate into ECs. So the rate of CD133 expression can be used to distinguish EPCs from ECs [10-13]. In this study, CD133 was highly expressed in the induced MSCs, which indicated that the MSCs could differentiate into endothelial ancestral cells.

At the beginning of induction, CD133 was highly expressed in EPCs. But CD133 decreased dramatically after 2 weeks and it is a single that the EPCs begin to differentiate into the ECs. So it is time to transplant the cells into the infarcted myocardium. What's more, the terminal differentiated ECs can not be transplanted successfully, so it is better to transplant the EPCs in stead of the ECs to regenerate and form the vessels [14]. Considering all of the above reasons, we chose the EPCs to transplant within 2 weeks of induction.

The rate of CD133 expression in our study is different from that of the others. The possible reasons are: 1) the methods to identify and purify the EPSc are not mature and CD133 expresses in the other cells as well; 2) the EPCs are instable. Its phenotype can change and its biologic activity can increase. All of these reasons can influence the results [15-17]; 3) the difference of experiment methods, animal genera and detection time can affect the results too.

5.2. The Effect of Cell Transplantation on the Myocardial Ischemia

Not only the singl-cell transplantation but also the associated-cell transplantation can improve the heart function (**Table 2**), increase the output of each beat, decrease the area of MI, prevent the ventricle remodeling and inhibit the apoptosis (**Table 3**).

The mechanism about the cell transplantation to treat MI is not very clear. We speculate the possible mechanisms are the following: 1) promoting the myocardial cells and the vessels to regenerate. Compared with the Cont group, the infarction was limited in the epicardial (Epi) layer in the cell transplantation groups, and there was seldom in the midmyocardial (M) layer or the endocardial (Endo) layer. It showed that the area was decreased after cell transplantation. Troponin I and CD34 antigen were expressed highly in the cell transplantation groups. These indicate that the cell transplantation can promote myocardial cells to regenerate and form the vessels in the M layer and the Endo layer. It is beneficial

Table 2. The effect of the cell transplantation on the heart function.

	The cont group		The CLCs group		The EPCS group		The Comb group	
	Pre	Post	Pre	Post	Pre	Post	Pre	Post
LVEDD (mm)	0.99 ± 0.01	1.53 ± 0.13	1.49 ± 0.11	1.24 ± 0.02※	1.35 ± 0.14	1.21 ± 0.09※	1.51 ± 0.23	1.01 ± 0.01※
LVESD (mm)	0.62 ± 0.32	1.23 ± 0.02	1..08 ± 0..09	0.98 ± 0.04※	1.03 ± 0.17	0.98 ± 0.12※	1.37 ± 0.19	1.11 ± 0.03※
LVPWH (cm)	0.21 ± 0.01	0.23 ± 0.02	0.27 ± 0.03	0.24 ± 0.02	0.23 ± 0.01	0.21 ± 0.01	0.28 ± 0.04	0.23 ± 0.03
FS (%)	37.51 ± 1.21	13.8 ± 0.36	27.43 ± 2.11	27.38 ± 3.12※	23.68 ± 1.25	26.98 ± 2.19※	20.62 ± 1.37	32.12 ± 3.41※
SV (ml)	2.13 ± 0.02	1.93 ± 0.02	1.97 ± 0.12	2.13 ± 0.09※	2.43 ± 0.11	3.40 ± 0.21※	2.64 ± 0.32	3.28 ± 0.21※
LVEF (%)	52.58 ± 3.12	32.49 ± 1.29	49.67 ± 1.24	53.22 ± 2.13※	51.42 ± 2.31	56.91 ± 2..04※	54.27 ± 1.29	62.61 ± 2.37※

Pre means pre-transplantation; Post means post-transplantation; LVEDD means the left ventricular end diastolic diameter; LVESD means the left ventricular end systole diameter; LVPWH means the left ventricular posterior wall hypertrophy; FS means the fractional shortening; SV means the stork volume; LVEF means the left ventricular ejection fraction. ※$P < 0.05$, post vs pre.

Table 3. The rate of necrosis in each group.

Group	The Cont group	The CLCs group	The EPCs group	The Comb group
Necrosis (%)	8.6 ± 0.94	6.94 ± 0.59※	6.4 ± 0.27※	4.63 ± 0.74※#

※$P < 0.05$, the cont group vs the cell transplantation groups; #$P < 0.05$, the associated cell transplantation vs the single cell transplantation.

for enhancing the contraction and left ventricular ejection fraction. Luciano injected the self stem cells into cardiac muscle of female Yorkshire pigs whose left anterior descending had been ligated [18]. He found that myocardial cells regenerated between the EPi layer and the Endo layer and the cells regenerated more than those in the control. Immunohistochemistry showed the regeneration-relative antigens, such as Ki-67 and c-kit, were expressed significantly in the cells. His experiment indicated that the cell regeneration is the main mechanism of the cell transplantation to treat MI; 2) inhibiting the apoptosis. This study shows the cell transplantation can inhibit the apoptosis and this is an important aspect of the cell transplantation. It is probably relative to the stem cell factor (SCF). Firstly, the myocardium interstitium fibroses and the inflammation take place after MI. Fibroblast and macrophage express SCF. MSCs have c-kit expressed at its surface, which is the ligand of SCF. When MSCs have been transplanted into the infarcted myocardium, c-kit connects with SCF and the latter can inhibit PIK3 and regulate phospholipase C (PPC) and apoptosis activated by PPC [19-21]. Secondly, the necrotic tissues can cause inflammation, tumor necrosis factor (TNF), transforming growth factor-β1 (TGF-β1). These factors can induce apoptosis receptors, such as Fas, TNF superfamily and TGF-β receptor, *et al.* These receptors connect with relevant ligands and activate the apoptosis induced by caspases superfamily. What's more, SCF can inhibit the apoptosis induced by TNF and TGF-β1 [22-24]; 3) the number of the transplanted cells. If the MSCs were induced and differentiated into CLCs and EPCs *in vivo*, the number of CLCs and EPCs is small and it will reduce the curative effect [25]. We can increase the number of the cells by inducing MSCs *in vitro*. And it is benefit to concentrate the cells by injecting them into the surrounding of the infarcted myocardium. This method is feasible in our experiment; 4) interfering in the ventricle remodeling. This study indicates that the heart function has been improved after the cell transplantation, such as, the LVEDD and the LVESD shortening, the output of each beat increasing, and so on. It is probably because the cell transplantation interferes in the ventricle remodeling. Its possible mechanism is that the cell transplantation inhibits the myocardium interstitial fibrosis. The researchers [26] transplanted the MSCs into the infarced myocardium of the rats and detected the expression of collagen I, II, matrix metalloproteinase and TGF-β1 by the means of immunohistochemistry, RT-PCR and in-situ hybridization. After one month, they found that the concentration of collagen I, II, matrix metalloproteinase and TGF-β1 decreased significantly in the MSCs group, however, extracellular matrix and TGF-β1 increased in the MI control group. TGF-β1 is the most important factor which can cause myocardium interstitial fibrosis so far. It can regulate the synthesis and the decomposition of extracellular matrix and promote the fibroblast regeneration. So the cell transplantation can prevent ventricle remodeling, but the thickness of the ventricle wall is not different between the Cont group and the cell transplantation group. It is probably because of the short time of observation [27].

In a conclusion, the heart function in the Cont group worsened gradually after MI. However, the heart function and the ventricle remodeling improved in the cell transplantation groups. Compared among the cell transplantation groups, the associated cell transplantation is superior to the single cell transplantation at the aspects of the heart function, necrosis and the area of MI. There is no difference between the CLCs group and the EPCs group considering the curative effect. Maybe it is because the CLCs regenerate the myocardial cells and increase the contraction, but do not improve the blood flow [28]. While the EPCs form the vessels and enhance the perfusion, but do not increase the contraction. The associated cell transplantation offer both the CLCs and the EPCs, so it can improve the contraction and the perfusion. It is better for the transplanted cells to survive and the hibernating myocardial cells and the stunning myocardial cells to recover. What's more, after the MSCs are induced, the receptors and the ligands at their surface change. They can react with some cytokine and inflammatory factors and take positive action in the inflammatory reaction, antagonize ischemia and hypoxia and improve the apoptosis caused by oxygen-derived free radicals [29]. And these effections are better in the associated cell transplantation than in the single cell transplantation. After the associated cell transplantation, CLCs and EPCs react with each other and lead EPCs to differentiate into the active myocardial cells, so it increases the number of the myocardial cells. It is more benefit to improve the heart contraction [30].

There are limitations in our study. Firstly, MSC can not differerntiate into CLCs abundantly very much after induced by 5-AZA. Secondly, it is not enough to determine the time of the EPCs transplantation by the concentratin of CD133. Thirdly, the cells have not been purified after induced and differentiated orientatedly [31].

REFERENCES

[1] Flynn, A., Chen, X., O'Connell, E., *et al.* (2012) A comparison of the efficacy of transplantation of bone marrow-derived mesenchymal stem cells and unrestricted somatic stem cells on outcome after acute myocardial infarction. *Stem Cell Research & Therapy*, **3**, 36-44. http://dx.doi.org/10.1186/scrt127

[2] Zeinaloo, A., Zanjani, K.S., Bagheri, M., *et al.* (2011) Intracoronary administration of autologous mesenchymal stem cells in a critically ill patient with dilated cardio-

myopathy. *Pediatric Transplantation*, **15**, E183-E186. http://dx.doi.org/10.1111/j.1399-3046.2010.01366.x

[3] Maureira, P., Marie, P.Y., Yu, F., *et al.* (2012) Repairing chronic myocardial infarction with autologous mesenchymal stem cells engineered tissue in rat promotes angiogenesis and limits ventricular remodeling. *Journal of Biomedical Science*, **19**, 93-99. http://dx.doi.org/10.1186/1423-0127-19-93

[4] Kim, S.W., Lee, D.W., Yu, L.H., *et al.* (2012) Mesenchymal stem cells overexpressing GCP-2 improve heart function through enhanced angiogenic properties in a myocardial infarction model. *Cardiovascular Research*, **95**, 495-506. http://dx.doi.org/10.1093/cvr/cvs224

[5] Kim, S.W., Lee, D.W., Yu, L.H., *et al.* (2012) Mesenchymal stem cells overexpressing GCP-2 improve heart function through enhanced angiogenic properties in a myocardial infarction model. *Cardiovascular Research*, **95**, 495-506. http://dx.doi.org/10.1093/cvr/cvs224

[6] Chi, N.H., Yang, M.C., Chung, T., *et al.* (2012) Cardiac repair achieved by bone marrow mesenchymal stem cells/silk fibroin/hyaluronic acid patches in a rat of myocardial infarction model. *Biomaterials*, **33**, 5541-5551. http://dx.doi.org/10.1016/j.biomaterials.2012.04.030

[7] Wang, T., Sun, S., Wan, Z., *et al.* (2012) Effects of bone marrow mesenchymal stem cells in a rat model of myocardial infarction. *Resuscitation*, **83**, 1391-1396. http://dx.doi.org/10.1016/j.resuscitation.2012.02.033

[8] Zheng, S.X., Weng, Y., Zhou, C., *et al.* (2012) Comparison of cardiac stem cells and mesenchymal stem cells transplantation on the cardiac electrophysiology in rats with myocardial infarction. *Stem Cell Reviews*, **4**, 1-11.

[9] Otto Beitnes, J., Oie, E., Shahdadfar, A., *et al.* (2012) Intramyocardial injections of human mesenchymal stem cells following acute myocardial infarction modulate scar formation and improve left ventricular function. *Cell Transplant*, **21**, 1697-1709. http://dx.doi.org/10.3727/096368911X627462

[10] Du, Y.Y., Yao, R., Hu, X.Q., *et al.* (2011) Dural modulation effects of mesenchymal stem cells implantation on myocardial collagen remodeling in a rat model of myocardial infarction. *Chinese Journal of Cardiovascular Diseases*, **39**, 840-846.

[11] Xie, X., Sun, A., Zhu, W., *et al.* (2012) Transplantation of mesenchymal stem cells preconditioned with hydrogen sulfide enhances repair of myocardial infarction in rats. *Tohoku Journal of Experimental Medicine*, **226**, 29-36. http://dx.doi.org/10.1620/tjem.226.29

[12] Shi, B., Liu, Z.J., Zhao, R.Z., *et al.* (2011) Effect of mesenchymal stem cells on cardiac function and restenosis of injured artery after myocardial infarction. *National Medical Journal of China*, **91**, 2269-2273.

[13] Mishra, P.K. (2008) Bone marrow-derived mesenchymal stem cells for treatment of heart failure: Is it all paracrine actions and immunomodulation? *Journal of Cardiovascular Medicine*, **9**, 122-128. http://dx.doi.org/10.2459/JCM.0b013e32820588f0

[14] Du, Y.Y., Yao, R., Pu, S., *et al.* (2012) Mesenchymal stem cells implantation increases the myofibroblasts congergating in infarct region in a rat model of myocardial infarction. *Chinese Journal of Cardiovascular Diseases*, **40**, 1045-1050.

[15] Wen, Z., Zheng, S., Zhou, C., *et al.* (2012) Bone marrow mesenchymal stem cells for post-myocardial infarction cardiac repair: microRNAs as novel regulators. *Journal of Cellular and Molecular Medicine*, **16**, 657-671. http://dx.doi.org/10.1111/j.1582-4934.2011.01471.x

[16] Nayan, M., Paul, A., Chen, G., *et al.* (2011) Superior therapeutic potential of young bone marrow mesenchymal stem cells by direct intramyocardial delivery in aged recipients with acute myocardial infarction: *In vitro* and *in vivo* investigation. *Journal of Tissue Engineering*, **11**, 211-223.

[17] Jin, J., Zhao, Y., Tan, X., *et al.* (2011) An improved transplantation strategy for mouse mesenchymal stem cells in an acute myocardial infarction model. *PLoS One*, **6**, e21005. http://dx.doi.org/10.1371/journal.pone.0021005

[18] Vassalli, G. and Moccetti, T. (2011) Cardiac repair with allogeneic mesenchymal stem cells after myocardial infarction. *Swiss Medical Weekly*, **141**, w13209.

[19] Carlson, S., Trial, J., Soeller, C., *et al.* (2011) Cardiac mesenchymal stem cells contribute to scar formation after myocardial infarction. *Cardiovascular Research*, **91**, 99-107. http://dx.doi.org/10.1093/cvr/cvr061

[20] Wen, Z., Zheng, S., Zhou, C., *et al.* (2011) Repair mechanisms of bone marrow mesenchymal stem cells in myocardial infarction. *Journal of Cellular and Molecular Medicine*, **15**, 1032-1043. http://dx.doi.org/10.1111/j.1582-4934.2010.01255.x

[21] Armiñán, A., Gandía, C., García-Verdugo, J.M., *et al.* (2010) Mesenchymal stem cells provide better results than hematopoietic precursors for the treatment of myocardial infarction. *Journal of the American College of Cardiology*, **55**, 2244-2053. http://dx.doi.org/10.1016/j.jacc.2009.08.092

[22] Hare, J.M., Traverse, J.H., Henry, T.D., *et al.* (2009) A randomized, double-blind, placebo-controlled, dose-escalation study of intravenous adult human mesenchymal stem cells (prochymal) after acute myocardial infarction. *Journal of the American College of Cardiology*, **54**, 2277-2086. http://dx.doi.org/10.1016/j.jacc.2009.06.055

[23] Li, Z., Guo, J., Chang, Q., *et al.* (2009) Paracrine role for mesenchymal stem cells in acute myocardial infarction. *Biological & Pharmaceutical Bulletin*, **32**, 1343-1346. http://dx.doi.org/10.1248/bpb.32.1343

[24] Mias, C., Lairez, O., Trouche, E., *et al.* (2009) Mesenchymal stem cells promote matrix metalloproteinase secretion by cardiac fibroblasts and reduce cardiac ventricular fibrosis after myocardial infarction. *Stem Cells*, **27**, 2734-2743. http://dx.doi.org/10.1002/stem.169

[25] Grauss, R.W., Winter, E.M., van Tuyn, J., *et al.* (2007) Mesenchymal stem cells from ischemic heart disease patients improve left ventricular function after acute myocardial infarction. *American Journal of Physiology, Heart and Circulatory Physiology*, **293**, H2438-H2447. http://dx.doi.org/10.1152/ajpheart.00365.2007

[26] Berger, S., Aronson, D., Lavie, P., *et al.* (2013) Endothelial progenitor cells in acute myocardial infarction and sleep-disordered breathing. *American Journal of Respi-*

ratory and Critical Care Medicine, **187**, 90-98. http://dx.doi.org/10.1164/rccm.201206-1144OC

[27] Kuliczkowski, W., Derzhko, R., Prajs, I., *et al.* (2012) Endothelial progenitor cells and left ventricle function in patients with acute myocardial infarction: Potential therapeutic considertions. *American Journal of Therapeutics*, **19**, 44-50. http://dx.doi.org/10.1097/MJT.0b013e3181e0cab3

[28] Schuh, A., Liehn, E.A., Sasse, A., *et al.* (2010) Transplantation of endothelial progenitor cells improves neovascularization and left ventricular function after myocardial infarction in a rat model. *Basic Research in Cardiology*, **103**, 69-77. http://dx.doi.org/10.1007/s00395-007-0685-9

[29] Lev, E.I., Kleiman, N.S., Birnbaum, Y., *et al.* (2005) Circulating endothelial progenitor cells and coronary collaterals in patients with non-ST segment elevation myocardial infarction. *Journal of Vascular Research*, **42**, 408-414. http://dx.doi.org/10.1159/000087370

[30] Mitchell, A.J., Sabondjian, E., Blackwood, K.J., *et al.* (2013) Comparison of the myocardial clearance of endothelial progenitor cells injected early versus late into reperfused or sustained occlusion myocardial infarction. *International Journal of Cardiovascular Imaging*, **29**, 497-504. http://dx.doi.org/10.1007/s10554-012-0086-5

[31] Jung, C., Florvaag, A., Oberle, V., *et al.* (2012) Positive effect of eplerenone treatment on endothelial progenitor cells in patients with chronic heart failure. *Journal of the Renin-Angiotensin-Aldosterone System*, **13**, 401-406. http://dx.doi.org/10.1177/1470320312447650

ABBREVIATIONS

MSC: mesenchymal stem cell
MI: myocardial infarction
EPC: endothelial progenitor cells
CLCs: cardiomyocycte-like cells
ECGS: endothelial cell growth supplements
LAD: left anterior descending
β-MHC: β-myosin heavy main
ECs: endothelial cells
PHO: phospholamban
ANP: atrial natriuretic polypeptide
LVESD: left ventricular end systole diameter
LVEDD: the left ventricular end diastolic diameter
LVPWH: the left ventricular posterior wall hypertrophy
FS: the fractional shortening
SV: the stork volume
LVEF: left ventricular ejection fractio
Cont group: the control group
CLC group: the cardiomyocyte-like cell group
EPC group: the endothelial progenitor cell group
Comb group: the combination group

18

Mesenchymal stem cell enhances chondral defects healing in horses*

Ana Lucia Miluzzi Yamada[1], Armando de Mattos Carvalho[2], Andrei Moroz[3], Elenice Deffune[4], Marcos Jun Watanabe[1], Carlos Alberto Hussni[1], Celso Antônio Rodrigues[1], Ana Liz Garcia Alves[1#]

[1]Department of Veterinary Surgery and Anesthesiology, School of Veterinary Medicine and Animal Science (FMVZ), UNESP, Universidade Estadual Paulista, Botucatu, Brazil; [#]Corresponding Author: anaalves@fmvz.unesp.br
[2]Faculty of Veterinary Medicine, Cuiabá University, Cuiabá, Brazil
[3]Department of Morphology, Institute of Biosciences, UNESP, Botucatu, Brazil
[4]Blood Center, School of Medicine, UNESP, Botucatu, Brazil

ABSTRACT

The purpose of this study was to evaluate the effect of intralesional Mesenchymal Stem Cells (MSC) on the treatment of experimentally induced articular chondral defects in horses, emphasizing the benefits of this application in veterinary medicine. Chondral defects were induced in the medial femoral trochlea of both hind limbs of four horses. Thirty days post induction; the horses were divided into two groups. The G1 was submitted to treatment with MSC and the G2 was the control group. Clinical evaluations, synovial fluid analysis and synovial Prostaglandin E_2 (PGE_2) assessment were performed prior to defects and fortnightly up to 120 and 150 days. Macroscopic, histopathological and histochemical evaluations were performed at the end of the experiment. The treatment with MSC reduced the intraarticular inflammatory process. The G1 showed lower PGE_2 concentrations in the synovial fluid and greater percentage of mononuclear cells and lower percentages of lymphocytes and neutrophils. The treatment improved the macro and microscopic aspects of repair tissue. No difference was observed in the scores of lameness between the G1 and G2. The use of MSC in the treatment of chondral defects minimized joint inflammation, as confirmed by synovial fluid analysis. The treatment resulted in an improved repair tissue, verified by macroscopic examination, histochemical and histopathological analysis.

Keywords: Arthroscopy; Cartilage; Equine; Lameness; Mesenchymal Stem Cells

1. INTRODUCTION

Osteoarthritis is defined as a disorder of the joints considering a group of disturbances that present a common result: progressive destruction of articular hyaline cartilage [1]. In adult specimens, the articular cartilage is devoid of innervation and organization and lymphatic vessels, which results in reduced inflow of blood progenitor cells and a limited reparatory mechanism [2,3]. Thus, the repair tissue formed in extensive injuries and superficial defects is composed exclusively of fibrocartilage, which avoids the morphological and functional recovery of the tissue, resulting in the progression of osteoarthritis [4,5].

Mesenchymal Stem Cells (MSC) are an important cell source that could assist in the treatment of chondral defects. They are easily harvested and own a high expansion capacity *in vitro* [5]. MSC are multipotent, adult cells capable of differentiating into all mesoderm tissues. They present fibroblastic morphology and should adhere to plastic, show osteogenic, adipogenic and chondrogenic differentiation and express surface markers [6,7]. The benefits resulting from the use of MSC in chondral defects and osteoarthritis, such as tropism for injured cartilage, paracrine activity, cellular differentiation and proliferation, predict good results and more effective treatments [8-10].

*This study was financially supported by the FAPESP (São Paulo Research Foundation) (2008/56360-7 and 2009/06059-1).

Satisfactory results have been achieved using stem cells in intraarticular injections, intralesional applications and within biocompatible scaffolds [11-14]. It is known that these cells are capable of secreting various bioactive molecules and are immunomodulatory and chemotactic. MSC also reduce inflammatory cell infiltrate and provide cellular support during chondral repair. However, in spite of presenting good results, MSC implantation still face failures in the application, maintenance of cellular phenotype and evidence of effectiveness, particularly in the long-term [7,8,15].

The present study observed the effects of intralesional application of MSC in fibrin glue in the treatment of chondral defects induced in horses, knowing the limited reparatory mechanism of chondral tissue, the inflammatory processes involved in osteoarthritis, the biological capabilities of this cell type and obstacles encountered in this type of treatment.

2. MATERIALS AND METHODS

2.1. Surgical Procedures

This study was approved by the Animal Experimentation Ethics Committee of the School of Veterinary Medicine and Animal Science, UNESP, Botucatu, São Paulo, Brazil, on December 17, 2008, under protocol 256/2008; which does not allow the euthanasia.

Eight patellofemoral joints of both hind limbs of four healthy horses were submitted to arthroscopic surgery [16] to produce a chondral defect. These defects were treated according to the group: Group G1 (four joints) were administered autologous implants of MSC in fibrin glue; G2 (four joints) constituted the experimental control group. The arthroscopic procedure for the induction of chondral defects was considered as day zero (D-0) of the experimental period. Then, the horses were anesthetized (general anesthesia by isoflurane inhalation) and placed in dorsal recumbency. A 10-mm-diameter defect was created in the proximal aspect of medial femoral trochlear ridge, using a motorized shaver drill and a Ferris-Smith forceps causing sufficient drilling to achieve the premeasured size. The defects were induced at sufficient depth to completely remove the articular cartilage and calcified cartilage, however without perforating the subchondral bone.

Following surgery, the horses received prophylactic antibiotics (Association of penicillin[1], 30.000 IU/kg q 72 hours IM for ten days) and anti-inflammatory medication (Phenylbutazone[2] 4, 4 mg/kg q 24h IV for two days) and local curative twice daily to control postoperative pain and to prevent infections. These animals remained confined in stalls until the end of the experiment.

[1]Antibiotic Vitalfarma, Vitalfarma Pharmaceutical Ltd., Minas Gerais, Brazil.

[2]Injectable Equipalazone, Phenylbutazone Marcolab, Rio de Janeiro, Brazil.

2.2. Mesenchymal Stem Cells

The MSC used in the experiment were extracted and cultured from adipose tissue harvested following an incision in a region located about 5 cm lateral to the midline of the tail base. A mean of 1.0 g of adipose tissue were collected for each horse in G1. The isolation and culture of stromal vascular fraction cells were performed according to the technique described for horses [6]. The dose used in the treatment was 10^7 cells per joint. The MSC characterization was performed after the third passage (40 days on average), by flow cytometry analysis. The markers used were mouse anti-rat CD90, mouse anti-horse CD13 and mouse anti-horse CD44 and CD45. The CD13 and CD44 markers are specific for equine species, while the CD90 and CD45 markers are from different species, such that any interspecies reaction would be observed. A secondary goat anti-mouse IgG-FITC marker was used. For negative control of the markers used in the samples, tests to calibrate flow cytometry were performed: cell fluorescence and fluorescence of the cells added to the secondary antibody were both read, in accordance with the technique already described [6]. MSC implantation in G1 horses was performed 30 days (D-30) following chondral defect induction (D-0) through intralesional application by arthroscopy. The acquisition of 3 ml platelet-poor plasma, which is rich in fibrinogen, was necessary to suspend the pellet of cultivated MSC and to make the fibrin glue. Therefore was added to the compound previously prepared 10% of bovine thrombin for development of fibrin glue gel, required to seal the implant within the induced chondral defect.

2.3. Laboratorial and Clinical Evaluations

Collection of synovial fluid from the patellofemoral joints for analyses was performed prior to defect induction and fortnightly up to day 120 and 150, in both groups. Analysis of synovial fluid was divided into four categories: physical, chemical and cytological examination and PGE_2 assessment. For the physical examination, synovial fluid appearance and viscosity were assessed at the time of collection. For the chemical analysis, the amount of protein, fibrinogen and glucose were evaluated with reagent strips[3]. For the cytological examination, overall and differential counts of nucleated cells were performed, leukocytes were quantified as percentages and the concentration of synovial PGE_2 was determined by enzyme immunoassay using a commercially available ELISA (Enzyme Linked Immunosorbent Assay) kit[4], in

[3]Combur 10-Test M, Cobas, Roche, Brazil.

accordance with the manufacturer's recommendations. Both groups were clinically evaluated at the same time that synovial fluid samples were collected. The scores of lameness in all horses of G1 and G2 were graded in scores from 0 to 5 [2] and the joints were inspected daily to verify the presence of inflammation and infection.

2.4. Morphological Evaluations

On D-150, both groups were submitted to macroscopic evaluation of the articular cartilage by arthroscopy. The articular surfaces of the medial femoral trochlea, the general appearance of the cartilage surface, repair tissue, cartilage erosion and fibrillation were all evaluated. At the same time, samples were collected to perform histopathological and histochemical analysis. For the histopathological analyses, sectioned samples were stained by the standard methods of Hematoxylin-Eosin (H.E.), and for the histochemical analyses the sample were stained by Picrosirius Red and Toluidine Blue. Analysis of the sections was performed under light microscope and polarizing microscope by a veterinary pathologist evaluator who was blinded to the sample groups. To evaluate tissue repair, the following aspects were considered: tissue morphology; matrix staining; structural integrity; the predominance of chondrocytes; and the presence and arrangement of collagen fibrils, considering the aspect of fibrosis.

2.5. Statistical Methods

For the numerical measurements was performed the "Two-Way Repeated Measures ANOVA" and the Mann-Whitney test. The means were compared by the Tukey test. For the measurements attributed scores, the non-parametric Kruskal-Wallis was used. When a statistically significant difference occurred, the Tukey test was used to compare median values. A value of $p < 0.05$ was considered significant.

3. RESULTS

On D-30, the joints were distended with CO_2 instead of sterile fluid, allowing the fibrin glue perfectly adhere along the borders and complete the entire place of chondral defects. The intralesional application of the treatments was performed with an 11G needle, model Komiyashiki. It has blunt tip and allowed adequate application of the gel compound in the gelling final stages. Thus, no obstructions of the needle were observed due to the treatment gelling. The use of 10% thrombin in the sample previously separated for treatment was adequate to achieve polymerization and adhesion of the fibrin glue with cells (**Figure 1**).

The mean of the initial mononuclear cells, obtained immediately following adipose tissue processing was 39.5×10^4 cells/mL. MSC following cultivation presented mean cell viability of 78% immediately prior to treatment application. A mean of 1.35×10^7 cells per joint were applied to G1 horses. The immunophenotypic characterization in the flow cytometry analysis revealed the mean of expression for CD13 and CD45 of 1.58% and 0.22%, respectively, which was considered negative. For CD90 and CD44, the mean expression of MSC was 98.5% and 68.5%, respectively, presenting as positive expression, confirming the characterization of these cells as MSC.

In the physical and chemical exams of synovial fluid, the appearance and glucose concentration showed no significant differences between the groups and times analyzed, varying within the normal range for the species. A decrease in viscosity occurred only after the surgical procedures, in both groups. Regarding protein and fibrinogen, when the treatments were compared, no statistical difference was observed ($p > 0.05$). Protein and fibrinogen concentrations were higher only after surgery.

In the cytological examination of synovial fluid there were differences between the treated and control groups. The values found for total nucleated cells in synovial fluid are demonstrated (**Table 1**). Concerning cytology, the results of mononuclear cells are showed in **Table 2**. The percentage of neutrophils (**Table 3**) and lymphocytes (**Table 4**) were lower in G1. Regarding PGE_2 quantification, lower values of PGE_2 occurred in G1 and greater in G2, but these were not statistically significant (**Table 5**).

No difference in lameness scores occurred between the groups, only between the times analyzed (**Table 6**). During inspection of the joints after surgical interventions, only mild signs of inflammation were observed, such as a slight increase in local volume and mild synovial effusion, pain during local palpation and an increase in temperature in both groups. These signs of inflammation presented remission up to day 4 or 5 following the arthroscopic procedures. No adverse clinical reactions were observed following treatment.

On D-150, G1 presented better macroscopic appearance of tissue repair compared with G2 (**Figure 2**). In the histopathological and immunohistochemical analyses (**Figure 3**), fibrocartilage formation was verified in all eight joints. The four joints from G2 only presented fibroblastic cells showing greater intensity of fibrosis. In G2, surrounding the repair tissue, in the area of transition between the newly formed tissue and the normal cartilage, the presence of dead chondrocytes and empty lacunae were observed. In the polarized images stained with Picrosirius Red, the prevalence of initial phase fibrosis

[4]Parameter™ PGE_2 assay kit from R&D Systems, Inc. Minneapolis, USA, distributed by LGC Biotecnologia, São Paulo, Brazil.

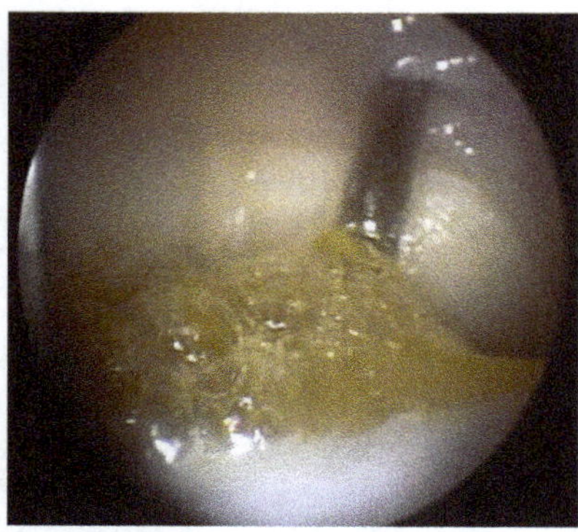

Figure 1. Arthroscopic image of application of treatment (D-30) with the MSC in fibrin glue at the injury site in G1.

Table 1. Mean total count of nucleated cells in the synovial fluid of both groups at different times during the experimental period.

Group	Days 0	15	30	45	60	75	90	120	150	X
G1	60.0	568.2	219.8	550.0	222.5	161.8	215.0	190.0	180.7	263.1
G2	70.0	877.5	161.2	550.0	151.5	146.2	289.5	685.0	175.0	345.1
X	65.0 B	722.9 A	190.5 AB	550.0 AB	187.0 AB	154.0 B	252.2 AB	437.5 AB	177.9 B	

Means followed by same capital letters along the row are not statistically different by the Tukey test ($p > 0.05$). Analysis of variance between treatments with repeated measurements over time (Two-way repeated measures ANOVA). Descriptive summary of the means (cells/μL). There was no statistical difference between treatments.

Table 2. Relative mean of mononuclear cells (%) in the synovial fluid of both groups at different times during the experimental period.

Group	Days 0	15	30	45	60	75	90	120	150	X
G1	98.0	96.5	96.5	93.2	62.0	68.0	74.0	81.0	61.0	**81.1 a**
G2	78.0	66.5	59.2	64.0	81.0	58.8	54.5	46.8	21.8	**58.9 b**
X	**88.0**	**81.5**	**77.9**	**78.6**	**71.5**	**63.4**	**64.2**	**63.9**	**41.4**	

Table 3. Relative mean of neutrophils (%) in the synovial fluid of both groups at different times during the experimental period.

Group	Days 0	15	30	45	60	75	90	120	150	X
G1	0.0 Ab	0.0 Ab	0.0 Aa	3.0 Aa	9.2 Aa	0.8 Aa	3.0 Aa	2.0 Aa	1.2 Aa	**2.1 a**
G2	10.0 Aa	14.0 Aa	5.0 Aa	2.5 Aa	3.0 Aa	7.8 Aa	3.8 Aa	10.0 Aa	1.2 Aa	**6.4 b**
X	**5.0**	**7.0**	**2.5**	**2.8**	**6.1**	**4.2**	**3.4**	**6.0**	**1.2**	

Table 4. Relative mean of lymphocytes (%) in the synovial fluid of both groups at different times during the experimental period.

Group	Days 0	15	30	45	60	75	90	120	150	X
G1	2.0	3.5	3.5	3.8	3.8	5.8	22.0	17.0	12.8	**8.2 a**
G2	14.2	19.5	10.8	8.5	16.0	30.8	3.5	17.2	27.0	**16.4 b**
X	**8.1**	**11.5**	**7.1**	**6.1**	**9.9**	**18.2**	**12.8**	**17.1**	**19.9**	

Means followed by same small letters down the column and capital letters along the row are not statistically different by the Tukey test ($p > 0.05$). Analysis of variance between treatments with repeated measurements over time (Two-way repeated measures ANOVA). Descriptive summary of the means in percentage.

was observed in all eight joints; however, G2 presented the highest quantity of fibrosis. In sections stained with Toluidine Blue, proteoglycan staining was moderate and irregular in the treated group, while toluidine blue staining was absent on all G2 slides.

4. DISCUSSION

Subchondral lesions were not used in this study. The drilling of subchondral bone induces the cell migration and passage of growth factors from the subchondral vasculature and bone marrow to the injury site, [7,10] such the perforation of the subchondral bone would significantly interfere with treatment evaluation, thus it is invariably avoided.

One of the criteria for MSC characterization is their capacity of expression of surface markers CD13, CD90 and CD44, together with the absence of expression of hematopoietic lineage markers, such as CD45 [6,17]. The inverse result of CD13 marker can be explained by different methods of MSC isolation, cell culture duration, the use of monoclonal antibodies detecting different epitopes of the same protein surface or by varying degrees of sensitivity used in cytometry flow analysis [6,17,18]. CD13 presented no reaction in this experiment, showing incompatibility with studies involving humans [18,19]; however, the results obtained from the other markers confirmed the immunophenotypic MSC characterization, so a therapeutic application was possible [6,20].

Concerning the laboratory analysis of synovial fluid, a reduction in viscosity following the arthroscopic procedures was expected. Joint inflammation caused by surgical aggression breaks the hyaluronate molecules, resulting in this change. The postsurgical reduction in viscosity should also be accompanied by an increase in overall cell count, which was verified during this experiment [12,21, 22]. Surgical aggression, even when minimally invasive, promotes different degrees of synovitis, which results in synovial effusion and the influx of proteins and fibri-

Table 5. Mean concentration of PGE_2 in the synovial fluid of both groups at different times during the experimental period.

Group	Days									X
	0	15	30	45	60	75	90	120	150	
G1	568.0 B	553.8 B	453.9 B	979.0 ABb	885.9 ABb	408.8 B	1558.3 A	940.8 ABb	364.2 Bb	**806.3**
G2	395.2 C	498.6 C	476.0 C	1472.7 ABa	1597.7 Aa	725.3 BC	855.2 ABCb	1405.9 ABa	870.9 ABCa	**921.9**
X	**481.6**	**526.2**	**465.0**	**1225.9**	**1241.8**	**567.1**	**1206.7**	**1173.4**	**617.5**	

Means followed by same small letters down the column and capital letters along the row are not statistically different by the Tukey test ($p > 0.05$). Analysis of variance between treatments with repeated measurements over time (Two-way repeated measures ANOVA). Descriptive summary of the means in pg/μL. There was no statistical difference between treatments.

Table 6. Median scores for lameness and p values of both groups at different times during the experimental period.

Group	Days									p
	0	15	30	45	60	75	90	120	150	
G1	0.0 Ba	1.0 ABa	2.0 Aa	2.0 Aa	2.0 Aa	2.0 Aa	1.5 Aa	1.5 Aa	1.5 Aa	**0.008**
G2	0.0 Ca	1.0 BCa	0.8 BCb	1.2 ABb	2.0 Aa	2.0 Aa	2.0 Aa	1.0 BCa	0.5 BCb	**<0.001**
p	**1.0**	**1.0**	**0.01**	**0.13**	**1.0**	**1.0**	**0.13**	**0.13**	**0.06**	

Means followed by same small letters down the column and capital letters along the row are not statistically different by the Tukey test ($p > 0.05$). Analysis of variance between treatments with repeated measurements over time (Two-way repeated measures ANOVA). Descriptive summary of the median of scores of lameness. There was no statistical difference between treatments.

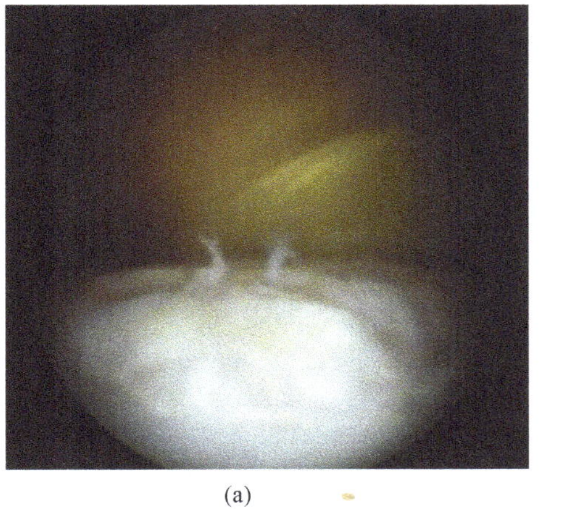
(a)

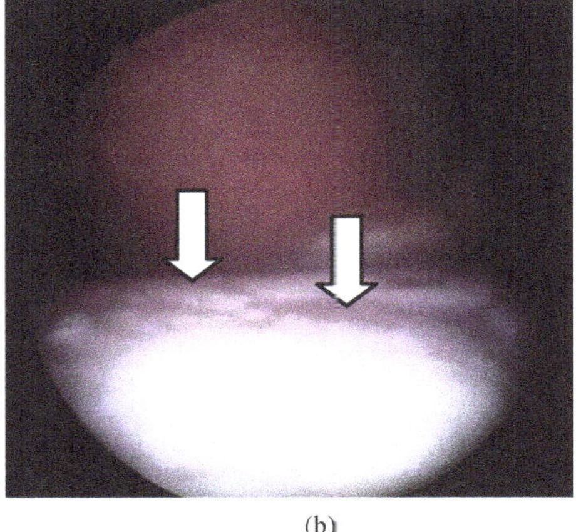
(b)

Figure 2. Arthroscopic images of the joints at D-150. Repair tissue completely filling the injury and proliferations in G1 (a). Filling failures, irregularities (arrows), minimal repair tissue formation and persistence of joint degradation in G2 (b).

nogen [2], as observed on D-15 and D-45.

Normal synovial fluid should present large quantities of mononuclear cells (>80%) derived from blood monocytes, synoviocytes and tissue macrophages. The decrease in mononuclear cell counts represents varying degrees of joint inflammation [22,23], which probably occurred in the four joints from G2. Neutrophils should constitute less than 10% of the total cell count in the synovial fluid, since higher percentages are a sure indication of joint inflammation [22,23]. In this study, G2 presented higher percentages of neutrophils and lymphocytes reflecting increased joint inflammation. It is known that MSC are capable of reducing lymphocyte activation and inflammatory infiltrate, which explains the lower quantity of inflammatory cells in G1 synovial fluid [7,8]. The G1 presented lower concentrations of PGE_2, even without the statistical differences. PGE_2 is an excellent indicator of the degree of joint inflammation, because it is sensitive and detected by ELISA, and is not correlated with the nucleated cell count. Quantification of PGE_2 is performed independently of leukocyte count, since it is released by synovial cells, chondrocytes and resident subchondral cells, but not neutrophils or mononuclear cells [24,25]. Administration of MSC, which are capable of inhibiting diverse inflammatory reactions and present great immunomodulatory action, explains the mild reduction in the PGE_2 concentration in G1 [8,26].

On D-15 and D-45, the lameness score was probably

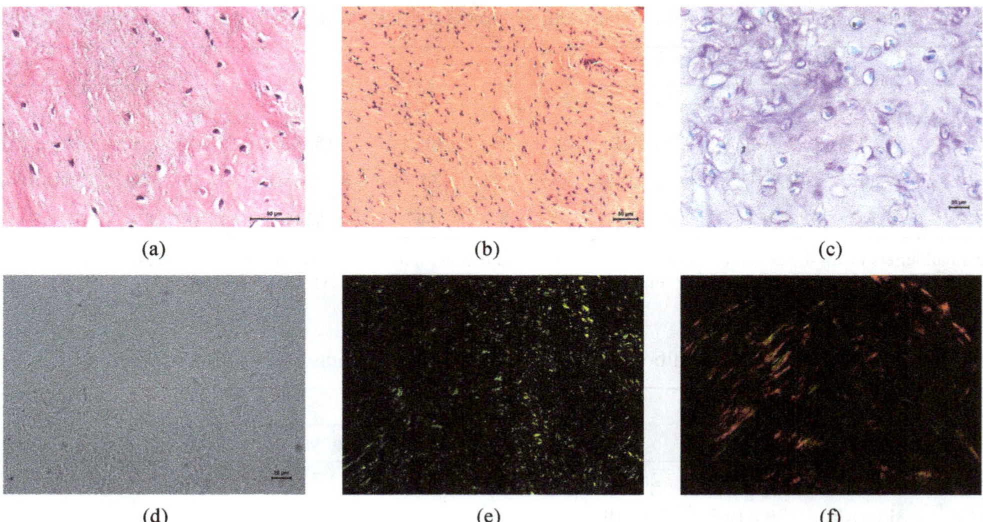

(a) (b) (c)

(d) (e) (f)

Figure 3. Photomicroscopy under natural light on D-150 (the end of experiment) of G1 (a) and G2 (b) stained by H.E., showing the formation of fibrocartilaginous tissue, with a predominance of chondrocytes in G1 (40× magnification in A and 20× magnification in B). Photomicroscopy under natural light of G1 (c) and G2 (d) stained by toluidine blue, showing irregular staining in G1 and no staining in G2 (40× magnification). Photomicroscopy under polarized light of G1 (e) and G2 (f) stained by Picrosirius Red, in which G2 presents thick fibers and predominance of yellow or red (type I collagen) and G1 presents finer fibers and predominance of green (type II collagen) (20× magnification).

not only influenced by the chondral defect created or imposed by the treatment, but also by painful stimulation of the joint capsule and synovial membrane inflammation, resulting from surgical manipulation [2,27]. The nonsignificant differences in lameness scores are contrasted by observations of a reduction in PGE_2 concentrations in synovial fluid in the G1 joints [9,28]. This fact seems to suggest that PGE_2 is not closely related to the degree of lameness or clinical manifestations of pain, but only with generalized joint inflammation [29]. We also observed that perhaps a larger number of animals for this experiment would prove most important differences in both the laboratory and clinical analysis. It was not possible to increase the number of animals due to limitations of the equine experimental model. These data are preliminary and important but more studies should be performed.

Analysis of the results obtained during macroscopic inspection of the lesions treated was in agreement with data reported in the literature, in which research involveing stem cells on the treatment of cartilage defects presented the formation of smooth white repair tissue that was apparently fibrous and well attached and completely filled, without failure of fill in the cartilage. Chondral lesions that were not submitted to treatment presented filling failure and persistent articular cartilage degradation [12,13,15]. Studies reported that lesions treated with stem cells present a lower rate of occurrence of erosions and fibrillations surrounding the lesion, lower rates of osteophytes, better macroscopic appearance and less articular cartilage degeneration [11,13]. The macroscopic findings for G1 joints showed a better repair tissue at six months.

The histopathological and histochemical improvement in G1 was a result of better alignment and cell proliferation and subsequent production of extracellular matrix, resulting from the chemotactic and paracrine actions of MSC that also constituted an adequate cell source [5,7, 30]. The increased production of fibrosis in the G2 joints, confirmed by sections stained with Picrosirius Red, prevented the samples of this group from staining with Toluidine Blue. The absence of Toluidine Blue stain in the control group was probably due to low cell density and, consequently, to lower extracellular matrix production. In spite of the irregular results regarding staining by Toluidine Blue in the treated group, a clear improvement in the response of this group was observed compared with untreated G2. Since there was no possibility of animals sacrifice, only samples harvested from the repair site, by arthroscopic, were examined.

Major obstacles to the success of cell therapy in relation to chondral defects have been reported in the literature. MSC can disperse from the implant site due to runoff and implant vehicle instability. Moreover, local inflammation may induce apoptosis because of the presence of nitric oxide, cytokines and metalloproteinases [7,31]. All these aspects are related to the findings reported for joints treated with MSC. The principal recommendations to solve these problems are the implantation of predifferentiated MSC, in scaffolds that permit adhesion and provide an adequate microenvironment, because they are biocompatible. Allied to this, the MSC should be administered with a cell source rich in growth factors that sustain their proliferation and differentiation [7,10].

We know that fibrin glue remains on the place of the lesion for approximately one week. However, we recognize in this study the difficulty of knowing exactly how long these cells persist in the local of implant, even if it can migrate, differentiate or proliferate. Nevertheless, through our results, we can conclude that the treatment of chondral lesions with MSC reduced the degree of joint inflammation, as verified by cytological analysis of synovial fluid. Morphological evaluations [32] have shown that experimental chondral defects treated with MSC had better aspect of the repair tissue compared with the control group. The morphology of G1 was closer to normal cartilage compared with controls, but it did not reduce the lameness scores. The correct use, investigations and defined objectives make this a promising therapy in the treatment of joint injuries in horses, constituting a therapeutic possibility for structural and functional restoration of damaged articular cartilage. The use of stem cells in the treatment of chondral defects was effective, immunomodulatory and helpful in the tissue repair development.

REFERENCES

[1] Schlueter, A.E. and Orth, M.W. (2004) Equine osteoarthritis: A brief review of the disease and its causes. *Equine and Comparative Exercise Physiology*, **1**, 221-231. http://dx.doi.org/10.1079/ECP200428

[2] Stashak, T.D. (2006) Adam's lameness in horse. 5th Edition, Roca, São Paulo.

[3] Brommer, H., Brama, P.A.J., Laasanen, M.S., Helminen, H.J., van Weeren, P.R. and Jurvelin, J.S. (2005) Functional adaptation of articular cartilage from birth to maturity under the influence of loading: A biomechanical analysis. *Equine Veterinary Journal*, **37**, 148-154. http://dx.doi.org/10.2746/0425164054223769

[4] McIlwraith, C.W. (2005) From arthroscopy to gene therapy—30 years of looking in joints. *51th Annual Convention of the American Association of Equine Practitioners*: *Proceedings of the American Association of Equine Practitioners*, Lexington.

[5] Coleman, C.M., Curtin, C., Barry, F.P., O'Flatharta, C. and Murphy, M. (2010) Mesenchymal stem cells and osteoarthritis: Remedy or accomplice? *Human Gene Therapy*, **21**, 1239-1250. http://dx.doi.org/10.1089/hum.2010.138

[6] Carvalho, A.M. (2009) Autologous implant of mesenchymal stem cells adipose derived in the treatment of experimental tendinitis in equine: Clinical evaluation, ultrasonography, histopathological and immunohistochemical. Dissertation, School of Veterinary Medicine and Animal Science, São Paulo State University, Botucatu.

[7] Vinatier, C., Mrugala, D., Jorgensen, C., Guicheux, J. and Noel, D. (2009) Cartilage engineering: A crucial combination of cells, biomaterials and biofactors. *Trends in Biotechnology*, **27**, 307-314. http://dx.doi.org/10.1016/j.tibtech.2009.02.005

[8] Nöth, F., Steinert, A.F. and Tuan, R.S. (2008) Technology Insight: Adult mesenchymal stem cells for osteoarthritis therapy. *Nature Clinical Practice Rheumatology*, **4**, 371-380.

[9] Frisbie, D.D., Kisiday, J.D., Kawcak, C.E., Werpy, N.M. and McIlwraith, C.W. (2009) Evaluation of adipose-derived stromal vascular fraction or bone marrow-derived mesenchymal stem cells for treatment of osteoarthritis. *Journal of Orthopaedic Research*, **27**, 1675-1680. http://dx.doi.org/10.1002/jor.20933

[10] Fortier, L., Potter, H.G., Rickey, E.J., Schanabel, L.V., Foo, L.F., Chong, L.R., Stokol, T., Cheethan, J. and Nixon, A.J. (2010) Concentrated bone marrow aspirate improves full-thickness cartilage repair compared with microfracture in equine model. *The Journal of Bone and Joint Surgery*, **92**, 1927-1937. http://dx.doi.org/10.2106/JBJS.I.01284

[11] Murphy, J.M., Fink, D.J., Hunziker, E.B. and Barry, F.P. (2003) Stem cell therapy in a caprine model of osteoarthritis. *Arthritis & Rheumatism*, 48, 3464-3474. http://dx.doi.org/10.1002/art.11365

[12] Wilke, M.M., Nydam, D.V. and Nixon, A.J. (2007) Enhanced early chondrogenesis in articular defect following arthroscopic mesenchymal stem cell implantation in a equine model. *Journal of Orthopaedic Research*, **25**, 914-925. http://dx.doi.org/10.1002/jor.20382

[13] McIlwraith, C.W., Frisbie, D.D., Kisiday, J.D., Kawcak, C.E., Werpy, N.M. and Rodkey, W.G. (2010) Use of bone marrow-derived culture-expanded mesenchymal stem cells to augment healing of chondral defects treated with microfracture. *Annual Convention of the American Association of Equine Practitioners*: *Proceedings of the American Association of Equine Practitioners*, Baltimore, 27-28.

[14] Carrade, D.D., Owens, D.S., Galuppo, L.D., Vidal, M.A., Ferraro, G.L., Librach, F., Buerchler, S., Friedman, M.S., Walker, N.J. and Borjesson, D.L. (2011) Clinicopathologic findings following intra-articular injection of autologous and allogeneic placentally derived equine mesenchymal stem cells in horses. *Cytotherapy*, **13**, 419-430. http://dx.doi.org/10.3109/14653249.2010.536213

[15] Raheja, L.F., Galuppo, L.D., Bowers-Lepore, J., Dowd, J.P., Tablin, F. and Yellowley, C.E. (2011) Treatment of bilateral medial femoral condyle articular cartilage fissures in a horse using bone marrow-derived multipotent mesenchymal stromal cells. *Journal of Equine Veterinary Science*, **31**, 147-154. http://dx.doi.org/10.1016/j.jevs.2010.12.009

[16] McIlwraith, C.W. (2005) Diagnostic and surgical arthroscopy in the horse. 3rd Edition,Mosby-Elsevier.

[17] Gimble, G.M. and Guilak, F. (2003) Adipose-derived adult stem cells: Isolation, characterization, and differentiation potential. *Cytotherapy*, **5**, 362-369.

http://dx.doi.org/10.1080/14653240310003026

[18] Schäffler, A. and Büchler, C. (2007) Concise review: Adipose tissue-derived stromal cells-basic and clinical implications for novel cell-based therapies. *Stem Cells*, **25**, 818-827. http://dx.doi.org/10.1634/stemcells.2006-0589

[19] Tapp, H., Hanley, E.N.J., Patt, J.C. and Grubber, H.E. (2009) Adipose-derived stem cells: Characterization and current application in orthopaedic tissue repair. *Experimental Biology and Medicine*, **234**, 1-9. http://dx.doi.org/10.3181/0805-MR-170

[20] Radcliffe, C.H., Flaminio, M.J.B.F. and Fortier, L.A. (2010) Temporal analysis of equine bone marrow aspirate during establishment of putative mesenchymal progenitor cell populations. *Stem Cells and Development*, **19**, 269-282. http://dx.doi.org/10.1089/scd.2009.0091

[21] Martins, E.A.N., Silva, L.C.L.C. and Baccarin, R.Y.A. (2007) Evaluation of the synovial fluid of the femuropatellar joint after experimental medial patellar desmotomy in horses. *Ciência Rural*, **37**, 784-788. http://dx.doi.org/10.1590/S0103-84782007000300028

[22] Steel, C.M. (2008) Equine synovial fluid analysis. *Veterinary Clinics of North America*: *Equine Practice*, **24**, 437-454. http://dx.doi.org/10.1016/j.cveq.2008.05.004

[23] Pozzobon, R., Brass, K.E., Fighera, R.A. and de la Corte, F. (2009) Physical, biochemical and cytological characteristics of synovial fluid with induced synovitis model in ponies. *Ciência Animal Brasileira*, **10**, 1303-1309.

[24] May, S.A., Hooke, R.E., Peremans, K.Y. and Verschooten, F. (1994) Prostaglandin E2 in equine joint disease. *Vlaams Diergeneesk Tijdschr*, **63**, 187-191.

[25] Bertone, A.L., Palmer, J.L. and Jones, J. (2001) Synovial fluid cytokines and eicosanoids as markers of joint disease in horse. *Veterinary Surgery*, **30**, 528-538. http://dx.doi.org/10.1053/jvet.2001.28430

[26] Peroni, J.F. and Borjesson, D.L. (2011) Anti-inflammatory and immunomodulatory activities of stem cells. *Veterinary Clinics of North America*: *Equine Practice*, **27**, 351-362. http://dx.doi.org/10.1016/j.cveq.2011.06.003

[27] Palmer, J.L. and Bertone, A.L. (1994) Joint structure, biochemistry and biochemical disequilibrium in synovitis and equine joint disease. *Equine Veterinary Journal*, **26**, 263-277. http://dx.doi.org/10.1111/j.2042-3306.1994.tb04386.x

[28] Frisbie, D.D. and Smith, R.K.W. (2010) Clinical update on the use of mesenchymal stem cells in equine orthopaedics. *Equine Veterinary Journal*, **42**, 86-89. http://dx.doi.org/10.2746/042516409X477263

[29] De Grauw, J.C., Van de Lest, C.H.A., Van Weeren, R., Brommer, H. and Brama, A.J. (2006) Arthrogenic lameness of the fetlock: Synovial fluid markers of inflammation and cartilage turnover in relation to clinical joint pain. *Equine Veterinary Journal*, **38**, 305-311. http://dx.doi.org/10.2746/042516406777749236

[30] Khan, W.S., Johnson, D.S. and Hardingham, T.E. (2009) The potential of stem cells in the treatment of knee cartilage defects. *The Knee*, 1-6.

[31] Kon, E., Mutini, A., Arcangeli, E., Delcogliano, M., Filardo, G., Aldini, N.N., Pressato, D., Quarto, R., Zaffagnini, S. and Marcacci, M. (2010) Novel nanostructured scaffold for osteochondral regeneration: Pilot study in horses. *Journal of Tissue Engineering and Regenerative Medicine*, **4**, 300-308. http://dx.doi.org/10.1002/term.243

[32] Hoemann, C., Kandel, R., Roberts, S., Saris, D.B.F., Creemers, L., Mainil Valet, P., Méthot, S., Hollander, A.P. and Buschmann, M.D. (2011) International cartilage repair society (ICRS) recommended guidelines for histological endpoints for cartilage repair studies in animal models and clinical trials. *Cartilage*, **2**, 153-172. http://dx.doi.org/10.1177/1947603510397535

Human umbilical cord blood-derived mononuclear cell transplantation for umbilical hernia and hepatic hydrothorax in primary biliary cirrhosis*

Ying-Mei Tang[1], Yun Zhang[2], Li-Ying You[1], Wei-Min Bao[3], Hong-Wei Wang[2], Jin-Hui Yang[1#], Xiang Hu[2†]

[1]Hepatology Center, The 2nd Affiliated Hospital of Kunming Medical College, Yunnan Research Center for Liver Diseases, Kunming, China; [#]Corresponding Author: scheldon_t@tom.com
[2]Shenzhen Beike Cell Engineering Research Institute, Shenzhen, China; [†]Corresponding Author: publication@beikebiotech.com
[3]Department of General Surgery, Yunnan Provincial 1st People's Hospital, Kunming, China

ABSTRACT

Cell therapy was proposed as a potential treatment intervention for liver cirrhosis recently due to the fact that the therapeutic protocol for primary biliary cirrhosis (PBC)-associated refractory umbilical hernia and hepatic hydrothorax is not well defined currently. We report herein the case of a 58-year-old woman who received routine treatments for PBC, which developed into an incarcerated hernia and uncontrolled hydrothorax. This subject's condition was significantly improved and maintained stable condition after receiving human umbilical cord blood-derived mononuclear cell (CBMC) transplantation. Consequently, this new strategy may be a potential treatment option for the refractory umbilical hernia and hydrothorax caused by PBC. However, sufficient data from large-scale controlled and double-blinded clinical trials are needed to further confirm the treatment efficacy and long-term safety before this cell transplantation can be used as a regular therapy for liver cirrhosis.

Keywords: Primary Biliary Cirrhosis (PBC); Umbilical Hernia; Hepatic Hydrothorax; Human Umbilical Cord Blood-Derived Mononuclear Cell (CBMC) Transplantation

1. INTRODUCTION

Primary biliary cirrhosis (PBC) is an immune-mediated chronic progressive inflammatory liver disease that leads to the destruction of small interlobular bile ducts, progressive cholestasis, and, eventually, fibrosis and cirrhosis of the liver, commonly necessitating liver transplantation [1,2]. PBC primarily affects women with a prevalence of up to 1 in 1000 women over 40 years of age [2]. Ursodeoxycholic acid (UDCA) is currently the only FDA-approved standard medical treatment for PBC. Up to 2/3 patients with PBC may have a normal life expectancy with appropriate doses of UDCA administration. However, 1/3 patients do not adequately respond to UDCA therapy and consequently may need additional medical therapy and/or liver transplantation, especially those in advanced stage [2,3]. New treatment interventions need to be explored for those patients with late-stage PBC due to the limitation of liver transplantation, hindered by the organ donor shortage and complications associated with rejection and immunosuppression. Recently, cell therapy has been proposed as a potential treatment intervention for liver cirrhosis.

We report herein one case diagnosed with PBC that developed into an incarcerated hernia and uncontrolled hydrothorax after routine treatments. Human umbilical cord blood-derived mononuclear cell (CBMC) transplantation was recommended for this subject's refractory condition because she refused surgical treatment. This subject was discharged from the hospital at one week following two cell transplantations and showed that liver function and general condition have improved. A six-month follow-up showed similar improvements. This preliminary data suggested CBMC transplantation may have beneficial effects on patients with late-stage liver cirrhosis and associated umbilical hernia and hydrothorax [4,5].

2. CASE REPORT

A 58-year-old woman was admitted to the 2nd Affiliated Hospital of Kunming Medical College with a 9-month history of abdominal distention and tachypnea on

*Xiang Hu is a shareholder of Shenzhen Beike Cell Engineering Research Institute. No other authors declare any competing interests.

December 23rd, 2010. Physical examination showed: poor general condition, slight scleral icterus, coarse breath sounds in left lung, absent breath sounds in right lower lung, abdominal distension and soft, umbilical protrusion on the abdominal wall, positive shifting dullness of abdomen, and edema on both lower extremities. Laboratory analysis revealed low levels of serum albumin (27 g/L; normal range is 35 - 55 g/L) and cholinesterase (1755 U/L; normal range is 3500 - 10,000 U/L), prolonged prothrombin time, positive test result of antimitochondrial antibodies (AMA)-M2. Liver biopsy observed destroyed middle and small bile ducts. No obstruction of large bile duct was found through magnetic resonance cholangiopancreatography (MRCP). X ray of chest showed a large amount of pleural effusion in the right chest and a few in the left side. B-ultrasound clued liver injury with reduced liver volume, widened portal and splenic veins, splenomegaly, and massive ascites. This subject was diagnosed with PBC based on above findings.

Therapy was initiated with orally administration of UDCA 25 mg/kg/day, spironolactone 100 mg/day and furosemide 40 mg/day. 25 g/day of human albumin was infused. Thoracentesis and drainage tube placed into the patient's right chest were operated in order to treat hydrothorax at two days after admission. A totally of 4100 ml of yellow turbid fluid was drained. The drainage tube was removed five days later when the shortness of breath was relieved. This subject's condition had been stable for the next month in the hospital with above treatments but aggravated with a large amount of pleural effusion, incarcerated umbilical hernia with part of the small intestine and ascites as contents and spontaneous bacterial peritonitis afterwards. In the following two months, surgical manual reduction to umbilical hernia, thoracentesis drainage and abdominal paracentesis were performed and antibiotics were administered to relieve the symptoms. This subject refused to receive surgical treatment.

Allogeneic CBMC transplantation was recommended as a further therapeutic option because umbilical hernia and hydrothorax were recurrent and gradually aggravated after routine treatment interventions. The treatment protocol and patient consent were approved by the local institutional review board of the 2nd Affiliated Hospital of Kunming Medical College under the auspices of the National Ministry of Health. The treatment procedure was clearly explained to this subject and her family members and the informed consent was obtained before each initiation of cell transplantations. Human umbilical cord blood (hUCB) was obtained from informed, healthy donors after normal spontaneous vaginal deliveries in according with the sterile procurement guidelines in the hospital. The procedure for CBMC preparation, including hUCB collection and mononuclear cell extraction, cultivation and harvest, was reported in a previous publication [6]. Two CBMC transplantations were performed and 5×10^7 CBMCs, containing 1.0% - 2.0% $CD34^+$ cells as determined by flow cytometry, were transfused per time. The first infusion was processed through the hepatic artery on April 6th, 2011 and another infusion through intravenous injection two weeks later. No adverse effect was observed during and after the cell transplantation.

Dramatic alleviation on abdomen pain, umbilical hernia and pleural effusion was shown following the first cell transplantation. The levels of serum albumin (33.5 g/L) and cholinesterase (5484 U/L) were significantly increased and the liver function was normal at six days after two cell transplantations. In addition, the general condition, including the complexion and appetite, was significantly improved. This subject was discharged at one week after two cell transplantations on a stable condition with no recurrence of umbilical hernia and pleural effusion. Orally administration of UDCA (250 mg, twice per day) was continued after discharge without other treatments. Six months after discharge, stable improvements were still observed on the general condition and liver function. This subject had good appetite and her weight had gained 7 kilograms. The levels of serum albumin (40 g/L) and cholinesterase (4800 U/L) remain the normal range. CT examination on November 23rd, 2011 showed a few pleural effusions in the right chest and a small amount of ascites.

3. DISCUSSION

Liver cirrhosis represents the final common pathological outcome for the majority of chronic liver diseases caused by a variety of factors, such as PBC. Umbilical hernia is a common complication in approximately 20% of patients with cirrhosis and uncontrolled ascites [7]. The umbilical hernia may develop into leakage, ulceration, rupture and incarceration that can be serious and cause around 30% of mortality rate [8]. Paracentesis applied to drainage ascites for reducing the pressure of abdominal cavity is not effective for majority patients and may lead to incarceration of the umbilical hernia due to the decreased tension. Surgery is a treatment option for incarcerated umbilical hernia but this is considered to be high risks with increased perioperative morbidity and mortality on cirrhotic patients with poor liver function [9]. Furthermore, the recurrence rate of umbilical hernia after surgical therapy is as high as 60% [10]. Therefore, there is currently no primary option to treat refractory umbilical hernias in patients with liver cirrhosis.

Hepatic hydrothorax occurs in 0.4% - 12.2% of cirrhotic patients [11]. Tube thoracostomy and mechanical pleurodesis are the standard treatment for recurrent symptomatic hydrothorax. Video-assisted thoracic surgery has also been used to control pleural effusion [12]. However, the therapeutic effects from above treatments are limited. In this case, umbilical hernias and hydrothorax were recurrent and uncontrolled by the conventional treatments. Consequently, this subject developed hernias incarceration, whereas the therapeutic protocol for cirrhosis-associated refractory umbilical hernia and hepatic hydrothorax has not been well defined.

Stem cell-based therapy is of potential value in tissue regeneration and replacement and represents a unique opportunity for the treatment of liver cirrhosis. To date, the most common source of stem cells is bone marrow and many studies proved that the bone marrow stem cells contribute functionally and significantly to liver fibrosis not only in animal models [4,13,14] but also in patients [5,15-17]. However, bone marrow aspiration for patients with liver cirrhosis, especially at the late-stage, is an invasive procedure with high risks due to their bleeding tendency and poor general condition. Alternatively, hUCB may be a preferable source for stem cell transplantation to safely treat non-hematopoietic conditions as CBMCs are easy to obtain and have greater proliferative capacity, primitive ontogeny, lower immunogenicity and lower risk of graft versus-host disease [18-21].

CBMCs are comprised of a heterogenous population of hematopoietic and mesenchymal stem cells, endothelial progenitor cells, and immature immunological cells, capable of differentiating into multiple cell lineages [4, 22]. One research group confirmed the differentiation of CBMCs into hepatocytes in three different ways, namely co-culture with injured liver cells, growth factor-assisted culture, and CBMC transplantation in animal models of liver injury [23]. Study results showed that transplanted hUCB-derived $CD34^+$ cells fused with hepatocytes of NOG mice without liver injury, lost their hematopoietic phenotype, and began hepatocyte-specific gene transcription [24]. It has been reported that umbilical cord blood does contain mesenchymal stem cells (MSCs), which were able to differentiate into hepatocyte-like cells under appropriate induction conditions, and can serve as an alternative source of MSCs to bone marrow [25,26]. In addition, recent studies demonstrated that the transplanted hUCB-derived stem cells successfully incorporated into the liver of recipient animals and differentiated into functional hepatocyte-like cells that expressed hepatocyte-specific markers [27-30].

Furthermore, the therapeutic effects of CBMC transplantation have been studied in animal cirrhotic models. The histopathology of liver tissue in cirrhotic rats was significantly improved by intrahepatically transplanted CBMCs through replacing the damaged hepatocytes and decomposing the surrounding collagen fiber, including the decrease of hepatocellular necrosis, inflammatory infiltration and fibroplasias, and the resolution of fibrosepta [31]. It has been suggested that infused hUCB-derived MSCs differentiated to hepatocyte-like cells and significantly reduced the expression of transforming growth factor b1 (TGF-b1), collagen type I and α-smooth muscle actin (α-SMA) to inhibit the fibrogenesis/cirrhogenesis and recover liver function in CCl4-induced cirrhotic rats [32]. Intrahepatical transplantation of hUCB-derived MSCs could significantly improve the survival of rats with acute hepatic necrosis and the underlying mechanisms involved may include the transdifferentiation of MSCs into hepatocyte-like cells and targeted migration of these cells to liver lesion sites [33]. It has also been showed that hUCB-derived MSCs could improve insulin resistance in rats with CCl4-induced liver cirrhosis, thereby contributing to glucose homeostasis [34]. In addition, transplantation of microencapsulated hepatic-like cells derived from umbilical cord blood cells could preliminarily alleviate the symptoms in rat models with acute hepatic failure, which may be related to the immunosuppressive and substitution effects and liver repair promotion of the transplanted cells [35]. These *in vivo* findings provide a rationale for the therapeutic benefit of CBMC transplantation on liver cirrhosis although the underlying mechanism need to be further investigated.

Encouragingly, the treatment results in this case study showed that CBMC transplantation was well tolerated by this subject with refractory umbilical hernias and hepatic hydrothorax caused by PBC. Although this subject's condition continued to deteriorate after routine treatments, remarkable improvements were observed shortly following CBMC transplantation without the intervention of diuretic and human serum albumin. Moreover, stable improvements of this subject's general condition and liver function were still observed at six months after the treatment.

In summary, umbilical hernia and hepatic hydrothorax are common complications of liver cirrhosis and the treatment remains difficult due to the increased risks following surgical interventions. This case report indicates that CBMC transplantation may represent a promising therapeutic strategy for liver cirrhosis and associated refractory umbilical hernia and hydrothorax. However, sufficient data from large-scale controlled and double-blinded clinical trials are needed to further confirm the treatment efficacy and long-term safety.

4. ACKNOWLEDGEMENTS

The project was supported by the Natural Science Foundation of Yunnan Province (2010CD170). We thank Feng Sha and Yan-ping Liang (Hepatology Center, the 2nd Affiliated Hospital of Kunming Medical College, Yunnan Research Center for Liver Diseases) for helping clinical data collection.

REFERENCES

[1] Poupon, R. (2010) Primary biliary cirrhosis: A 2010 update. *Journal of Hepatology*, **52**, 745-758. doi:10.1016/j.jhep.2009.11.027

[2] Hohenester, S., Oude-Elferink, R.P. and Beuers, U. (2009) Primary biliary cirrhosis. *Seminars in Immunopathology*, **31**, 283-307. doi:10.1007/s00281-009-0164-5

[3] Kaplan, M.M. and Gershwin, M.E. (2005) Primary biliary cirrhosis. *The New England Journal of Medicine*, **353**, 1261-1273. doi:10.1056/NEJMra043898

[4] Zhao, D.C., Lei, J.X., Chen, R., Yu, W.H., Zhang, X.M., Li, S.N. and Xiang, P. (2005) Bone marrow-derived mesenchymal stem cells protect against experimental liver fibrosis in rats. *World Journal of Gastroenterology*, **11**, 3431-3440.

[5] Terai, S. and Sakaida, I. (2011) Autologous bone marrow cell infusion therapy for liver cirrhosis patients. *Journal of Hepato-Biliary-Pancreatic Sciences*, **18**, 23-25. doi:10.1007/s00534-010-0305-1

[6] Yang, W.Z., Zhang, Y., Wu, F., Min, W.P., Minev, B., Zhang, M., Luo, X.L., Ramos, F., Ichim, T.E., Riordan, N.H. and Hu, X. (2010) Safety evaluation of allogeneic umbilical cord blood mononuclear cell therapy for degenerative conditions. *Journal of Translational Medicine*, **8**, 75. doi:10.1186/1479-5876-8-75

[7] Eker, H.H., van Ramshorst, G.H., de Goede, B., Tilanus, H.W., Metselaar, H.J., de Man, R.A., Lange, J.F. and Kazemier, G. (2011) A prospective study on elective umbilical hernia repair in patients with liver cirrhosis and ascites. *Surgery*, **150**, 542-546. doi:10.1016/j.surg.2011.02.026

[8] Lemmer, J.H., Strodel, W.E., Knol, J.A. and Eckhauser, F.E. (1983) Management of spontaneous umbilical hernia disruption in the cirrhotic patient. *Annals of Surgery*, **198**, 30-34. doi:10.1097/00000658-198307000-00006

[9] Garrison, R.N., Cryer, H.M., Howard, D.A. and Polk, H.C. Jr. (1984) Clarification of risk factors for abdominal operations in patients with hepatic cirrhosis. *Annals of Surgery*, **199**, 648-655. doi:10.1097/00000658-198406000-00003

[10] Belghiti, J. and Durand, F. (1997) Abdominal wall hernias in the setting of cirrhosis. *Seminars in Liver Disease*, **17**, 219-226. doi:10.1055/s-2007-1007199

[11] Gordon, F.D., Anastopoulos, H.T. and Crenshaw, W. (1997) The successful treatment of symptomatic, refracttory hepatic hydrothorax with transjugular intrahepatic portosystemic shunt. *Hepatology*, **25**, 1366-1369. doi:10.1002/hep.510250611

[12] Park, S.Z., Shrager, J.B. and Allen, M.S. (1997) Treatment of refractory, nonmalignant thydrothorax with a pleurovenous shunt. *The Annals of Thoracic Surgery*, **63**, 1777-1779. doi:10.1016/S0003-4975(97)00131-8

[13] Russo, F.P., Alison, M.R., Bigger, B.W., Amofah, E., Florou, A., Amin, F., Bou-Gharios, G., Jeffery, R., Iredale, J.P. and Forbes, S.J. (2006) The bone marrow functionally contributes to liver fibrosis. *Gastroenterology*, **130**, 1807-1821. doi:10.1053/j.gastro.2006.01.036

[14] Oyagi, S., Hirose, M., Kojima, M., Okuyama, M., Kawase, M., Nakamura, T., Ohgushi, H. and Yagi, K. (2006) Therapeutic effect of transplanting HGF-treated bone marrow mesenchymal cells into CCl4-injured rats. *Journal of Hepatology*, **44**, 742-748. doi:10.1016/j.jhep.2005.10.026

[15] Amer, M.E., El-Sayed, S.Z., El-Kheir, W.A., Gabr, H., Gomaa, A.A., El-Noomani, N. and Hegazy, M. (2011) Clinical and laboratory evaluation of patients with end-stage liver cell failure injected with bone marrow-derived hepatocyte-like cells. *European Journal of Gastroenterology & Hepatology*, **23**, 936-941. doi:10.1097/MEG.0b013e3283488b00

[16] Peng, L., Xie, D.Y., Lin, B.L., Liu, J., Zhu, H.P., Xie, C., Zheng, Y.B. and Gao, Z.L. (2011) Autologous bone marrow mesenchymal stem cell transplantation in liver failure patients caused by hepatitis B: Short-term and long-term outcomes. *Hepatology*, **54**, 820-828. doi:10.1002/hep.24434

[17] Kim, J.K., Park, Y.N., Kim, J.S., Park, M.S., Paik, Y.H., Seok, J.Y., Chung, Y.E., Kim, H.O., Kim, K.S., Ahn, S.H., Kim, Y., Kim. M.J., Lee, K.S., Chon, C.Y., Kim, S.J., Terai, S., Sakaida, I. and Han, K.H. (2010) Autologous bone marrow infusion activates the progenitor cell compartment in patients with advanced liver cirrhosis. *Cell Transplantation*, **19**, 1237-1246. doi:10.3727/096368910X506863

[18] Broxmeyer, H.E., Douglas, G.W., Hangoc, G., Cooper, S., Bard, J., English, D., Arny, M., Thomas, L. and Boyse, E.A. (1989) Human umbilical cord blood as a potential source of transplantable hematopoietic stem/progenitor cells. *Proceedings of the National Academy of Sciences of the USA*, **86**, 3828-3832. doi:10.1073/pnas.86.10.3828

[19] Schoemans, H., Theunissen, K., Maertens, J., Boogaerts, M., Verfaillie, C. and Wagner, J. (2006) Adult umbilical cord blood transplantation: A comprehensive review. *Bone Marrow Transplantation*, **38**, 83-93. doi:10.1038/sj.bmt.1705403

[20] Stanevsky, A., Goldstein, G. and Nagler, A. (2009) Umbilical cord blood transplantation: Pros, cons and beyond. *Blood Reviews*, **23**, 199-204. doi:10.1016/j.blre.2009.02.001

[21] Yang, W.Z., Zhang, Y., Wu, F., Zhang, M., Cho, S.C., Li, C.Z., Li, S.H., Shu, G.J., Sheng, Y.X., Zhao, N., Tang, Y., Jiang, S., Jiang, S., Gandjian, M., Ichim, T.E. and Hu, X. (2011) Human umbilical cord blood-derived mononuclear cell transplantation: Case series of 30 subjects with hereditary ataxia. *Journal of Translational Medicine*, **9**, 65. doi:10.1186/1479-5876-9-65

[22] Teramoto, K., Asahina, K., Kumashiro, Y., Kakinuma, S., Chinzei, R., Shimizu-Saito, K., Tanaka, Y., Teraoka, H. and Arii, S. (2005) Hepatocyte differentiation from embryonic stem cells and umbilical cord blood cells. *Journal of Hepato-Biliary-Pancreatic Surgery*, **12**, 196-202. doi:10.1007/s00534-005-0980-5

[23] Zhang, F.T., Fang, J.Z., Yu, J., Wan, H.J., Ye, J., Long, X., Yin, M.J. and Huang, C.Q. (2006) Conversion of mononuclear cells from human umbilical cord blood into heap-

tocyte-like cells. *Academic Journal of Second Military Medical University*, in Chinese, **21**, 358-364.

[24] Fujino, H., Hiramatsu, H., Tsuchiya, A., Niwa, A., Noma, H., Shiota, M., Umeda, K., Yoshimoto, M., Ito, M., Heike, T. and Nakahata, T. (2007) Human cord blood CD34+ cells develop into hepatocytes in the livers of NOD/SCID/γ_c^{null} mice through cell fusion. *The FASEB Journal*, **21**, 3499-3510. doi:10.1096/fj.06-6109com

[25] Lee, O.K., Kuo, T.K., Chen, W.M., Lee, K.D., Hsieh, S.L. and Chen, T.H. (2004) Isolation of multipotent mesenchymal stem cells from umbilical cord blood. *Blood*, **103**, 1669-1675. doi:10.1182/blood-2003-05-1670

[26] Hong, S.H., Gang, E.J., Jeong, J.A., Ahn, C., Hwang, S.H., Yang, I.H., Park, H.K., Han, H. and Kim, H. (2005) In vitro differentiation of human umbilical cord blood-derived mesenchymal stem cells into hepatocyte-like cells. *Biochemical and Biophysical Research Communications*, **330**, 1153-1161. doi:10.1016/j.bbrc.2005.03.086

[27] Moon, Y.J., Yoon, H.H., Lee, M.W., Jang, I.K., Lee, D.H., Lee, J.H., Lee, S.K., Lee, K.H., Kim, Y.J. and Eom, Y.W. (2009) Multipotent progenitor cells derived from human umbilical cord blood can differentiate into hepatocyte-like cells in a liver injury rat model. *Transplantation Proceedings*, **41**, 4357-4360. doi:10.1016/j.transproceed.2009.08.053

[28] Sun, Y., Xiao, D., Zhang, R.S., Cui, G.H., Wang, X.H. and Chen, X.G. (2007) Formation of human hepatocyte-like cells with different cellular phenotypes by human umbilical cord blood-derived cells in the human-rat chimeras. *Biochemical and Biophysical Research Communications*, **357**, 1160-1165. doi:10.1016/j.bbrc.2007.04.087

[29] Kakinuma, S., Tanaka, Y., Chinzei, R., Watanabe, M., Shimizu-Saito, K., Hara, Y., Teramoto, K., Arii, S., Sato, C., Takase, K., Yasumizu, T. and Teraoka, H. (2003) Human umbilical cord blood as a source of transplantable hepatic progenitor cells. *Stem Cells*, **21**, 217-227. doi:10.1634/stemcells.21-2-217

[30] Nonome, K., Li, X.K., Takahara, T., Kitazawa, Y., Funeshima, N., Yata, Y., Xue, F., Kanayama, M., Shinno, E., Kuwae, C., Saito, S., Watanabe, A. and Sugiyama, T. (2005) Human umbilical cord blood-derived cells differentiate into hepatocyte-like cells in the Fas-mediated liver injury model. *American Journal of Physiology Gastrointestinal and Liver Physiology*, **289**, 1091-1099. doi:10.1152/ajpgi.00049.2005

[31] Bassiouny, A.R., Zaky, A.Z., Abdulmalek, S.A., Kandeel, K.M., Ismail, A. and Moftah, M. (2011) Modulation of AP-endonuclease1 levels associated with hepatic cirrhosis in rat model treated with human umbilical cord blood mononuclear stem cells. *International Journal of Clinical and Experimental Pathology*, **4**, 692-707.

[32] Jung, K.H., Shin, H.P., Lee, S., Lim, Y.J., Hwang, S.H., Han, H., Park, H.K., Chung, J.H. and Yim, S.V. (2009) Effect of human umbilical cord blood-derived mesenchymal stem cells in a cirrhotic rat model. *Liver International*, **29**, 898-909. doi:10.1111/j.1478-3231.2009.02031.x

[33] Shi, L.L., Liu, F.P. and Wang, D.W. (2011) Transplantation of human umbilical cord blood mesenchymal stem cells improves survival rates in a rat model of acute hepatic necrosis. *American Journal of the Medical Sciences*, **342**, 212-217. doi:10.1097/MAJ.0b013e3182112b90

[34] Jung, K.H., Uhm, Y.K., Lim, Y.J. and Yim, S.V. (2011) Human umbilical cord blood-derived mesenchymal stem cells improve glucose homeostasis in rats with liver cirrhosis. *International Journal of Oncology*, **39**, 137-143. doi:10.3892/ijo.2011.1016

[35] Zhang, F.T., Wan, H.J., Li, M.H., Ye, J., Yin, M.J., Huang, C.Q. and Yu, J. (2011) Transplantation of microencapsulated umbilical-cord-blood-derived hepatic-like cells for treatment of hepatic failure. *World Journal of Gastroenterology*, **17**, 938-945. doi:10.3748/wjg.v17.i7.938

20

CD133 and CD24 expression in renal tissue of patients affected by autosomal dominant polcystic kidney disease

Daniele Lodi*, Giulia Ligabue, Fabrizio Cavazzini, Valentina Lupo, Gianni Cappelli, Riccardo Magistroni*

Department of Medicine and Medical Specialties, Division of Nephrology Dialysis and Transplantation, University of Modena and Reggio Emilia, Modena, Italy; *Corresponding Authors: lele.lodi@alice.it, rmagistroni@unimore.it

ABSTRACT

Background: Autosomal dominant polycystic kidney disease is a condition mainly characterized by the progressive development and enlargement of cysts in each kidney. In this process a high rate of proliferation and apoptosis of tubular cells has been documented and interpreted as a futile attempt of tissue repair. In consideration of the role of stem cells in reparative processes we investigated the presence and localization of CD133 + CD24+ renal progenitors in renal ADPKD tissue and cells. Methods: Two normal kidneys and two ADPKD kidneys were examined. CD133 and CD24 expression was investigated by confocal microscopy and immunoblotting. Furthermore cystic isolated cells and cultured immortalized cells were characterized. Results: CD133 and CD24 have the same localization in ADPKD tissues and in normal kidneys: expression is restricted to a subset of epithelial cells (PEC) of Bowman's capsule and to tubular cells in a focal and segmental pattern. Furthermore, in ADPKD tissue, cysts diffusely express CD133 and CD24. According to a quantitative analysis in ADPKD tissue CD133 + CD24 + cells are statistically more expressed in tubules ($p < 0.001$) and less expressed in the Bowman's capsule ($p = 0.0016$) compared to the same localizations in control tissue. Conclusions: CD133 and CD24 antigens, typically expressed by renal epithelial progenitors, are more expressed in ADPKD tubules and highly expressed in ADPKD cysts. Whether CD133 and CD24 expression would signify renal progenitor recruitment or alternatively an expression pattern of the dedifferentiation of ADPKD cells remains unclear.

Keywords: Renal Stem Cells; CD133; CD24; ADPKD

1. INTRODUCTION

Autosomal Dominant Polycystic Kidney Disease (ADPKD) can arise from mutations in either PKD1 (85% of affected patients) or PKD2 (15% of affected patients) genes with clinically indistinguishable manifestations [1]. ADPKD affects over 1:1000 of the worldwide population and it causes 1:3000 hospitalization. ADPKD is asymptomatic in about 50% of subjects with pkd genes mutated [2]. It is a systemic disease associated with renal failure, intracranial arterial aneurysms, cardiac valvular defects, colonic diverticulosis and cyst formation in other organs such as the liver, spleen and pancreas. Nevertheless ADPKD gives mainly renal manifestations: the patients develop renal cysts which progressively lead to disruption of renal parenchyma, interstitial fibrosis, cellular infiltration and loss of functional nephrons. Renal degeneration finally progresses to end-stage renal disease [1].

PKD1 (located on chromosome 16) codes for a large transmembrane protein of 460 KDa involved in the control of calcium permeation and cell-cell/matrix interaction. PKD2 (located on chromosome 4) codes for a calcium channel of about 110 KDa. The polycystin 1 and 2 (the proteins were coded by PKD1 and PKD2 genes) collaborate together in a functional complex [3,4].

Previous studies have demonstrated a high rate of proliferation and apoptosis in the cysts of ADPKD patients4 and this phenomenon has been interpreted as an unproductive attempt of tissue reparation. In this scenario a likely involvement of renal progenitors can be hypothesized.

Sagrinati *et al.* identified, in human adult kidneys, a subset of Parietal Epithelial Cells (PECs) in the Bowman's capsule that revealed self-renewal potential and high cloning efficiency. This subset of PECs exhibits co-expression of stem cell markers CD24 and CD133 and absence of lineage-specific markers. Under appropriate culture conditions, individual clones of CD24 + CD133 + PEC could be induced to generate mature, functional, tubular cells with phenotypic features of proximal and/or distal tubules [5].

ADPKD is characterized by expansion of cysts and tubular hyperplasia in the context of a sustained proliferative and apoptotic process. In this brief report we explored the pathologic features of presumptive renal progenitor cells in ADPKD renal tissue trying to explain the nature of their involvement in the disease: tissue repair or increase of cystic lesions.

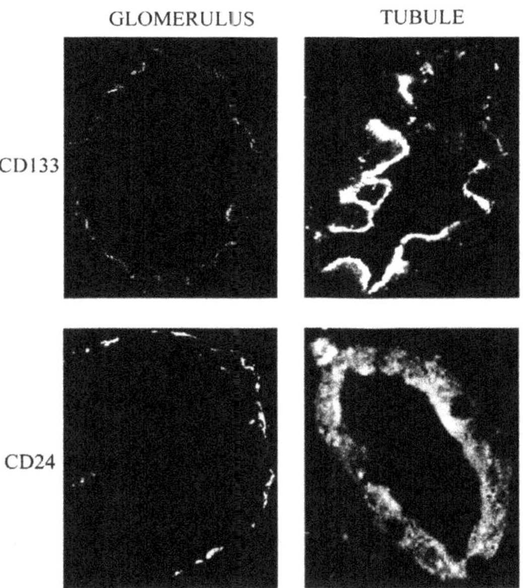

Figure 1. CD133 and CD24 expression in normal kidney. The first lane shows tissue expression of CD133 in Bowman's capsules and tubules. CD133 is expressed in a subset of PEC in the Bowman's capsule and in the luminal side of positive tubular cells. The second lane shows tissue expression of CD24 in Bowman's capsules and tubules. CD24 is expressed in a subset of PEC in the Bowman's capsule and in the cytoplasm of tubular cells.

2. RESULTS

2.1. Expression of CD133 and CD24 in Normal and ADPKD Kidney

In normal kidney at the glomerular level the confocal microscopic analysis shows that CD133 and CD24 are co-expressed by a subset of parietal epithelial cells (PEC) in the Bowman's capsule (**Figure 1**: on line publication): CD24 has a generalized and diffuse presentation, CD133 is generalized and segmental. At tubular level the distribution of the expression of both CD133 and CD24 is focal and global. In the normal kidney specimen the overall intensity of CD24 + cells have the similar median value compared to CD133 + cells but the distribution of the intensity for the CD24 + cells is larger (**Figure 2(a)**: on line publication). In the ADPKD kidney specimen the overall intensity of CD133 is higher, but not statistically significant, than the intensity of CD24 + cells (**Figure 2(b)**: on line publication). It is interesting to note that at cellular level CD133 is polarized to the luminal side of the tubular cell surface as well to the urinary space side in positive PECs, whereas CD24 is not clearly polarized but shows a diffuse distribution at the membrane and cytoplasm level (**Figure 1**: on line publication).

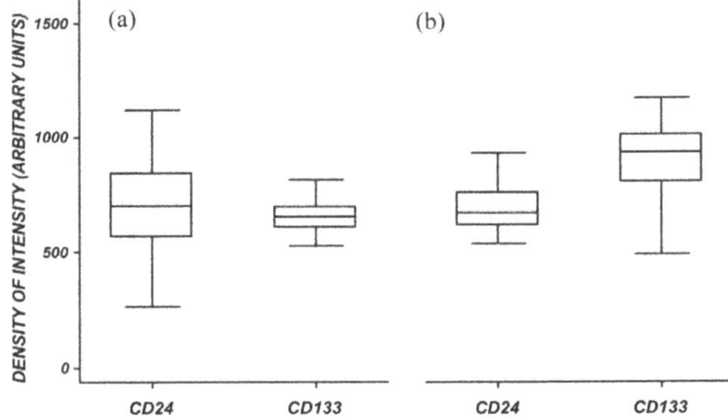

Figure 2. Morphometric analysis of CD24 and CD133 global expression (a) in normal kidney and (b) in ADPKD kidney. (a) In normal tissue, CD24 and CD133 the median expression is similar, even though CD24 intensity has a larger distribution than CD133; (b) In ADPKD tissue, CD133 expression is higher than that of CD24.

Analysis of confocal microscopy of ADPKD kidneys revealed that CD133 and CD24 were expressed in a subset of glomerular (**Figures 3(a)-(c)**) and tubular (**Figures 3(d)-(f)**) cells and they showed the same tissue of normal kidney [5]: CD133 presents a generalized and segmental pattern while CD24 is generalized and diffuse in the Bowman's capsule. The expression of both CD133 and CD24 is focal and global in the tubules.

The cysts of ADPKD samples showed a segmental co-expression pattern of CD133 and CD24. CD24 has a generalized distribution in the samples while CD133 is segmental. The cells of large cysts show a flatted morphology and a co-localization of CD133 and CD24 can be appreciated in some segments (**Figures 3(g)-(i)**).

The quantitative comparison between normal kidney and ADPKD kidney revealed an increased CD133 expression in tubules while glomerular expression appears

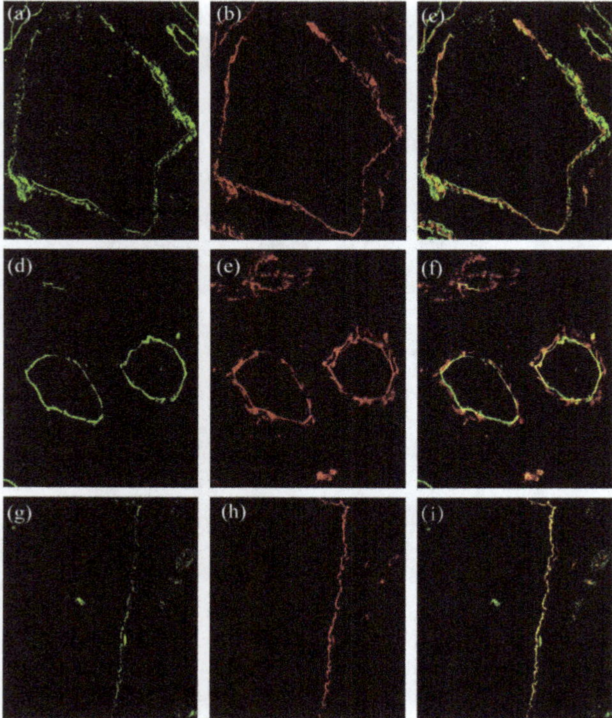

Figure 3. CD133 and CD24 expression in ADPKD samples. The first lane shows glomerular expression of CD133 (a) and CD24 (b). CD133 and CD24 are co-localized and co-expressed by a subset of PEC in the Bowman's capsule (c). The second lane shows tubular expression of CD133 (d) and CD24 (e). CD133 and CD24 are co-expressed in these tubules (f). The third lane shows cystic expression of CD133 (g) and CD24 (h). CD133 and CD24 are co-localized and co-expressed by the cystic cells (i).

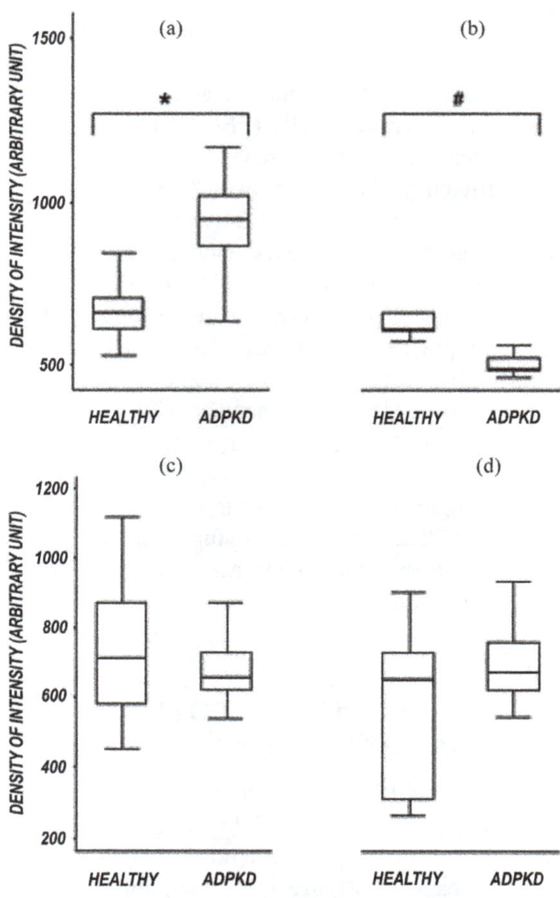

Figure 4. Morphometric analysis of CD133 and CD24 expression in tubules and glomerula of normal kidney and ADPKD kidney. CD133 expression is higher in ADPKD tubules than in normal tubules ($^{*}p < 0.001$). (a) CD133 expression is reduced in ADPKD glomerula compared to normal glomerula ($^{\#}p = 0.0016$); (b) CD24 expression is not statistically different in both normal tubules vs ADPKD tubules (c) and normal glomerula vs ADPKD glomerula (d) comparison.

reduced in ADPKD samples (**Figure 4**). After image analysis Mann-Whitney test resulted statistically significant for these comparisons (ADPKD tubules vs Normal tubules: $z = -7.681$ $p < 0.001$; ADPKD Glomerula vs Normal Glomerula: $z = 3.162$ $p = 0.0016$). CD 24 expression in glomerular and tubules does not show quantitative difference between normal and ADPKD samples (**Figure 4**).

2.2. Expression of CD133 and CD24 in Cultured Cells

Cells deriving from the cystic wall of ADPKD tissue were scraped and expanded in culture. The epithelial nature of these cells was confirmed by cytocheratin immunohistochemical characterization (**Figure 5** and **Table 1**: on line publication). In the subsequent analyses were used the clones of isolated cells that showed the complete expression of the cytokeratins (CAM 5.2, CK 7, MNF 116) usually expressed by cystic cells in tissue specimens.

Isolated cystic cells show a characteristic expression

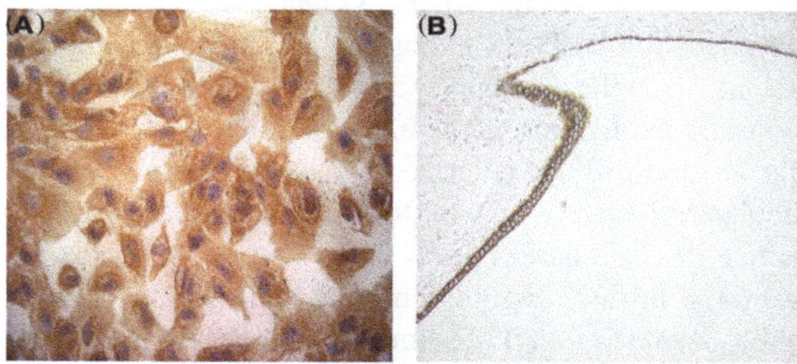

Figure 5. Example of cytokeratin expression (CK 7) in cultured cystic cells and in cyst. Immunohistochemical analysis reveals that both cultured cystic cells (A) and cystic epithelium (B) express CK 7.

pattern for CD133 and CD24 (**Figures 6(A)-(C)**: on line publication). CD133 is localized on the cellular membrane (**Figure 6(A)**: on line publication) while CD24 is globally diffused in the cytoplasm (**Figure 6(B)**: on line

Table 1. Immunohistochemical analysis of cytokeratin expression in ADPKD tissue. (1) Focal and global distribution; (2) Focal and segmental distribution.

	CAM 5.2	CK 7	CK 20	MNF 116
Bowman's Capsule	-	+ (2)	-	+ (2)
Tubules	+ (1)	+ (1)	-	+ (1)
Cysts	+ (2)	+ (2)	-	+ (2)

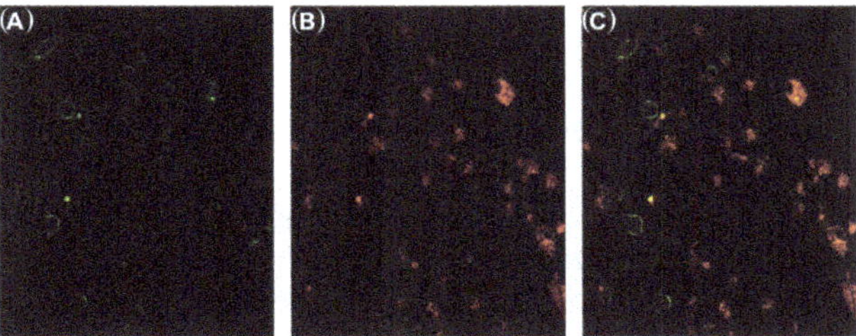

Figure 6. CD133 and CD24 expression in cystic cells in colture. CD133 is closely expressed by the cellular membrane (A). CD24 is expressed in the cytoplasm (B). CD133 and CD24 are co-expressed by the cystic cells (C).

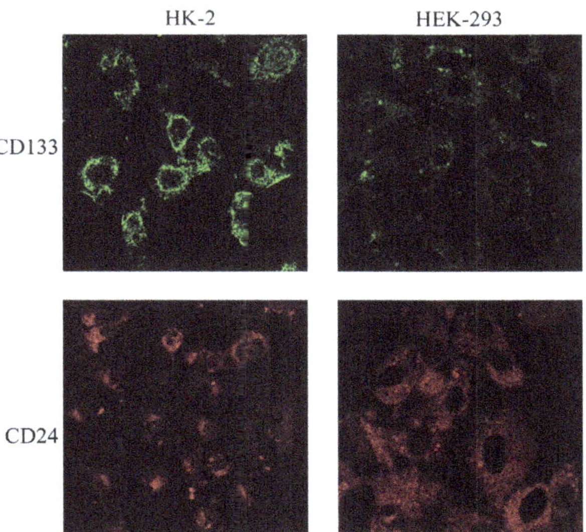

Figure 7. CD133 and CD24 expression in cellular lines. HK-2 show a similar antigen-expression pattern to cystic cells: CD133 is localized on the cellular membrane and CD24 is localized in the cytoplasm. HEK-293 have a diffused and low cellular expression of CD133 and CD24.

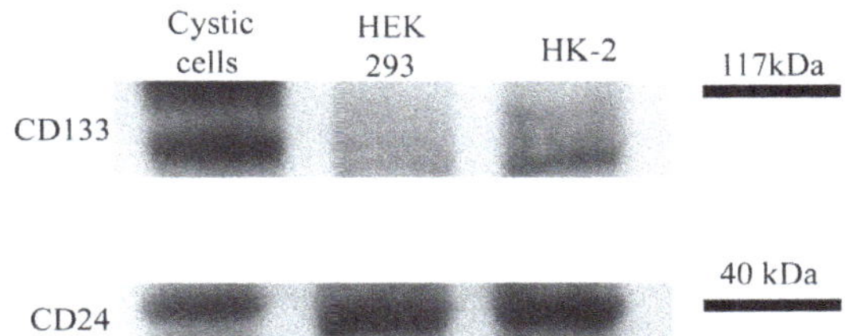

Figure 8. Western blot analysis of CD133 and CD24 expression in untreated HEK-293, HK-2 and cystic cells. Cystic cells express the highest amount of CD133 whereas HEK-293 the lowest. CD24 amount is similar in the three populations.

publication). The expression of CD24 is more diffuse while few cells are CD133+; only a small subset of isolated cystic cells are both CD133 and CD24 positive.

The same expression pattern is appreciable in HK-2 cell line while in HEK-293 cell line this peculiar pattern is lacking, both antigens presenting a cytoplasmic distribution (**Figure** 7: on line publication).

By western blot analysis CD133 is highly expressed by cystic cells, HK-2 presents an intermediate level of expression while HEK-293 cell line shows an almost absent expression (**Figure 8**). Analogous amounts of CD24 can be detected in the three cellular populations (**Figure 8**).

3. DISCUSSION

The high rate of proliferation and apoptosis of cystic cells is a well known phenomenon in ADPKD [4]. It has been interpreted as an unsuccessful proliferative repair response of abnormal tubular cells degenerating into cyst formation. The abnormal behavior of the tubule in ADPKD patients origins from genetic ablation of a critical function of the polycystin proteins and primary cilia [6,7]. This system is supposed to act as a sensor for renal injury monitoring the urinary intratubular flux. According to this model an abnormal constitutive activation of this pathway in ADPKD leads to the futile (proliferative) attempt to repair an essentially non existing injury [4].

In this scenario where proliferation and renal tissue repair are active we could speculate a possible role for renal progenitors. The target of our report has been an explorative analysis of surface antigens related to stemness in ADPKD tissue. A multipotent progenitor cell population constituted by CD24+ and CD133+ parietal epithelial cells (PECs), in adult human glomerula has been described. In this report a murine model of acute renal failure caused by glycerol induced rhabdomiolysis has been generated and injection of CD24+ and CD133+ PECs differentiated into tubular cells significantly ameliorating kidney damage 5. CD133 is a pentaspan transmembrane glycoprotein suspected to have a role in maintaining stem cell properties by suppressing differentiation and promoting proliferation. CD133 expression is also associated to several types of cancer [8-10]. CD133 function is not clear but its presence on early and undifferentiated cells is suggestive of a growth factor receptor, and the presence of five tyrosine residues on the 50-aa cytoplasmic tail may indicate that the protein is phosphorylated in response to ligand binding and triggers a signal transduction [11]. CD24 is a sialoglycoprotein expressed on mature granulocytes [12], B and T lymphocyte subsets [13,14], normal and cancer stem cells

[15,16]. The protein is anchored via a glycosyl phosphatidylinositol to cell surface. It acts as adhesion molecule and is involved in cell migration and signal transduction.

In our specimens we could appreciate the presence of a rich CD24+ and CD 133+ cell population. In ADPKD the distribution of these cells is qualitatively similar to normal tissue with the notable exception of a significant expression in cystic cells. Quantitatively CD 133+ cell population appears globally increased in ADPKD tissue. In particular we found a statistically significant increase of CD133 expression in tubules while glomerular expression appears reduced in ADPKD compared to control tissue. In this scenario the speculative hypothesis of an active migration of progenitors from the glomerular "niche" [17] to the tubule interstitial compartment is intriguing.

The abundant presence of CD133+ and CD24+ cells in ADPKD renal tissue sustains the hypothesis of an important role of this cell population in the disease. Inflammation and tubular damage are common features of ADPKD and CD133+ and CD24+ cells could likely play a role in the reparative process. Furthermore the diffuse presence of these elements in the cystic wall suggest that they could contribute to cystic expansion and disease progression. Anyway as far as now no evidence is available to sustain the hypothesis that CD133+ and CD24+ cystic cells are progenitors migrated into the cystic wall rather than the alternative hypothesis that they represent dedifferentiated [18] tubular cells that express "*de novo*" CD133 and CD24.

The expression of CD133 and CD24 is maintained in cystic cells isolated and cultured in vitro. Furthermore we evaluated the expression of these antigens in two tubular immortalized cellular lines, HEK293 and HK2.

4. CONCLUSION

In conclusion we demonstrated an abundant population of CD133+ CD24+cells in renal tissue obtained from ADPKD patients. This cell population is present in the cystic wall and abundant in tubules, which conversely seems to be reduced in ADPKD glomerula in comparison to normal tissue. The role of this cells was not clear yet, but it could be interesting to evaluate more cases of ADPKD, in different stages (from asymptomatic to late stage), and clarify if CD133+ CD24+cells were prognostic factors for a poorer or better evolution of the disease. Additionally, we cannot univocally conclude that the CD133 + CD24 + cystic cells represent migrated renal progenitors rather than tubular dedifferentiated cells 18, but with a deeper biomarker analysis we could understand their origin and their hypothetical migration. Knowing this element will be important to understand more in detail pathophysiology of ADPKD and find new target to delay the progression of the disease.

5. MATERIAL AND METHODS

5.1. Antibodies

CD133 monoclonal (293C3) antibody for immunofluorescence was provided by Miltenyi Biotec (Miltenyi Biotec, Bergisch Gladbach, Germany). CD133 monoclonal (W6B9C1) antibody for Western blot was provided by Miltenyi Biotec (Miltenyi Biotec, Bergisch Gladbach, Germany). CD24 monoclonal (SN3) antibody was provided by Santa Cruz (Santa Cruz Biotechnology Inc., Santa Cruz CA, USA). PKD1 rabbit polyclonal (H-260) antibody was provided by Santa Cruz (Santa Cruz Biotechnology Inc., Santa Cruz CA, USA). Goat anti mouse IgG2b-Alexa 568 conjugate, goat anti mouse IgG2b-Alexa 633 conjugate, goat anti mouse IgG1-Alexa 568 conjugate, goat anti rabbit IgG-Rhod conjugate, goat anti mouse IgG-HRP conjugate were used as secondary antibodies. Cytokeratins monoclonal (CAM 5.2, CK7 [RCK105], CK20 [SPM140] and MNF 116) antibody was provided by Becton Dickinson (only CAM 5.2) (Becton Dickinson, CA, USA) and Abcam (the others) (Abcam, Cambridge, UK).

5.2. Tissues

Normal kidney fragments were obtained from a cadaveric kidney donor. The kidney was not suitable for transplantation due to the incidental discovery of a neoplastic nodule of 5 cm at the lower pole upon macroscopic examination. The pathologic examination diagnosed a clear cell carcinoma (grade 2 according to Fuhrman classification; T1bN0M0 according to the International Union Against Cancer classification); the lower pole was excised and the remaining parenchyma was used in the following procedures. The remaining parenchyma did not reveal any evidence of clear cell carcinoma.

Polycystic kidney tissue was obtained from 2 ADPKD patients underwent to nephrectomy in preparation for receiving renal transplantation. All procedures were preceded by the approval of our Local Ethical Committee on human experimentation and informed consent was obtained from the patients.

5.3. Culture

Human Kidney 2 cells (HK-2) were maintained in DMEM F-12 (Invitrogen/GIBCO, Cralsbad, California) supplementated with 10% FBS (PAA laboratories GmbH, Pasching, Austria), 2000 U/ml penicillin (PAA laboratories GmbH, Pasching, Austria), 2000 ug/ml streptomycin (PAA laboratories GmbH, Pasching, Austria), and 20 mM L-glutamine (Invitrogen/GIBCO, Cralsbad, California).

Human Embryonic Kidney 293 cells (HEK-293) were maintained in DMEM (Invitrogen/GIBCO, Cralsbad,

California) supplementated with 5% FBS (PAA laboratories GmbH, Pasching, Austria), 2000 U/ml penicillin (PAA laboratories GmbH, Pasching, Austria), 2000 ug/ml streptomycin (PAA laboratories GmbH, Pasching, Austria), and 20 mM L-glutamine (Invitrogen/GIBCO, Cralsbad, California).

HK-2 and HEK-293 were grown two weeks and medium was changed every two days. After every week, cells were washed with PBS (PAA laboratories GmbH, Pasching, Austria) and were trypsinizated (Invitrogen/GIBCO, Cralsbad, California). Cells harvested were, in part, seeded on chambers slides and the others were used to extract proteins.

Cystic cells were obtained by fragments of renal cysts deprived of external membrane. Each cyst was picked up, was divided in some little fragments and were digested by collagenase (Invitrogen/GIBCO, Cralsbad, California) for one hours. Every pieces of a single cysts were seeded on a plate, previously treated by collagene type I (Invitrogen/GIBCO, Cralsbad, California), the same medium used for HK-2.

5.4. Immunofluorescence

Three-micrometer frozen kidney samples mounted on Super Frost Plus slides (Menzel-Gläser, Thermo Scientific, Waltham, MA) were cut by a cryostat (Leica 1720, Leica Mycrosystems, Heerbrog, Germany). The sections, or cellular spots, were fixed with PFA for 10 min, washed with PBS. Slides were coated (3% Bovine Serum Albumin in PBS buffer) for 1 h at 20°C. Slides were incubated by primary antibody for 1 h at 37°C, washed with PBS and successively incubated by secondary antibody for 1 h at 20°C. Primary and secondary antibodies were diluted in coating solution. Slides were closed with Vectashield® Mounting Medium with DAPI (Vector Laboratories, Inc., Burlingame, CA, USA). Tissue samples, or cells, were examined by immunofluorescence microscopy (Olympus BX41 Microscopy). Laser Confocal images were obtained with Leica TCS SP2 (Leica Microsystems, Heerbrog, Germany).

5.5. Immunohistochemical

The same type of sample mounted on slides used for immunofluorescence analysis was handled for immunohistochemical evaluation. Slides were coated (3% Bovine Serum Albumin in PBS buffer) for 1 h at 20°C. Slides were incubated by primary antibody over night at 4°C, washed with PBS and successively incubated by secondary antibody (conjugated horse radish peroxidise) by for 30 min at 20°C. Hydrogen peroxide and diaminobenzidine (DAB) (SIGMA-ALDRICH, St. Louis, MO, USA) were used to obtain chromogen reaction. Olympus BX41 microscope was used to evaluate the samples.

5.6. Image Analysis

Images of immunoflucrescence-marked kidney were sampled by an acquisition system composed by Olympus BX41 microscope, Olympus XC30 and CELL B 3.0 analysis image processing (Olympus Europa GmbH, Hamburg Germany). Images were saved in tagged image file format (.tiff). The files were analyzed with Inspector Matrox (Matrox Electronic System Ltd., Quebec Canada). ROI (region of interest) defines a portion of image that contains areas to analyze. ROI of each renal component (tubules, glomeruli and cysts) were sampled and converted in a list of single grey tone amount, from white (highest value) to black (zero). Background fluorescence was obtained sampling spot of negative structure, such mesangium or negative tubules, in every image.

5.7. Statistical Analysis

Total brightness/positive area ratio was calculated for each ROI. The following analysis of expression were performed: CD24+ in tubules of normal tissue, CD24+ in glomeruli of normal tissue, CD24+ in tubules of ADPKD samples, CD24+ in glomeruli of ADPKD samples, CD24+ in cysts of ADPKD samples, CD133+ in tubules of normal samples, CD133 + in glomeruli of normal tissue, CD133+ in tubules of ADPKD samples, CD133 + in glomeruli of ADPKD samples, CD133 + in cysts of ADPKD samples. Normal and ADPKD tissue components were compare by Mann-Whitney test. Results were considered statistically significant for $p < 0.01$. All statistical analysis were performed with the software SPSS Statistics 19.0.1 (IBM corporation, New York, USA).

5.8. Western Blot Analysis

Total proteins were extracted from cellular pellets with Triton X-100 based lysis buffer. Proteins were loaded on SDS-PAGE (3% stacking, 7.5% resolving), previously denatured with 4X Reducing Loading Buffer (200mM TrisHCl, 20% β-Mercapto Ethanol, 8% SDS, 0.4% Bromofenol Blue, 40% glycerol). After SDS-PAGE run and transblot, nitrocellulose membranes were previously incubated by antibodies anti-CD133 and anti-CD24 and subsequently by horse radish peroxidise conjugated secondary antibodies. The detection was obtained by exposition of radiological plates to peroxidise substrate activated by the enzyme.

6. DISCLOSURES

The authors certify that there is no conflict of interest with any financial organization regarding the material discussed in the manuscript.

7. ACKNOWLEDGEMENTS

This study was supported by the Research Program "Regione-Università 2007-2009-Innovative Research" granted by the Regional Sanitary Service of Emilia Romagna, Italy.

REFERENCES

[1] Chang, M.Y. and Ong, A.C. (2008) Autosomal dominant polycystic kidney disease: Recent advances in pathogenesis and treatment. *Nephron Physiology*, **108**, 1-7. http://dx.doi.org/10.1159/000112495

[2] Wei, W., Hackmann, K., Xu, H., Germino, G. and Qian, F. (2007) Characterization of cis-autoproteolysis of polycystin-1, the product of human polycystic kidney disease 1 gene. *Journal of Biological Chemistry*, **282**, 21729-21737. http://dx.doi.org/10.1074/jbc.M703218200

[3] Delmas, P., Padilla, F., Osorio, N., Coste, B., Raoux, M. and Crest, M. (2004) Polycystins, calcium signaling, and human diseases. *Biochemical and Biophysical Research Communications*, **322**, 1374-1383. http://dx.doi.org/10.1016/j.bbrc.2004.08.044

[4] Weimbs, T. (2007) Polycystic kidney disease and renal injury repair: Common pathways, fluid flow, and the function of polycystin-1. *American Journal of Physiology, Renal Physiology*, **293**, F1423-F1432. http://dx.doi.org/10.1152/ajprenal.00275.2007

[5] Sagrinati, C., Netti, G.S., Mazzinghi, B., *et al.* (2006) Isolation and characterization of multipotent progenitor cells from the Bowman's capsule of adult human kidneys. *Journal of the American Society of Nephrology*, **17**, 2443-2456. http://dx.doi.org/10.1681/ASN.2006010089

[6] Rodat-Despoix, L. and Delmas, P. (2009) Ciliar functions in the nephron. *Pflugers Archiv*, **458**, 179-187. http://dx.doi.org/10.1007/s00424-008-0632-0

[7] Praetorius, H.A. and Spring, K.R. (2003) The renal cell primary cilium functions as a flow sensor. *Current Opinion in Nephrology and Hypertension*, **12**, 517-520. http://dx.doi.org/10.1097/00041552-200309000-00006

[8] Tirino, V., Desiderio, V., Paino, F., *et al.* (2011) Human primary bone sarcomas contain CD133+ cancer stem cells displaying high tumorigenicity *in vivo*. *FASEB Journal*, **25**, 2022-2030.

[9] Lorico, A. and Rappa, G. (2011) Phenotypic heterogeneity of breast cancer stem cells. *Journal of Oncology*, **2011**, 135039. http://dx.doi.org/10.1155/2011/135039

[10] Janikova, M., Skarda, J., Dziechciarkova, M., *et al.* (2010) Identification of CD133+/nestin+ putative cancer stem cells in non-small cell lung cancer. *Biomedical Papers of the Medical Faculty of the University Palacky, Olomouc, Czechoslovakia*, **154**, 321-326. http://dx.doi.org/10.5507/bp.2010.048

[11] Miraglia, S., Godfrey, W., Yin, A.H., *et al.* (1997) A novel five-transmembrane hematopoietic stem cell antigen: Isolation, characterization, and molecular cloning. *Blood*, **90**, 5013-5021.

[12] Kobayashi, S.D., Voyich, J.M., Whitney, A.R. and DeLeo, F.R. (2005) Spontaneous neutrophil apoptosis and regulation of cell survival by granulocyte macrophage-colony stimulating factor. *Journal of Leukocyte Biology*, **78**, 1408-1418. http://dx.doi.org/10.1189/jlb.0605289

[13] Vlkova, M., Fronkova, E., Kanderova, V., *et al.* (2010) Characterization of lymphocyte subsets in patients with common variable immunodeficiency reveals subsets of naive human B cells marked by CD24 expression. *Journal of Immunology*, **185**, 6431-6438. http://dx.doi.org/10.4049/jimmunol.0903876

[14] Berga-Bolanos, R., Drews-Elger, K., Aramburu, J. and Lopez-Rodriguez, C. (2010) NFAT5 regulates T lymphocyte homeostasis and CD24-dependent T cell expansion under pathologic hypernatremia. *Journal of Immunology*, **185**, 6624-6635. http://dx.doi.org/10.4049/jimmunol.1001232

[15] Jiang, W., Sui, X., Zhang, D., *et al.* (2011) CD24: A novel surface marker for PDX1-positive pancreatic progenitors derived from human embryonic stem cells. *Stem Cells*, **29**, 609-607.

[16] Myung, J.H., Gajjar, K.A., Pearson, R.M., Launiere, C.A., Eddington, D.T. and Hong, S. (2011) Direct measurements on CD24-mediated rolling of human breast cancer MCF-7 cells on E-selectin. *Analytical Chemistry*, **83**, 1078-1083. http://dx.doi.org/10.1021/ac102901e

[17] Romagnani, P. and Kalluri, R. (2009) Possible mechanisms of kidney repair. *Fibrogenesis & Tissue Repair*, **2**, 3. http://dx.doi.org/10.1186/1755-1536-2-3

[18] Ong, A.C. and Harris, P.C. (2005) Molecular pathogenesis of ADPKD: The polycystin complex gets complex. *Kidney International*, **67**, 1234-1247. http://dx.doi.org/10.1111/j.1523-1755.2005.00201.x

Pretreatment with antioxidants prevent bone injury by improving bone marrow microenvironment for stem cells

Lingling Xian[1,2], Michael Lou[1], Xiangwei Wu[1,2], Bing Yu[1], Frank Frassica[1], Mei Wan[1], Lijuan Pang[1,2], Chunyi Wen[3], Erik Tryggestad[4], John Wong[4], Xu Cao[1*]

[1]Department of Orthopaedic Surgery, School of Medicine, Johns Hopkins University, Baltimore, USA;
[*]Corresponding Author: xcao11@jhmi.edu
[2]Shihezi Medical College, Shihezi University, Shihezi, China
[3]Department of Orthopaedics, University of Hong Kong, Hong Kong, China
[4]Radiation Oncology Medical Physics, School of Medicine, Johns Hopkins University, Baltimore, USA

ABSTRACT

Irradiation induces bone injury by generating free radicals that adversely affect the microenvironment for Mesenchymal stem cells (MSCs) and damages bone marrow blood vessels. We wished to investigate the efficacy of antioxidant administration in protecting stem cell microenvironments and promoting bone marrow vasculature recovery after radiation treatment. The antioxidant ascorbic acid was administered 3 times at a dosage: 150 mg/kg/day to experimenttal groups 3 days before targeted radiation by a unique Small Animal Radiation Research Platform (SARRP). Histological staining indicated that antioxidant treated mice had less severe bone marrow damage 1 week after irradiation with substantial marrow cellular recovery 4 weeks later. Flow cytometry analysis showed that antioxidant administration was correlated with a rebound in MSC quantity in bone marrow. Anti-oxidant treatment was also observed to allow for better vasculature retention and recovery through angiographic imaging. Our data suggests that pre-treatment with ascorbic acid serves to improve bone marrow microenvironments for bone marrow stem cells after radiation treatment.

Keywords: Irradiation; Bone Injury; Stem Cells; Microenvironment; Antioxidant

1. INTRODUCTION

Radiation therapy has been widely utilized in the clinical setting to treat a variety of malignancies such as gliomas of the brain, prostate tumors, lung carcinomas, lymphoma, gynecologic cancers, and breast cancers [1-3]. Ionizing radiation damages bone tissue resulting in bone density loss and an increased risk of fractures [4,5]. Bone insufficiency can be as high as 45% amongst female patients post-radiation treatments for cervical cancers [6]. Animal models suggest substantial loss of trabecular bone after irradiation [7]. Currently, few preventive steps are taken to ensure maximized recovery after radiation treatment.

Ionizing radiation creates oxidative stress by generating free radicals and reactive oxygen species that damage major cellular components such as proteins, membranes, and nucleic acids [8]. Hematopoietic stem cell sensitivity to radiation is well documented [9]. However, the response and sensitivity of MSCs to radiation is not well studied. MSCs differentiation fates include osteogenic and adipogenic lineages, hence their involvement in bone remodeling and repair [1,10]. Bone marrow cells experience high sensitivity to the effects of ionizing radiation as demonstrated in murine animal models [11]. Irradiation creates oxidative cellular damage, along with resulting in marrow microenvironment changes weeks after administration [1]. Therefore, curbing the pervasiveness of damage from free radicals would be an effective strategy for clinical recovery post-treatment.

Damaging free radicals arising from irradiation in the bone microenvironment affects bone marrow stem cell viability [1]. Damage to bone marrow vasculatures, major stem cell niches, likely affects the recovery of MSCs in the irradiated areas. In this study, we investigated the effects of antioxidant administration on bone marrow stem cells and residing microenvironment after irradiation. The Small Animal Research Radiation Platform (SARRP) we utilized allows for precise radiation administration with resolution up to 1 mm [12]. Our findings suggest that administration of the antioxidant ascorbic acid lessened the extent of radiation damage of bone marrow micro-environments for stem cells, and improves recovery prognosis.

2. MATERIALS AND METHODS

2.1. Mice

8-week-old c57BL/6 male mice were given per os (p.o.) ascorbic acid at doses of 0, and 150 mg/kg/day 3 days before irradiation. The irradiation procedure was done as previously reported [1]. Briefly, a clinically applicable dose rate of (4 Gy min^{-1}) was delivered using 225 kVp with a 3.0 mm focal spot with up to a 13 mA beam current. Irradiation was given once per day for 5 days, wit the total dose at 20 Gys. All animals were maintained in the animal facility of the Johns Hopkins University School of Medicine. The experimental protocol was reviewed and approved by the Institutional Animal Care and Use Committee of the Johns Hopkins University, Baltimore MD, USA.

2.2. Histochemistry and Histomorphometric Analysis

At the time of sacrifice, proximal and distal femora of mice 1 week and 4 weeks post-irradiation treated or untreated with ascorbic acid were resected and fixed in 10% buffered formalin for 48 hours, decalcified in 10% ethylenediamine tetraacetic acid (EDTA) (pH 7.4) for 20 days, and embedded in paraffin. 4-μm-thick longitude-nally oriented sections of bone including the metaphysis and diaphysis were processed for hematoxylin and eosin (H&E) staining. Sections were microphotographed to perform histomorphometric measurements on the highlighted areas of the bone displayed on the digitalized image. Quantitative histomorphometric analysis was conducted in a blinded fashion with OsteoMeasure XP Software (OsteoMetrics, Inc., Decatur, GA, USA). 2-dimensional parameters of trabecular bone were measured in a 2 mm square, one-mm distal to the lowest point of the growth plate in the trabecular bone.

2.3. CFU-F and CFU-Ob Assays

At the time of sacrifice, the femurs were cut in half, into proximal and distal pieces, and bone marrow from medullary cavities were collected individually. Cell number was determined after removal of red blood cells with Zapoglobin (Coulter Corp.). For assays of CFU-F and CFU-Ob number, 1×10^6 murine marrow cells were plated into six well plates in 2 mL α-MEM supplemented with glutamine (2 mM az), penicillin (100 U/mL), streptomycin sulfate (100 μg/mL), and 20% lot-selected FBS. Duplicate cultures were established. After 2 - 3 hr of adhesion, unattached cells were removed, and 2.5×10^6 irradiated guinea pig feeder cells (provided by Dr. Bren-dan J. Canning) were added to the cultivation medium of adherent cultures immediately after washing. On day 14, cultures were fixed and stained with 0.5% crystal violet. Colonies containing 50 or more cells were noted. For CFU-Ob assay, the cells were cultured with osteogenic medium (10% FBS, 10^{-7} M dexamethasone, 10 mM β-glycerol phosphate and 50 μM ascorbate-2-phos phate) for 21 days and analyzed with alizarin red staining. The colony-forming efficiency was determined by number of colonies per 10^6 marrow cells plated.

2.4. Fluorescence-Activated Cell Sorting (FACS) Analysis

Cell aliquots isolated from bone marrow were incubated for 20 minutes at 4˚C with phycoerythrin (PE)-, fluorescein isothiocyanate (FITC)-, peridinin chlorophyll protein (Per CP)-, and allophycocyanin (APC)-conjugated antibodies against mouse Sca-1, CD29, CD45, and CD11b (Bio-legend). Acquisition was performed on a fluorescence-activated cell sorting (FACS) Aria model (BD Biosciences), and analysis was performed using a FACS DIVE software version 6.1.3 (BD Biosciences).

2.5. Measurement of Lipid Oxidation

Peripheral venous blood was drawn into syringes containing preservative-free heparin (25 U/mL, Gibco, Life Technologies, Gaithersburg, MD) and centrifuged at 3500 rpm for 10 minutes at 5˚C - 10˚C to isolate the plasma. Bone marrow samples were collected into preservative-free heparinized saline (25 U/mL). And centrifuged at 3500 rpm for 10 min at 5˚C - 10˚C to isolate bone marrow plasma. Plasma lipid oxidation was assessed by determining the level of Thiobarbituric Acid Reactive Substances (TBARS) using a TBARS assay kit (zep-tometrix).

2.6. Micro-CT Angiography Analysis

Blood vessels in long bone were imaged by contrast-enhanced micro-CT angiography. The thoracic cavity was opened after the animals were anesthetized. The vasculature was flushed with 0.9% normal saline solution containing heparin sodium (100 U/mL) through a needle inserted into the left ventricle, and then pressure fixed with 10% neutral buffered formalin. After that, the vessels were flushed again using heparinized saline solution. Finally, the vasculature was perfused with a radiopaque silicone rubber compound containing lead chromate (Microfil MV-122; Flow Tech). The corpses were stored at 4˚C overnight for contrast agent polymerization. Mouse femurs were dissected from the bodies and soaked for 4 days in 10% neutral buffered formalin to ensure complete tissue fixation. Specimens were subsequently treated for 48 hours in a formic acid-based solution (Cal-Ex II) for decalcification in order to visualize the vasculature inside bone. Images were obtained using a high-resolution micro-CT imaging system (5.7-μm isotropic voxel size) (Skyscan 1172, Kontich, Belgium). Isotropic voxel size for the scans is 5.5 μm. X-ray voltage of 50 kV and 200 μA were applied for image acquisition. After standardized reconstruction by a modified Feldkamp algorithm via SkyScan recon software, the datasets were analyzed using SkyScan CT-analyser software. The vasculature was then examined with ANT™ software (SkyScan) by the following parameters: Vessel volume/tissue volume, vessel number and vessel thickness.

2.7. Statistics

Data were presented as the mean ± SEM and analyzed using an one-way analysis of variance (ANOVA) followed by Dunnett's test.

3. RESULTS

3.1. Effects of Antioxidant Administration on Bone Marrow Microenvironment after Local Irradiation

The SARRP device was utilized to provide an accurate delivery of radiation at 1 mm resolution with additional aid provided by micro-CT and X-ray imaging. C57BL/6 mice were irradiated at the left distal (LD) half of the femur (**Figure 1(a)**) with a dosage of 4 Grays once a day for 5 consecutive days with the cumulative amount of radiation exposure at 20 Grays. In order to examine the effects of anti-oxidant administration on MSCs and vascular changes post-irradiation, the antioxidant ascorbic acid or Vitamin C was orally given at 150 mg/kg/day 3

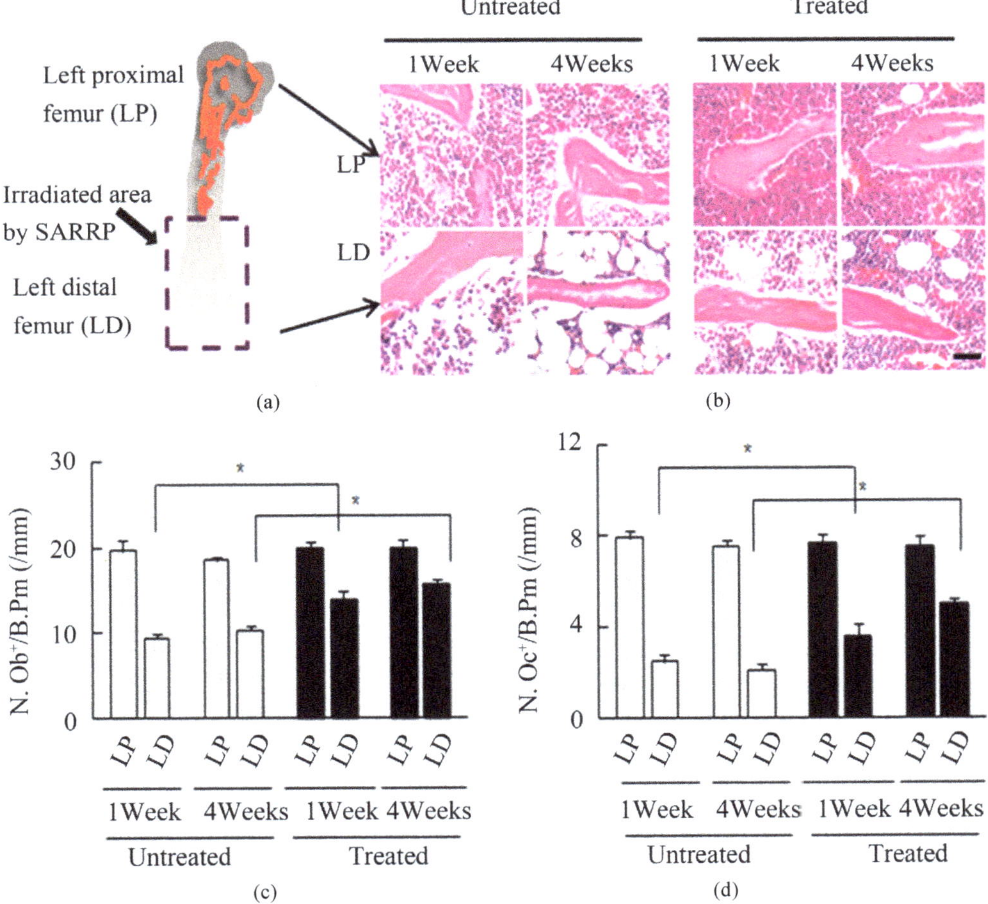

Figure 1. H&E-staining and bone histomorphometric analysis of trabecular bone from the ascorbic acid treated or untreated c57BL/6 male mice 1 week and 4 weeks post-local irradiation; (a) Model of local irradiation on left distal femur; (b) Light micrographs of H&E-staining on trabecular bone sections from proximal and distal femora of mice 1 week and 4 weeks post-irradiation treated or untreated with ascorbic acid. LP: Left proximal femur, LD: Left distal femur, Scale bar: 50 μm; (c) Number of osteoblasts per bone perimeter ($N.Ob^+/B.Pm$); (d) Number of osteoclasts per bone perimeter ($N.Oc^+/B.Pm$). Data represent the mean ± SEM; n = 10; $^*p < 0.05$.

days before irradiation. The control group received no ascorbic acid. The left proximal (LP) femur area did not receive direct radiation. Histological staining indicated that the amount of radiation damage was extensive in the LD femoral areas at 1 week and this damage was also found at 4 weeks after radiation treatment (**Figure 1(b)**). Significant bone marrow cell ablation and irradiation induced adipogenesis can be observed in the LD antioxidant untreated mice even 4 weeks after radiation. The LD antioxidant treated mice had less severe damage 1 week after irradiation with substantial marrow cellular recovery at 4 weeks (**Figure 1(b)**). The results suggest that irradiation damages the bone marrow microenvironment and antioxidant treatment may be able to lessen the extent of that damage.

We analyzed the effects of irradiation and antioxidant treatment on bone cells with histomorphometry. Our results indicated that osteoblast and osteoclast cell number were significantly lower in the left distal femoral sections (LD) 1 and 4 weeks after irradiation when compared with proximal femoral controls (LP) (**Figures 1(c)** and **(d)**). The mice showed increased numbers of osteoclast and osteoblast cells when treated with the antioxidant in 1 week and 4 weeks post-treatment in comparison to their untreated counterparts (**Figures 1(c)** and **(d)**). The results support that treatment with antioxidants elevated the level of bone cells 1 week and 4 weeks after irradiation.

3.2. Effects of Antioxidant Administration on MSCs Potential Post-Irradiation

Bone Marrow Mesenchymal Stem Cells (BMSCs) were isolated from the Right Distal (RD), Right Proximal (RP), Left Distal (LD), and Left Proximal (LP) quadrants. A CFU-Fibroblast (CFU-F) assay was then conducted to examine the effects of irradiation on BMSCs. In the antioxidant untreated left femur isolates (LD and LP), none to very few numbers of cells were colony forming even 4 weeks after irradiation. However, in the antioxidant treated isolates, viable colony forming cells were observed at 1 and 4 weeks post irradiation. CFU-F counts in antioxidant treated LD and LP isolates were significantly higher than their untreated counterparts (**Figures 2(a)** and **(c)**). We performed a CFU-Osteoblast (CFU-Ob) assay visualized via alizarin red staining to assess the differentiation potential of BMSC isolates. With antioxidant treatment, differentiated cells obtained from both LD and LP isolates have significantly elevated CFU-Ob counts (**Figures 2(b)** and **(d)**). Of note, LP cell numbers are affected despite that quadrant not having gone through direct radiation exposure. The assays suggest that radiation damage is extensive; affecting BMSCs away from the local site of radiation and antioxidant administration appears to improve the number and also the differentiation potential of BMSCs in bone marrow 1 and 4 weeks post-radiation.

Previous studies have established that $CD29^+$ $Sca1^+$ $CD45^-$ $CD11b^-$ cells in the bone marrow stroma belong to a subset of MSCs in circulation [13]. Local detection of $CD29^+$ $Sca1^+$ $CD45^-$ $CD11b^-$ MSCs isolated from irradiated mice showed a very significant drop in MSCs from LD antioxidant treated, untreated and LP treated and untreated 1 week after irradiation (**Figure 2(e)**). However, in LP antioxidant treated groups 4 weeks post irradiation, MSC numbers have recovered substantially to levels matching our contralateral controls-RD, RP (**Figure 2(e)**). A similar increase in cell number was also observed for LD antioxidant treated mice as well. Overall, antioxidant treated groups in the LP and LD allowed for significantly higher MSC counts than untreated groups. These results support that administration of ascorbic acid allowed for increased MSC numbers locally following irradiation.

3.3. Antioxidants Reduce Free Radical Levels from Local Irradiation

Oxidative stress from radiation damage was monitored utilizing a thiobarbituric acid reactive substances assay (TBARS) with bone marrow isolates from antioxidant treated, and untreated subsets with all four quadrants (LD, LP, RD, RP) present. TBARS assessed the consequences of lipid peroxidation and malondialdehyde levels specifically [1]. In antioxidant untreated mice, LD TBARS levels remained high and relatively unchanged from 1 and 4 weeks after irradiation (**Figure 3(a)**). In the not directly irradiated LP area, TBARS levels were increased at 1 week and decreased to the basal level at 4 weeks indicating that free radicals diffused ipsilaterally to the proximal femur resulting in MSCs damage. Noticeably, LP antioxidant treated mice had no significant elevation in TBARS levels even 1 week after irradiation. Similarly, LD antioxidant treated mice showed significantly decreased TBARs levels compared to LD untreated mice (**Figure 3(a)**). TBARS analysis conducted with peripheral blood plasma showed higher levels 1 week after radiation in circulation in the antioxidant untreated group. Antioxidant treated mice demonstrated little to no increase of TBARS in blood plasma after irradiation (**Figure 3(b)**). Our results demonstrate that irradiation generates free radicals, whose levels decrease after antioxidants are administered.

3.4. Antioxidant Treatment on MSC Vascular Niche Preservation

Bone vasculature is a crucial component in the formation and remodeling of bone. Micro-phil perfused femurs

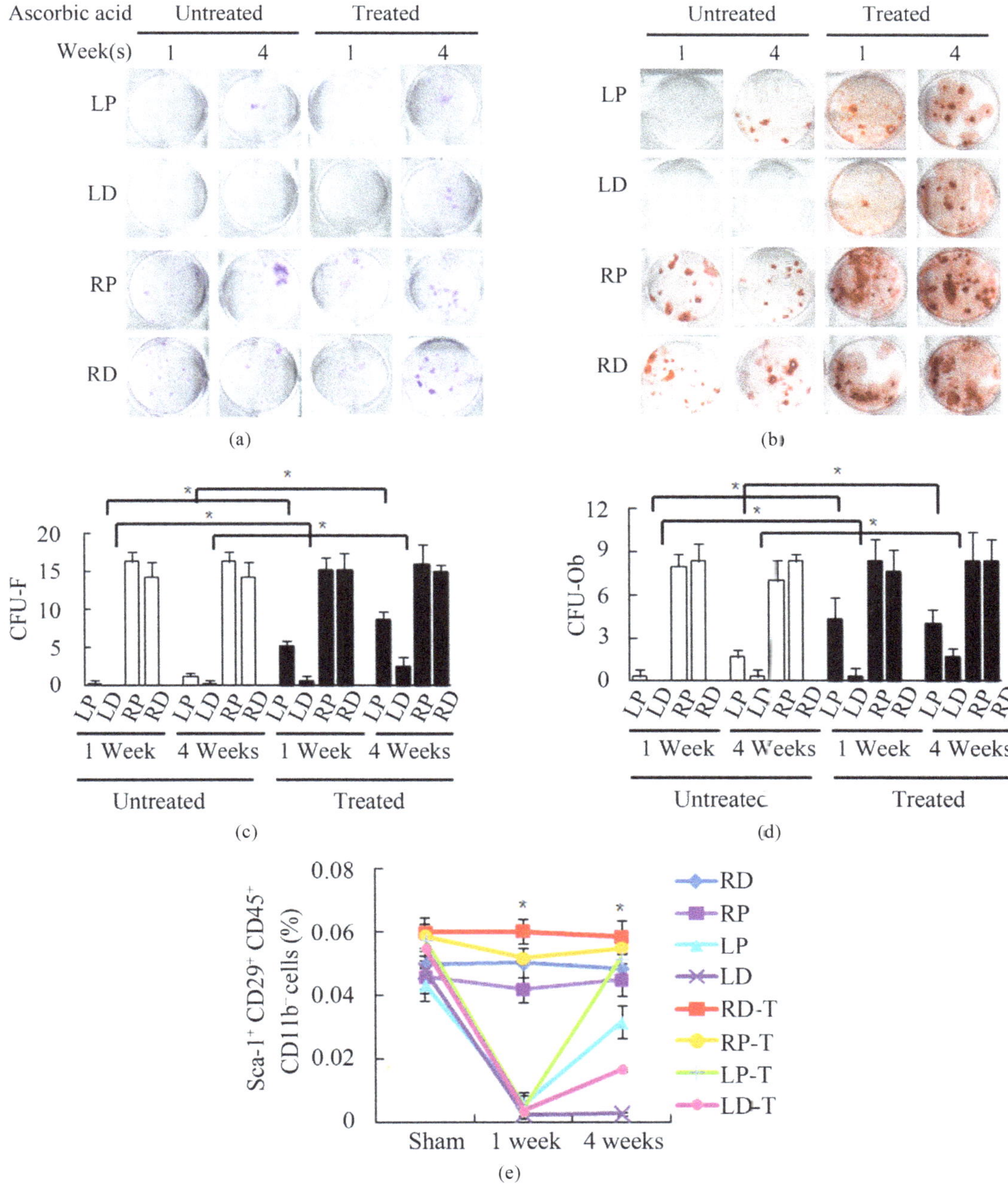

Figure 2. Antioxidant effects on irradiation induced mesenchymal stem cells change in bone marrow. (a) (b) Colonies formed from harvested femur bone marrow of mice as indicated in CFU-F and CFU-Ob assays (1×10^5 bone marrow nucleated cells were plated into six-well plates); (c) (d) The colony-forming efficiency was determined by number of colonies per 10^5 marrow cells plated. Data represent the mean ± SEM of triplicate cultures of bone marrow nucleated cells from five individual mice, $^*p < 0.05$; (e) FACS analysis of sorted Sca-1^+, CD29^+, CD45^- and CD11b^- cells from bone marrow cell suspension obtained from mice. LP: Left proximal femur; LD: Left distal femur; RP: Right proximal femur; RD: Right distal femur. Data represent the mean ± SEM; n = 10; $^*p < 0.05$.

were imaged utilizing 3-dimensional micro-CT and analyzed for parameters after irradiation. 1 week postirradiation, LD sites showed almost complete vasculature ablation (**Figure 4(a)**). However, in the antioxidant treated mice, there was more intact vasculature compared to the untreated mice in the left femur as a whole (**Figure 4(a)**). Morphometric results assessing vessel volume, thickness, and number yielded similar results suggesting that mice treated with antioxidants typically had more intact vasculature and suggested more vasculature re-

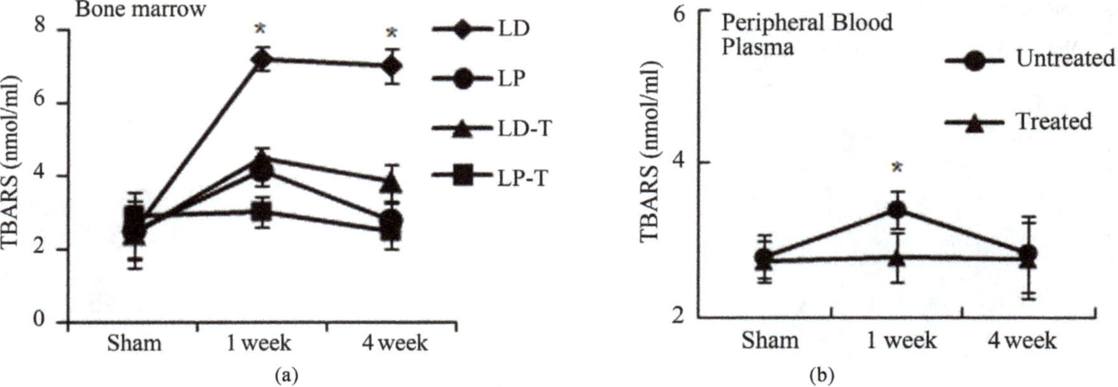

Figure 3. Antioxidant prevent the production of free radicals by local irradiation. Free radicals were assessed in both bone marrow (a) and peripheral blood (b); Pre-irradiation, and 1 week and 4 weeks post-irradiation detected by thiobarbituric acid reactive substances (TBARS) assay. LP: Left proximal femur; LD: Left distal femur; LP-T: Left proximal femur from mice treated with ascorbic acid; LD-T: Left distal femur from mice treated with ascorbic acid. Data represent the mean ± SEM; n = 10; $^{*}p < 0.05$.

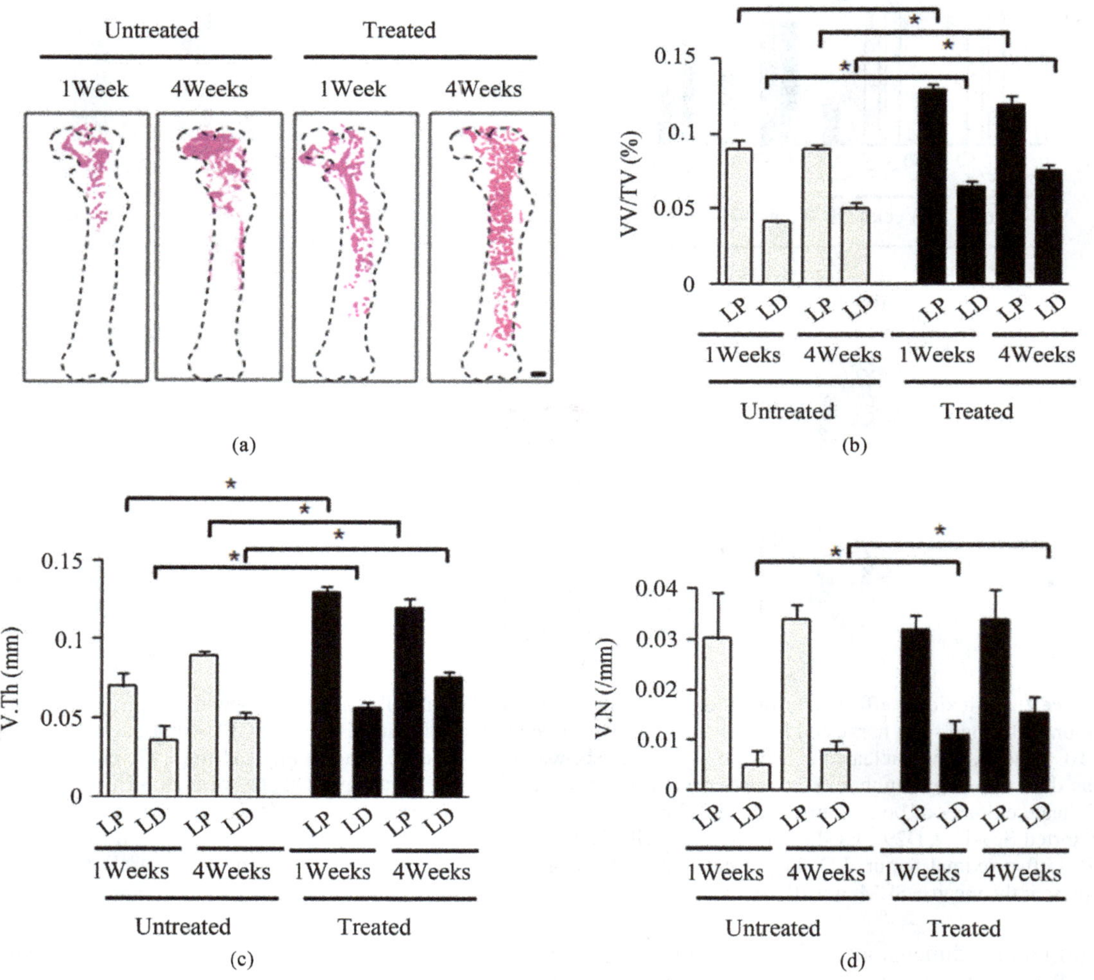

Figure 4. Effects of antioxidant on irradiation induced bone marrow angiogenesis. (a) Representative 3-dimensional μCT images of femora from the mice after local irradiation. Scale bar: 1 mm ((b)-(d)); Quantitative μCT angiography analysis. Vascular volume fraction (VV/TV) (b); Vascular thickness (V.Th) (c); and Vascular number (V.N) (d) were measured. Data represent the mean ± SEM; n = 10; $^{*}p < 0.05$.

covery compared to their untreated counterparts in the left femur (**Figures 4(b)-(d)**). Vasculatures in the LD and LP antioxidant treated mice were more numerous, thicker, and had higher volume compared to the untreated group (**Figures 4(b)-(d)**). These data suggested that antioxidant administration is correlated with vasculature retention and recovery after irradiation.

4. DISCUSSION

Irradiation induces bone injury by producing free radicals that adversely affect the stem cell microenvironment for MSCs while damaging bone marrow blood vessels [1]. Improving bone marrow microenvironment and accelerating vasculogenesis could be therapeutically useful for patients to minimize radiation-induced bone injury. The aim of this study was to investigate the efficacy of antioxidant treatment in protecting bone marrow stem cells and promoting bone marrow vasculature recovery after radiation treatment.

Previous studies have shown that ascorbic acid acts as a protective agent against radiation and is involved in maintaining human fibroblast survival, DNA double stranded break repair, and sister chromatid exchanges [14]. Pretreatment with ascorbic acid may effectively prevent radiation-induced irreversible gastrointestinal damage (GI syndrome) by down-regulating apoptosis associated genes [15]. Improved survival as a result of a high antioxidant diet has been attributed to a reduction in radiation-induced oxidative stress and apoptosis of bone marrow hematopoetic stem cells [16]. The effects of antioxidant on MSCs survival and repopulation are still unclear. We found that histological analysis in ascorbic acid treated mice showed alleviated bone marrow microenvironment damage and substantial cellular repopulation 1 and 4 weeks after radiation. CFU-F and CFU-Ob assays indicated more active MSCs existing in both the LP and LD femurs in ascorbic acid treated mice. Our evidence suggests that administration of antioxidants reduced the effects of free radical damage and ROS, thus allowing better MSCs survival and recovery.

Several studies reported that MSCs reside in a perivascular niche, and bone marrow vasculature is a critical component of bone tissue and functions in maintenance of MSCs [17]. We found that high retention of the vasculature associating with antioxidant treatment is correlated with improved bone marrow recovery following irradiation. Reduction of free radical levels by ascorbic acid may contribute to the alleviation of vascular injury following irradiation. However, the mechanisms still need to be further investigated.

Our study suggests that administration of antioxidants prior to radiation exposure may initially limit the extent of radiation damage by allowing vasculature retention and higher MSCs survival. Such effects could therefore shorten the recovery time by allowing for earlier cellular repopulation of the radiated bone marrow. Previous studies have suggested that a diet high in antioxidants may improve patient prognosis following radiation treatments for cancer [18]. In this study, we provide suggestive evidence through *in vivo* analysis of the bone marrow itself. Furthermore, bone insufficiency could be correlated with bone marrow MSCs depletion from direct and indirect effects of radiation [1]. It could be proposed that retention of bone marrow MSCs provided by taking preventive antioxidants could function as a therapeutic approach to reducing the side effects on bone tissue following irradiation.

5. ACKNOWLEDGEMENTS

This project was supported by National Institutes of Health Grant AR 053973 (XC).

REFERENCES

[1] Cao, X., Wu, X., Frassica, D., Yu, B., Pang, L., Xian, L., Wan, M., Lei, W., Armour, M., Tryggestad, E., Wong, J., Wen, C.Y., Lu, W.W. and Frassica, F.J. (2011) Irradiation induces bone injury by damaging bone marrow microenvironment for stem cells. *Proceedings of the National Academy of Sciences of USA*, **108**, 1609-1614. doi:10.1073/pnas.1015350108

[2] Ng, A.K., Bernardo, M.V., Weller, E., Backstrand, K., Silver, B., Marcus, K.C., Tarbell, N.J., Stevenson, M.A., Friedberg, J.W. and Mauch, P.M. (2002) Second malignancy after Hodgkin disease treated with radiation therapy with or without chemotherapy: Long-term risks and risk factors. *Blood*, **100**, 1989-1996. doi:10.1182/blood-2002-02-0634

[3] Taghian, A., de Vathaire, F., Terrier, P., Le, M., Auquier, A., Mouriesse, H., Grimaud, E., Sarrazin, D. and Tubiana, M. (1991) Long-term risk of sarcoma following radiation treatment for breast cancer. *International Journal of Radiation Oncology, Biology and Physics*, **21**, 361-367. doi:10.1016/0360-3016(91)90783-Z

[4] Hopewell, J.W. (2003) Radiation-therapy effects on bone density. *Medical and Pediatric Oncology*, **41**, 208-211. doi:10.1002/mpo.10338

[5] Baxter, N.N., Habermann, E.B., Tepper, J.E., Durham, S.B. and Virnig, B.A. (2005) Risk of pelvic fractures in older women following pelvic irradiation. *The Journal of the American Medical Association*, **294**, 2587-2593. doi:10.1001/jama.294.20.2587

[6] Kwon, J.W., Huh, S.J., Yoon, Y.C., Choi, S.H., Jung, J.Y., Oh, D. and Choe, B.K. (2008) Pelvic bone complications after radiation therapy of uterine cervical cancer: Evaluation with MRI. *American Journal of Roentgenology*, **191**, 987-994. doi:10.2214/AJR.07.3634

[7] Wernle, J.D., Damron, T.A., Allen, M.J. and Mann, K.A. (2010) Local irradiation alters bone morphology and increases bone fragility in a mouse model. *Journal of Biomechanics*, **43**, 2738-2746. doi:10.1016/j.jbiomech.2010.06.017

[8] Clutton, S.M., Townsend, K.M., Walker, C., Ansell, J.D. and Wright, E.G. (1996) Radiation induced genomic instability and persisting oxidative stress in primary bone marrow cultures. *Carcinogenesis*, **17**, 1633-1639. doi:10.1093/carcin/17.8.1633

[9] Down, J.D., Boudewijn, A., van Os, R., Thames, H.D. and Ploemacher, R.E. (1995) Variations in radiation sensitivity and repair among different hematopoietic stem cell subsets following fractionated irradiation. *Blood*, **86**, 122-127.

[10] Jaiswal, R.K., Jaiswal, N., Bruder, S.P., Mbalaviele, G., Marshak, D.R. and Pittenger, M.F. (2000) Adult human mesenchymal stem cell differentiation to the osteogenic or adipogenic lineage is regulated by mitogen-activated protein kinase. *Journal of Biologic Chemistry*, **275**, 9645-9652. doi:10.1074/jbc.275.13.9645

[11] Senn, J.S. and McCulloch, E.A. (1970) Radiation sensitivity of human bone marrow cells measured by a cell culture method. *Blood*, **35**, 56-60.

[12] Deng, H., Kennedy, C.W., Armour, E., Tryggestad, E., Ford, E., McNutt, T., Jiang, L. and Wong, J. (2007) The small-animal radiation research platform (SARRP): Dosimetry of a focused lens system. *Physics in Medicine and Biology*, **52**, 2729-2740. doi:10.1088/0031-9155/52/10/007

[13] Tang, Y., Wu, X., Lei, W., Pang, L., Wan, C., Shi, Z., Zhao, L., Nagy, T.R., Peng, X., Hu, J., Feng, X.,Van Hul, W., Wan, M. and Cao, X. (2009) TGF-beta1-induced migration of bone mesenchymal stem cells couples bone resorption with formation. *Nature Medicine*, **15**, 757-765. doi:10.1038/nm.1979

[14] Fujii, Y., Kato, T.A., Ueno, A., Kubota, N., Fujimori, A. and Okayasu, R. (2010) Ascorbic acid gives different protective effects in human cells exposed to X-rays and heavy ions. *Mutation Research*, **699**, 58-61.

[15] Yamamoto, T., Kinoshita, M., Shinomiya, N., Hiroi, S., Sugasawa, H., Matsushita, Y., Majima, T., Saitoh, D. and Seki, S. (2010) Pretreatment with ascorbic acid prevents lethal gastrointestinal syndrome in mice receiving a massive amount of radiation. *Journal of Radiation Research* (*Tokyo*), **51**, 145-156. doi:10.1269/jrr.09078

[16] Wambi, C., Sanzari, J., Wan, X.S., Nuth, M., Davis, J., Ko, Y.H., Sayers, C.M., Baran, M., Ware, J.H. and Kennedy, A.R. (2008) Dietary antioxidants protect hematopoietic cells and improve animal survival after total-body irradiation. *Radiation Research*, **169**, 384-396. doi:10.1667/RR1204.1

[17] Greenberger, J.S. and Epperly, M. (2009) Bone marrow-derived stem cells and radiation response. *Seminars in Radiation Oncology*, **19**, 133-139. doi:10.1016/j.semradonc.2008.11.006

[18] Brown, M.S., Buchanan, R.B. and Karran, S.J. (1980) Clinical observations on the effects of elemental diet supplementation during irradiation. *Clinical Radiology*, **31**, 19-20. doi:10.1016/S0009-9260(80)80075-4

Temporal epigenetic modifications differentially regulate ES cell-like colony formation and maturation

Jong S. Rim[1*], Karen L. Strickler[1*], Christian W. Barnes[1], Lettie L. Harkins[1], Jaroslaw Staszkiewicz[1], Jeffrey M. Gimble[2], Gregory H. Leno[3], Kenneth J. Eilertsen[1,2*]

[1]NuPotential Inc., Baton Rouge, USA; [*]Corresponding Authors: jsrnupotential@laetc.com, kjenupotential@laetc.com
[2]Stem Cell Biology Laboratory, Pennington Biomedical Research Center, Baton Rouge, USA
[3]Department of Anatomy & Cell Biology, Carver College of Medicine, University of Iowa, Iowa City, USA

ABSTRACT

Human somatic cells can be directly reprogrammed to induced pluripotent stem (iPS) cells by forced expression of the transcription factors Oct4, Sox2, and either Klf4 and cMyc or Nanog and Lin28, using virus-based systems. However, low reprogramming efficiency and the potential for deleterious virus-induced genomic modification limit the clinical potential of this technology. Recent reports indicate, however, that the generation of iPS cells can be enhanced by the addition of synthetic small molecules, including epigenetic modulators. In this report, we demonstrate that the epigenetic modifiers Valproic Acid (VPA) and 5-azacytidine activate the reciprocal transcriptional regulation of endogenous pluripotency transcription factor genes in human dermal fibroblasts and that VPA alone can directly activate endogenous Oct4 in the absence of transgenes. Moreover, using human adipose cells, we demonstrate that histone deacetylase inhibition, prior to reprogramming factor transfection, increases embryonic stem (ES) cell-like colony formation ~2 - 3 fold. In addition, DNA methyltransferase (DNMT) inhibition during human ES cell culture promotes maturation of reprogrammed somatic cells, increasing the yield ~4 fold. These data provide proof of principle that reprogramming efficiency can be improved by inhibiting specific repressive epigenetic regulatory components at the levels of ES cell-like colony formation and maturation. In addition, these studies raise the interesting possibility that a more efficient small molecule-based reprogramming system may provide a superior alternative to current virus-based approaches.

Keywords: Epigenetic Modification; Somatic Cell Reprogramming

1. INTRODUCTION

Forced expression of the transcription factors Oct4, Sox2, and either Klf4 and cMyc or Nanog and Lin28 can transform differentiated somatic cells into induced pluripotent stem (iPS) cells. In many respects, iPS cells are the functional equivalent of pluripotent embryonic stem (ES) cells [1-3] and therefore, hold enormous research and clinical potential. For example, iPS cells may facilitate mechanistic studies for degenerative diseases, drug discovery and toxicity testing. Indeed, several reports have described and validated "disease-in-a-dish" model systems [4-8]. The prospect for clinical application is limited, however, by reprogramming inefficiency and safety issues associated with viral vector transduction.

The efficiency of iPS cell production is influenced by the reprogramming strategy employed. Indeed, the number and combinations of transcription factors, the origin and developmental stage of the recipient cell, the method of transduction, and the use of small molecule epigenetic modifiers all play a role in determining the degree of iPS cell formation and colony maturation. Several general conclusions can be drawn from these studies. First, expression of pluripotency-related transcription factors while silencing p53 improves reprogramming efficiency [9,10]. Second, somatic cells from early development stages have greater reprogramming potential than mature cells [2]. Third, more efficient transfection methods, such as the polycistronic lentiviral system, improves reprogramming [11]. Finally, exposure to small molecule epigenetic modifiers also increases iPS cell production [12].

Reprogramming strategies are also being developed that address the safety concerns raised by the widely used virus-based reprogramming platforms. These include the use of non-integrating plasmids and mRNA [10,13-15], miRNA [16], excisable transposons [17,18], and proteins [19,20]. Identification of a small molecule or a cocktail of small molecules, to reprogram cells also promises to provide safer iPS cells and enhance opportunities for scalability ([21-24] see review, [25]).

Although the molecular mechanisms involved in somatic cell reprogramming are not well defined, it is clear that epigenetic modification has proven to be critical for de-differentiation of somatic cells. The most well studied example is promoter specific DNA de-methylation and histone acetylation. These changes are required for the re-expression of pluripotency-related genes that are silenced during animal development [26]. Recent genome-wide mapping of target promoters for Oct4, Sox2, Klf4 and c-myc, as well as Nanog, Dax1, Rex1, Zpf281, and Nac1 factors, has provided a more detailed and global understanding of the pluripotent epigenome in mouse ES cells [27]. Among the more than 6000 target gene promoters analyzed, two categories emerged with respect to transcription factor binding and promoter activity. First, target promoters bound by four or fewer factors are repressed while those associated with a higher factor density are active. Remarkably, the transcriptional network of ES cells includes auto- and reciprocal-transcriptional regulation as well as protein-protein interactions that contribute to regulate pluripotency gene expression.

We hypothesize that epigenetic modification directly activates an endogenous pluripotent transcription network resulting in the increased efficiency of transcription factor-based somatic cell reprogramming. In this report, we used two epigenetic modifying agents, an inhibitor of DNA methyltransferase (DNMT) and a histone deacetylase (HDAC) inhibitor, to begin to test this hypothesis. We found that both DNMT and HDAC inhibitors activate the endogenous reprogramming factor transcription network in human dermal fibroblasts. In addition, we demonstrated that exposure of human preadipocytes to an HDAC inhibitor, prior to transfection, increases the induction of initial ES-like colony formation and that exposure to a DNMT inhibitor after transfection, facilitates iPS colony maturation.

2. MATERIALS AND METHODS

2.1. Cell Culture

Human dermal fibroblasts from adult, neonatal and fetal origin (Cell Applications Inc., San Diego, CA) were cultured with fibroblast growth medium (Cell Applications) at 37°C, 5% CO_2 in a humidified incubator. Human preadipocytes (Cell Applications) were maintained with preadipocyte growth medium (Cell Applications) or Dulbecco's modified Eagle medium (DMEM) supplemented with 10% FBS, 50 U/ml penicillin and 50 μg/ml streptomycin at 37°C, 5% CO_2 in a humidified incubator. Human adipose derived adult stem cells (Stem Cell Biology Laboratory, Pennington Biomedical Research Center, Baton Rouge, LA) were maintained with DMEM supplemented with 10% FBS, 50 U/ml penicillin and 50 μg/ml streptomycin at 37°C, 5% CO_2 in a humidified incubator. The human adipose derived stem cells were obtained from subjects undergoing elective surgery with written informed consent under a protocol reviewed and approved by the Pennington Biomedical Research Center Institutional Review Board (PBRC #23040). Cell culture medium was supplemented with 5 mM VPA (Sigma), 5 μM 5-azacytidine (Sigma), 1 μM TSA (Sigma), 5 μM Scriptaid (BioMol) or 25 - 100 μM Zebularine (Sigma, concentrations as indicated in the figure) for the treatment as indicated. Adipose cell derived iPS (AdiPS-Ctl, AdiPS-TSA) cells were generated from human preadipocytes (Cell Applications) or human adipose derived adult stem cells as described in the paper, and maintained on an irradiated mouse embryonic fibroblast (MEF) feeder layer from ATCC (Manassas, VA) or on Matrigel coated cell culture plates (BD Biosciences) with mTeSR1 hES culture medium (StemCell Technology). Mel-1 human ES cells were purchased from Millipore (Temecula, CA) and maintained on MEF feeder layer (ATCC, Manassas, VA) with mTeSR1 hES culture medium (StemCell Technology).

2.2. Lentiviral Transduction and Generation of AdiPS Cells

High titer lentivirus, overexpressing human Oct4 or Nanog proteins, was purchased from System Biosciences (San Diego, CA). The day before lentiviral transfection, human dermal fibroblasts were trypsinized, counted, and seeded in 6-well plates at a density of 4×10^5 cells/well. The next day, culture medium was replaced with prewarmed medium containing 3 μg/ml polybrene (Sigma) and 5 MOI of lentivirus. Eighteen hours later, culture medium was changed with fresh fibroblast growth medium or treated with histone deacetylase inhibitor (HDACi) or DNA methyltransferase inhibitor (DNMTi). After 7 days treatment, total RNA was isolated for gene expression analysis. High titer polycistronic lentivirus STEMCCA (Oct4, Sox2, Klf4, c-Myc) (Millipore, Temecula, CA) were transfected into human preadipocytes. Briefly, 10^5 human preadipocytes that had been cultured with or without HDACi and/or DNMTi, were transfected with 75 MOI of STEMCCA lentivirus overnight. Lentiviral infection was repeated the next day, and culture medium was changed with fresh preadipocyte growh medium. When the cells reached confluence, they were trypsinized, counted and seeded on a prepared MEF feeder layer at a density of 5×10^4 cells with mTeSR1 medium (StemCell Technology) supplemented with 10 μM ROCK inhibitor (ROCKi) (Stemgent).

2.3. Quantitative Realtime RT-PCR

Total RNA was prepared from cultures using Trizol Reagent (Life Technology) and the RNeasy Mini RNA isolation kit (Qiagen) with DNase I digestion. Total RNA (1 μg) from each sample was subjected to oligo (dT)-primed reverse transcription (Invitrogen) to generate cDNA. Quantitative PCR to measure mRNA expression levels was performed with Taqman gene expression assays (Applied Biosystems) using a 7300 real-time PCR system in the genomic core facility at Pennington Biomedical Research Center. Expression levels were compared to known standard samples and were normalized to GAPDH.

2.4. Immunofluorescence and Alkaline Phosphatase Staining

Cells were fixed with 4% paraformaldehyde in PBS for 10 min, and incubated for 1 hr with antibodies specific for pluripotency markers Oct4, Nanog, Sox2 (Abcam) and TRA1-60 (Millipore). After washing three times with PBS, cells were incubated for 1 hr with fluorescent conjugated secondary antibody (Invitrogen). Nuclei were detected by DAPI staining (Vector shield). Alkaline Phosphatase staining was performed using the Alkaline Phosphatase Staining kit (Stemgent).

2.5. *In Vitro* Differentiation

Human AdiPS cells cultured on MEF feeder layers were treated with dispase (StemCell Technology) and transferred to Matrigel coated plates (BD Biosciences) with mTeSR1 culture medium. When attached AdiPS colonies started to contact each other, spontaneous differentiation was initiated by changing medium with Dulbecco's modified Eagle medium (DMEM) supplemented with 10% FBS, 50 U/ml penicillin and 50 ug/ml streptomycin. Continuously beating (heart) cells were observed by microscopy.

2.6. Teratoma Formation

For *in vivo* teratoma formation, human AdiPS cells were collected with cell recovery solution (BD Biosciences). After washing with ice cold PBS, cells were resuspended at 4×10^6 cells/ml in PBS and mixed with BD matrigel matrix HC (BD Biosciences) in a final volume of 0.5 ml on ice for each injection. Cell suspensions were injected subcutaneously in athymic nude mice using a 23G needle. Six weeks after the injection, tumors were surgically dissected and each teratoma was evaluated by H&E staining. Experiments involving vertebrate animals were approved by Pennington Biomedical Research Center's Institutional Animal Care and Use Committee (A3677-01, protocol #624) and conformed to or exceeded NIH standards.

2.7. Bisulfite Sequencing

DNA was isolated and purified by DNeasy Blood and Tissue kit (Qiagen). Bisulfite conversion was performed using the EZ DNA Methylation kit (Zymo Research). Converted DNA was amplified by PCR using primers for Oct3/4 or Nanog as follows: Oct4 forward primer: 5'-GTTAGAGGTTAAGGTTAGTGGGTG

Oct4 reverse primer: 5'-AAACCTTAAAAACTTAACCAAATCC

Nanog forward primer: 5'-TGGTTAGGTTGGTTTTAAATTTTTG

Nanog reverse primer: 5'-AACCCACCCTTATAAATTCTCAATTA

Dlk1 #1 forward primer: 5'-GTTTTTTTGTTTTTGTTGGTTTT

Dlk1 #1 reverse primer: 5'-ACTAAAAATCTCACACATCCCCTAC

Dlk1 #2 forward primer: 5'-AGTTGTATTTGGGTGAATGGATTAT

Dlk1 #2 reverse primer: 5'-AAAACAAAAAAACCAAACAAAAAAC

Dlk1 #3 forward primer: 5'-TTTAATAGGAGAGGGTGGAGATGTA

Dlk1 #3 reverse primer: 5'-CCTTACCTAAAATCACAAATCAAAAA.

PCR products were cloned into *E. coli* using the TOPO TA cloning kit (Invitrogen). Ten clones of each sample were verified by sequencing with SP6 and T7 primers.

2.8. Low Density Microarray

Human TaqMan® low density stem cell pluripotency arrays (TLDA) which contain 96 embryonic stem cell and post-implantation/differentiated tissue genes, and endogenous control genes were purchase from ABI (Applied Biosystems, Foster City, CA). Total RNA was isolated using an RNeasy RNA Isolation Kit (Qiagen, Valencia, CA), qualified, and quantified by spectrometry, and 50 ng total RNA was reverse transcribed to cDNA using the High Capacity cDNA Archive Kit (Applied Biosystems). TLDA qRT-PCR was performed as follows: for each sample, 100 μl of the sample-specific PCR mix (including 5 μl cDNA) was pipetted into the sample wells of the Micro Fluidic Card. The card was centrifuged, sealed, and run on the Applied Biosystem's 7900HT Sequence Detection System using the manufacturer's SDS 2.3 software. Relative quantification, using the $\Delta\Delta$ C_T method, was performed to determine fold changes in gene expression, relative to endogenous control, in reprogrammed stem cells compared to a baseline.

3. RESULTS

3.1. Activation of the Endogenous Reprogramming Factor Network by Inhibition of Histone Deacetylase or DNA Methyltransferase

Differentiation silences pluripotency gene transcription during development and thereby, limits the genomic potential of the cell. This is partly due to epigenetic modifications of promoter regions by DNA methylation and histone modification. Thus, it stands to reason that the acquisition of pluripotency during cell reprogramming should also involve epigenetic modifications that enable pluripotency gene expression. To test this hypothesis, we first determined whether or not treatment of adult human dermal fibroblasts (HDFa) with epigenetic modulators increased expression of the pluripotency gene, Oct4. We found that increased mRNA expression of the endogenous Oct4 gene occurred after only three days of treatment with the histone deacetylase (HDAC) inhibitor, valproic acid (VPA, 5 mM), and to a lesser extent, with the DNA methyltransferase (DNMT) inhibitor, zebularine (**Figure 1(a)**, 25 μM, 50 μM, 100 μM). The effect of zebularine on expression was concentration dependent. Surprisingly, however, differences in expression between control and zebularine-treated samples were not significant until day 7 of the incubation at a zebularine concentration of 100 mM (**Figure 1(a)**). Oct4 mRNA levels remained elevated through 7 days of treatment with either inhibitor. However, expression levels of the endogenous Oct4 gene were much lower than the levels of ectopic expression achieved following transduction of HDFa cultures with a lentivirus expressing the human Oct4 gene (**Figure 1(b)**).

To determine the effects of VPA, and a second DNMT inhibitor, 5-azacytidine (5-aza), on ectopic expression of Oct4 and Nanog genes, we isolated mRNA from drug-treated HDFa cultures following Oct4 or Nanog lentivirus transduction. We then performed real-time RT-PCR using a gene specific primer and probes as described in Materials and Methods. We found that both VPA- and 5-aza-treated Oct4 lentivirus-infected cells had higher levels of Oct4 expression than that observed in control, VPA- or 5-aza-treated non-infected, and non-treated Oct4-lentivirus infected cultures (**Figure 1(c)**). However, the absolute level of Oct4 mRNA expressed following induction was still one-third lower than that observed in human embryonic stem (hES) cells grown under standard conditions (data not shown). Results similar to those in HDFa cells were also observed in human dermal fibroblasts isolated from neonatal (HDFn) and fetal (HDFf) tissues.

This trend was also revealed with the transcription factor, Nanog. Specifically, VPA and 5-aza treatments each increased Nanog mRNA expression relative to control cultures (**Figure 1(d)**). In addition, VPA- and 5-aza-treatment of cultures infected with Nanog lentivirus induced Nanog expression relative to control, VPA- or 5-aza-treated non-infected, and untreated Nanog lentivirus infected cultures (**Figure 1(d)**). However, unlike Oct4 expression, the absolute level of Nanog expression was 10-fold higher than the levels observed in hES cells. Taken together, these results suggest that the epigenetic modifiers, VPA and 5-azacytidine, activate the auto-transcriptional regulation of pluripotency transcription factors Oct4 and Nanog in somatic cells.

We also observed a slight induction of Oct4 (**Figure 2(a)**) and Nanog (**Figure 2(b)**) mRNA levels in Nanog- and Oct4-lentivirus-infected HDFa cells, respectively, following VPA and 5-azaC treatments. Similarly, the low levels of endogenous Sox2 that are normally observed in HDFf cells were increased by overexpression of Oct4 or Nanog and 5-azaC treatment (**Figure 2(c)**) However, VPA treatment did not significantly increase Sox2 expression (**Figure 2(c)**). These data suggest that the epigenetic modifiers, VPA and 5-azaC, also activate the reciprocal transcriptional regulation of the endogenous pluripotency transcription factors in somatic cells.

3.2. Induction of ES Cell-Like Colony Formation by Pre-Treatment of Human Preadipocytes with an HDAC Inhibitor

The VPA- and 5-azaC-induced expression of Oct4 and Nanog genes raises the interesting possibility that epigenetic modification, prior to lentivirus transduction, may facilitate the reprogramming of somatic cells. Adult human adipose stem cells can be reprogrammed to iPS cells more rapidly and efficiently than human fetal skin fibroblasts [28] and therefore, we chose to use this system for our studies. Our experimental strategy is outlined in **Figure 3(a)**. We first treated human pre-adipocytes with various HDAC inhibitors (HDACi) below their cell cycle inhibitory concentrations. Pre- (Day 7) and post-treated (Day 2) cells are shown in **Figure 3(b)** (left panel) and illustrate the change in cell density and morphology during HDACi treatment. These pre-treated cells were then transfected with lentivirus containing mouse Oct4, Sox2, Klf4 and cMyc cDNAs. Lentiviral transfection was repeated the next day and when the transfected cells reached confluence, they were split and transferred onto mouse embryonic fibroblast feeder layers. Colonies were initially apparent 9 days post-infection (Day 9) and each contained approximately 30 - 40 cells that displayed typical hES morphology (**Figure 3(b)**, right panel). By day13, tightly packed colonies with defined boundaries

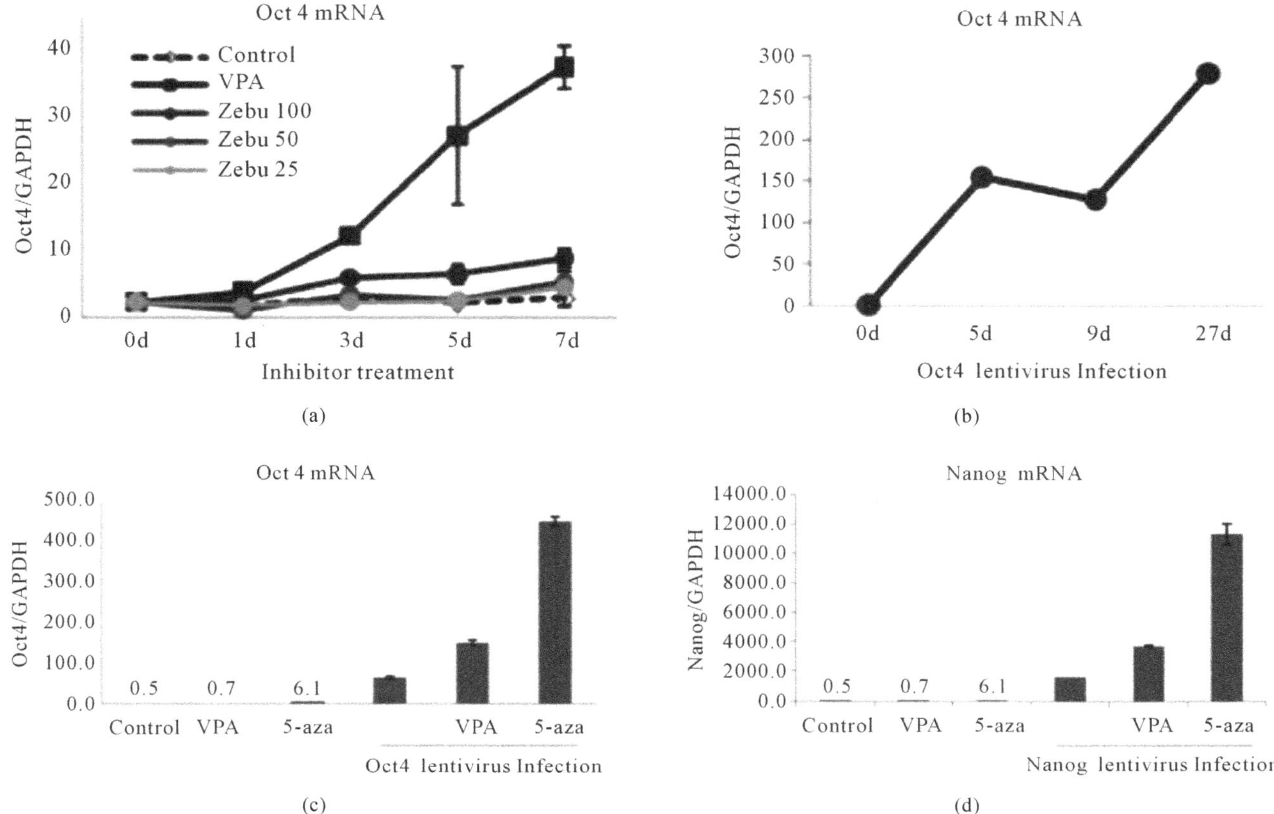

Figure 1. Induced expression of the Oct4 and Nanog genes in human dermal fibroblasts. (a) Analysis of Oct4 mRNA expression in adult human dermal fibroblasts (HDFa) following treatment with HDAC and DNMT inhibitors. Primary cultures from HDFa were treated with the HDAC inhibitor, Valproic acid (VPA, 5 mM), or the DNMT inhibitor, zebularine (25 μM, 50 μM, 100 μM), as indicated. Quantitative realtime RT-PCR was performed as described in Materials and Methods. mRNA levels were compared to known standard samples and were normalized to GAPDH. Results are mean values (+/–SEM, $n = 5$). One-way ANOVA demonstrated a significant difference ($p < 0.05$) between the control and the treatment; (b) Analysis of Oct4 mRNA expression in HDFa cells following Oct4 lentivirus transfection. HDFa were transfected with lentivirus and isolated RNA was subjected to quantitative RT-PCR. mRNA levels were compared to known standard samples and normalized to GAPDH. Results are mean values (+/-SEM, $n = 3$); (c) Expression of Oct4 mRNA in HDfa cells subjected to Oct4-expressing lentivirus infection and HDAC or DNMT inhibition. HDFa cells were transfected with or without Oct4 lentivirus and treated for 7 days with VPA (5 mM) or the DNMT inhibitor, 5-azacytidine (5-aza, 5 μM)) as indicated prior to RNA isolation. Total RNA was isolated and subjected to quantitative RT-PCR. Expression levels were compared to known standard samples and normalized to GAPDH. Results are mean values (+/–SEM, $n = 3$). mRNA levels for Control, VPA and 5-aza samples are also presented in numerical form for comparison to lentivirus-infected samples. One-way ANOVA demonstrated a significant difference ($p < 0.05$) between the control and treatments; (d) Analysis of Nanog mRNA expression in HDFa cells following Nanog lentivirus transfection. HDFa were transfected with lentivirus expressing Nanog and isolated RNA was subjected to quantitative RT-PCR. mRNA levels were compared to known standard samples and normalized to GAPDH. Results are mean values (+/–SEM, $n = 3$). mRNA levels for Control, VPA and 5-aza samples are also presented in numerical form for comparison to lentivirus-infected samples. One-way ANOVA demonstrated a significant difference ($p < 0.05$) between the control and the TSA colonies.

were observed and the number of colonies in each well was determined. TSA pre-treatment resulted in a more than 2-fold increase in colony formation relative to untreated control cultures (**Figure 3(c)**). Similar results were observed when comparing Scriptaid- and VPA-pretreated cultures with their respective un-treated control cultures (data not shown).

AdiPS-Ctl and AdiPS-TSA cell lines were obtained by clonal expansion of the control and TSA colonies, respectively (**Figure 3(b)**, right panel). Cells were characterized with respect to alkaline phosphatase staining, a marker for early ES cell formation, Oct4/TRA1-60 (red/green) and Sox2/TRA1-60 (red/green) combination staining and by the formation of embryoid bodies (EB) (**Figure 3(d)**). TRA1-60 is a surface marker for matured iPS cells [29] and embryoid bodies represent the earliest stages of differentiation and embryo development *in vitro*. ES cell-like colonies from pre-treated cultures were in-

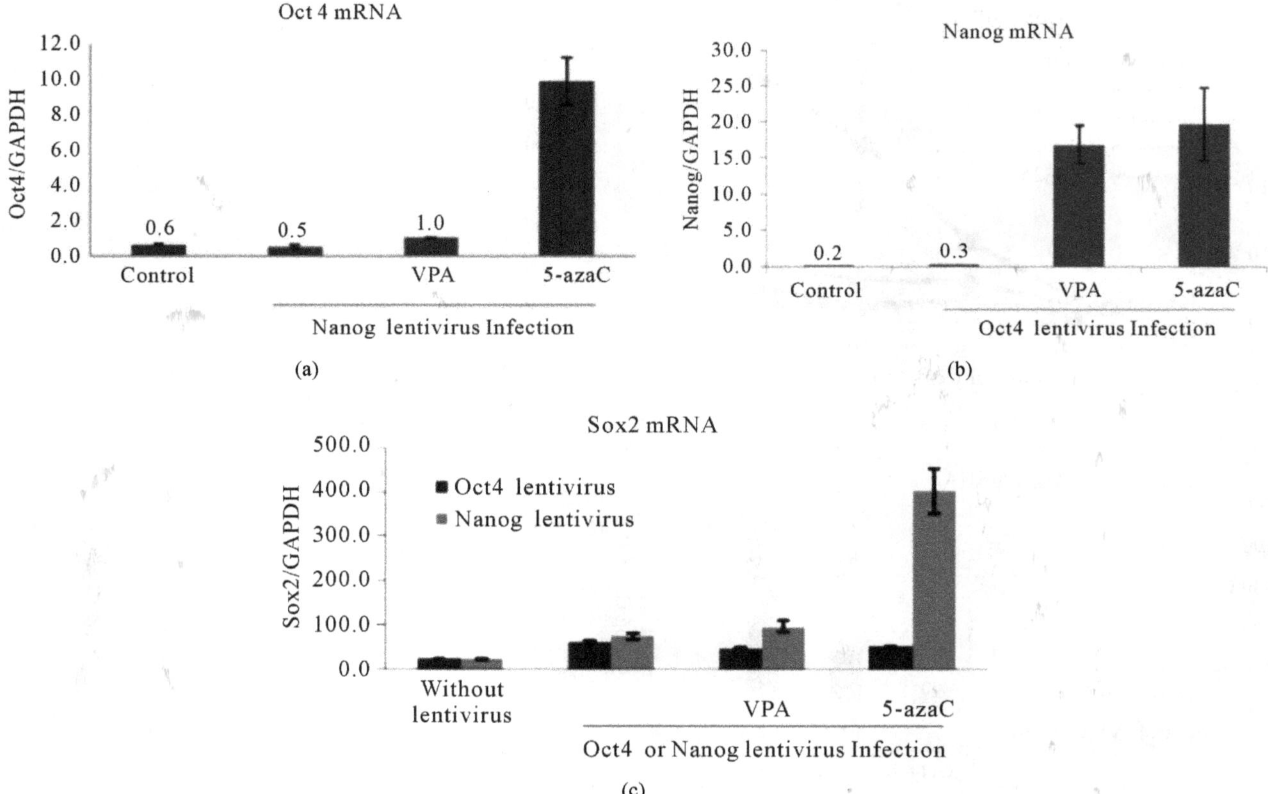

Figure 2. Reciprocal activation of endogenous pluripotency factor genes in Oct4 or Nanog lentivirus-infected HDF cells by treatment with HDAC or DNMT inhibitors. (a) Expression of Oct4 mRNA in HDFa cells subjected to Nanog-expressing lentivirus infection and HDAC or DNMT inhibition. HDFa cells were transfected with or without Nanog lentivirus and treated with VPA or 5-azacytidine as indicated. Total RNA was isolated and subjected to quantitative RT-PCR. Expression levels were compared to known standard samples and normalized to GAPDH. Results are mean values (+/–SEM, $n = 3$). One-way ANOVA demonstrated a significant difference ($p < 0.05$) between the control and the treatment; (b) Expression of Nanog mRNA in HDFa cells subjected to Oct4-expressing lentivirus infection and HDAC or DNMT inhibition. HDFa cells were transfected with or without Oct4 lentivirus and treated with VPA or 5-azacytidine as indicated. Results are mean values (+/–SEM, $n = 3$). One-way ANOVA demonstrated a significant difference ($p < 0.05$) between the control and the treatment; (c) Expression of Sox2 mRNA in HDFa cells subjected to Oct4- or Nanog-expressing lentivirus infection and HDAC or DNMT inhibition. HDFa cells were transfected with or without Oct4 lentivirus and treated with VPA or 5-azacytidine as indicated. Dark bars indicate Sox2 mRNA levels in Oct4 lentivirus infected cells and the light bars Sox2 levels in Nanog-expressing lentivirus-infected cells.

distinguishable from control colonies with respect to the parameters analyzed. Thus, HDACi treatment increases the formation of colonies that are grossly similar to control colonies.

Realtime RT-PCR also revealed a 10^3 - 10^4-fold increase in Oct4 and Nanog mRNA levels between preadipocyte and AdiPS-Ctl or AdiPS-TSA cells (**Figure 3(e)**, top panel) consistent with the expected changes associated with cell reprogramming. In addition, bisulfite sequencing demonstrated extensive demethylation (open circles) of the promoter regions of Oct4 and Nanog genes in AdiPS-Ctl or AdiPS-TSA cells relative to preadipocyte colonies (**Figure 3(e)**, bottom panel).

We next compared pluripotency marker gene expression levels in AdiPS cells with the levels in preadipocyte and hES cells (Mel-1) by low density microarray. As expected, both AdiPS-Ctl and AdiPS-TSA cells showed similar gene expression patterns to Mel-1 hES cells and strikingly different profiles than preadipocyte cells (**Figure 3(f)**). Expression of ectopic pluripotency genes was not detected in established AdiPS cell lines (data not shown). These data suggest that AdiPS clonal cell lines more closely resemble hES cells than their preadipocyte progenitors with respect to pluripotency gene expression.

To determine if AdiPS cells display functional similarities to hES cells, we next conducted *in vitro* and *in vivo* differentiation experiments. Human AdiPS cells were first transferred to Matrigel plates and treated with high-serum, low growth factor medium for 3 to 4 weeks. Live-image microscopy revealed beating cardiomyocytes (white arrows) (**Figure 4(a)**). AdiPS cells were also injected into the interscapular region of athymic Nude mice

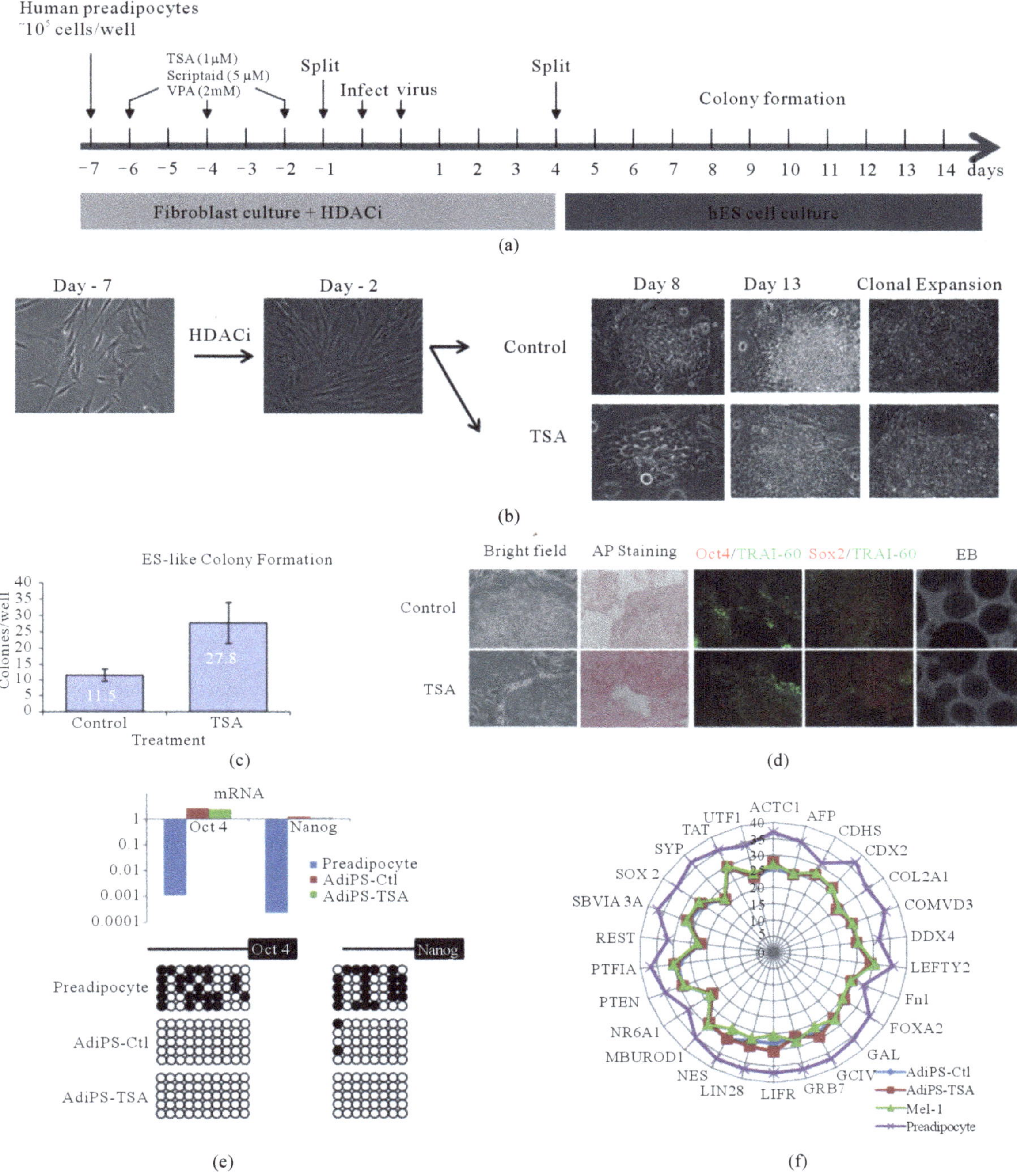

Figure 3. Characterization of adipose induced pluripotent stem (AdiPS) cells produced by pre-treatment of preadipocytes with epigenetic modulators. (a) Experimental strategy for production of AdiPS cells; (b) Left Panel: Preadipocytes treated with HDAC inhibitors (HDACi). Images show and increase in cell density and changes in cell morphology during treatment. Right Panel: ES cell-like colonies from control and TSA-treated cultures showing well-defined boundaries; (c) The mean number of ES cell-like colonies formed in TSA-treated and untreated control cultures; (d) Analysis of morphology and immunostaining for the pluripotency marker (Oct4, Sox2) and matured iPS/ES cells (TRA1-60) in control and TSA-treated AdiPS cells. Embryoid bodies (EB). Alkaline phosphatase (AP); (e) Top panel: Oct4 and Nanog mRNA expression levels in preadipocytes and in control adipose-derived iPS cell (AdiPS-Ctl) and TSA-treated adipose-derived iPS cell (AdiPS-TSA) cultures. Bottom panel: DNA methylation status of Oct4 and Nanog promoter regions from human preadipocyte, AdiPS-Ctl and AdiPS-TSA cells. Open circles: unmethylated CpG dinucleotides; closed circles; methylated CpG dinucleotides; (f) Low density microarray analysis comparing pluripotency gene expression in preadipocyte, hES cell (Mel-1), AdiPS-Ctl and AdiPS-TSA cells. Values indicate relative quantitation by the $\Delta\Delta$ C_T method.

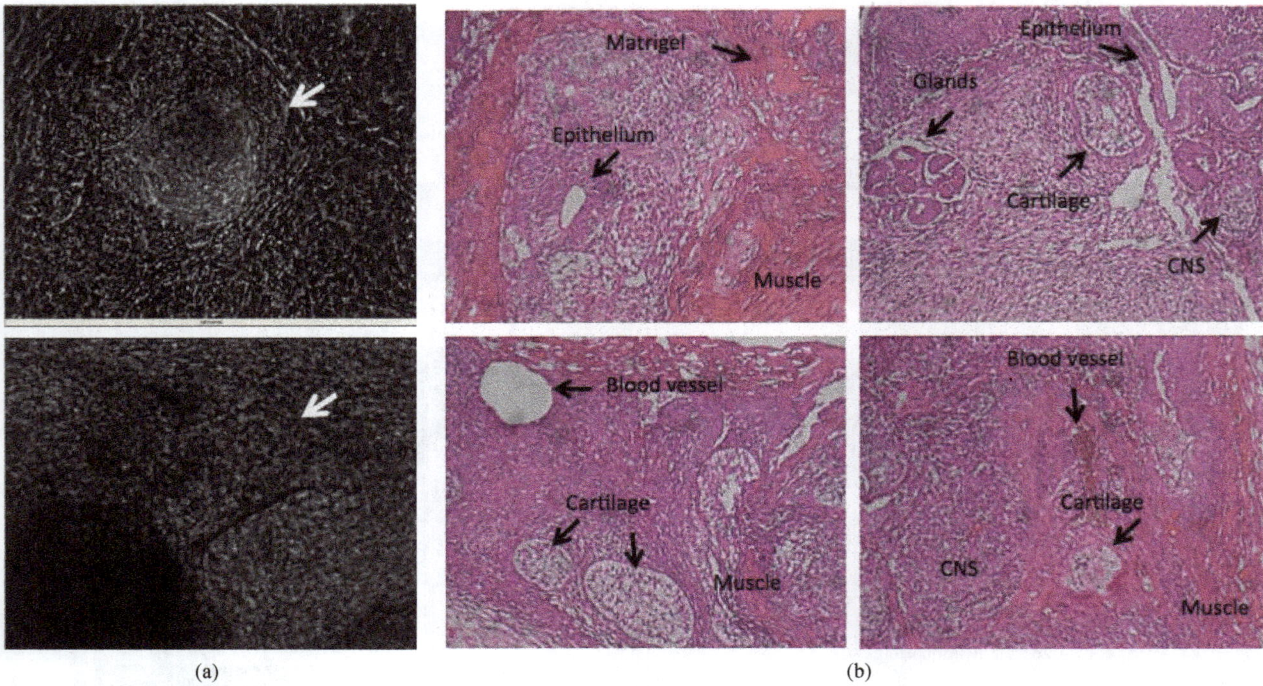

Figure 4. Differentiation of AdiPS cells *in vitro* and *in vivo*. (a) Morphology of beating cardiomyocytes. Human AdiPS cells were transferred onto a Matrigel plate and treated with high serum/low growth factor medium for 3 to 4 weeks. Live images of *in vitro*-generated beating cardiomyocytes (white arrows) were captured by microscopy; (b) Morphology of formed teratomas. Human AdiPS cells were injected into athymic nude mice and after 6 to 7 weeks, samples were collected and stained with hemotoxylin-eosin (H&E). These four panels represent different sections through a teratoma illustrating tissues of all three embryonic germ layers as indicated; epithelium, muscle, cartilage, glands, central nervous system (CNS).

to assess their capacity for teratoma formation. Teratoma masses were observed 6 - 7 weeks after injection and H&E staining demonstrated tissues representing all three germ layers (**Figure 4(b)**). Comparison of preadipocytes with human adipose-derived adult stem cells, isolated from subcutaneous fat, was indistinguishable with respect to their responses to HDAC inhibitor pre-treatment (data not shown).

The expression status of the Dlk1-Dio3 imprinted gene cluster reflects the potential for production of high-grade chimaeras and their viability [30]. Interestingly, HDAC inhibitor treatment reactivates Dlk1-Dio3 expression within partially reprogrammed cells resulting in the establishment of fully reprogrammed mouse iPS cells. High levels of Dlk1 (also known as Pref1) mRNA have also been detected in mouse preadipocytes and these levels dramatically decrease during adipocyte differentiation [31]. Therefore, we sought to determine the effect of the HDAC inhibitor, TSA, on the Dlk1 gene in our human AdiPS cells. Both types of AdiPS cells and hES cells were found to express high levels of Dlk1 mRNA as compared to human preadipocytes (**Figure 5(a)**). However, AdiPS-TSA cells had higher levels of *Dlk*1 gene expression than AdiPS-Ctl cells. The promoter region of the imprinted Dlk1 gene harbors hemimethylated CpG dinucleotides [32]. This region also contains a CTCF insulator binding motif (CCGCnnGGnGGg/tC) as indicated by the box in **Figure 5(b)**. Analysis of this region using bisulfite sequencing revealed differential hemimethylation of CpG dinucleotides between preadipocytes, hES cells and our AdiPS cells in the region of the CTCF binding site (**Figures 5(c)** and **(d)**). Specifically, human preadipocytes showed higher levels of hemi-methylation than Mel-1, AdiPS-Ctl and AdiPS cells (**Figure 5(d)**). These results agree well with published reports [30] and suggest that pretreatment of human preadipocytes with a broad range HDAC inhibitor such as TSA, might improve the quality of reprogrammed cells.

3.3. Induction of ES Cell-Like Colony Maturation by Post-Treatment of Cells with an HDAC Inhibitor

It has been shown that only a small percentage of ES cell-like colonies become fully reprogrammed and acquire hES cell characteristics such as pluripotency and self-renewal. Thus, colony formation alone is necessary, but not sufficient, for pluripotentcy of ES-like cells. The acquisition of pluripotency and self-renewal has been termed colony maturation and we next sought to determine how post-treatment of lentivirus-transfected cells

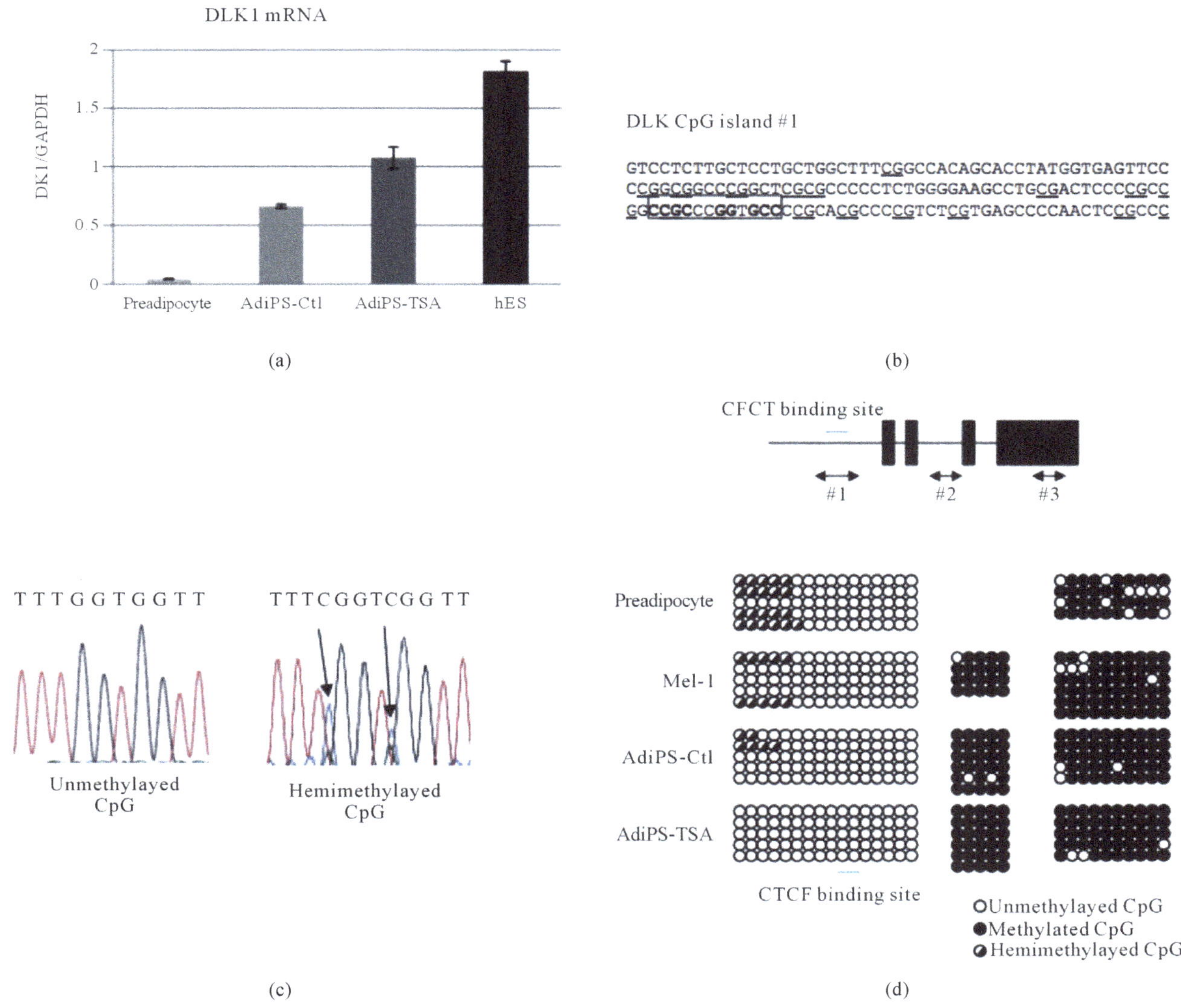

Figure 5. Dlk1 mRNA expression and DNA methylation of the Dlk1 promoter. (a) Dlk1 mRNA levels from human preadipocytes, hES cells and AdiPS cells (AdiPS-Ctl, AdiPS-TSA) were determined by Real-time RT-PCR and expression was normalized to GAPDH; (b) Nucleotide sequence of the Dlk1 promoter. CpG dinucleotides are underlined and the putative CTCF binding site is shown within the box; (c) Representative chromatograms of unmethylated and hemimethylated CpG dinuleotides within the Dlk1 gene promoter; (d) DNA methylation status of the human Dlk1 gene. Analysis of three genomic regions (#1 - #3) by bisulfite sequencing. Black boxes and horizontal line denote exons and introns, respectively. Empty circles, unmethylated CpG dinucleotides; filled circles, methylated CpG dinucleotides; half-filled circles, hemimethylated CpG dinucleotides.

with the epigenetic modifier, zebularine, affects this process. Our experimental strategy is outlined in **Figure 6(a)**. TSA (1 μM) or zebularine (50 μM) pre-treated human preadipocytes were transfected with lentivirus as previously described (see **Figure 3(a)**). One day after transferring to a mouse embryonic fibroblast feeder layer, hES culture medium was supplemented with zebularine as indicated. Colonies were first visible 3 days later (**Figure 6(b)**). These colonies were tracked through clonal expansion and cell lines were established (**Figure 6(b)**) as described in our earlier experiment (see **Figure 3(a)**). Tightly packed colonies growing on the feeder layer were stained with alkaline phosphatase (AP), and double immunostained for Sox2/TRA1-60 (red/green) (**Figure 6(c)**), markers for colony formation and maturation, respectively. The percentage of positive colonies in each treatment group is shown in **Figure 6(d)**. All treatment regimens produced colonies that were positive for AP. However, only 50% - 60% of the colonies from cells pretreated with TSA or Zeb stained positive for Sox2. More colonies from cells pretreated with zebularine (Zeb) showed TRA1-60 staining (~22%) than control (Ctl) colonies (8%) or colonies from cells pretreated with TSA (8%). Moreover, zebularine post-treatment increased the

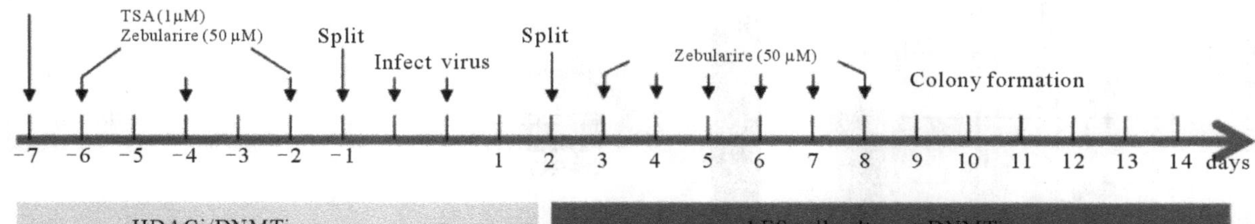
Human preadipocytes
~10⁵ cells/well
TSA(1μM)
Zebularire (50 μM)
Split
Infect virus
Split
Zebularire (50 μM)
Colony formation
−7 −6 −5 −4 −3 −2 −1 1 2 3 4 5 6 7 8 9 10 11 12 13 14 days
HDACi/DNMTi
hES cell culture + DNMTi

(a)

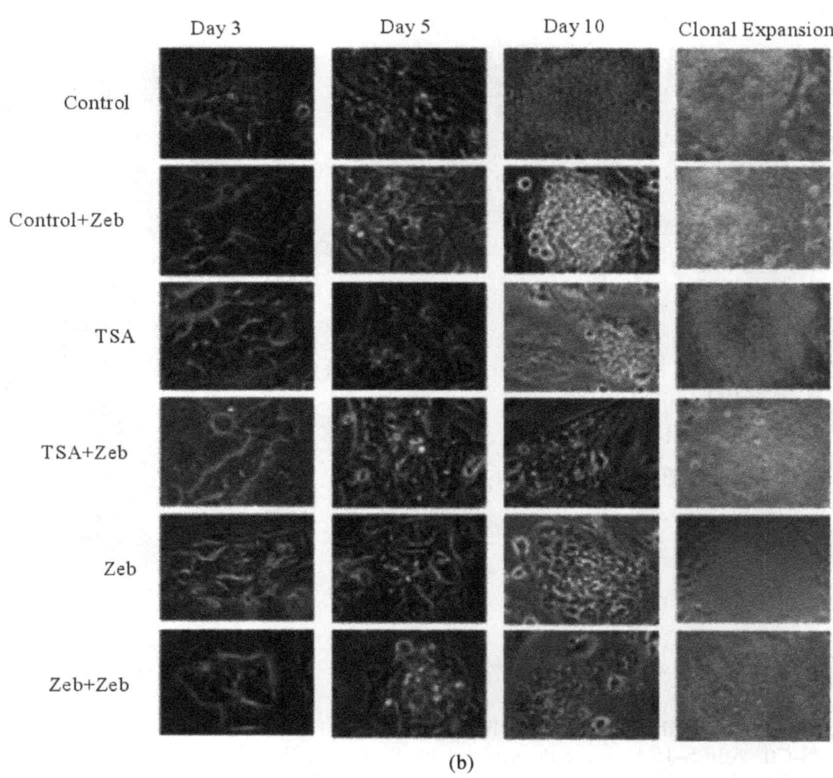
Day 3
Day 5
Day 10
Clonal Expansion
Control
Control+Zeb
TSA
TSA+Zeb
Zeb
Zeb+Zeb

(b)

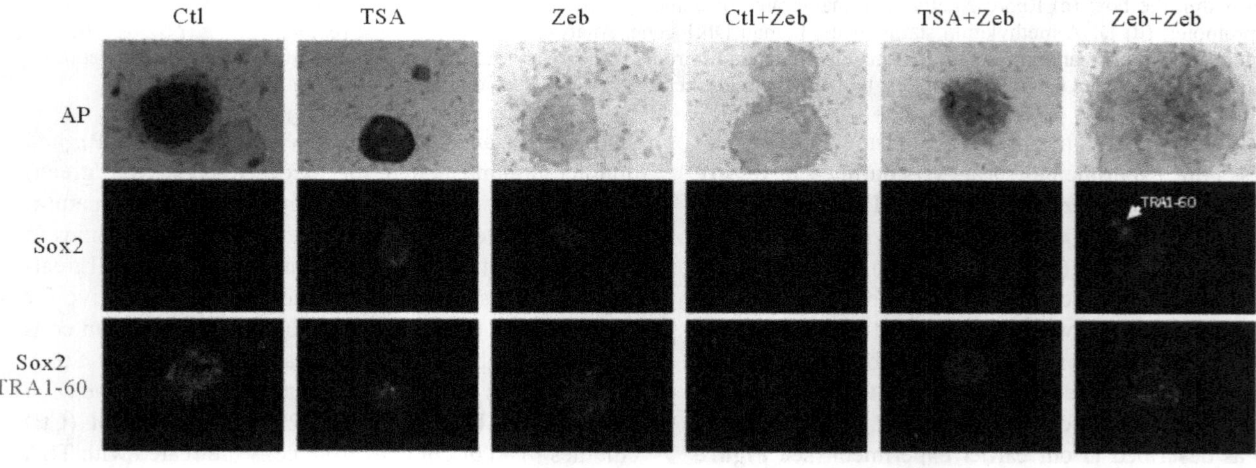
Ctl
TSA
Zeb
Ctl+Zeb
TSA+Zeb
Zeb+Zeb
AP
Sox2
Sox2
TRA1-60
TRA1-60

(c)

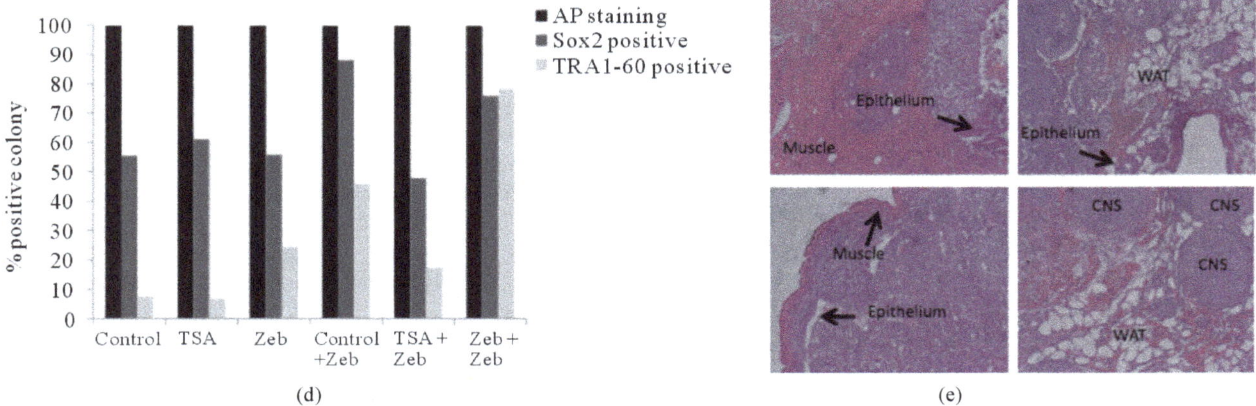

Figure 6. Characterization of adipose induced pluripotent stem (AdiPS) cells produced by pre- and post-treatment of preadipocytes with epigenetic modulators. (a) Experimental scheme for AdiPS cell production; (b) Morphological progression of ES cell-like colony formation in preadipocytes treated with the epigenetic modulators, TSA (1 μM) and/or zebularine (50 μM); (c) Examples of ES cell-like colonies stained for alkaline phosphatase (AP), Sox2 and Sox2/TRA1-60; (d) The percentage of positive-staining colonies observed in each experimental group is shown in **Figure 6(c)**; (e) Teratoma formation in nude mice following AdiPS cell injection. All three embryonic germ layers are visible by hematoxylin-eosin (H&E) staining; epithelium, muscle, white adipocytes (WAT), central nervous system (CNS).

number of both Sox2 (88%) and TRA1-60 (42%) expressing colonies as compared to colonies from cells pretreated with TSA (50% - 60% Sox2 and 8% TRA1-60) or zebualrine (50% - 60% Sox2 and 22% TRA1-60). Somewhat surprisingly, colonies from cells pretreated with TSA and subsequently post treated with zebularine had reduced Sox2 (~42%) and TRA1-60 (18%) expression compared to colonies from cells only post-treated with zebularine. In contrast, pretreatment and post-treatment of cells with zebularine resulted in greater than 75% of the colonies staining positive for Sox2 and TRA1-60. Realtime RT-PCR of established AdiPS cell lines confirmed that Sox2 (or Oct4 or Nanog) immunostaining was not due to ectopic gene expression (data not shown). Established AdiPS cells were also injected into Nude mice to assess their potential for teratoma formation. All three germ layers were present in the recovered tissue masses indicating teratoma formation (**Figure 6(e)**).

4. DISCUSSION

We have generated human adipose tissue-derived iPS (AdiPS) cells from primary preadipocytes and adipose-derived adult stem cells using epigenetic modulation combined with lentivirus-induced pluripotency factor expression. Our results demonstrate three important points. First, treatment of cells with HDAC or DNMT inhibitors, either before or after lentivirus transfection, increases pluripotency factor expression. These data sug- gest that epigenetic modification may activate both the auto-transcriptional and the reciprocal transcriptional regulation pathways of the endogenous pluripotency factors, Oct4 and Nanog, in adult human cells. Second, epigenetic modulation of adipose tissue-derived cells, before lentivirus-induced pluripotency factor expression, increases the efficiency of ES cell-like colony formation. Third, DNMT inhibition, both before and after ES cell-like colony formation, increases the efficiency of colony maturation. Taken together, these data raise the interesting possibility that selective, small molecule-based epigenetic modulation may promote pluripotency transcription factor expression and in turn, provide a more efficient means for iPS cell production.

Adipose tissue is likely to be an excellent source for cell reprogramming for at least two reasons. First, adipose tissue, like bone marrow, maintains adult mesenchymal stem cells that can differentiate toward the osteogenic, adipogenic, neurogenic, myogenic, and chondrogenic lineage [33-35]. Second, it has been demonstrated that adipose derived stem cells express high levels of pluripotent transcription factors such as Oct4, Sox2, Rex1, Klf4, cMyc, and Esrrβ [28,35]. Therefore, these cells may provide a more favorable template for reprogramming to ES-like cells due to their greater plasticity for reprogramming coupled with their broader differentiation potential relative to non-adipose-derived tissue sources. Moreover, adipose cells may also provide an avenue for creating model "disease-in-a-dish" systems that exploit natural variations among fat depots associated with divergent metabolic responses.

Numerous groups are attempting to bypass viral vector-mediated reprogramming factor over-expression as a cell reprogramming strategy. Recent alternative strategies include targeting the activation of self-renewal while inhibiting differentiation by controlling cell-signaling pathways. Approaches include inhibitors of MEK [36], GSK [37], ROCK [36], and TGFβ [38]. In addition, p53 inhibition has been reported to improve reprogramming [39] as well as the application of a Ca^{2+} channel activator [40]. Inhibitors of epigenetic modifications that target DNMT [12,40], HDAC [12], lysine methylase [37], and HMT [40] enable more efficient viral-based reprogramming through single-factor (Oct4) or dual-factor (Oct4 and Sox2) over-expression [38,41]. Recently, Yuan and colleagues reported that the protein, arginine methylatransferase inhibitor (AMI-5), in combination with a TGFβ inhibitor, enabled Oct4 single-factor induced reprogramming of mouse embryonic fibroblasts [24]. These and other results indicate that a pure chemical-based reprogramming strategy for somatic cells is indeed, feasible.

5. CONCLUSION

In this study, we identified multiple effects of small molecule epigenetic modulators on somatic cell reprogramming. Primarily, we found that HDAC inhibition, prior to reprogramming factor transfection, increases ES cell-like colony formation up to 3-fold as compared to non-treated controls. Furthermore, DNMT inhibition before and after reprogramming factor induction promotes maturation of partially reprogrammed cells and yields ~4-fold more mature colonies than the control group. Thus, our data demonstrate that small molecule-based epigenetic modulation can be used to augment existing virus-based reprogramming regimens. In addition, our work here may also provide valuable information regarding the development of virus-independent, small molecule-based reprogramming strategies that target restrictive epigenetic modifications that are established during differentiation.

6. ACKNOWLEDGEMENTS

The authors thank Dr. David Burk and Ms. Susan Newman for technical advice. This work was funded by the Louisiana Board of Regents Industrial Ties Program Grant LEQSF (2008-11)-RD-B-06 and by NIH Small Business Innovation Research grant (1 R43 HL104977). We also acknowledge the use of Genomics, Cell Biology and Imaging Core facilities that are supported, in part, by COBRE (NIH P20- RR021945) and NORC (NIH 1P30-DK072476) center grants from the NIH.

REFERENCES

[1] Takahashi, K. and Yamanaka, S. (2006) Induction of pluripotent stem cells from mouse embryonic and adult fibroblast cultures by defined factors. *Cell*, **126**, 663-676. doi:10.1016/j.cell.2006.07.024

[2] Park, I.-H., Arora., N., Huo, H.G., Maherali, N., Ahfeldt, T., Shimamura, A., Lensch, M.W., Cowan, C., Hochedlinger, K. and Daley, G. Q. (2008) Disease-Specific induced pluripotent stem cells. *Cell*, **134**, 1-10. doi:10.1016/j.cell.2008.07.041

[3] Yu, J.Y., Vodyanik, M.A., Smuga-Otto, K., Antosiewicz-Bourget, J., Frane, J.L., Tian, S., Nie, J., Jonsdottir, G.A., Ruotti, V., Stewart, R., Slukvin, I.I. and Thomson, J.A. (2007) Induced pluripotent stem cell lines derived from human somatic cells. *Science*, **318**, 1917-1920. doi:10.1126/science.1151526

[4] Meng, X.L., Shen, J.S., Kawagoe, S., Ohashi, T., Brady, R.O., *et al.* (2010) Induced pluripotent stem cells derived from mouse models of lysosomal storage disorders. *Proceedings of the National Academy of Sciences of the USA*, **107**, 7886-7891. doi:10.1073/pnas.1002758107

[5] Ebert, A.D., Yu, J.Y., Rose, F.F. Jr., Mattis, V.B., Lorson, C.L., *et al.* (2009) Induced pluripotent stem cells from a spinal muscular atrophy patient. *Nature*, **457**, 277-280.

[6] Lee, G., Papapetrou, E.P., Kim, H., Chambers, S.M., Tomishima, M.J., *et al.* (2009) Modelling pathogenesis and treatment of familial dysautonomia using patient-specific iPSCs. *Nature*, **461**, 402-406.

[7] Rashid, S.T., Corbineau, S., Hannan, N., Marciniak, S.J., Miranda, E., *et al.* (2010) Modeling inherited metabolic disorders of the liver using human induced pluripotent stem cells. *The Journal of Clinical Investigation*, **120**, 3127-3136. doi:10.1172/JCI43122

[8] Zhang, N., An, M.C., Montoro, D., Ellerby, L.M. (2010) Characterization of human huntington's disease cell model from induced pluripotent stem cells. *PLoS Currents*, **2**, RRN1193. doi:10.1371/currents.RRN1193

[9] Zhao, T. and Xu, Y. (2010) p53 and stem cells: New developments and new concerns. *Trends in Cell Biology*, **20**, 170-175. doi:10.1016/j.tcb.2009.12.004

[10] Yu, J.Y., Hu, K.J., Smuga-Otto, K., Tian, S.L., Stewart, R., Slukvin, I.I. and Thomson, J.A., (2009) Human induced pluripotent stem cells free of vector and transgene sequences. *Science*, **10**, 797-801. doi:10.1126/science.1172482

[11] Sommer, C.A., Stadtfeld, M., Murphy, G.J., Hochedlinger, K., Kotton, D.N., *et al.* (2009) Induced pluripotent stem cell generation using a single lentiviral stem cell cassette. *Stem Cells*, **27**, 543-549. doi:10.1634/stemcells.2008-1075

[12] Huangfu, D.W., Maehr, R., Guo, W.J., Eijkelenboom, A., Snitow, M., Chen, A.E. and Melton, D.A. (2008) Induction of pluripotent stem cells by defined factors is greatly improved by small-molecule compounds. *Nature Biotechnology*, **26**, 795-797.

[13] Okita, K., Nakagawa, M., H., Hong, Ichisaka, T. and Yamanaka, S., (2008) Generation of mouse induced pluripotent stem cells without viral vectors. *Science*, **322**, 949-953. doi:10.1126/science.1164270

[14] Warren, L., Manos, P.D., Ahfeldt, T., Loh, Y.-H., Li, H., *et al.* (2010) Highly efficient reprogramming to pluripotency and directed differentiation of human cells with synthetic modified mRNA. *Cell Stem Cell*, **7**, 618-630. doi:10.1016/j.stem.2010.08.012

[15] Yakubov, E., Rechavi, G., Rozenblatt, S. and Givol, D.

(2010) Reprogramming of human fibroblasts to pluripotent stem cells using mRNA of four transcription factors. *Biochemical and Biophysical Research Communications*, **394**, 189-193. doi:10.1016/j.bbrc.2010.02.150

[16] Anokye-Danso, F., Trivedi, C.M., Juhr, D., Gupta, M., Cui, Z., *et al.* (2011) Highly efficient miRNA-mediated reprogramming of mouse and human somatic cells to pluripotency. *Cell Stem Cell*, **8**, 376-388. doi:10.1016/j.stem.2011.03.001

[17] Woltjen, K., Michael, I.P., Mohseni, P., Desai, R., Mileikovsky, M., *et al.* (2009) *piggy*Bac transposition reprograms fibroblasts to induced pluripotent stem cells. *Nature*, **458**, 766-770.

[18] Kaji, K., Norrby, K., Paca, A., Mileikovsky, M., Mohseni, P., *et al.* (2009) Virus-Free induction of pluripotency and subsequent excision of reprogramming factors. *Nature*, **458**, 771-775.

[19] Kim, D., Kim, C.-H, Moon, J.-I., Chung, Y.-G., Chang, M.-Y., Han, B.-S., Ko, S., Yang, E., Cha, K.Y., Lanza, R. and Kim, K.-S. (2009) Generation of human induced pluripotent stem cells by direct delivery of reprogramming proteins. *Cell Stem Cell*, **4**, 472-476. doi:10.1016/j.stem.2009.05.005

[20] Zhou, H.Y., Wu, S.L., Joo, J.Y., Zhu, S.Y., Han, D.W., Lin, T.X., Trauger, S., Bien, G., Yao, S., Zhu, Y., Siuzdak, G., Scholer, H.R., Duan, L.X. and Ding, S. (2009) Generation of induced pluripotent stem cells using recombinant proteins. *Cell Stem Cell*, **4**, 381-384.

[21] Zhu, S.Y., Li, W.L., Zhou, H.Y., Wei, W.G., Ambasudhan, R., *et al.* (2010) Reprogramming of human primary somatic cells by OCT4 and chemical compounds. *Cell Stem Cell*, **7**, 651-655. doi:10.1016/j.stem.2010.11.015

[22] Li, Y., Zhang, Q., Yin, X., Yang, W., Du, Y., *et al.* (2011) Generation of iPSCs from mouse fibroblasts with a single gene, Oct4, and small molecules. *Cell Research*, **21**, 196-204. doi:10.1038/cr.2010.142

[23] Chen, J.K., Liu, J., Yang, J.Q., Chen, Y., Chen, J., *et al.* (2011) BMPs functionally replace Klf4 and support efficient reprogramming of mouse fibroblasts by Oct4 alone. *Cell Research*, **21**, 205-212. doi:10.1038/cr.2010.172

[24] Yuan, X., Wan, H., Zhao, X., Zhu, S., Zhou, Q., *et al.* (2011) Combined chemical treatment enables Oct4-induced reprogramming from mouse embryonic fibroblasts. Stem Cells, **29**, 549-553. doi:10.1002/stem.594

[25] Zhu, S., Wei, W. and Ding, S. (2011) Chemical strategies for stem cell biology and regenerative medicine. *Annual Review of Biomedical Engineering*, **13**, 73-90.

[26] Jaenisch, R. and Young, R. (2008) Stem cells, the molecular circuitry of pluripotency and nuclear reprogramming. *Cell*, **132**, 567-582. doi:10.1016/j.cell.2008.01.015

[27] Kim, J., Chu, J.L., Shen, X.H., Wang, J.L. and Orkin, S.H. (2008) An extended transcriptional network for pluripotency of embryonic stem cells. *Cell*, **132**, 1049-1061. doi:10.1016/j.cell.2008.02.039

[28] Sun, N., Panetta, N.J., Gupta, D.M., Wilson, K.D., Lee, A., *et al.* (2009) Feeder-Free derivation of induced pluripotent stem cells from adult human adipose stem cells. *Proceedings of the National Academy of Sciences of the USA*, **106**, 15720-15725. doi:10.1073/pnas.0908450106

[29] Chan, E.M., Ratanasirintrawoot, S., Park, I.-H., Manos, P.D., Loh, Y.-H., *et al.* (2009) Live cell imaging distinguishes bona fide human iPS cells from partially reprogrammed cells. *Nature Biotechnology*, **27**, 1033-1037.

[30] Stadtfeld, M., Apostolou, E., Akutsu, H., Fukuda, A., Follett, P., *et al.* (2010) Aberrant silencing of imprinted genes on chromosome 12qF1 in mouse induced pluripotent stem cells. *Nature*, **465**, 175-181.

[31] Sul, H.S., Smas, C., Mei, B. and Zhou, L. (2000) Function of pref-1 as an inhibitor of adipocyte differentiation. *International Journal of Obesity and Related Metabolic Disorders*, **24**, 15-19.

[32] Wylie, A.A., Murphy, S.K., Orton, T.C. and Jirtle, R.L. (2000) Novel imprinted DLK1/GTL2 domain on human chromosome 14 contains motifs that mimic those implicated in IGF2/H19 regulation. *Genome Research*, **10**, 1711-1718. doi:10.1101/gr.161600

[33] Zuk, P.A., Zhu, M., Ashjian, P., De Ugarte, D.A., Huang J.I., *et al.* (2002) Human adipose tissue is a source of multipotent stem cells. *Molecular Biology of the Cell*, **13**, 4279-4295. doi:10.1091/mbc.E02-02-0105

[34] Zuk, P.A., Zhu, M., Mizuno, H., Huang, J., Futrell, J.W., *et al.* (2001) Multilineage cells from human adipose tissue: implications for cell-based therapies. *Tissue Engineering*, **7**, 211-228. doi:10.1089/107632701300062859

[35] Izadpanah, R., Trygg, C., Patel, B., Kriedt, C., Dufour, J., Gimble, J.M. and Bunnell, B.A. (2006) Biologic properties of mesenchymal stem cells derived from bone marrow and adipose tissue. *Journal of Cellular Biochemistry*, **99**, 1285-1297. doi:10.1002/jcb.20904

[36] Lin, T.X., Ambasudhan, R., Yuan, X., Li, W.L., Hilcove, S., *et al.* (2009) A chemical platform for improved induction of human iPSCs. *Nature Methods*, **6**, 805-808.

[37] Li, W.L., Zhou, H.Y., Abujarour, R., Zhu, S.Y., Joo, Y.J., *et al.* (2009) Generation of human-induced pluripotent stem cells in the absence of exogenous Sox2. *Stem Cells*, **27**, 2992-3000. doi:10.1002/stem.240

[38] Ichida, J.K., Blanchard, J., Lam, K., Son, E.Y., Chung, J.E., *et al.* (2009) A small-molecule inhibitor of tgf-β signaling replaces Sox2 in reprogramming by inducing Nanog. *Cell Stem Cell*, **5**, 491-503. doi:10.1016/j.stem.2009.09.012

[39] Esteban, M.A., Wang, T., Qin, B.M., Yang, J.Y., Qin, D.J., *et al.* (2010) Vitamin C enhances the generation of mouse and human induced pluripotent stem cells. *Cell Stem Cell*, **6**, 71-79. doi:10.1016/j.stem.2009.12.001

[40] Shi, Y., Desponts, C., Do, J.T., Hahm, H.S., Scholer, H.R., *et al.* (2008) Induction of pluripotent stem cells from mouse embryonic fibroblasts by Oct4 and Klf4 with small-molecule compounds. *Cell Stem Cell*, **3**, 568-574. doi:10.1016/j.stem.2008.10.004

[41] Huangfu, D.W., Osafune, K., Maehr, R., Guo, W.J., Eijkelenboom, A., Chen, S.B., Muhlestein, W. and Melton, D.A. (2008) Induction of pluripotent stem cells from primary human fibroblasts with only Oct4 and Sox2. *Nature Biotechnology*, **26**, 1269-1275.

23

Adipose-derived stem cell therapy for severe muscle tears in working German shepherds: Two case reports

S. Gary Brown[1], Robert J. Harman[2], Linda L. Black[2]

[1]Veterinary Orthopedic and Surgery Service, Western University of Health Sciences, Pomona, USA; gary@vetortho.com
[2]Vet-Stem Inc., Poway, USA; LBlack@Vet-Stem.com

ABSTRACT

Injuries to muscle in the elite athlete are common and may be responsible for prolonged periods of loss of competitive activity. The implications for the athlete, his/her coach and team may be catastrophic if the injury occurs at a critical time in the athlete's diary. Imaging now plays a crucial role in diagnosis, prognostication and management of athletes with muscle injuries. This article discusses the methods available to clinicians and radiologists that are used to assess skeletal muscle injury. The spectrum of muscle injuries sustained in the elite athlete population is both discussed and illustrated.

Keywords: Adipose-Derived; Stem Cell; Dog; Muscle

1. INTRODUCTION

Muscle injuries occur frequently in athletic dogs and athletes [1]. Traditional therapies, such as non-steroidal anti-inflammatory administration, rest, antioxidant therapy and physical therapy have generally not been helpful in preventing fibrosis and permanent muscle contracture, which leads to functional impairment. Similar findings occur in human medicine in that similar suggested treatments for muscle injury are generally not sufficient to enhance muscle regeneration and prevent fibrosis [2].

Depending on their severity, muscle strains may be categorized into three grades [1]: Grade 1 is a mild strain with damage to individual muscle fibers with no hematoma formation; Grade 2 is a more extensive tear, with increased muscle fiber involvement, with no complete rupture [3], localized swelling and heat and slight lameness; and Grade 3 is a complete rupture of a muscle with major disruption of the muscle fibers and hematoma formation, palpable disruption, and significant pain [1].

Inflammation, the hallmark of acutely injured muscle [4], initiates a rapid invasion of the muscle by inflammatory cell populations that can persist for days to weeks. The inflammation phase is followed, and partially coexists with the muscle repair, regeneration, and growth phases. Neutrophils migrate to injured muscle followed by macrophages that remove damaged myofibers [5] and secrete factors that are chemotactic for muscle precursor cells [6]. Macrophages have also been implicated in muscle damage via the release of nitric oxide and through promotion of membrane damage in non-diseased muscle [4]. Although new muscle fibers regenerate after injury, the healing progress is very slow and can lead to fibrosis and functional impairment [6].

Biological approaches to enhance muscle regeneration and prevent fibrosis are being investigated in animal models and human medicine [6]. Because of the lack of therapeutic options that decrease fibrosis, significant efforts are being made to improve the current treatment of skeletal muscle injury using a regenerative medicine approach [2]. Matziolus *et al.* demonstrated that autologous bone marrow-derived cells enhance muscle strength following skeletal muscle crush injury in rats [7]. The same group later reported that rats with severe skeletal muscle injury treated with mesenchymal stem cells responded in a dose dependent manner with an increasing logarithmic response in muscle contractile force as the dose of MSCs was increased [8]. Muscle derived stem cells used in skeletal muscle injury in mice promote angiogenesis and decrease fibrosis [9]. Merritt and colleagues used MSC-seeded extracellular matrix (ECM) to treat skeletal muscle injury in rats. This group demonstrated that the implanted MSC-seeded ECM had more blood vessels and regenerating skeletal myofibers than the ECM without cells ($p < 0.05$). There is ample literature to support the use of adult stem cells in the treatment of muscle injury.

Adipose-derived stem cells (ADSC) have been the focus of recent reviews [10] and studies [9,11-13]. Autologous ADSCs have been used in veterinary medicine since 2003. However, there are no reports to our knowledge of treatment with ADSCs or other stem cells, in dogs with muscle injury. Two working, male German shepherd dogs presented for acute semitendinosus muscle injuries in one or both hind limbs. The surgeon confirmed the clinical diagnosis of muscle tear using ultrasound. At that time, approximately 60 grams of fat was harvested from the falciform ligament in each, and the ADSC (stromal vascular fraction) extracted by Vet-Stem, Inc. (Poway, CA) [11]. Forty-eight hours later, the dogs were placed under anesthesia and the ADSC aliquot was injected with a 22 gauge needle by digital palpation directly into the muscle, both intralesional and paralesional, and intravenously. Follow-up ultrasound evaluations were performed six to ten weeks after stem cell therapy. Muscle biopsy was not performed because of potential increased morbidity in a clinical case. New needle biopsy techniques might be considered in the future. MRI was not available in this practice. Outcome measurements for the case reports included owner assessments (visual assessment of dog's improvement in affected tasks) and surgeon assessments (flexibility and agility from normal to very severe) before and at end of treatment period, and the ability of the dog to return to work.

2. CASE REPORTS

Cris, a four-year-old male German shepherd police dog, became suddenly lame while training. Five days later, the owner reported that the dog's lameness had improved but that the dog's gait remained abnormal. Cris presented at that time bearing less weight on the left rear limb with a slight circumduction gait. On palpation, the distal two-thirds of the left semitendinosus muscle was swollen at the mid belly region with a palpable dimple. Sonography revealed poorly defined hypoechoic region in the distal two-thirds of the left semitendinosus muscle 8.1 mm wide × 30.8 mm long. These findings are compatible with a focal tear in the left semitendinosus muscle with an area of central hemorrhage and/or edema consistent with a grade 3 tear (**Figure 1**). No abnormalities were seen in the right semitendinosus muscle. At that time, the surgeon prescribed Previcox (227 mg 5 days/week) and antioxidant therapy (Niacinamide, 50 mg/day; Sam-E, 225 mg/day; Vitamin E, 200 IU/day; 3V Caps, 1 cap/day; and Omega Mint, 1/day) and the dog was prescribed cage rest for two weeks.

After two weeks, Cris had not responded to traditional therapy and the owner elected to treat with stem cells. After fat collection and stem cell isolation as previously described [11], the surgeon injected approximately 4.7 million ADSCs into the muscle injury site. Approximately 4.7 million cells were injected intravenously (IV). Antioxidant therapy was continued. Cris was walked each day for one month then began light training. Sonographic examination at 82 days post injection revealed significant reduction in lesion size, 11 mm wide × 15 mm long (**Figure 2(a)**-pre, **(b)**-post) and an increased number of fibers coursing through this area that appeared organized and oriented in the same plane as the normal muscle. Clinically the dog was normal with no lameness or gait abnormalities. On the owner evaluation, Cris improved from moderately affected before therapy to normal within 19 weeks after therapy. The surgeon's evaluation of Cris revealed him to have severely affected flexibility and moderately affected agility before therapy that improved to normal 19 weeks after the stem cell injection. Telephone conversation 21 months post injection reveals that he was in service and completely normal.

Jago, an eight-year-old male German shepherd police

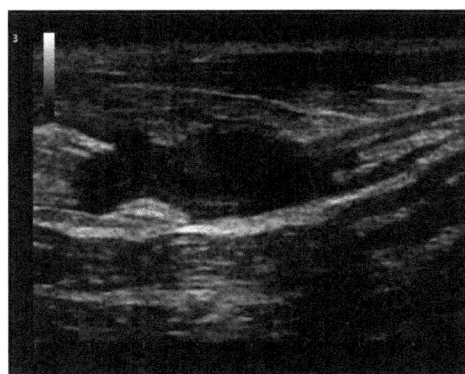

(a)

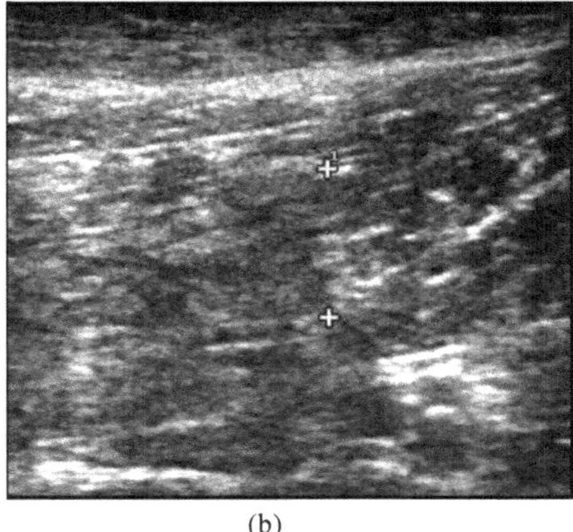

(b)

Figure 1. (a) Ultrasound scan of Cris left ST muscle tear before treatment: An 8 mm wide and 30 mm long poorly defined hypoechoic area is noted in the distal two thirds of the ST muscle compatible with a muscle tear; (b) Cris 82 days after treatment: The lesion is poorly defined with an iso-echoic area that measured 11 mm wide and 15 mm in length. An increase in fiber numbers is noted that are oriented in the same plane as the normal muscle.

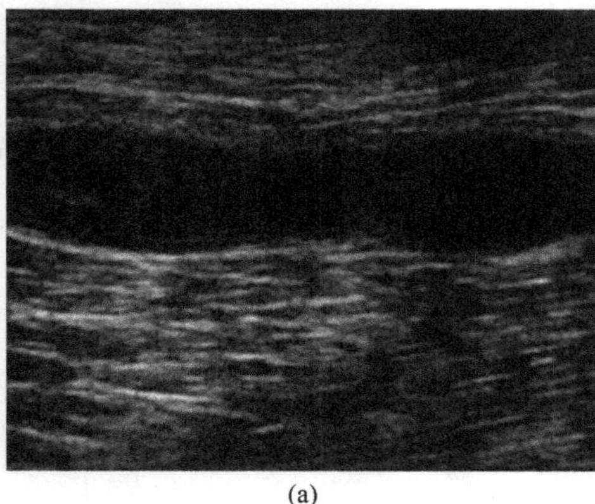

(a)

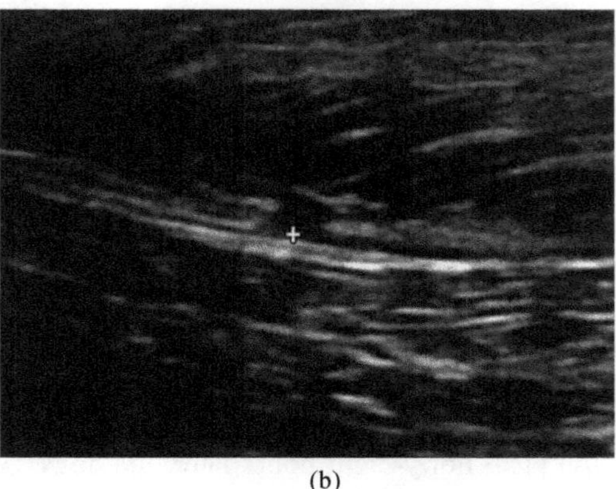

(b)

Figure 2. (a) Jago sonogram before treatment. A 9 mm wide × 6 cm long hypoechoic area exists in the cranial aspect of the right semitendinosus muscle consistent with a muscle tear. Generalized disruption of the muscle fiber pattern with no organized hyperechoic areas suggestive of scarring; (b) 11 weeks after ADSC treatment. The previously seen hypoechoic area decreased in size to measure 5 mm wide × 2.4 cm in length. An increase in fiber pattern development with fibers running parallel to the orientation of the muscle was observed.

dog, was injured during a suspect apprehension and presented seven days after injury with moderate to severe lameness and semitendinosus tenderness and swelling. Both rear limbs were affected. He was diagnosed clinically and sonographically with a grade 2.5 acute on chronic injury to his right semitendinosus muscle as demonstrated by ultrasound (**Figure 2(a)**-pre) and a grade 1 acute on chronic injury to his left semitendinosus muscle (not shown). The right muscle was about 30 percent enlarged on palpation and the dog had a circumduction gait in the right rear limb. The left muscle had no palpable enlargement, was not tender to palpation, and he had no gait abnormality, but had a history of stiffness. Jago was treated with 7.5 million ADSC in each muscle lesion and administered 3.8 million cells IV. He underwent physical therapy and antioxidant therapy, and was prescribed deracoxib (37.5 mg SID). Jago underwent one month of a progressively increased walking regimen prior to resuming light training at 105 days.

Twenty-two (22) weeks after injection Jago was markedly improved. His surgeon scores for agility and flexibility improved from severely affected to mildly affected. His owner evaluations were markedly improved. Jago competed in a two-day police dog competition and placed second in protection and third place in obedience 22 weeks post ADSC injection.

3. DISCUSSION

The beneficial effects of ADSC therapy in muscle injury are likely explained by the local secretion of cytokines and growth factors [14-16]. Natsu *et al.* treated skeletal muscle laceration with bone marrow-derived MSCs, and the muscle improved functionally without evidence of fusion or differentiation of the injected cells suggesting that mechanisms other than differentiation were responsible for the benefit seen [16]. ADSCs are also immunomodulatory, which may play a therapeutic role [17,18].

4. CONCLUSION

ADSC therapy enhanced muscle healing and prevented fibrosis in these clinical cases, similar to the reported literature in laboratory animals. The dogs returned to their previous training and occupations with a functional gait and no lameness. This is the first report of using stem cells in dogs to treat skeletal muscle injury. Further controlled clinical trials are necessary for the complete evaluation of the therapeutic benefit of ADSC therapy in canine muscle injuries.

5. ACKNOWLEDGEMENTS

The authors wish to thank Dr. David Detweiller, ACVR, for performing the sonograms and for his evaluations and comments. We thank Karen Lavrischeff, RVT for her editorial assistance.

REFERENCES

[1] Lee, J.C., *et al.* (2012) Imaging of muscle injuries. *British Journal of Radiology*, 2012. doi:10.1259/bjr/84622172

[2] Quintero, A., Wright, V., Fu, F., *et al.* (2009) Stem cells for the treatment of skeletal muscle injury. *Clinics in Sports Medicine*, **28**, 1-11. doi:10.1016/j.csm.2008.08.009

[3] Lewis, D., Shelton, D., Piras, A., *et al.* (1997) Gracilis or semitendinosus myopathy in 18 dogs. *Journal of the American Animal Hospital Association*, **33**, 177-188.

[4] Tidball, J. (2005) Inflammatory processes in muscle injury and repair. *American Physiological Society American Journal of Physiology—Regulatory, Integrative and Com-*

parative Physiology, **288**, 345-353.

[5] Hannafin, J.A., Pedowitz, R.A., Hidaka, C., *et al.* (1994) Pathophysiology and healing of musculoskeletal tissues. In: Griffin, L.Y., Ed., *Orthopaedic Knowledge Update: Sports Medicine*, American Academy of Orthopaedic, Rosemont, 17-33.

[6] Fukushima, K., Badlani, N., Usas, A., *et al.* (2001) The use of an antifibrosis agent to improve muscle recovery after laceration. *The American Journal of Sports Medicine*, **29**, 394-402.

[7] Matziolis, G., Winkler, T., Schaser, K., Wiemann, M., *et al.* (2006) Autologous bone marrow-derived cells enhance muscle strength following skeletal muscle crush injury in rats. *Tissue Engineering*, **12**, 361-367. doi:10.1089/ten.2006.12.361

[8] Winkler, T., von Roth, P., Matziolis, G., *et al.* (2009) Dose-response relationship of mesenchymal stem cell transplantation and functional regeneration after severe skeletal muscle injury in rats. *Tissue Engineering*, **15**, 487-494. doi:10.1089/ten.tea.2007.0426

[9] Ota, S., Uehara, K., Nozaki, M., *et al.* (2011) Intramuscular transplantation of muscle-derived stem cells accelerates skeletal muscle healing after contusion injury via enhancement of angiogenesis. *The American Journal of Sports Medicine*, **9**, 1912-1922. doi:10.1177/0363546511415239

[10] Gimble, J., Bunnell, B., Chiu, E., *et al.* (2011) Concise Review: Adipose-derived stromal vascular fraction cells and stem cells: Let's not get lost in translation. *Stem Cells*, **29**, 749-754. doi:10.1002/stem.629

[11] Black, L., Gaynor, J., Gahring, D., *et al.* (2007) Effect of adipose-derived mesenchymal stem and regenerative cells on lameness in dogs with chronic osteoarthritis of the coxofemoral joints: A randomized, double-blinded, multicenter, controlled trial. *Veterinary Therapeutics*, **8**, 272-284.

[12] Dahlgren, L.A. (2006) Use of adipose derived stem cells in tendon and ligament injuries. *Proceedings of American College of Veterinary Surgeons—Veterinary Symposium Equine and Small Animal*, **35**, E5.

[13] Nixon, A., Dahlgren, L., Haupt, J., *et al.* (2008) Effect of adipose-derived nucleated cell fractions on tendon repair in a collagenase-induced tendinitis model. *American Journal of Veterinary Research*, **69**, 1-10. doi:10.2460/ajvr.69.7.928

[14] Caplan, A. and Diego, C. (2011) The MSC: An injury drugstore. *Cell Stem Cell*, **9**, 11-15. doi:10.1016/j.stem.2011.06.008

[15] Kilroy, G., Foster, S., Wu, X., *et al.* (2007) Cytokine profile of human adipose-derived stem cells: Expression of angiogenic, hematopoietic, and pro-inflammatory factors. *Journal of Cellular Physiology*, **212**, 702-709. doi:10.1002/jcp.21068

[16] Natsu, K., *et al.* (2004) Allogeneic bone marrow-derived mesenchymal stromal cells promote the regeneration of injured skeletal muscle without differentiation into myofibers. *Tissue Engineering*, **10**, 1093-1112. doi:10.1089/ten.2004.10.1093

[17] Le Blanc, K. (2006) Mesenchymal stromal cells: Tissue repair and immune modulation. *Cytotherapy*, **8**, 559-561.

[18] McIntosh, K., Zvonic, S., Garrett, S., *et al.* (2006) The immunogenicity of adipose derived cells: Temporal changes *in vitro*. *Stem Cells*, **24**, 1246-1253. doi:10.1634/stemcells.2005-0235

24

Investigation of VEGF and PDGF signals in vascular formation by 3D culture models using mouse ES cells

Hitomi Hosoe[1], Yuri Yamamoto[1], Yusuke Tanaka[1], Mami Kobayashi[2], Nana Ninagawa[2], Shigeko Torihashi[1,2*]

[1]Department of Physical Therapy, Nagoya University School of Health Sciences, Nagoya, Japan;
[*]Corresponding Author: storiha@met.nagoya-u.ac.jp
[2]Department of Health Sciences, Nagoya University Graduate School of Medicine, Nagoya, Japan

ABSTRACT

Vascular formation *in vivo* involves several processes and signal cascades subsequently occurring in the embryo. Several models by ES cells have been reported for analysis *in vitro*. We show here a 3D culture system using collagen gel (AteloCell) as a simple and useful system for investigating vascular formations and analyzing the roles of factors *in vivo*. Although VEGF and PDGF are growth factors with multi-potentials for vascular formation, their sequential roles have not been elucidated. We investigated the effects of VEGF and PDGF B signals for vascular formation by a 3D culture system that embedded embryoid bodies (EBs) from ES cells into a collagen gel. After embedding EBs in the collagen gel with a medium containing VEGF, EBs gave off CD105 immunopositive vessels as the initial step of vasculogenesis. When the factor in the culture medium for EBs was switched from VEGF to PDGF B after 5 days of culture, the morphological features of vessels varied, suggesting the occurrence of vascular-type differentiation. After 11 days of 3D culture, vessels in both groups cultured with VEGF alone and switching to VEGF B at day 5 showed Flk-1 immunoreactivity. Some blood vessels cultured with PDGF B after day 5 expressed either EphrinB2 (arteriole marker) or Flt-4 (lymphatic marker) immunoreactivity, but vessels cultured with VEGF alone exhibited neither of them. Vessels cultured with these two factors could not differentiate into a venous type. The present study indicates that VEGF is the initial signal for vasculogenesis, and that PDGF B is probably involved in vascular diversification.

Keywords: Vasculogenesis; Angiogenesis; VEGF; PDGF; ES Cells; 3D Culture Model; Collagen Gel

1. INTRODUCTION

ES cells with pluripotency have been used to investigate the vascular formations involving primitive blood vessel formation, the differentiation of endothelial cells with a lumen, the assembly into cord-like structure, and the differentiation of vascular types. Early investigations *in vitro* used embryoid bodies (EBs) that resembled developing embryos in a 2D culture system [1]. Instead of 2D growths of vessels, 3D cultures showed a further similarity to vasculogenesis *in vivo*. Although Matrigel provide a useful material for 3D culture, several unqualified inclusions have interfered with a critical analysis [2-4]. The AteloCell, a highly purified and cutting off antigenic region of type I collagen proved more suitable than Matrigel for a 3D culture, and has been commonly used recently [5-7]. We used AteloCell collagen gel and embedded EBs completely into it in our model. Therefore, all blood vessels protruding from EBs expanded 3 dimensionally, similar to those in the embryo. Because the initiation of vasculogenesis involves several signal cascades and processes subsequently occur in the embryo, it still remained unclear and is worthy of investigation using a 3D culture system *in vitro*.

VEGF is well known as a key factor for both vasculogenesis as well as angiogenesis [8-11]. PDGF B is also a critical factor for the development of blood vessels [12,13]. Both factors independently participate in several steps of vascular formation. However, sequential usage of VEGF and PDGF B promoted angiogenesis in the myocardium following infarction [14]. Therefore, a combination of those two growth factors would produce non prospective effects on the blood vessel development that actually occurs in vascular formation *in vivo*. In the present study, we employed a 3D culture model using collagen gel, and analyzed the subsequent participation of two factors *i.e.*, VEGF and PDGF B in a vascular formation. Our findings indicate that VEGF initiated vasculogenesis, and PDGF B may have been involved in the differentiation of vascular types.

2. MATERIALS AND METHODS

2.1. Culture of Mouse ES Cells (M-ESCs)

Mouse ES cells (M-ESCs: G4-2; carrying the enhanced green fluorescent protein—EGFP—gene under the control of cytomegalovirus/chicken β-actin promoter) were expanded in the culture medium termed ES-DMEM. That is, Dulbecco's modified Eagle's medium (Sigma; St. Louis, MO; www.sigma-aldrich.com) with 0.1 mM non-essential amino acids (GIBCO; Carlsbad, CA; www.invitrogen.com), 100 mM sodium pyruvate (GIBCO), 100 mM 2-mercaptoethanol (Sigma), and 0.5% antibiotic-antimycotic (GIBCO) containing 10% fetal bovine serum (FBS; Biological Industries, Kibbuiz, Israel; www.bioind.com). For the expansion of M-ESCs, 1,000 U/mL of leukemia inhibitory factor (LIF; Chemicon, Temecula, CA; www.millipore.com) was added to ES-DMEM.

2.2. Induction to Mesodermal Cells and Preparation of 3D Culture

ES cells were changed to ES-DMEM (without LIF) to form embryoid bodies (EBs). About 660 cells in each well of a Micro Sphere array (MSCW1-CA600, STEM Biomethod http://stem-biomethod.co.jp) were compacted to form EBs for 2 days and treated with 10 - 3 mM all-trans retinoic acid (RA: R2625, Sigma) for 1 day. After 2 days of rinsing by ES-DMEM, EBs were embedded into collagen gel (AteloCell, DME-02; KOKEN Tokyo, www.kokenmpc.co.jp). About 30 EBs in each 35-mm dish (BD Falcon; www.bd.com) were mounted in 1 mL of collagen gel and incubated at 37˚C for one hour. After the solidifying of collagen gel, 1.5 mL of culture medium was added. At that moment, the date of 3D culture was designated as Day 0.

2.3. Medium Condition

From days 0 to 4, some EBs termed VEGF+ were incubated in ES-DMEM with 50 ng/mL of VEGF (VEGF A; mBA-165, Santa Cruz Biotech, Santa Cruz, CA.; www.scbt.com). As a control, EBs cultured with ES-DMEM alone were termed VEGF–. After day 5, EBs switched the medium from ES-DMEM with VEGF to ES-DMEM with 50 ng/mL of PDGF B (PDGF-BB, 100 - 14B PeproTech. Rocky Hill NJ.; www.peprotech.com) and were designated a PDGF B group (**Figure 1**). After day 5, EBs that continued to be cultured with VEGF were subsequently termed VEGF+. All culture samples were incubated at 37˚C with 5% CO2, and the medium was changed every other day.

2.4. Fluorescent Immunostaining

Samples in 3D culture were fixed with 4% paraformaldehyde in PBS for 10 minutes. After washing with PBS, the samples were treated with blocking solution containing 10% normal goat or donkey serum and 0.3% triton X-100 in PBS for 15 minutes. Some samples were frozen and sectioned (6 µm thickness) by a Cryostat (CM1510, Leica; Nussloch Germany; www.hbu.de). Samples and sections were incubated with the first antibody followed by a brief rinse with PBS and were treated with Alexa-labeled secondary antibody. The antibodies used are listed in **Table 1**, and first antibodies were incubated at 4˚C for 12 hours. The secondary antibodies were diluted 400 times and used for 30 min. They were rinsed with PBS, then stained with DAPI (1:1000, KPL Gaithersburg MD; www.kpl.com) for 3 min followed by a mounting with FluoromountTM (DBS, Pleasanton, CA; www.dibisys.com). Samples were observed using a fluorescent microscope, BZ-9000 (Keyence Osaka Japan; www.keyence.co.jp). Statistical analysis was carried out using a BZ-II analyzer (Keyence).

Table 1. Antibodies for fluorescent immunostaining.

Antibody (IgG)	Origin		Dilution
PECAM-1 (Goat)	sc-1506	Santa Cruz Biotech	1:50
EphrinB2 (Goat)	AF496	R&D system; Minneapolis MN; www.RnDSystems.com	1:50
Flt-4 (Rabbit)	53493	AnaSpec; San Jose. CA; www.anaspec.com	1:100
Flk-1 (Rabbit)	ab39256	abcam; Tokyo Japan; www.abcam.co.jp	1:100
PDGFR-β (Rabbit)	Ab-1	Thermo; Fremount CA; www.thermo.com	1:200
Eph receptor B4 (Rat)	ab73259	abcam	1:100
PROX1 (Mouse)	M05	Abmova; Taipei Taiwan; www.abnova.com.tw	1:80
CD105 (Rat)	MAB1320	R&D	1:100

Secondary antibodies: Alexa Fluor 594 donkey anti-goat IgG (A11058. Mo- lecular Probes, Leiden, Netherlands; www.probes.com), Alexa Fluor 594 goat anti-rabbit IgG (A11012), Alexa Fluor 594 goat anti-rat IgG (A11007), Alexa Fluor 594 goat anti-mouse IgG (A11005) and Alexa Fluor 488 donkey anti(A11006), Alexa Fluor 350 goat anti-rat IgG (A21093).

2.5. Morphological Analysis

EBs or vessels (budding) from VEGF+, VEGF–, and PDGF B groups were randomly chosen. From days 1 to 4, the number of EBs with budding was counted with three 35 mm culture dishes in each group. The length of 10 buddings was measured every 5 EBs in three dishes. On day 11, the length, thickness and number of branches of 10 vessels for every 5 EBs in three dishes were counted. Vessel thickness was measured at the mid-portion of the vessels from EB to their tips. Student *t*-tests were used to examine the results. Data are presented as mean ± SD. A significance level of $p < 0.05$ was chosen.

2.6. Gene Expression Profiling Using Real-Time PCR

Functional genes were analyzed using a mouse angiogenesis RT2 ProlilerTM PCR array (PAMM-024A; SA Bioscience, Frederick, MD, www.SABiosciences.com). EBs at day 0 and samples of either VEGF+ or PDGF B at day 11 were collected from 3D culture dishes (**Figure 1**). EBs and protruding vessels with small amounts of surrounding collagen gel were taken from the dishes and crushed using an ultrasound-sonic pulverizer for 30 second at 4˚C (Handy sonic; Tomy Seiko Tokyo, http://bio.tomys.co.jp). Subsequently, total mRNAs from these samples were extracted by an RNeasy micro kit (Qiagen, Valencia, CA; www.quiagen.com) according to the manufacturer's instructions. RNAs were immediately reverse-transcripted to cDNA by SuperScriptTM II (Qiagen). Using real-time PCR, 84 genes involved in modulating the biological processes of angiogenesis were analyzed following the manufactures instructions. Sample cDNAs were poured into 96-well plates and processed using a personal real-time PCR system (Mx3000p Stratagene; La Jolla. CA: www.stratagene.com). PCR was amplified to 40 cycles at 95˚C for 15 seconds and 60˚C for 60 seconds.

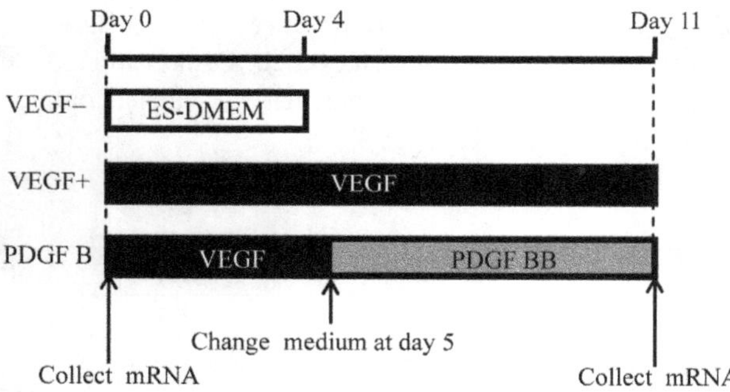

Figure 1. Schema of experimental groups and time schedule. The day when embryoid bodies (EBs) were embedded into AteloCell collagen gel as 3D culture was designated as Day 0. VEGF– group was cultured in the ES-DMEM for 4 days. VEGF+ group was incubated in the medium containing VEGF until day 11. PDGF B group was incubated with the medium containing VEGF that was switched to new one including PDGF B instead of VEGF at day 5. For PCR array, mRNAs were collected from EBs on day 0 and from samples of VEGF+ and PDGF B on day 11.

3. RESULTS

3.1. First Step of Vasculogenesis by VEGF

At day 1, some EBs sprouted a small number of short buds. The number of EBs with budding was higher in VEGF+ than that of VEGF–. On day 2, VEGF+ increased the EBs with budding, and the number of those EBs was remarkably higher than those of VEGF–. However, on days 3 and 4, VEGF– rapidly increased those EBs with processes growing from their buds. The difference in the number of EBs with budding between VEGF+ and VEGF– became smaller. Although the length of processes budding from EBs in both VEGF+ and VEGF– increased, it was longer in VEGF+ than that in VEGF– (**Figure 2**). To determine whether or not processes in VEGF+ and VEGF– were blood vessels, the expression of blood vessel marker proteins was examined by immuno-histochemistry. EBs at day 0 expressed Flt-1 (VEGF receptor 1) but not PDGF receptor β (data not shown). The processes of VEGF+ exhibited CD105 immunoreactivity by day 4, but after longer incubation they all showed both CD105 and PECAM 1 by day 11 (**Figure 3**). On the other hand, processes of VEGF– on day 4 expressed CD105, but did not show PECAM1 by day 11 (data not shown).

3.2. Effects of PDGF B

At day 5, half of the dishes embedding EBs were switched from a medium with VEGF to one containing PDGF B, and were termed the PDGF B group (**Figure 1**). After that, EBs of both VEGF+ and PDGF B groups increased blood vessels gradually (**Figures 4(a)-(d)**). At day 11, morphological features of the vessels differed between the two groups. Vessels of VEGF+ became longer and their average number of branches was higher than those of the PDGF B. Vessels of VEGF+ were thin and branched frequently to make a network or meshwork. The distribution area of vessels was more extensive than that of the PDGF B group (**Figures 4(e)-(f)**). On the other hand, many vessels of PDGF B thickened, and were shorter in the length than those in VEGF+ (**Figure 4(g)**). PDGF B altered the morphological features of the vessels, suggesting that it induced a differentiation of vessel types.

3.3. Expression of Vessel-Type Markers

Expression of marker proteins was examined by immuno-histochemistry on day 11 to identify the type of

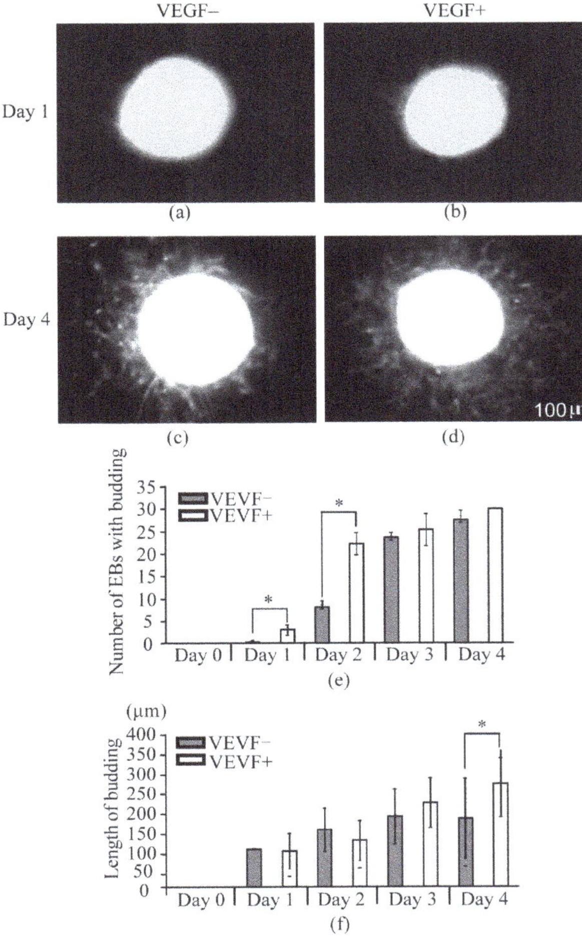

Figure 2. EBs with budding processes and their morphological alteration in VEGF− and VEGF+ groups EBs with budding processes in VEGF− and VEGF+ were demonstrated by EGFP fluorescent on day 1((a), (b)) and day 4 ((c), (d)), and their numerical data were summarized in graphs E and F. The total number of EBs with processes was counted in three 35 mm-dishes of VEGF+ and VEGF− groups (e). The length of the processes was measured in 10 processes of every 5 EBs in three dishes randomly chosen (f). Scale bar (100 μm) is common in (a)-(d). Data are presented as mean ±SD. $^{*}p < 0.05$.

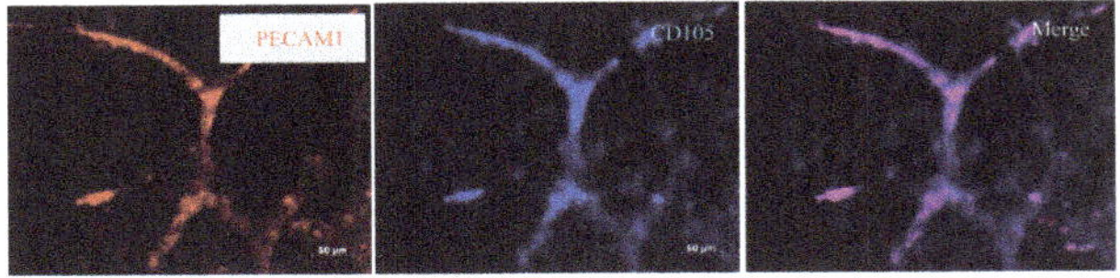

Figure 3. Expression of blood vessel markers. The processes of VEGF+ showed both CD105 and PECAM 1 (endothelial markers) immunoreactivity on day 11. Scale bar is 50 μm.

vessels. All vessels expressed PECAM 1 in both the VDGF+ and PDGF B groups. Vessels in the PDGF B group exhibited either Ephrin-B2, Flt-4 or PROX1 immunoreactivity, whereas none of VEGF+ expressed them **(Figures 5(a)-(c))**. Ephb4, a marker of veins, was ex-

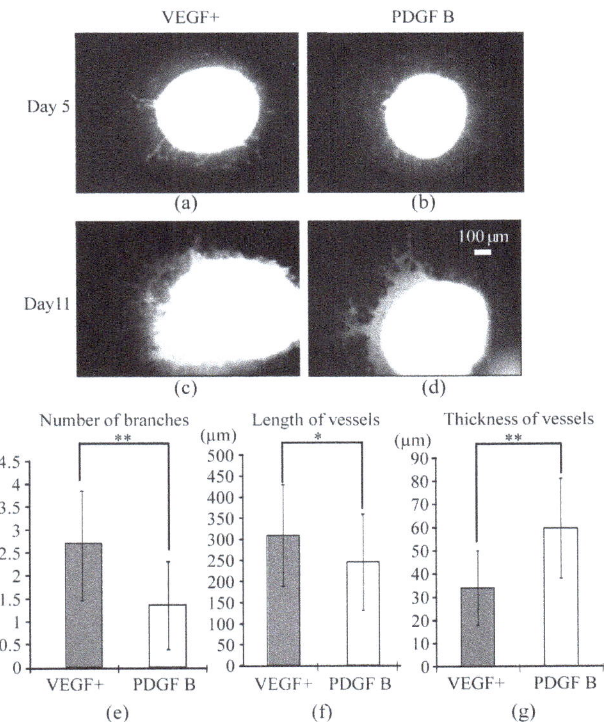

Figure 4. Morphological feature of vessels in VEGF+ and PDGF B. EBs and vessels in VEGF+ and PDGF B were demonstrated by EGFP fluorescent on day 5 (a, b) and day 11 (c, d), and their numerical data were summarized in graphs E, F and G. On day 11, the number of branches, length and thickness of vessels were counted on 10 vessels for every 5 EBs in three dishes of VEGF+ and PDGF B groups respectively. Scale bar (100 μm) is common in A-D. Data are presented as mean ± SD. $^{*}p < 0.05$, $^{**}p < 0.01$.

pressed in neither the VEGF+ nor PDGF B groups (data not shown). Blood vessels in both groups were Flk-1-immunopositive. In the cross sections, Flk 1-positive endothelium formed tubular structures with a lumen at the center of the epithelium. Not all but some of the Flk-1 positive epithelium also showed CD105 (**Figure 5(d)**).

3.4. Expression of mRNAs in Vessels

Expression profiles of mRNA in vessels of the VEGF+ and PDGF B groups were also analyzed by PCR array. A total of 84 genes involved in angiogenic factors that included growth factors and receptors, adhesion molecules, proteases, their inhibitors, matrix proteins, transcription factors and others were compared to both groups of vessels, and were calibrated with mRNA from EBs on day 0. Quite different expression profiles are summarized in **Table 2**. Important genes are shown in **Figure 6(a)**. As shown by the immuno-histochemistry, Ephb4 was low in both VEGF+ and PDGF B supporting protein levels. *Pdgf a* was expressed at a very low level in both vessels.

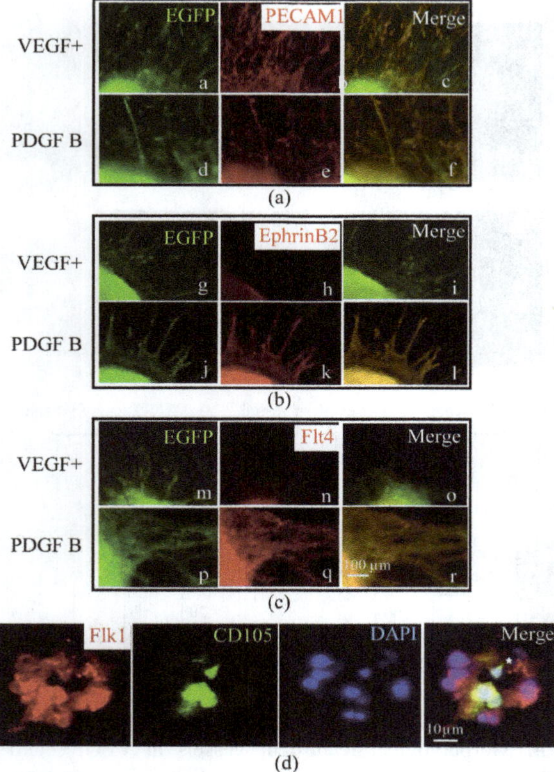

Figure 5. Immunofluorescent analysis of vessel types and existence of the lumen in the vessel at day 11. Common marker of blood vessels, PECAM1 was expressed in both VEGF+ and PDGF B as shown in (a) (a - f). In panel (b), arterial marker ephrin B2 was expressed in PDGF B (j - l), but not in VEGF+ (g - i). In panel (c), Lymphatic vessel marker flt4 was expressed in PDGF B (p - r), but not in VEGF+ (m - o). Scale bar (100 μm) is common in (a)-(c). In the cross section of blood vessels in (d), flk1 immunopositive endothelial cells surround the lumen (asterisk) and some endothelium also showed CD105 immunoreactivity.

Although VEGF was not added to the media of PDGF B after day 5, the mRNA of *Vegf a* was higher in BDGF B than that of VEGF+. Several mRNAs showed contradictory expression patterns. The number of mRNAs that increased expression intensity from EBs at day 0 was higher in PDGF B than that of VEGF+ (**Figure 6(b)**). Furthermore, the increases of the mRNA in PDGF B were more prominent than those of VEGF+. The word "data" is plural, not singular.

4. DISCUSSION

4.1. Three-Dimensional Culture in Collagen Gel

Our 3D culture system presents an environment more analogous to vascular formation *in vivo* than 2D culture. EBs were embedded in a collagen gel that avoided inclusion of the unknown materials involved in Matrigel.

Table 2. Genes showed considerable different expressions.

gene	VEGF+	PDGF B
Angptl	−1.10	4.14
Bai1	9.46	26.69
Ccl2	2.52	8.99
Tymp	7.96	3.16
Epas1	5.95	10.84
Flt1	9.08	3.86
Fzd5	11.17	3.50
Hand2	5.59	1.37
Itgav	1.68	5.73
Npr1	−2.28	1.86
Plg	13.29	4.16
Tbx1	6.07	1.60
Tbx4	3.37	13.91
Tgfb2	2.40	7.05
Tgfb3	1.66	8.68
Tgfbr1	−1.17	5.06
Thbs1	−1.53	3.31
Vegfa	7.79	12.54

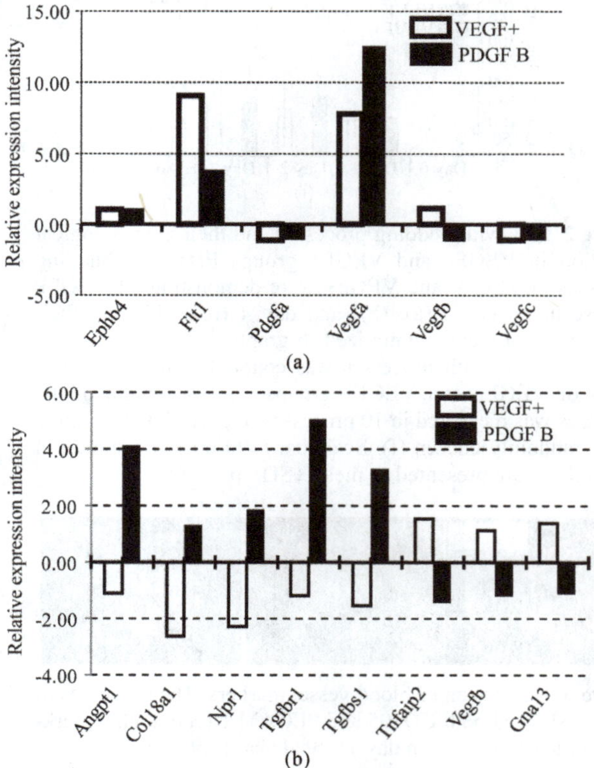

Figure 6. Expression profile of mRNAs in VEGF and PDGF B. Relative expression intensities of mRNAs in VEGF+ and PDGF B are summarized in two graphs (a) and (b). The value of EBs on day 0 is used as a calibrator and indicated as 1.00. Important genes for vessel types and factors are shown in (a). Contradictory expression pattern is shown in (b).

Therefore, we were able to simply compare the potency of two factors, VEGF and BDGF B. Before embedding into collagen gel, ES cells were treated for 2 days with RA during the formation of EBs. This short treatment with RA is important to induce cells into mesodermal lineage expressing VEGF receptor, Flk-1 [15]. Longer treatment with RA leads to a neuronal lineage (data not shown) [16].

4.2. VEGF Initiates Vasculogenesis

When EBs were cultured with VEGF (VEGF+), they protruded processes earlier than EBs without VEGF (VEGF–). Although EBs in VEGF– sprouted processes slightly later than VEGF+, the number of their processes showed a similarity to those of VEGF+ at day 4. The processes from both groups of EBs expressed CD105 immunoreactivities at day 4, while VEGF+ also expressed PECAM1 at day 11. These observations confirmed that the processes induced by VEGF were blood vessels. A previous report by Seifert *et al.* described VEGF as having no effect on ES cells in the differentiation of endothelial cells of blood vessels [17]. They added VEGF (30 ng/mL) directly to ES cells when they began to differentiate due to the withdrawal of LIF. Their ES cells had never been pretreated with RA. Thus, VEGF as shown here was able to initiate vasculogenesis on the mesodermal lineage cells by the treatment with RA. EBs in VEGF– protruded processes slightly later than VEGF+. EBs induced to mesodermal cells by RA that could produce VEGF by themselves, and provided it endogenously for vasculogenesis[7,13]. Perhaps EBs in VEGF– were initiated to vasculogenesis by a small amount of VEGF originally involved in ES-DEME [5,18].

4.3. Vascular Diversification by PDGF B Signal

PDGF B has been described as a multiple player in vasculogenesis and angiogenesis. It works on the maturation of blood vessels to develop mural cells/pericytes, angiogenic sprouting, and an increase in VEGF signals through VEGF A; VEGF receptor 2 [6,7,12,13]. However, an effective role for the differentiation of vessel types has not been well investigated.

Our present data indicate that PDGF B rather than VEGF induced the differentiation of vessels. After switching the medium at day 5, the shape of vessels was altered in PDGF B, when the vessels became thick, short and less branched. In fact, Angpt 1 (Angiopoietin 1) mRNA which regulates the blood vessel caliber was extremely up-regulated in PDGF B (**Figure 6(b)**). The markers of vessel types were revealed by immunostaining. Although the vessels in both VEGF+ and PDGF B expressed PECAM 1 (a blood vessel marker), only vessels in PDGF B showed immunoreactivities of either Eph B2 (an arterial marker) or Flt4 (a lymphatic marker). That was also confirmed by an mRNA expression profile by a PCR array (**Table 2**). A variety of mRNAs increased their expression in PDGF B (**Figure 6(b)**). Although VEGF had never been added to the culture medium of the PDGF B group, the mRNA of *Vegf a* was higher in the PDGF B group than that of VEGF+. After the activation of vasculogenesis by VEGF, vessels in PDGF B were able to produce VEGF on their own [7,13]. On the other hand, VEGF failed to induce the generation of PDGF B by day 11. Our results imply that the differentiation of vessel types requires a PDGF B signal in addition to VEGF. Cao *et al.* described PDGF B-induced lymphangiogenesis that had the potential to grow lymphatic vessels in their system using mouse cornea [19]. PDGF B stimulated both MAP kinase activity and cell motility [12]. Our morphological data support their findings that PDGF B induced the differentiation of lymphatic vessels, though their underlying molecular mechanisms have not been clarified.

Arterial-venous specifications have not been fully elucidated. Recently, notch and β-catenin signaling, in addition to VEGF, have been postulated an effective for arterial specifications [20]. Yamamizu *et al.* and others have described cAMP as also being involved in the arterial fate. When such signals are blocked, the arterial fate alters to a venous one under the influence of VEGF, which basically induces venous characteristics in vascular progenitors [21-23]. Our findings have been somewhat controversial. Neither VEGF+ nor PDGF B induced venous differentiation. Probably an unknown signal except for VEGF will be required in our system to differentiate into venous vessels. In the present study, PDGF B showed the potential to differentiate into arterial and lymphatic type vessels. As shown in **Table 2**, PDGF B increased the TGF-β family that might be implicated in such vascular specification [24,25]. Further investigation is warranted.

In summary, our 3D culture system using mouse ES cells and collagen gel is both simple and useful, and provides an analytical model for investigating vascular formation. The present study indicates that VEGF is the initial signal for vasculogenesis, and PDGF B is probably involved in vascular diversification.

5. ACKNOWLEDGEMENTS

We wish to thank Dr. H. Niwa (RIKEN, Kobe Japan) for his generous gift of mouse ES cells. This work was supported by Grants-in-Aid for Scientific Research Japan (S) and (B).

REFERENCES

[1] Wang, Z., Cohen, K., Shao, Y., Mole, P., Dombkowski, D.

and Scadden, D.T. (2004) Ephrin receptor, EphB4, regulates ES cell differentiation of primitive mammalian hemangioblasts, blood, cardiomyocytes, and blood vessels. *Blood*, **103**, 100-109. doi:10.1182/blood-2003-04-1063

[2] Gerecht-Nir, S., Ziskind, A., Cohen, S. and Itskovitz-Eldor, J. (2003). Human embryonic stem cells as an *in vitro* model for human vascular development and the induction of vascular differentiation. *Laboratory Investigation*, **83**, 1811-1120. doi:10.1097/01.LAB.0000106502.41391.F0

[3] Nakagami, H., Nakagawa, N., Takeya, Y., Kashiwagi, K., Ishida, C., Hayashi, S., Aoki, M., Matsumoto, K., Nakamura, T., Ogihara, T. and Morishita, R. (2006) Model of vasculogenesis from embryonic stem cells for vascular research and regenerative medicine. *Hypertension*, **48**, 112-119. doi:10.1161/01.HYP.0000225426.12101.15

[4] Boyd, N.L., Dhara, S.K., Rekaya, R., Godbey, E.A., Hasneen, K., Rao, R.R., West III, F.D., Gerwe, B.A. and Stice, S.L. (2007) BMP4 promotes formation of primitive vascular networks in human embryonic stem cell-derived embryoid bodies. *Experimental Biology and Medicine* (*Maywood*), **232**, 833-843.

[5] Feraud, O., Cao, Y. and Vittet, D. (2001) Embryonic stem cell-derived embryoid bodies development in collagen gels recapitulates sprouting angiogenesis. *Laboratory Investigation*, **81**, 1669-1681. doi:10.1038/labinvest.3780380

[6] Lindskog, H., Athley, E., Larsson, E., Lundin, S., Hellström, M. and Lindahl, P. (2006) New insights to vascular smooth muscle cell and pericyte differentiation of mouse embryonic stem cells *in vitro*. *Arteriosclerosis, Thrombosis, and Vascular Biology*, **26**, 1457-1464. doi:10.1161/01.ATV.0000222925.49817.17

[7] Magnusson, P.U., Looman, C., Ahgren, A., Wu, Y., Claesson-Welsh, L. and Heuchel, R.L. (2007) Platelet-Derived growth factor receptor-beta constitutive activity promotes angiogenesis *in vivo* and *in vitro*. *Arteriosclerosis, Thrombosis, and Vascular Biology*, **27**, 2142-2149. doi:10.1161/01.ATV.0000282198.60701.94

[8] Yurugi-Kobayashi, T., Itoh, H., Yamashita, J., Yamahara, K., Hirai, H., Kobayashi, T., Ogawa, M., Nishikawa, S., Nishikawa, S.-I. and Nakao, K. (2003). Effective contribution of transplanted vascular progenitor cells derived from embryonic stem cells to adult neovascularization in proper differentiation stage. *Blood*, **101**, 2675-2678. doi:10.1182/blood-2002-06-1877

[9] Coultas, L., Chawengsaksophak, K. and Rossant, J. (2005) Endothelial cells and VEGF in vascular development. *Nature*, **438**, 937-945.

[10] Lanner, F., Sohl, M. and Farnebo, F. (2007) Functional arterial and venous fate is determined by graded VEGF signaling and notch status during embryonic stem cell differentiation. *Arteriosclerosis, Thrombosis, and Vascular Biology*, **27**, 487-493. doi:10.1161/01.ATV.0000255990.91805.6d

[11] Ferrari, G., Cook, B.D., Terushkin, V., Pintucci, G. and Mignatti, P. (2009) Transforming growth factor-beta 1 (TGF-beta1) induces angiogenesis through vascular endothelial growth factor (VEGF)-mediated apoptosis. *Journal of Cellular Physiology*, **219**, 449-458. doi:10.1038/npre.2008.1758.1

[12] Thommen, R., Humar, R., Misevic, G., Pepper, M.S., Hahn, A.W., John, M. and Battegay, E.J. (1997) PDGF-BB increases endothelial migration on cord movements during angiogenesis *in vitro*. *Journal of Cellular Biochemistry*, **64**, 403-413. doi:10.1002/(SICI)1097-4644(19970301)64:3<403::AID-JCB7>3.0.CO;2-Z

[13] Lange, S., Heger, J., Euler, G., Wartenberg, M., Piper, H.M. and Sauer, H. (2009) Platelet-Derived growth factor BB stimulates vasculogenesis of embryonic stem cell-derived endothelial cells by calcium-mediated generation of reactive oxygen species. *Cardiovascular Research*, **81**, 159-168. doi:10.1093/cvr/cvn258

[14] Hao, X., Silva, E.A., Månsson-Broberg E.A., Grinnemo, K-H., Siddiqui, A.J., Dellgren, G., Wärdell E., Brodin, L.Å., Mooney, D.J. and Sylvén, C. (2007) Angiogenic effects of sequential release of VEGF-A165 and PDGF-BB with alginate hydrogels after myocardial infarction. *Cardiovascular Research*, **75**, 178-185. doi:10.1016/j.cardiores.2007.03.028

[15] Stavridis, M.P., Collins, B.J. and Storey, K.G. (2010) Retinoic acid orchestrates fibroblast growth factor signalling to drive embryonic stem cell differentiation. *Development*, **137**, 881-890. doi:10.1242/dev.043117

[16] Elizalde, C., Campa, V.M., Caro, M., Schlangen, K., Aransay, A.M., Del Mar Vivanco, M. and Kypta, R.M. (2010) Distinct roles for wnt-4 and wnt-11 during retinoic acid-induced neuronal differentiation. *Stem Cells*, **29**, 141-153. doi:10.1002/stem.562

[17] Seifert, T., Stoelting, S., Wagner, T. and Peters, S.O. (2008) Vasculogeneic maturation of E14 embryonic stem cells with evidence of early vascular endothelial growth factor independency. *Differentiation*, **76**, 857-867. doi:10.1111/j.1432-0436.2008.00271.x

[18] Kawamura, H., Li, X., Harper, S.J., Bates, D.O. and Claesson-Welsh, L. (2008) Vascular endothelial growth factor (VEGF)-A165b is a weak *in vitro* agonist for VEGF receptor-2 due to lack of coreceptor binding and deficient regulation of kinase activity. *Cancer Research*, **68**, 4683-4692. doi:10.1158/0008-5472.CAN-07-6577

[19] Cao, R., Björndahl, M.A., Religa, P., Clasper, S., Garvin, S., Galter D., Meister, B., Ikomi, F., Tritsaris, K., Dissing, S., Ohhashi, T., Jackson, D.G., and Cao, Y. (2004) PDGF-BB induces intratumoral lymphangiogenesis and promotes lymphatic metastasis. *Cancer Cell*, **6**, 333-345. doi:10.1016/j.ccr.2004.08.034

[20] Yamashita, J.K. (2007) Differentiation of arterial, venous, and lymphatic endothelial cells from vascular progenitors. *Trends in Cardiovascular Medicine*, **17**, 59-63. doi:10.1016/j.tcm.2007.01.001

[21] You, L.R., Lin, F.J., Lee, C.T., DeMayo, F.J., Tsai, M.J. and Tsai, S.Y. (2005) Suppression of Notch signalling by the COUP-TFII transcription factor regulates vein identity. *Nature*, **435**, 98-104.

[22] Herbert, S.P., Huisken, J., Kim, T.N., Feldman, M.E., Houseman, B.T., Wang, R.A., Shokat, K.M. and Stainier, D.Y. (2009) Arterial-Venous segregation by selective cell sprouting: An alternative mode of blood vessel formation.

Science, **326**, 294-298. doi:10.1126/science.1178577

[23] Yamamizu, K., Matsunaga, T., Uosaki, H., Fukushima, H., Katayama, S., Hiraoka-Kanie, M., Mitani, K. and Yamashita, J.K. (2010) Convergence of Notch and beta-catenin signaling induces arterial fate in vascular progenitors. *Journal of Cell Biology*, **189**, 325-338.

[24] Seki, T., Hong, K.H. and Oh, S.P. (2006) Nonoverlapping expression patterns of ALK1 and ALK5 reveal distinct roles of each receptor in vascular development. *Laboratory Investigation*, **86**, 116-129. doi:10.1038/labinvest.3700376

[25] Kokudo, T., Suzuki, Y., Yoshimatsu, Y., Yamazaki, T., Watabe, T. and Miyazono, K. (2008) Snail is required for TGFbeta-induced endothelial-mesenchymal transition of embryonic stem cell-derived endothelial cells. *Journal of Cell Science*, **121**, 3317-3324. doi:10.1242/jcs.028282

Benefits of dedifferentiated stem cells for neural regeneration

Yinda Tang[1,2,3#], Wen Xu[4#], Haiying Pan[1,2], Shiting Li[3], Yong Li[1,2*]

[1]Department of Pediatric Surgery, School of Medicine, University of Texas, Houston, USA;
[*]Corresponding Author: Yong.Li.1@uth.tmc.edu
[2]Center for Stem Cell and Regenerative Medicine, The University of Texas Health Science Center at Houston, Houston, USA
[3]Department of Neurosurgery, Shanghai Xinhua Hospital, School of Medicine, Shanghai Jiao Tong University, Shanghai, China
[4]Center for Neuroscience, University of Pittsburgh, Pittsburgh, USA

ABSTRACT

Dedifferentiation, as one of the mechanisms rerouting cell fate, regresses cells from a differentiated status to a more primitive one. Due to its potential of amplifying the stem/progenitor cell pool and reproducing sizable and desirable cellular elements, it has been attended in the field of regenerative medicine, which will hopefully provide novel therapeutic strategies for currently incurable diseases, such as varieties of central nervous system (CNS) diseases and injuries. In this article, we will first discuss naturally occurring and experimentally induced dedifferentiation, and then set forth principles in stem-cell based therapy in the neural field; beyond that, we will introduce two recent studies that show dedifferentiated stem cells contribute to neural regeneration. Moreover, we also present our recent research results of dedifferentiated muscle stem cells for neurogenic differentiation study *in vitro*. Further work will be conducted to elucidate the mechanism underlying the dedifferentiation process to facilitate the development of new strategies in regenerative medicine.

Keywords: Dedifferentiation; Neural Stem Cells; Muscle Stem Cells; Neurogenesis; Regenerative Medicine

1. DEDIFFERENTIATION, A POTENTIAL APPROACH INVOLVED IN REGENERATIVE MEDICINE

The ability of animals to regenerate lost tissues is a dramatic and poorly understood aspect of biology. The sources of the new cells and the routes to these regenerative phenomena have been sought after for decades. Dedifferentiation, which is one process involved in natural regeneration, refers to the reversion of a terminally differentiated cell back to a less differentiated stage within its own lineage as part of regenerative process. It was first used to describe ascidian stolon regeneration in 1902 [1] but there was little evidence for this concept besides cellular morphology. Since then, intensive studies have been carried out in this field and accumulating evidence of this naturally occurring process has emerged from lower organisms as well as from mammalian tissues; this evidence will shed light on the basic mechanism underlying regeneration and aid in conceiving new strategies in regenerative medicine.

In non-mammalian vertebrate species, complete regeneration of zebrafish heart following ventricle amputation can be achieved by dedifferentiation of cardiomyocytes through disassembling the sarcomeric contractile apparatus, which contains a large proportion of terminally differentiated cells that physically impede cytokinesis [2-9]. Another intensively studied case is the blastema formation after limb amputation in the urodele amphibians. Shortly after limb amputation, cells adjacent to the wound dedifferentiate and form a blastema that consists of undifferentiated cells, which subsequently proliferate and eventually redifferentiate to create all the components of the lost limb [10-17]. In mammals, evidence of dedifferentiation has also been observed. In the case of peripheral nerve injury, Schwann cells are capable of dedifferentiating and proliferating when they lose contact with the axon that they are myelinating [18-21]. Astrocytes, another type of mature glial cell, can upregulate proteins that are characteristic of neural stem cells (NSCs) and re-enter the cell cycle after brain injury [22-30]. As determined *in vitro*, a fraction of these reactive astrocytes also shows long-term self-renewal and multipotency by forming neurospheres [22]. Another recent study showed that reversion of spermatogonia to germline stem cells

#Authors contribute as the first author.

occurs in the murine spermatogenic compartment [31-33]. Most recently, using an ingenious cre/lox system, our research demonstrated for the first time that dedifferentiation of skeletal muscle cells to early progenitor cells, including myoblasts and muscle-derived stem cells (MDSCs), occurs in an injured mouse model *in vivo* and can enhance cell proliferation and myogenesis [34].

In addition to the evidence demonstrating that dedifferentiation takes place naturally under certain stresses in a wide spectrum of species, recent studies have also clearly shown that this process can be achieved by experimental induction. After treatment with the extract isolated from regenerating newt limbs, mouse myotubes reduce the expression of the myoblast determination genes MyoD and myogenin, and subsequently dedifferentiate and proliferate [35]. Similarly, another group has shown that small chemical molecules can dedifferentiate lineage-committed myoblasts to multipotent mesenchymal progenitor cells, which can further go through adipogenesis and osteogenesis to generate fat cells and bone cells, respectively [36,37]. There are also examples of more dramatic dedifferentiation induction resulting in even pluripotency. A plethora of differentiated cell types can be induced to undergo an almost complete reprogramming through overexpression of a cocktail of transcripttion factors, generating induced pluripotent stem cells (iPS cells) [38-42], which can be argued as the ultimate form of dedifferentiation by a broader definition, that is, a developmental event involving reduction in the molecular and/or functional properties of a differentiated cell type. According to this paradigm, cells might be "formatted" through dedifferentiation to a primitive status and then re-differentiate towards a new lineage to generate new types of cells. This lineage switch initiated through dedifferentiation makes it possible to use cell types that are relatively accessible and numerous in order to replace lost cell types that are scarcer and difficult to obtain through the progenitor cells of their own lineage. Given this possibility, some promising strategies might be conceived for the cell-based therapy for intractable diseases in certain organs and systems, such as the injured or degenerated central nervous system (CNS).

2. REGENERATION IN CNS: NEURAL STEM CELLS AND ADULT NEUROGENESIS

With respect to other organs, the CNS shows structural peculiarities, and owing to the relative lack of recovery from CNS injury, the dogmatic view of a "fixed, ended and immutable" neural tissue in mammals has been prevalent since the early 1900s [43-45]. The word "regeneration" in neuroscience was originally restricted to axonal regeneration by surviving cell bodies after injury [46-48]. Along with early emerging evidence of ongoing cell division in adult mammalian brain [49-51], technical advances such as the use of the S-phase marker Bromodeoxyuridine (BrdU) [52-54], the development of immunocytochemical reagents that could identify the phenotype of various neural cells [55-57], and more recently, the delicate manipulation of genetic methods for cell labeling and mutation, have led to an explosion of research in the field [58-60]. After Reynolds and Weiss showed in 1992 that precursor cells could be isolated from the forebrain and differentiate into neurons *in vitro* [61], neural stem cells (NSCs) have been characterized as self-renewing, proliferative and multipotent for the different neuroectodermal lineages of the CNS, including the multitude of neuronal and glial subtypes [62,63]. Since then, the meaning of the word "regeneration" in CNS could be extended from axonogenesis and synaptogenesis to the replacement of lost cells with newly generated elements coming from stem/progenitor cells, *i.e.*, adult neurogenesis. Such a possibility for cell renewal theoretically brings our nervous system into the context of regenerative medicine. However, before developing new strategies to figure out efficacious therapeutic approaches, it is a crucial point to determine how NSCs and adult neurogenesis provide the CNS with regenerative potential.

Adult neurogenesis is regulated by physiological and pathological activities at all levels, including the proliferation of adult neural stem cells or progenitors, differentiation and fate determination of progenitor cells, and the survival, maturation, and integration of newborn neurons. In normal conditions, adult neurogenesis has consistently been found to be restricted within two small germinal layer-derived areas, e.g., the Subventricular zone (SVZ) of the lateral ventricles and the Subgranular zone (SGZ) in the dentate gyrus of hippocampus [64-67]. In the remaining CNS parenchyma, local progenitor cells might support a "potential" neurogenesis, which in spite of their proliferative capacity and retention of potentialities *in vitro*, they do not perform neurogenesis *in vivo* [68,69]. Meanwhile, other studies believe that some local parenchymal progenitors actually sustain spontaneous neurogenesis *in vivo*. For example, in rodents and even some non-human primates, some newly generated neocortical neurons have been found [70-72], as well as some neurons of the piriform cortex originating from Ng^{2+} progenitor cells [73-75]. Thus, whether neurogenesis occurs in areas outside of the two widely accepted "neurogenic regions" remains controversial [76,77].

After unraveling the neurogenic potential in normal adult mammalian CNS, the question of how the neural stem/progenitor cells behave in different injury/pathological contexts need to be addressed. Although topographically restricted, neurogenic sites in mammalian brain that are active throughout life can react to injury [78-81], and adult neurogenesis may also be substantially augmented in neurodegenerative diseases [82,83]. For instance, experiments carried out in rodent models of stroke revealed that reactive neurogenesis does occur from the SVZ, leading to increased cell production and migration of neuronal precursors to the lesion site [79,80]. In addition to reactive neurogenesis from stem cell-containing "neurogenic regions", accumulating evidence indicates that different paradigms of brain lesion can induce neurogenic events from the local progenitors resident in normally "non-neurogenic sites", including the neocortex [84-86], striatum [87-89], amygdale [90], hypothalamus [89,91,92], substantianigra [93,94] and brainstem [95-97]. For example, local progenitors that are in a relatively quiescent state in layer I of the rat cerebral cortex were activated after ischemia, giving rise to new cortical interneurons [86]. These examples support the hypothesis that the mature CNS parenchyma may retain a latent stem/progenitor cell potential that is normally inhibited *in vivo*, but that, if properly evoked, might be exploited *in situ* for cell replacement.

3. STRATEGIES AND CHALLENGES FOR NEURAL REGENERATION WITH STEM CELLS

Given their ability to generate neuronal and glial cells in response to damage, neural stem cells are believed to play a core role in cell-based therapy for various neurobiological disorders, ranging from acute injury such as brain trauma and stroke, to chronic neurodegenerative diseases including Alzheimer's Disease (AD) and Parkinson's Disease (PD), all of which are characterized by neuronal loss. As described above, it can be concluded that the brain has an endogenous regenerative potential and that in some pathological conditions, it becomes more permissive. Based on this point, one conceivable strategy for neural regeneration is to enhance the endogenous neurogenesis *in situ* [73,78,85,86,98,99]. The advantage of this approach is that it takes advantage of the intrinsic potential of endogenous neural stem/progenitor cells, and as a result, is less invasive and has fewer side effects in comparison with strategies relying on cellular transplantation [100-103], which will be discussed later. However, in most cases, such neurogenic potential cannot be utilized in a successful way. First, the magnitude of the neurogenic response to injury appears small, and it remains unclear as to what extent this is, because new neurons fail to develop at a sufficiently rapid rate versus cell death prior to sufficient integration into the host environment. In one case of brain injury, the great majority of the newborn cells survive < 1 month, and fail to replace lost neuronal populations and to restore damaged neuronal circuits [104]. Newly born neurons could replace only 0.2% of the dead striatal neurons in another rat cerebral ischemia model [79]. The exact mechanism for this overall inability of the endogenous stem cell compartment to promote full and long-lasting neural regeneration remains unclear. Recent data suggest that an altered neurogenic niche, including various overlapping local interactions between growth factors [105-108], extracellular proteins [109,110], metalloproteases [111-113], neurotransmitters [108,114,115], and angiogenesis [116-118], can be responsible for this failure. Even if enhanced cellular survival can be achieved, there are still significant impediments to neural maturation and integration, such as glial scar formation [119,120], cell death [121,122], inflammation [123,124] and aging [125, 126], all of which are topics of an open field of research. Although encouraging results from various experiments involving the administration of neurotrophin [127-129] or anti-inflammatory drugs [130-132] have shown some evidence that functional recovery is related to enhanced endogenous neurogenesis, the road ahead is still rocky and full of obstacles.

Paralleling this new understanding of endogenous neurogenesis, much progress has been made in the area of exogenous neuronal transplantation [100-103]. Early transplantation of embryonic midbrain tissue to the brain was first performed for PD and Huntington's disease (HD) in animal models as well as human clinical applications [133-136]. However, these experiments demonstrated a limited efficacy, along with other problems such as tissue availability and ethical questions. Today, it seems possible to achieve such therapeutic effects by using various sources of stem cells, due to their ability to replace the lost tissue as well as their "bystander" effects like neuroprotection and immunomodulation [101]. NSCs can be extracted directly from fetal or adult tissue via the dissection and digestion of CNS regions. In serum-free cultures with Epidermal growth factor (EGF) and Fibroblast growth factor 2 (FGF2), they can proliferate and spontaneously differentiate into both neuronal and glial cells after withdrawal of growth factors [61,137]. This possibility of stable expansion and *in vitro* differentiation into desired neural cells makes human NSCs an attractive cell source for transplantation strategies. Fetal-tissue-derived NSCs are the only source of stem-cell-derived neural cells that have entered the clinical arena for treatment of Neuronal ceroidlipofuscinosis (NCL, Batten's disease) [138] and Pelizaeus-Merzbacher disease (PMD). Application of oncogene-immortalized NSCs [139] are also approved in a phase I clinical trial in the United Kingdom for stroke therapy. Results so far have been favorable and encouraging. Autologous NPCs obtained at the site of focal damage would be an even more attractive option since they avoid immunogenicity, al logenicity and ethical issues related to NSCs from other sources above [140]. The risk of tumor formation cannot be excluded and the long-term safety of such cells remains to be determined [141].

Embryonic stem cells (ESCs) are derived from blastocysts during the 16 cell stage and have an almost unlimited capacity to self-renew [142]. They can be expanded for many years and differentiated into neural stem or precursor cells and subsequently into brain cells, which makes them a feasible exogenous source [143-146]. On the other hand, ESCs also bear considerable teratogenic potential after implantation into host tissue, although protocols for inducing them into relatively pure differenttiated population before transplantation have been developed [147]. Immunosupression is also needed. In addition, immense ethical concerns exist regarding the use of human ESCs as well as government restrictions that continue to limit clinical applications [148].

The generation of iPS cells is considered the main breakthrough in regenerative medicine [38-42]. As mentioned in the first section in this article, these cells are reprogrammed via a thorough reversion from a terminal stageback to a pluripotent status, which can be considered a complete dedifferentiation. By re-differentiating along a neural lineage, such cells offer another autologous source that is ethically acceptable and eliminates the risk of immunological complications. However, these cells are also under risk of tumor formation, and safety cannot yet be guaranteed [149]. In addition, differences seem to remain between ESCs and iPS cells that render the differentiation of the latter cells into mature neurons much more difficult [150-152]. Therefore, their clinical application does not seem feasible in the near future. Most recently, induced neurons (iN) have been obtained by reprogramming adult somatic cells directly into mature neurons without the intermediate step of iPS cells [153-159]. Future studies are necessary to show whether it is possible to generate such specific neurons that are sufficiently mature for transplantation and also lack the risk of tumor formation.

Additionally, it has been shown that terminal neural differentiation can also be seen with non-CNS-derived multipotent somatic stem cells, such as mesenchymal stem cells (MSCs) [160,161], muscle stem cells (MuSCs) [162-164], placental cord blood stem cells [165,166], skin stem cells [167] and adipose derived stem cells [168,169]. These cells are relatively numerous and easy to collect from patients, presenting another autologous source without immune reaction. It is also possible that these stem cells provide trophic support to damaged neural tissue and as a result, enhances the endogenous approach [170]. However, the proof of functional neurons derived from MSCs has not been provided. Although there are already some ongoing clinical trials that show some possible clinical improvement [171], many questions concerning how to enhance their survival and the potential of neural differentiation remain to be addressed.

In summary, two main therapeutic strategies have been developed in neural regeneration. Exploring the potentialities of resident, endogenous adult stem/progenitor cells is an ideal approach for the future. In parallel, an intense effort has been made to produce stem/progenitor cells that could be used as transplantation tools so as to replace lost elements in pathologies. Immune reaction and ethical controversy are the primary issues related to the allogeneic approach of mainly utilizing embryonic/ fetal oriented cells, while the powerful iPS cells cannot avoid the risk of tumor formation and genetic instability. Figuring out how to enhance the survival, migration and neural differentiation potential of non-neural somatic stem cells will be the problem that needs to be resolved before these accessible autologous resources can be clinically applied.

4. DEDIFFERENTIATED SOMATIC STEM CELLS, A BETTER SOLUSTION?

Addressing the last point summarized above, we here introduce two lines of evidence that show dedifferentiation might contribute to the resolution. One is from our work that focuses on muscle stem cells (MuSCs), and the other one published most recently is related to mesenchymal stem cells (MSCs) [172]. They start from distinct approaches of induction of dedifferentiation, but they arrive at the same conclusion that dedifferentiated MuSCs or MSCs present improved neural regenerative potential.

4.1. Dedifferentiation-Reprogrammed MSCs

Hsiao Chang Chan and his group used a culture induction to perform dedifferentiation [172]. After establishing monoclonal MSC clones from primary rat bone marrow MSCs, they first initiated neuronal differentiation by transferring the clones into neuronal induction media and then returned them to stem cell characteristics by withdrawal of the induction media and reincubation in serum. These cells are considered dedifferentiated MSCs (De-MSCs). First, compared with uncommitted MSCs, De-MSCs are demonstrated to represent a previously undescribed distinct population of stem cells with several distinguishing features. Apart from the morphological and phenotypical similarity and the potential for multilineage differentiation into osteoblasts, adipocytes and chondrocytes, De-MSCs exhibit a predisposition to the neuronal lineages as demonstrated by both genetic and functional assays. Global gene expression profiling and PCR data show that dedifferentiated cells express increased levels of both neurogenesis-related genes and growth factors. The increase of nestin- and musashi-positive cells in De-MSCs suggests that these cells carry additional neuronal potentiality that is ready to be activated under appropriate conditions, which is representative of an immature neural phenotype, most likely neural stem/progenitor cells. Taken together, De-MSCs appear to represent a distinct population of stem cells with a higher potential for re-differentiation into neurons compared to their original counterparts.

Next, they asked the question of whether or not De-MSCs have significant advantages over undifferentiated MSCs with respect to proliferation and survival. Indeed, proliferating cellular nuclear antigen (PCNA) staining confirmed that De-MSCs proliferated vigorously at 24 hours after dedifferentiation occurred and indicated this might be a result of acute reentry into the cell cycle. De-MSCs also exhibited a survival advantage over undifferentiated MSCs under conditions of hydrogen peroxide (H_2O_2) oxidative stress, as demonstrated by FACS sorting analysis of Annexin-V/propidium iodide staining after H_2O_2 treatment. More importantly, they have found that De-MSCs maintained their anti-apoptotic properties after *in vitro* culture and passaging. Increased expression of bcl-2 family proteins was observed and appeared to play a role in the anti-apoptotic action. All of these results explained the observation of an increase in viable cells in De-MSCs compared to the uncommitted MSCs during the *in vitro* differentiation and dedifferentiation process and demonstrated that De-MSCs are advanced in cell survival and proliferation.

They went further to demonstrate the therapeutic advantage of De-MSCs *in vivo* in a rat model of neonatal hypoxic-ischemic brain damage (HIBD) via lateral ventricular transplantation of fluorescent cells isolated from GFP-transgenic animal. On day 7, GFP expression could only be detected in De-MSCs group, indicating improved cell survival. Moreover, a number of the surviving GFP-De-MSCs were found outside of the injection site, indicating migration of the cells. Immunostaining revealed that some GFP-positive De-MSCs expressed differentiated neuronal markers NF-M or MAP2, indicating neuronal differentiation from the De-MSCs *in vivo*. Of note, they also showed that the better survival of De-MSCs might lie in their greater ability to promote angiogenesis in the ischemic region. Finally, shuttle box tests confirmed a more significant improvement of functional recovery of HIBD animals after De-MSCs treatment. Taken together, these results indicated that De-MSCs had survival and neuronal differentiation advantages over undifferentiated MSCs under both *in vitro* and *in vivo* conditions. This makes them a promising cellular source in therapeutic strategies based on autologous transplantation for neural regeneration.

4.2. Update Study of Muscle Cell Dedifferentiation for Neurogenic Differentiation

As mentioned at the beginning of our discussion on dedifferentiation, various studies in the amphibian limb regeneration field have demonstrated that dedifferentiation plays the core role by which the multipotent stem cells are generated via the formation of the "blastema" that consequently regenerates the entire limb [10-17]. However, the occurrence of this process in mammalian skeletal muscle has been questioned, partially due to the contamination of other endogenous progenitor cells which might not be excluded using regular cell isolation techniques, leaving the possibility that they are the source of dedifferentiation rather than the terminally differentiated cells [173,174]. Therefore, as recently reported, we developed a conditional transgenic model based on cre/lox-β-galactosidase (gal) system to specifically and effectively isolate differentiated myofibers both *in vitro* and *in vivo* to obtain the purified source [34]. Using this model, we have successfully determined the superior myogenesis potential of the injury-induced dedifferentiated muscle stem cells (De-MuSCs) that were dedifferentiated from β-gal positive multinuclear myofibers in comparison with the non-injury counterpart. Moreover, some β-gal and CD31 (a marker for endothelial cells) dual positive signals were also found in the blood vasculation, raising the question of whether these De-MuSCs-could advantageously contribute to differentiation down other lineages, such as neurogenesis [34]. In the present experiment, we explored further with our previous novel cre/lox model in order to address this question.

De-MuSCs were obtained as previously described [34]. Briefly, Muscle Creatine Kinase-cre muscle derived cells (MCK-cre MDCs) and ROSA-lox-β-gal MDCs were implanted into the gastrocnemius (GM) muscles of SCID mice via intramuscular injection of equal populations. Three weeks later, a laceration injury was created at the cell implantation site in the GMs. Four days after injury, β-gal positive cells were isolated by flow cytometry. The pre-plate technique was then applied to isolate and expand the β-gal positive slow adhering cells (*i.e.*, PP5 and PP6), which were convectively demonstrated to be De-MuSCs. We used primary mouse myoblasts, a muscle progenitor cell, as the control counterpart.

After isolation, both cell lines were kept in muscle cell growth media for one week before being transferred into NSC media for the induction of neurosphere proliferation. For further neural differentiation analysis, single cells were transferred into neural differentiation media. Cultured in NSC media, De-MuSCs successfully presented neural stem/progenitor characteristics. By day 3 in NSC media, some De-MuSCs had aggregated to form neurosphere-like structures that floated in suspension (**Figure 1(c)**), a hallmark of the structure of NSCs or neural progenitor cells, while control cells showed no signs of forming these special structures (**Figure 1(a)**). By day 6, the majority of the De-MuSCs were floating as spheres (**Figure 1(d)**), while the control cells still retained muscle cell morphology and stayed attached to the flask (**Figure 1(b)**).

The phenotype of the cells within the De-MuSCs derived neurosphere was analyzed by immunocytochemistry with typical neural markers. These spheres stained positive for Nestin, a marker for neural progenitor/stem cells, as well as the markers for more mature neural lineage cells: Glial fibrilllary acidic protein (GFAP) for astrocytes, CNPase for oligodentrocytes and Neurofilament (NFm) for neurons. EdU was detected in a select group of cells in each neurosphere (**Figures 2(a)-(d)**), indicating the proliferative status of these cells when cultured with mitotic reagents EGF and bFGF.

RT-PCR was performed on De-MuSCs and myoblasts, under both non-induced and NSC medium-induced conditions to detect changes that occurred on a transcripttional level. Within the non-induced group, the control cells had higher mRNA levels of myogenin compared to the De-MuSCs (**Figure 3**). In the induced group, both the control cells and De-MuSCs had lost myogenin mRNA expression (**Figure 3**). Meanwhile, nestin expression increased significantly for control cells and only slightly for MuSCs after NSC media induction (**Figure 3**). The expression of the stem cell marker Sca-1, which was absent in control cells and low in De-MuSCs at the beginning, increased for both cell types after NSC medium induction (**Figure 3**).

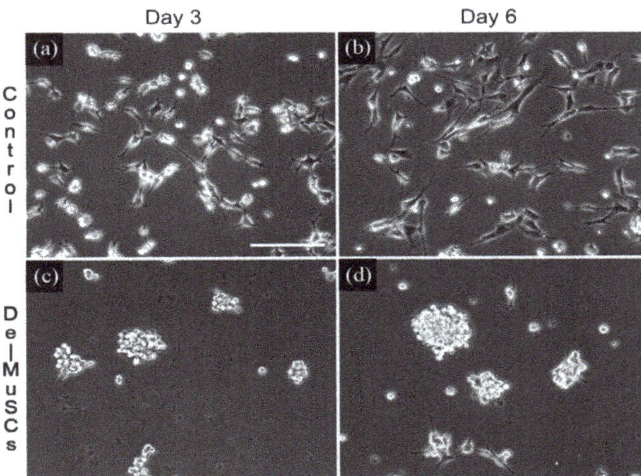

Figure 1. Results show that De-MuSCs Commit to Neural Lineage. Neurosphere-like structures were formed by De-MuSCs cultured in NSC proliferative media. De-MuSCs began to aggregate on day 3 (c) and presented morphology and architecture resembling that of neurosphere by day 6 (d), while the control primary myoblasts showed no signs of forming these structures (a)-(b) during these time period (3 and 6 days).

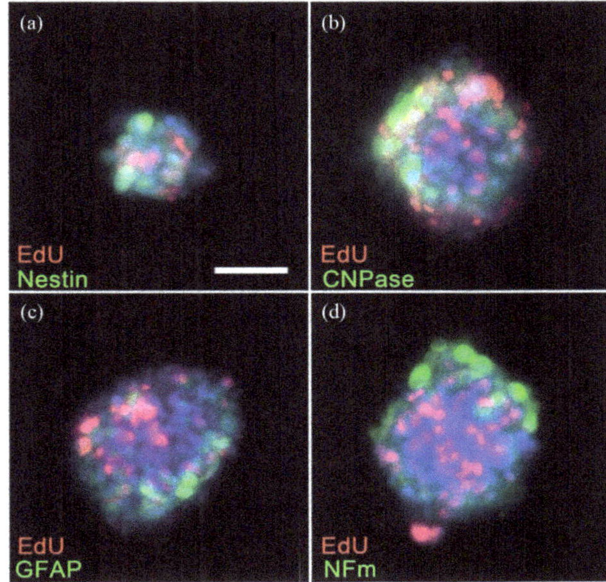

Figure 2. Immunocytochemistry showed the neural phenotype and proliferative status of the cells in the spheres that derived from De-MuSCs. On the fifth day after culturing in the NSC medium, these spheres stained positive for Nestin, a marker of neural progenitor/stem cells (a), as well as for other markers of mature neural cells, such as GFAP, NFm and CNPase (b)-(d). Mitosis assay performed 2 hours after EdU administration demonstrated the proliferative status of the cells in these spheres (a)-(d).

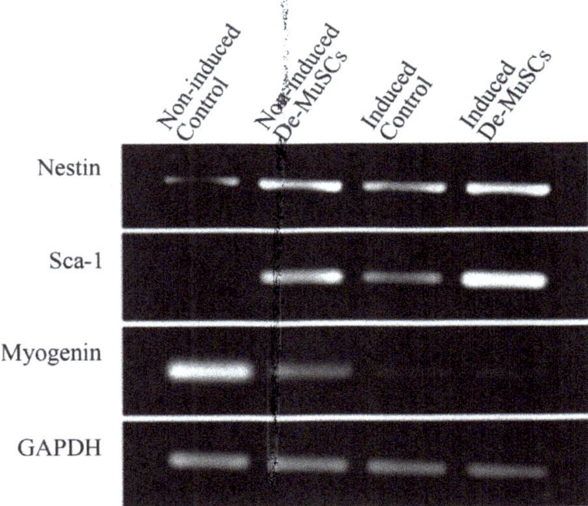

Figure 3. RT-PCR explored the alteration of the cell profile during culture with NSC medium. At the transcriptional level, the stem cell related markers Nestin and Sca-1 increased in both control cells and De-MuSCs after induction, although the De-MuSCs maintained a greater level. Meanwhile, the expression of Myogenin gradually decreased.

As for neural differentiation (ND) induction, the De-MuSCs but not the myoblasts successfully differentiated into neural lineage cells. After 3 days in ND media, cells which were solely positive for NFM and possessed long, thin projections that resembled neuronal processes were observed. These cells were EdU negative, indicating their postmitotic status (**Figure 4(a)**). After 8 days, although some of the cells were positive for α-smooth muscle actin (α-SMA), which might count for myofibroblast differentiation, the NFM positive cells were still detectable (**Figure 4(b)**). Meanwhile, other glial markers such as GFAP, CNPase were also positive in a subgroup of the cells, further suggesting the multiple potential of the De-MuSCs for neural differentiation.

In summary, our results potentially showed that De-MuSCs successfully formed neurosphere-like structures that contained neural stem/progenitor cells within NSC medium culture. RT-PCR confirmed that they were endowed with the capacity of differentiating along the neural lineage while they gradually lost myogenic potential. After being transferred into ND medium, De-MuSCs presented with neuronal morphology and immunophenotype, confirming they became terminally differentiated neuron-like cells. Since our data implies that De-MuSCs have the potential to commit to the neural lineage, they may be able to aid recovery from neurological diseases by providing an easily accessible cell source for neural regeneration.

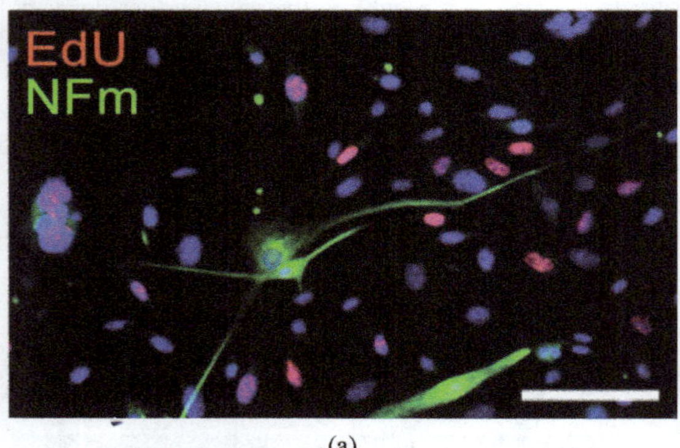

(a)

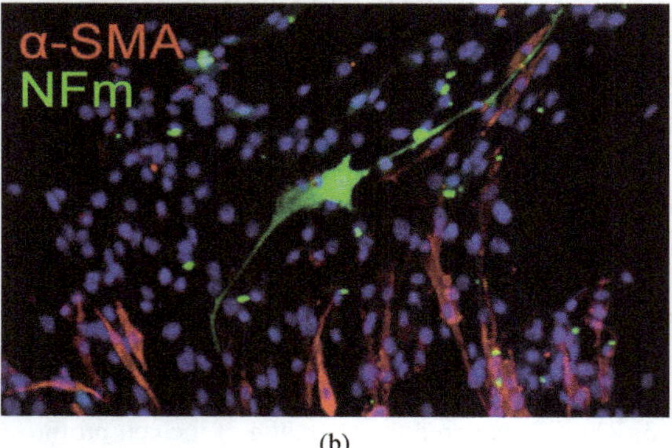

(b)

Figure 4. De-MuSCs differentiated into neuron-like cells after induction within ND medium. After 3 days in ND medium culture, some cells which were solely positive for NFm and possessed long, thin projections that resembled neuronal processes were observed. These cells were EdU negative, indicating their post-mitotic status (a); Eight days later, some of the cells began expressing for α-smooth muscle actin (α-SMA), while there still scattered some NFm positive cells reminded scattered among the population (b).

Taken together, the two studies above indicate that through various approaches, lineage committed somatic stem cells can be further dedifferentiated to a more primitive status, such as De-MSCs and De-MuSCs, which appear to have survival, proliferation, migration and neuronal differentiation advantages over their original counterparts under both *in vitro* and *in vivo* conditions. Because of the aforementioned characteristics as well as their accessibility, substantial population, and autologous orientation, they provide hope for finding a novel treatment strategy with improved therapeutic efficacy.

5. CONCLUSION

Regenerative medicine carries the responsibility of tackling various neurological diseases with limited treatment efficacies. Stem cell-based therapy can restore neural function by either enhancing the endogenous neurogenesis that is normally quiescent or replacing the lost cellular elements via exogenous transplantation of stem cell-derived cells. Dedifferentiation, as one significant approach involved in naturally occurring regeneration and experimental reprogramming, gives us more insight into these strategies. Among a variety of theoretically available cellular sources, dedifferentiated somatic stem cells with enhanced survival, proliferation, migration and neural differentiation in addition to easy accessibility and low tendency of tumor formation may offer an optimal solution. We introduced a recent study that depicted the advantages of De-MSCs along with our preliminary results that showed the remarkable superiority of De-MuSCs in neural regeneration. The detailed characterization of this novel stem cell population and the precise mechanism behind their beneficial effects still remain unclear, so further investigation must be conducted before the benefits of these stem cells can be clinically applied. However, the insight into dedifferentiation that we have already gained will bring us one step closer to finding effective bedside treatments for neurological disease.

REFERENCES

[1] Driesch, H. (1902) Studien über das regulationsvermögen der organismen. 6. Die restitution der Clavellina lepadiformis. *Archiv für Entwicklungs mechanik*, **14**, 247-287. doi:10.1007/BF02162039

[2] Poss, K.D., Wilson, L.G. and Keating, M.T. (2002) Heart regeneration in zebrafish. *Science*, **298**, 2188-2190. doi:10.1126/science.1077857

[3] Jopling, C. (2010) Zebrafish heart regeneration occurs by cardiomyocyte dedifferentiation and proliferation. *Nature*, **464**, 606-609. doi:10.1038/nature08899

[4] Kikuchi, K. (2010) Primary contribution to zebrafish heart regeneration by gata4+ cardiomyocytes. *Nature*, **464**, 601-605. doi:10.1038/nature08804

[5] Raya, A. (2003) Activation of Notch signaling pathway precedes heart regeneration in zebrafish. *Proceedings of the National Academy of Sciences of USA*, **100**, 11889-11895. doi:10.1073/pnas.1834204100

[6] Sleep, E. (2010) Transcriptomics approach to investigate zebrafish heart regeneration. *Journal of Cardiovasc Medicine*, **11**, 369-380. doi:10.2459/JCM.0b013e3283375900

[7] Lien, C.L., Schebesta, M., Makino, S., Weber, G.J. and Keating, M.T. (2006) Gene expression analysis of zebrafish heart regeneration. *PLoS Biology*, **4**, e260. doi:10.1371/journal.pbio.0040260

[8] Lepilina, A. (2006) A dynamic epicardial injury response supports progenitor cell activity during zebrafish heart regeneration. *Cell*, **127**, 607-619. doi:10.1016/j.cell.2006.08.052

[9] Ahuja, P., Sdek, P. and MacLellan, W.R. (2007) Cardiac myocyte cell cycle control in development, disease, and regeneration. *Physiological Reviews*, **87**, 521-544. doi:10.1152/physrev.00032.2006

[10] Brockes, J.P. and Kumar, A. (2002) Plasticity and reprogramming of differentiated cells in amphibian regeneration. *Nature Reviews Molecular Cell Biology*, **3**, 566-574. doi:10.1038/nrm881

[11] Echeverri, K., Clarke, J.D. and Tanaka, E.M. (2001) *In vivo* imaging indicates muscle fiber dedifferentiation is a major contributor to the regenerating tail blastema. *Developmental Biology*, **236**, 151-164. doi:10.1006/dbio.2001.0312

[12] Odelberg, S.J., Kollhoff, A. and Keating, M.T. (2000) Dedifferentiation of mammalian myotubes induced by msx1. *Cell*, **103**, 1099-1109. doi:10.1016/S0092-8674(00)00212-9

[13] Brockes, J.P. and Kumar, A. (2005) Appendage regeneration in adult vertebrates and implications for regenerative medicine. *Science*, **310**, 1919-1923. doi:10.1126/science.1115200

[14] Lo, D.C., Allen, F. and Brockes, J.P. (1993) Reversal of muscle differentiation during urodele limb regeneration. *Proceedings of the National Academy of Sciences of USA*, **90**, 7230-7234. doi:10.1073/pnas.90.15.7230

[15] Kumar, A., Velloso, C.P., Imokawa, Y. and Brockes, J.P. (2004) The regenerative plasticity of isolated urodele myofibers and its dependence on MSX1. *PLoS Biology*, **2**, e218. doi:10.1371/journal.pbio.0020218

[16] Kragl, M. (2009) Cells keep a memory of their tissue origin during axolotl limb regeneration. *Nature*, **460**, 60-65. doi:10.1038/nature08152

[17] Nye, H.L., Cameron, J.A., Chernoff, E.A. and Stocum, D.L. (2003) Regeneration of the urodele limb: A review. *Developmental Dynamics*, **226**, 280-294. doi:10.1002/dvdy.10236

[18] Chen, Z.L., Yu, W.M. and Strickland, S. (2007) Peripheral regeneration. *Annual Review of Neuroscience*, **30**, 209-233. doi:10.1146/annurev.neuro.30.051606.094337

[19] Woodhoo, A. (2009) Notch controls embryonic Schwann cell differentiation, postnatal myelination and adult plasticity. *Nature Neuroscience*, **12**, 839-847. doi:10.1038/nn.2323

[20] Mirsky, R. (2008) Novel signals controlling embryonic Schwann cell development, myelination and dedifferentiation. *Journal of the Peripheral Nervous System*, **13**, 122-135. doi:10.1111/j.1529-8027.2008.00168.x

[21] Monje, P.V., Soto, J., Bacallao, K. and Wood, P.M. (2010) Schwann cell dedifferentiation is independent of mitogenic signaling and uncoupled to proliferation: Role of cAMP and JNK in the maintenance of the differentiated state. *The Journal of Biological Chemistry*, **285**, 31024-31036. doi:10.1074/jbc.M110.116970

[22] Buffo, A. (2008) Origin and progeny of reactive gliosis: A source of multipotent cells in the injured brain. *Proceedings of the National Academy of Sciences of USA*, **105**, 3581-3586. doi:10.1073/pnas.0709002105

[23] Pekny, M. and Nilsson, M. (2005) Astrocyte activation and reactive gliosis. *Glia*, **50**, 427-434. doi:10.1002/glia.20207

[24] Brown, A.M. and Ransom, B.R. (2007) Astrocyte glycolgen and brain energy metabolism. *Glia*, **55**, 1263-1271. doi:10.1002/glia.20557

[25] Pekny, M. and Pekna, M. (2004) Astrocyte intermediate filaments in CNS pathologies and regeneration. *The Journal of Pathology*, **204**, 428-437. doi:10.1002/path.1645

[26] Schmid-Brunclik, N., Burgi-Taboada, C., Antoniou, X., Gassmann, M. and Ogunshola, O.O. (2008) Astrocyte responses to injury: VEGF simultaneously modulates cell death and proliferation. *American Journal of Physiology —Regulatory, Integrative and Comparative Physiology*, **295**, R864-R873. doi:10.1152/ajpregu.00536.2007

[27] Seri, B., Garcia-Verdugo, J.M., McEwen, B.S. and Alvarez-Buylla, A. (2001) Astrocytes give rise to new neurons in the adult mammalian hippocampus. *Journal of Neuroscience*, **21**, 7153-7160.

[28] Lang, B. (2004) Astrocytes in injured adult rat spinal cord may acquire the potential of neural stem cells. *Neuroscience*, **128**, 775-783. doi:10.1016/j.neuroscience.2004.06.033

[29] Buffo, A., Rolando, C. and Ceruti, S. (2010) Astrocytes in the damaged brain: Molecular and cellular insights into their reactive response and healing potential. *Biochemical Pharmacology*, **79**, 77-89. doi:10.1016/j.bcp.2009.09.014

[30] Sofroniew, M.V. and Vinters, H.V. (2010) Astrocytes: Biology and pathology. *Acta Neuropathologica*, **119**, 7-35. doi:10.1007/s00401-009-0619-8

[31] Barroca, V., Lassalle, B., Coureuil, M., Louis, J.P., Le Page, F., Testart, J., Allemand, I., Riou, L. and Fouchet, P. (2009) Mouse differentiating spermatogonia can generate germinal stem cells *in vivo*. *Nature Cell Biology*, **11**, 190-196. doi:10.1038/ncb1826

[32] Brawley, C. and Matunis, E. (2004) Regeneration of male

germline stem cells by spermatogonial dedifferentiation *in vivo*. *Science*, **304**, 1331-1334. doi:10.1126/science.1097676

[33] Nakagawa, T., Sharma, M., Nabeshima, Y., Braun, R.E. and Yoshida, S. (2010) Functional hierarchy and reversebility within the murine spermatogenic stem cell compartment. *Science*, **328**, 62-67. doi:10.1126/science.1182868

[34] Mu, X., Peng, H., Pan, H., Huard, J. and Li, Y. (2011) Study of muscle cell dedifferentiation after skeletal muscle injury of mice with a Cre-Lox system. *PloS One*, **6**, Article ID e16699. doi:10.1371/journal.pone.0016699

[35] McGann, C.J., Odelberg, S.J. and Keating, M.T. (2001) Mammalian myotube dedifferentiation induced by newt regeneration extract. *Proceedings of the National Academy of Sciences of USA*, **98**, 13699-13704. doi:10.1073/pnas.221297398

[36] Rosania, G.R., Chang, Y.T., Perez, O., Sutherlin, D., Dong, H., Lockhart, D.J. and Schultz, P.G. (2000) Myoseverin, a microtubule-binding molecule with novel cellular effects. *Nature Biotechnology*, **18**, 304-308. doi:10.1038/73753

[37] Chen, S., Zhang, Q., Wu, X., Schultz, P.G. and Ding, S. (2004) Dedifferentiation of lineage-committed cells by a small molecule. *Journal of the American Chemical Society*, **126**, 410-411. doi:10.1021/ja037390k

[38] Takahashi, K. and Yamanaka, S. (2006) Induction of pluripotent stem cells from mouse embryonic and adult fibroblast cultures by defined factors. *Cell*, **126**, 663-676. doi:10.1016/j.cell.2006.07.024

[39] Okita, K., Ichisaka, T. and Yamanaka, S. (2007) Generation of germline-competent induced pluripotent stem cells. *Nature*, **448**, 313-317. doi:10.1038/nature05934

[40] Takahashi, K., Tanabe, K., Ohnuki, M., Narita, M., Ichisaka, T., Tomoda, K. and Yamanaka, S. (2007) Induction of pluripotent stem cells from adult human fibroblasts by defined factors. *Cell*, **131**, 861-872. doi:10.1016/j.cell.2007.11.019

[41] Park, I.H., Zhao, R., West, J.A., Yabuuchi, A., Huo, H., Ince, T.A., Lerou, P.H., Lensch, M.W. and Daley, G.Q. (2008) Reprogramming of human somatic cells to pluripotency with defined factors. *Nature*, **451**, 141-146. doi:10.1038/nature06534

[42] Yu, J., Vodyanik, M.A., Smuga-Otto, K., Anto0- siewicz-Bourget, J., Frane, J.L., Tian, S., Nie, J., Jonsdottir, G.A., Ruotti, V., Stewart, R., *et al*. (2007) Induced pluripotent stem cell lines derived from human somatic cells. *Science*, **318**, 1917-1920. doi:10.1126/science.1151526

[43] Ramon y Cajal, S. (1913) Degeneration and regeneration of the nervous system. Oxford University Press, London.

[44] Colucci-D'Amato, L., Bonavita, V. and di Porzio, U. (2006) The end of the central dogma of neurobiology: Stem cells and neurogenesis in adult CNS. *Neurological Sciences*, **27**, 266-270. doi:10.1007/s10072-006-0682-z

[45] Gross, C.G. (2000) Neurogenesis in the adult brain: Death of a dogma. *Nature Reviews Neuroscience*, **1**, 67-73. doi:10.1038/35036235

[46] Davies, S.J., Fitch, M.T., Memberg, S.P., Hall, A.K., Raisman, G. and Silver, J. (1997) Regeneration of adult axons in white matter tracts of the central nervous system. *Nature*, **390**, 680-683.

[47] Nishio, T. (2009) Axonal regeneration and neural network reconstruction in mammalian CNS. *Journal of Neurology*, **256**, 306-309. doi:10.1007/s00415-009-5244-x

[48] Liu, K., Tedeschi, A., Park, K.K. and He, Z. (2011) Neuronal intrinsic mechanisms of axon regeneration. *Annual Review of Neuroscience*, **34**, 131-152. doi:10.1146/annurev-neuro-061010-113723

[49] Altman, J. and Das, G.D. (1965) Autoradiographic and histological evidence of postnatal hippo campal neurogenesis in rats. *The Journal of Comparative Neurology*, **124**, 319-335. doi:10.1002/cne.901240303

[50] Altman, J. (1969) Autoradiographic and histological studies of postnatal neurogenesis. IV. Cell proliferation and migration in the anterior forebrain, with special reference to persisting neurogenesis in the olfactory bulb. *The Journal of Comparative Neurology*, **137**, 433-457. doi:10.1002/cne.901370404

[51] Altman, J. (1963) Autoradiographic investigation of cell proliferation in the brains of rats and cats. *The Anatomical Record*, **145**, 573-591. doi:10.1002/ar.1091450409

[52] Miller, M.W. and Nowakowski, R.S. (1988) Use of bromodeoxyuridine-immunohistochemistry to examine the proliferation, migration and time of origin of cells in the central nervous system. *Brain Research*, **457**, 44-52. doi:10.1016/0006-8993(88)90055-8

[53] Taupin, P. (2007) Protocols for studying adult neurogenesis: Insights and recent developments. *Regenerative Medicine*, **2**, 51-62. doi:10.2217/17460751.2.1.51

[54] Gould, E., Reeves, A.J., Graziano, M.S. and Gross, C.G. (1999) Neurogenesis in the neocortex of adult primates. *Science*, **286**, 548-552. doi:10.1126/science.286.5439.548

[55] Lendahl, U., Zimmerman, L.B. and McKay, R.D. (1990) CNS stem cells express a new class of intermediate filament protein. *Cell*, **60**, 585-595. doi:10.1016/0092-8674(90)90662-X

[56] Mullen, R.J., Buck, C.R. and Smith, A.M. (1992) NeuN, a neuronal specific nuclear protein in vertebrates. *Development*, **116**, 201-211.

[57] Bonfanti, L. (2006) PSA-NCAM in mammalian structural plasticity and neurogenesis. *Progress in Neurobiology*, **80**, 129-164. doi:10.1016/j.pneurobio.2006.08.003

[58] Dhaliwal, J. and Lagace, D.C. (2011) Visualization and genetic manipulation of adult neurogenesis using transgenic mice. *European Journal of Neuroscience*, **33**, 1025-1036. doi:10.1111/j.1460-9568.2011.07600.x

[59] Yamaguchi, M., Saito, H., Suzuki, M. and Mori, K. (2000) Visualization of neurogenesis in the central nervous system using nestin promoter-GFP transgenic mice. *NeuroReport*, **11**, 1991-1996. doi:10.1097/00001756-200006260-00037

[60] Imayoshi, I., Sakamoto, M. and Kageyama, R. (2011) Genetic methods to identify and manipulate newly born neurons in the adult brain. *Frontiers in Neuroscience*, **5**, 64. doi:10.3389/fnins.2011.00064

[61] Reynolds, B.A. and Weiss, S. (1992) Generation of neurons and astrocytes from isolated cells of the adult mam-

malian central nervous system. *Science*, **255**, 1707-1710. doi:10.1126/science.1553558

[62] Gage, F.H. (2000) Mammalian neural stem cells. *Science*, **287**, 1433-1438. doi:10.1126/science.287.5457.1433

[63] Temple, S. (2001) The development of neural stem cells. *Nature*, **414**, 112-117. doi:10.1038/35102174

[64] Ming, G.L. and Song, H. (2011) Adult neurogenesis in the mammalian brain: Significant answers and significant questions. *Neuron*, **70**, 687-702. doi:10.1016/j.neuron.2011.05.001

[65] Ming, G.L. and Song, H. (2005) Adult neurogenesis in the mammalian central nervous system. *Annual Review of Neuroscience*, **28**, 223-250. doi:10.1146/annurev.neuro.28.051804.101459

[66] Kempermann, G. and Gage, F.H. (2000) Neurogenesis in the adult hippocampus. *Novartis Foundation Symposium*, **231**, 220-235, 235-241, 302-226.

[67] Alvarez-Buylla, A. and Garcia-Verdugo, J.M. (2002) Neurogenesis in adult subventricular zone. *The Journal of Neuroscience*, **22**, 629-634.

[68] Shihabuddin, L.S., Horner, P.J., Ray, J. and Gage, F.H. (2000) Adult spinal cord stem cells generate neurons after transplantation in the adult dentate gyrus. *The Journal of Neuroscience*, **20**, 8727-8735.

[69] Horner, P.J., Power, A.E., Kempermann, G., Kuhn, H.G., Palmer, T.D., Winkler, J., Thal, L.J. and Gage, F.H. (2000) Proliferation and differentiation of progenitor cells throughhout the intact adult rat spinal cord. *The Journal of Neuroscience*, **20**, 2218-2228.

[70] Dayer, A.G., Cleaver, K.M., Abouantoun, T. and Cameron, H.A. (2005) New GABAergic interneurons in the adult neocortex and striatum are generated from different precursors. *The Journal of Cell Biology*, **168**, 415-427. doi:10.1083/jcb.200407053

[71] Gould, E., Reeves, A.J., Graziano, M.S. and Gross, C.G. (1999) Neurogenesis in the neocortex of adult primates. *Science*, **286**, 548-552. doi:10.1126/science.286.5439.548

[72] Gould, E., Vail, N., Wagers, M. and Gross, C.G. (2001) Adult-generated hippocampal and neocortical neurons in macaques have a transient existence. *Proceedings of the National Academy of Sciences of USA*, **98**, 10910-10917. doi:10.1073/pnas.181354698

[73] Richardson, W.D., Young, K.M., Tripathi, R.B. and McKenzie, I. (2011) NG2-glia as multipotent neural stem cells: Fact or fantasy? *Neuron*, **70**, 661-673. doi:10.1016/j.neuron.2011.05.013

[74] Rivers, L.E., Young, K.M., Rizzi, M., Jamen, F., Psachoulia, K., Wade, A., Kessaris, N. and Richardson, W.D. (2008) PDGFRA/NG2 glia generate myelinating oligodendrocytes and piriform projection neurons in adult mice. *Nature Neuroscience*, **11**, 1392-1401. doi:10.1038/nn.2220

[75] Guo, F., Maeda, Y., Ma, J., Xu, J., Horiuchi, M., Miers, L., Vaccarino, F. and Pleasure, D. (2010) Pyramidal neurons are generated from oligodendroglial progenitor cells in adult piriform cortex. *The Journal of Neuroscience*, **30**, 12036-12049. doi:10.1523/JNEUROSCI.1360-10.2010

[76] Gould, E. (2007) How widespread is adult neurogenesis in mammals? *Nature Reviews Neuroscience*, **8**, 481-488. doi:10.1038/nrn2147

[77] Breunig, J.J., Arellano, J.I., Macklis, J.D. and Rakic, P. (2007) Everything that glitters isn't gold: A critical review of postnatal neural precursor analyses. *Cell Stem Cell*, **1**, 612-627. doi:10.1016/j.stem.2007.11.008

[78] Nakatomi, H., Kuriu, T., Okabe, S., Yamamoto, S., Hatano, O., Kawahara, N., Tamura, A., Kirino, T. and Nakafuku, M. (2002) Regeneration of hippocampal pyramidal neurons after ischemic brain injury by recruitment of endogenous neural progenitors. *Cell*, **110**, 429-441. doi:10.1016/S0092-8674(02)00862-0

[79] Arvidsson, A., Collin, T., Kirik, D., Kokaia, Z. and Lindvall, O. (2002) Neuronal replacement from endogenous precursors in the adult brain after stroke. *Nature Medicine*, **8**, 963-970. doi:10.1038/nm747

[80] Thored, P., Arvidsson, A., Cacci, E., Ahlenius, H., Kallur, T., Darsalia, V., Ekdahl, C.T., Kokaia, Z. and Lindvall, O. (2006) Persistent production of neurons from adult brain stem cells during recovery after stroke. *Stem Cells*, **24**, 739-747. doi:10.1634/stemcells.2005-0281

[81] Kernie, S.G. and Parent, J.M. (2010) Forebrain neurogenesis after focal ischemic and traumatic brain injury. *Neurobiology of Disease*, **37**, 267-274. doi:10.1016/j.nbd.2009.11.002

[82] Enciu, A.M., Nicolescu, M.I., Manole, C.G., Muresanu, D.F., Popescu, L.M. and Popescu, B.O. (2011) Neuroregeneration in neurodegenerative disorders. *BioMedCentral Neurology*, **11**, 75. doi:10.1186/1471-2377-11-75

[83] Winner, B., Kohl, Z. and Gage, F.H. (2011) Neurodegenerative disease and adult neurogenesis. *European Journal of Neuroscience*, **33**, 1139-1151. doi:10.1111/j.1460-9568.2011.07613.x

[84] Jiang, W., Gu, W., Brannstrom, T., Rosqvist, R. and Wester, P. (2001) Cortical neurogenesis in adult rats after transient middle cerebral artery occlusion. *Stroke*, **32**, 1201-1207. doi:10.1161/01.STR.32.5.1201

[85] Magavi, S.S., Leavitt, B.R. and Macklis, J.D. (2000) Induction of neurogenesis in the neocortex of adult mice. *Nature*, **405**, 951-955. doi:10.1038/35016083

[86] Ohira, K., Furuta, T., Hioki, H., Nakamura, K.C., Kuramoto, E., Tanaka, Y., Funatsu, N., Shimizu, K., Oishi, T., Hayashi, M., *et al.* (2010) Ischemia-induced neurogenesis of neocortical layer 1 progenitor cells. *Nature Neuroscience*, **13**, 173-179. doi:10.1038/nn.2473

[87] Benraiss, A., Chmielnicki, E., Lerner, K., Roh, D. and Goldman, S.A. (2001) Adenoviral brain-derived neurotrophic factor induces both neostriatal and olfactory neuronal recruitment from endogenous progenitor cells in the adult forebrain. *The Journal of Neuroscience*, **21**, 6718-6731.

[88] Van Kampen, J.M., Hagg, T. and Robertson, H.A. (2004) Induction of neurogenesis in the adult rat subventricular zone and neostriatum following dopamine D3 receptor stimulation. *European Journal of Neuroscience*, **19**, 2377-2387. doi:10.1111/j.0953-816X.2004.03342.x

[89] Pencea, V., Bingaman, K.D., Wiegand, S.J. and Luskin, M.B. (2001) Infusion of brain-derived neurotrophic factor

into the lateral ventricle of the adult rat leads to new neurons in the parenchyma of the striatum, septum, thalamus, and hypothalamus. *The Journal of Neuroscience*, **21**, 6706-6717.

[90] Park, J.H., Cho, H., Kim, H. and Kim, K. (2006) Repeated brief epileptic seizures by pentylenetetrazole cause neurodegeneration and promote neurogenesis in discrete brain regions of freely moving adult rats. *Neuroscience*, **140**, 673-684. doi:10.1016/j.neuroscience.2006.02.076

[91] Kokoeva, M.V., Yin, H. and Flier, J.S. (2005) Neurogenesis in the hypothalamus of adult mice: Potential role in energy balance. *Science*, **310**, 679-683. doi:10.1126/science.1115360

[92] Migaud, M., Batailler, M., Segura, S., Duittoz, A., Franceschini, I. and Pillon, D. (2010) Emerging new sites for adult neurogenesis in the mammalian brain: A comparative study between the hypothalamus and the classical neurogenic zones. *European Journal of Neuroscience*, **32**, 2042-2052. doi:10.1111/j.1460-9568.2010.07521.x

[93] Zhao, M., Momma, S., Delfani, K., Carlen, M., Cassidy, R.M., Johansson, C.B., Brismar, H., Shupliakov, O., Frisen, J. and Janson, A.M. (2003) Evidence for neurogenesis in the adult mammalian substantia nigra. *Proceedings of the National Academy of Sciences of USA*, **100**, 7925-7930. doi:10.1073/pnas.1131955100

[94] Van Kampen, J.M. and Robertson, H.A. (2005) A possible role for dopamine D3 receptor stimulation in the induction of neurogenesis in the adult rat substantia nigra. *Neuroscience*, **136**, 381-386. doi:10.1016/j.neuroscience.2005.07.054

[95] Zheng, Y., Begum, S., Zhang, C., Fleming, K., Masumura, C., Zhang, M., Smith, P. and Darlington, C. (2011) Increased BrdU incorporation reflecting DNA repair, neuronal dedifferentiation or possible neurogenesis in the adult cochlear nucleus following bilateral cochlear lesions in the rat. *Experimental Brain Research*, **210**, 477-487. doi:10.1007/s00221-010-2491-0

[96] Charrier, C., Coronas, V., Fombonne, J., Roger, M., Jean, A., Krantic, S. and Moyse, E. (2006) Characterization of neural stem cells in the dorsal vagal complex of adult rat by *in vivo* proliferation labeling and *in vitro* neurosphere assay. *Neuroscience*, **138**, 5-16. doi:10.1016/j.neuroscience.2005.10.046

[97] Fagerlund, M., Jaff, N., Danilov, A.I., Peredo, I., Brundin, L. and Svensson, M. (2011) Proliferation, migration and differentiation of ependymal region neural progenitor cells in the brainstem after hypoglossal nerve avulsion. *Restorative Neurology and Neuroscience*, **29**, 47-59.

[98] Okano, H., Sakaguchi, M., Ohki, K., Suzuki, N. and Sawamoto, K. (2007) Regeneration of the central nervous system using endogenous repair mechanisms. *Journal of Neurochemistry*, **102**, 1459-1465. doi:10.1111/j.1471-4159.2007.04674.x

[99] Robel, S., Berninger, B. and Gotz, M. (2011) The stem cell potential of glia: Lessons from reactive gliosis. *Nature Reviews Neuroscience*, **12**, 88-104. doi:10.1038/nrn2978

[100] Benchoua, A. and Onteniente, B. (2011) Intracerebral transplantation for neurological disorders. Lessons from developmental, experimental, and clinical studies. *Frontiers in Cellular Neuroscience*, **6**, 2.

[101] Martino, G. and Pluchino, S. (2006) The therapeutic potential of neural stem cells. *Nature Reviews Neuroscience*, **7**, 395-406. doi:10.1038/nrn1908

[102] Schouten, J.W., Fulp, C.T., Royo, N.C., Saatman, K.E., Watson, D.J., Snyder, E.Y., Trojanowski, J.Q., Prockop, D.J., Maas, A.I. and McIntosh, T.K. (2004) A review and rationale for the use of cellular transplantation as a therapeutic strategy for traumatic brain injury. *Journal of Neurotrauma*, **21**, 1501-1538. doi:10.1089/neu.2004.21.1501

[103] Enzmann, G.U., Benton, R.L., Talbott, J.F., Cao, Q. and Whittemore, S.R. (2006) Functional considerations of stem cell transplantation therapy for spinal cord repair. *Journal of Neurotrauma*, **23**, 479-495. doi:10.1089/neu.2006.23.479

[104] Liu, F., You, Y., Li, X., Ma, T., Nie, Y., Wei, B., Li, T., Lin, H. and Yang, Z. (2009) Brain injury does not alter the intrinsic differentiation potential of adult neuroblasts. *The Journal of Neuroscience*, **29**, 5075-5087. doi:10.1523/JNEUROSCI.0201-09.2009

[105] Guillemot, F. and Zimmer, C. (2011) From cradle to grave: The multiple roles of fibroblast growth factors in neural development. *Neuron*, **71**, 574-588. doi:10.1016/j.neuron.2011.08.002

[106] Chaichana, K., Zamora-Berridi, G., Camara-Quintana, J. and Quinones-Hinojosa, A. (2006) Neurosphere assays: Growth factors and hormone differences in tumor and nontumor studies. *Stem Cells*, **24**, 2851-2857. doi:10.1634/stemcells.2006-0399

[107] Bath, K.G. and Lee, F.S. (2010) Neurotrophic factor control of adult SVZ neurogenesis. *Developmental Neurobiology*, **70**, 339-349.

[108] Hagg, T. (2009) From neurotransmitters to neurotrophic factors to neurogenesis. *The Neuroscientist*, **15**, 20-27. doi:10.1177/1073858408324789

[109] Barros, C.S., Franco, S.J. and Muller, U. (2011) Extracellular matrix: Functions in the nervous system. *Cold Spring Harbor Perspectives in Biology*, **3**, Article ID: a005108. doi:10.1101/cshperspect.a005108

[110] Busch, S.A. and Silver, J. (2007) The role of extracellular matrix in CNS regeneration. *Current Opinion in Neurobiology*, **17**, 120-127. doi:10.1016/j.conb.2006.09.004

[111] Yong, V.W. (2005) Metalloproteinases: Mediators of pathology and regeneration in the CNS. *Nature Reviews Neuroscience*, **6**, 931-944. doi:10.1038/nrn1807

[112] Candelario-Jalil, E., Yang, Y. and Rosenberg, G.A. (2009) Diverse roles of matrix metalloproteinases and tissue inhibitors of metalloproteinases in neuroinflammation and cerebral ischemia. *Neuroscience*, **158**, 983-994. doi:10.1016/j.neuroscience.2008.06.025

[113] Cunningham, L.A., Wetzel, M. and Rosenberg, G.A. (2005) Multiple roles for MMPs and TIMPs in cerebral ischemia. *Glia*, **50**, 329-339. doi:10.1002/glia.20169

[114] Platel, J.C., Stamboulian, S., Nguyen, I. and Bordey, A. (2010) Neurotransmitter signaling in postnatal neurogenesis: The first leg. *Brain Research Reviews*, **63**, 60-71. doi:10.1016/j.brainresrev.2010.02.004

[115] O'Keeffe, G.C., Barker, R.A. and Caldwell, M.A. (2009) Dopaminergic modulation of neurogenesis in the subventricular zone of the adult brain. *Cell Cycle*, **8**, 2888-2894. doi:10.4161/cc.8.18.9512

[116] Shen, Q., Goderie, S.K., Jin, L., Karanth, N., Sun, Y., Abramova, N., Vincent, P., Pumiglia, K. and Temple, S. (2004) Endothelial cells stimulate self-renewal and expand neurogenesis of neural stem cells. *Science*, **304**, 1338-1340. doi:10.1126/science.1095505

[117] Yang, X.T., Bi, Y.Y. and Feng, D.F. (2011) From the vascular microenvironment to neurogenesis. *Brain Research Bulletin*, **84**, 1-7. doi:10.1016/j.brainresbull.2010.09.008

[118] Quaegebeur, A., Lange, C. and Carmeliet, P. (2011) The neurovascular link in health and disease: Molecular mechanisms and therapeutic implications. *Neuron*, **71**, 406-424. doi:10.1016/j.neuron.2011.07.013

[119] Rolls, A., Shechter, R. and Schwartz, M. (2009) The bright side of the glial scar in CNS repair. *Nature Reviews Neuroscience*, **10**, 235-241. doi:10.1038/nrn2591

[120] Silver, J. and Miller, J.H. (2004) Regeneration beyond the glial scar. *Nature Reviews Neuroscience*, **5**, 146-156. doi:10.1038/nrn1326

[121] Okouchi, M., Ekshyyan, O., Maracine, M. and Aw, T.Y. (2007) Neuronal apoptosis in neurodegeneration. *Antioxidants & Redox Signaling*, **9**, 1059-1096. doi:10.1089/ars.2007.1511

[122] Bauer, S. and Patterson, P.H. (2005) The cell cycle-apoptosis connection revisited in the adult brain. *The Journal of Cell Biology*, **171**, 641-650. doi:10.1083/jcb.200505072

[123] Carpentier, P.A. and Palmer, T.D. (2009) Immune influence on adult neural stem cell regulation and function. *Neuron*, **64**, 79-92. doi:10.1016/j.neuron.2009.08.038

[124] Russo, I., Barlati, S. and Bosetti, F. (2011) Effects of neuroinflammation on the regenerative capacity of brain stem cells. *Journal of Neurochemistry*, **116**, 947-956. doi:10.1111/j.1471-4159.2010.07168.x

[125] Kuhn, H.G., Dickinson-Anson, H. and Gage, F.H. (1996) Neurogenesis in the dentate gyrus of the adult rat: Age-related decrease of neuronal progenitor proliferation. *Journal of Neurochemistry*, **16**, 2027-2033.

[126] Driscoll, I., Howard, S.R., Stone, J.C., Monfils, M.H., Tomanek, B., Brooks, W.M. and Sutherland, R.J. (2006) The aging hippocampus: A multi-level analysis in the rat. *Neuroscience*, **139**, 1173-1185. doi:10.1016/j.neuroscience.2006.01.040

[127] Cao, Q., He, Q., Wang, Y., Cheng, X., Howard, R.M., Zhang, Y., DeVries, W.H., Shields, C.B., Magnuson, D.S., Xu, X.M., *et al.* (2010) Transplantation of ciliary neurotrophic factor-expressing adult oligodendrocyte precursor cells promotes remyelination and functional recovery after spinal cord injury. *Journal of Neurochemistry*, **30**, 2989-3001. doi:10.1523/JNEUROSCI.3174-09.2010

[128] Hayon, Y., Dashevsky, O., Shai, E., Varon, D. and Leker, R.R. (2012) Platelet microparticles promote neural stem cell proliferation, survival and differentiation. *Journal of Molecular Neuroscience*, **47**, 659-665.

[129] Bambakidis, N.C., Petrullis, M., Kui, X., Rothstein, B., Karampelas, I., Kuang, Y., Selman, W.R., Lamanna, J.C. and Miller, R.H. (2012) Improvement of neurological recovery and stimulation of neural progenitor cell proliferation by intrathecal administration of sonic hedgehog. *Journal of Neurosurgery*, **116**, 1114-1120. doi:10.3171/2012.1.JNS111285

[130] Ekdahl, C.T., Claasen, J.H., Bonde, S., Kokaia, Z. and Lindvall, O. (2003) Inflammation is detrimental for neurogenesis in adult brain. *Proceedings of the National Academy of Sciences of USA*, **100**, 13632-13637. doi:10.1073/pnas.2234031100

[131] Edwards, P., Arango, M., Balica, L., Cottingham, R., El-Sayed, H., Farrell, B., Fernandes, J., Gogichaisvili, T., Golden, N., Hartzenberg, B., *et al.* (2005) Final results of MRC CRASH, a randomised placebo-controlled trial of intravenous corticosteroid in adults with head injury-outcomes at 6 months. *The Lancet*, **365**, 1957-1959. doi:10.1016/S0140-6736(05)66552-X

[132] Monje, M.L., Toda, H. and Palmer, T.D. (2003) Inflammatory blockade restores adult hippocampal neurogenesis. *Science*, **302**, 1760-1765. doi:10.1126/science.1088417

[133] Madrazo, I., Drucker-Colin, R., Diaz, V., Martinez-Mata, J., Torres, C. and Becerril, J.J. (1987) Open microsurgical autograft of adrenal medulla to the right caudate nucleus in two patients with intractable Parkinson's disease. *The New England Journal of Medicine*, **316**, 831-834. doi:10.1056/NEJM198704023161402

[134] Bachoud-Levi, A.C., Gaura, V., Brugieres, P., Lefaucheur, J.P., Boisse, M.F., Maison, P., Baudic, S., Ribeiro, M.J., Bourdet, C., Remy, P., *et al.* (2006) Effect of fetal neural transplants in patients with Huntington's disease 6 years after surgery: A long-term follow-up study. *The Lancet Neurology*, **5**, 303-309. doi:10.1016/S1474-4422(06)70381-7

[135] Freed, C.R., Greene, P.E., Breeze, R.E., Tsai, W.Y., DuMouchel, W., Kao, R., Dillon, S., Winfield, H., Culver, S., Trojanowski, J.Q., *et al.* (2001) Transplantation of embryonic dopamine neurons for severe Parkinson's disease. *The New England Journal of Medicine*, **344**, 710-719. doi:10.1056/NEJM200103083441002

[136] Olanow, C.W., Goetz, C.G., Kordower, J.H., Stoessl, A.J., Sossi, V., Brin, M.F., Shannon, K.M., Nauert, G.M., Perl, D.P., Godbold, J., *et al.* (2003) A double-blind controlled trial of bilateral fetal nigral transplantation in Parkinson's disease. *Annals of Neurology*, **54**, 403-414. doi:10.1002/ana.10720

[137] Johe, K.K., Hazel, T.G., Muller, T., Dugich-Djordjevic, M.M. and McKay, R.D. (1996) Single factors direct the differentiation of stem cells from the fetal and adult central nervous system. *Genes & Development*, **10**, 3129-3140. doi:10.1101/gad.10.24.3129

[138] Tamaki, S.J., Jacobs, Y., Dohse, M., Capela, A., Cooper, J.D., Reitsma, M., He, D., Tushinski, R., Belichenko, P.V., Salehi, A., *et al.* (2009) Neuroprotection of host cells by human central nervous system stem cells in a mouse model of infantile neuronal ceroid lipofuscinosis. *Cell Stem Cell*, **5**, 310-319. doi:10.1016/j.stem.2009.05.022

[139] Miljan, E.A. and Sinden, J.D. (2009) Stem cell treatment of ischemic brain injury. *Current Opinion in Molecular*

Therapeutics, **11**, 394-403.

[140] Zhu, J., Zhou, L. and XingWu, F. (2006) Tracking neural stem cells in patients with brain trauma. *The New England Journal of Medicine*, **355**, 2376-2378. doi:10.1056/NEJMc055304

[141] Amariglio, N., Hirshberg, A., Scheithauer, B.W., Cohen, Y., Loewenthal, R., Trakhtenbrot, L., Paz, N., Koren-Michowitz, M., Waldman, D., Leider-Trejo, L., *et al.* (2009) Donor-derived brain tumor following neural stem cell transplantation in an ataxia telangiectasia patient. *PLoS Medicine*, **6**, Article ID e1000029. doi:10.1371/journal.pmed.1000029

[142] Evans, M. (2011) Discovering pluripotency: 30 years of mouse embryonic stem cells. *Nature Reviews Molecular Cell Biology*, **12**, 680-686. doi:10.1038/nrm3190

[143] Soundararajan, P., Lindsey, B.W., Leopold, C. and Rafuse, V.F. (2007) Easy and rapid differentiation of embryonic stem cells into functional motoneurons using sonic hedgehog-producing cells. *Stem Cells*, **25**, 1697-1706. doi:10.1634/stemcells.2006-0654

[144] Lee, H., Shamy, G.A., Elkabetz, Y., Schofield, C.M., Harrsion, N.L., Panagiotakos, G., Socci, N.D., Tabar, V. and Studer, L. (2007) Directed differentiation and transplantation of human embryonic stem cell-derived motoneurons. *Stem Cells*, **25**, 1931-1939. doi:10.1634/stemcells.2007-0097

[145] Kriks, S., Shim, J.W., Piao, J., Ganat, Y.M., Wakeman, D.R., Xie, Z., Carrillo-Reid, L., Auyeung, G., Antonacci, C., Buch, A., *et al.* (2011) Dopamine neurons derived from human ES cells efficiently engraft in animal models of Parkinson's disease. *Nature*, **480**, 547-551.

[146] Weick, J.P., Liu, Y. and Zhang, S.C. (2011) Human embryonic stem cell-derived neurons adopt and regulate the activity of an established neural network. *Proceedings of the National Academy of Sciences of USA*, **108**, 20189-20194. doi:10.1073/pnas.1108487108

[147] Doi, D., Morizane, A., Kikuchi, T., Onoe, H., Hayashi, T., Kawasaki, T., Motono, M., Sasai, Y., Saiki, H., Gomi, M., *et al.* (2012) Prolonged maturation culture favors a reduction in the tumorigenicity and the dopaminergic function of human esc-derived neural cells in a primate model of parkinson's disease. *Stem Cells*, **30**, 935-945.

[148] Guhr, A., Kurtz, A., Friedgen, K. and Loser, P. (2006) Current state of human embryonic stem cell research: An overview of cell lines and their use in experimental work. *Stem Cells*, **24**, 2187-2191. doi:10.1634/stemcells.2006-0053

[149] Plath, K. and Lowry, W.E. (2011) Progress in understanding reprogramming to the induced pluripotent state. *Nature Reviews Genetics*, **12**, 253-265. doi:10.1038/nrg2955

[150] Kim, K., Doi, A., Wen, B., Ng, K., Zhao, R., Cahan, P., Kim, J., Aryee, M.J., Ji, H., Ehrlich, L.I., *et al.* (2010) Epigenetic memory in induced pluripotent stem cells. *Nature*, **467**, 285-290. doi:10.1038/nature09342

[151] Bilic, J. and Izpisua Belmonte, J.C. (2012) Concise review: Induced pluripotent stem cells versus embryonic stem cells: Close enough or yet too far apart? *Stem Cells*, **30**, 33-41. doi:10.1002/stem.700

[152] Schwartz, P.H., Brick, D.J., Stover, A.E., Loring, J.F. and Muller, F.J. (2008) Differentiation of neural lineage cells from human pluripotent stem cells. *Methods*, **45**, 142-158. doi:10.1016/j.ymeth.2008.03.007

[153] Vierbuchen, T., Ostermeier, A., Pang, Z.P., Kokubu, Y., Sudhof, T.C. and Wernig, M. (2010) Direct conversion of fibroblasts to functional neurons by defined factors. *Nature*, **463**, 1035-1041. doi:10.1038/nature08797

[154] Caiazzo, M., Dell'Anno, M.T., Dvoretskova, E., Lazarevic, D., Taverna, S., Leo, D., Sotnikova, T.D., Menegon, A., Roncaglia, P., Colciago, G., *et al.* (2011) Direct generation of functional dopaminergic neurons from mouse and human fibroblasts. *Nature*, **476**, 224-227. doi:10.1038/nature10284

[155] Kim, J., Efe, J.A., Zhu, S., Talantova, M., Yuan, X., Wang, S., Lipton, S.A., Zhang, K. and Ding, S. (2011) Direct reprogramming of mouse fibroblasts to neural progenitors. *Proceedings of the National Academy of Sciences of USA*, **108**, 7838-7843. doi:10.1073/pnas.1103113108

[156] Yang, N., Ng, Y.H., Pang, Z.P., Sudhof, T.C. and Wernig, M. (2011) Induced neuronal cells: How to make and define a neuron. *Cell Stem Cell*, **9**, 517-525. doi:10.1016/j.stem.2011.11.015

[157] Marro, S., Pang, Z.P., Yang, N., Tsai, M.C., Qu, K., Chang, H.Y., Sudhof, T.C. and Wernig, M. (2011) Direct lineage conversion of terminally differentiated hepatocytes to functional neurons. *Cell Stem Cell*, **9**, 374-382. doi:10.1016/j.stem.2011.09.002

[158] Son, E.Y., Ichida, J.K., Wainger, B.J., Toma, J.S., Rafuse, V.F., Woolf, C.J. and Eggan, K. (2011) Conversion of mouse and human fibroblasts into functional spinal motor neurons. *Cell Stem Cell*, **9**, 205-218. doi:10.1016/j.stem.2011.07.014

[159] Pang, Z.P., Yang, N., Vierbuchen, T., Ostermeier, A., Fuentes, D.R., Yang, T.Q., Citri, A., Sebastiano, V., Marro, S., Sudhof, T.C., *et al.* (2011) Induction of human neuronal cells by defined transcription factors. *Nature*, **476**, 220-223.

[160] Wislet-Gendebien, S., Wautier, F., Leprince, P. and Rogister, B. (2005) Astrocytic and neuronal fate of mesenchymal stem cells expressing nestin. *Brain Research Bulletin*, **68**, 95-102. doi:10.1016/j.brainresbull.2005.08.016

[161] Krabbe, C., Zimmer, J. and Meyer, M. (2005) Neural transdifferentiation of mesenchymal stem cells: A critical review. *Acta Pathologica, Microbiologica et Immunologica*, **113**, 831-844. doi:10.1111/j.1600-0463.2005.apm_3061.x

[162] Romero-Ramos, M., Vourch, P., Young, H.E., Lucas, P.A., Wu, Y., Chivatakarn, O., Zaman, R., Dunkelman, N., el-Kalay, M.A. and Chesselet, M.F. (2002) Neuronal differentiation of stem cells isolated from adult muscle. *Journal of Neuroscience Research*, **69**, 894-907. doi:10.1002/jnr.10374

[163] Kondo, T., Case, J., Srour, E.F. and Hashino, E. (2006) Skeletal muscle-derived progenitor cells exhibit neural competence. *NeuroReport*, **17**, 1-4. doi:10.1097/01.wnr.0000192732.00535.ff

[164] Alessandri, G., Pagano, S., Bez, A., Benetti, A., Pozzi, S.,

Iannolo, G., Baronio, M., Invernici, G., Caruso, A., Muneretto, C., *et al.* (2004) Isolation and culture of human muscle-derived stem cells able to differentiate into myogenic and neurogenic cell lineages. *The Lancet*, **364**, 1872-1883. doi:10.1016/S0140-6736(04)17443-6

[165] Herranz, A.S., Gonzalo-Gobernado, R., Reimers, D., Asensio, M.J., Rodriguez-Serrano, M. and Bazan, E. (2010) Applications of human umbilical cord blood cells in central nervous system regeneration. *Current Stem Cell Research & Therapy*, **5**, 17-22. doi:10.2174/157488810790442822

[166] Slovinska, L., Novotna, I., Kubes, M., Radonak, J., Jergova, S., Cigankova, V., Rosocha, J. and Cizkova, D. (2011) Umbilical cord blood cells $CD133^+/CD133^-$ cultivation in neural proliferation media differentiates towards neural cell lineages. *Archives of Medical Research*, **42**, 555-562. doi:10.1016/j.arcmed.2011.10.003

[167] Amoh, Y., Kanoh, M., Niiyama, S., Hamada, Y., Kawahara, K., Sato, Y., Hoffman, R.M. and Katsuoka, K. (2009) Human hair follicle pluripotent stem (hfPS) cells promote regeneration of peripheral-nerve injury: An advantageous alternative to ES and iPS cells. *Journal of Cellular Biochemistry*, **107**, 1016-1020. doi:10.1002/jcb.22204

[168] Kwon, E.B., Lee, J.Y., Piao, S., Kim, I.G. and Ra, J.C. (2011) Comparison of human muscle-derived stem cells and human adipose-derived stem cells in neurogenic trans-differentiation. *Korean Journal of Urology*, **52**, 852-857. doi:10.4111/kju.2011.52.12.852

[169] Locke, M., Feisst, V. and Dunbar, P.R. (2011) Concise review: Human adipose-derived stem cells: Separating promise from clinical need. *Stem Cells*, **29**, 404-411. doi:10.1002/stem.593

[170] Salem, H.K. and Thiemermann, C. (2010) Mesenchymal stromal cells: Current understanding and clinical status. *Stem Cells*, **28**, 585-596.

[171] Cox, C.S. Jr., Baumgartner, J.E., Harting, M.T., Worth, L.L., Walker, P.A., Shah, S.K., Ewing-Cobbs, L., Hasan, K.M., Day, M.C., Lee, D., *et al.* (2011) Autologous bone marrow mononuclear cell therapy for severe traumatic brain injury in children. *Neurosurgery*, **68**, 588-600. doi:10.1227/NEU.0b013e318207734c

[172] Liu, Y., Jiang, X., Zhang, X., Chen, R., Sun, T., Fok, K.L., Dong, J., Tsang, L.L., Yi, S., Ruan, Y., *et al.* (2011) Dedifferentiation-reprogrammed mesenchymal stem cells with improved therapeutic potential. *Stem Cells*, **29**, 2077-2089. doi:10.1002/stem.764

[173] Raff, M. (2003) Adult stem cell plasticity: Fact or artifact? *Annual Review of Cell and Developmental Biology*, **19**, 1-22. doi:10.1146/annurev.cellbio.19.111301.143037

[174] Wagers, A.J. and Weissman, I.L. (2004) Plasticity of adult stem cells. *Cell*, **116**, 639-648. doi:10.1016/S0092-8674(04)00208-9

26

The CD133/1⁺ cell subset from human subcutaneous adult fat retains hemogenic potential

Camila Santos de Moraes[1], Paulo Roberto Albuquerque Leal[2], Daniel Fabiano Ferreira[3], Fernando Serra[3], Eliana Abdelhay[4], Claudia Sondermann Freitas[1*]

[1]Experimental Medicine Program, Research Coordination, National Cancer Institute of Rio de Janeiro, Rio de Janeiro, Brazil; [*]Corresponding author: csondermannf@yahoo.com.br
[2]Plastic Surgery, Cancer Hospital I, National Cancer Institute of Rio de Janeiro, Rio de Janeiro, Brazil
[3]Pedro Ernesto Hospital, Rio de Janeiro State University, Rio de Janeiro, Brazil
[4]Bone Marrow Transplantation Unit, National Cancer Institute of Rio de Janeiro, Rio de Janeiro, Brazil

ABSTRACT

Research has shown that cells from adult fat tissue can effect long-term blood reconstitution. Fat-derived multipotentiality was ascribed to CD34$^+$ perivascular populations from its prominent microvasculature, that represent mostly non-hemogenic, mesenchymal cells, although this tissue contains a CD34$^+$45$^+$ subset committed to a hemogenic fate. Here, in order to analyze cell subsets presenting hemogenic capabilities within fat, CD133/1$^+$ cells and pericytes, the latter defined by CD140b (PDGFRb, Platelet-Derived Growth Factor Receptor Beta) expression, were immunomagnetically selected from stromal-vascular fractions (SVF). *In vitro* Colony Forming Unit (CFU) assays were negative for CD140b$^+$ pericytes and positive for CD133/1$^+$ cells when a prolonged CFU assay was performed, revealing fat as another store of primitive progenitors that retain hemogenic potential.

Keywords: Adipose Tissue-Derived Stem Cells; CD133; Hematogenesis; Hemangioblast; Pericyte

1. INTRODUCTION

Adult tissues aside from bone marrow (BM) figure as alternative sources of multipotent cells, representing complex mixtures of stem and progenitor subsets, either committed or not to particular differentiation fates [1,2]. In this context, subcutaneous fat contains large quantities of cells with multipotential capabilities [3], available for numerous therapeutic purposes [4], including long-term blood reconstitution, as was shown in mouse models [5, 6].

Fat-derived multipotentiality has been ascribed to CD34$^+$ pericytes [7], among a multiplicity of cell subsets surrounding microvessels [8,9]. However, in this tissue, only the committed CD34$^+$45$^+$ subset presents hemogenic potential, the majority of the CD34$^+$ pool representing non-hemogenic mesenchymal stem cells [10], resembling the CD34$^+$ stroma of fetal bone marrow [11].

In its glycosylated form, surface expressed CD133/1 (AC133) is considered a marker of "stemness" [12,13]. Among progenitors from BM and umbilical cord blood (UCB), CD133 marks a primitive hemogenic subset [14,15], as well as microvasculature-forming endothelial precursor cells (EPC) [16]. Bipotent hemogenic and endothelial progenitors in adult tissues were reported as "adult hemangioblasts" [17], putatively reminiscent from development. The vascular origin of hematogenesis in the embryo has been shown to represent a transdifferentiation event, the blood cells arising directly from endothelial cells of the dorsal aorta [18]. In adults, circulating EPC coexpress CD133, CD34 and VEGFR (Vascular Endothelium Growth Factor Receptor) [19]. It seemed plausible that in fat, which plasticity requires constant neovasculogenesis, EPC at diverse stages would be strongly represented, some of which are putatively CD133$^+$.

In fact, the presence of bipotent hemogenic and endothelial progenitors in fat has been reported, defined by VEGFR expression. Surprisingly, however, these did not relate to CD34 nor CD133 expression [20]. On the other hand, development models point to pericytes as derived from EPC, which are committed under the control of VEGF [21].

Taken together, these findings raise some ambiguity among the potentialities of fat-derived adult progenitors. Here, our group intended to search for cells presenting hemogenic properties within fat subcutaneous tissues, focusing on two cell subsets defined using the surface markers CD133/1 and CD140b (PDGFRb), the latter a marker of pericytes [7,22].

2. METHODS

2.1. Processing Human Lipoaspirates

Human subcutaneous fat tissues were obtained following informed consent, in accordance with the Ethics Committees from both institutions involved (CEP-HUPE 2311, CEP-INCA 42/09). Nonobese women (median weight 62 kg) submitted to elective aesthetic surgeries were donors of abdomen or hip lipoaspirates, extracted following the injection of saline plus epinephrine 1:500,000, without local anesthetic, but under general anesthesia or spinal block. Aspirates from 60 mL sterile syringes were extensively washed by centrifugation with phosphate-buffered saline (PBS), during which fat tissue pieces floated while blood contaminants pelleted and were discarded. Tissue was digested with collagenase type 1A (Sigma-Aldrich, USA) at a final concentration of 0.25 mg/mL in PBS, for 1h at 37˚C, blocked with complete culture medium (DMEM with 10% FBS, GIBCO, Life Tech, USA), and centrifuged at 800 × g for 10 min, in order to collect the pelleted stromal-vascular fraction (SVF)

Fresh SVF cell suspensions were submitted to positive selection through immunomagnetic columns (Miltenyi Biotech, Germany) after incubation with the following Miltenyi bead-conjugated antibodies (Ab): anti-human CD133/1; anti-human CD34; anti-human CD45; goat anti-mouse IgG, as a secondary Ab following primary purified anti-human CD140b (Pharmingen, BD Biosciences, USA).

2.2. CFU Assays

The selected cells (10^4 - 10^5) were suspended in Iscove's Medium (GIBCO) with 2% FBS (Hyclone SH30070.03, Thermo Sci, USA), mixed with semisolid medium with hematopoietic cytokines (Methocult GF 04434, StemCell Tech, USA) (containing Bovine Serum Albumin, 2-Mercaptoethanol, Recombinant Human (rh) Stem Cell Factor, rh GM-CSF, rh IL-3, and rh Erythropoietin), and dispensed onto 35 mm plastic culture plates for the CFU assay. After 2 - 3 weeks colonies were counted, and classified according to standard morphologic parameters as erythroid progenitors (BFU-E), granulocyte-macrophage progenitors (CFU-GM) and mixed granulocyte, erythroid, macrophage and megakaryocyte progenitors (CFU-GEMM). Positive controls for this assay were run in parallel, using $CD34^+$ positively-selected cells from UCBs, obtained following informed consent of the parents of neonates at the Laranjeiras Perinatal Clinic, Rio de Janeiro, after project approval by the Board of the institution, in accordance with the ethical regulations. UCB mononuclear cells were separated by density gradient (Histopaque 1077, Hybri-Max, Sigma), suspended in 12.5% DMSO in complete medium and stored in liquid nitrogen at −196˚C until use.

Colonies from each experiment were harvested as a pool, cells washed with PBS containining 2% FCS and processed for cytofluorometric analysis as follows. After incubation with FcR Blocking Reagent Human (Miltenyi) for 15 min at 8˚C, plus 20 min with the monoclonal antibodies Phycoerithrin (PE)-conjugated anti-human Glycophorin A, and Fluorescein Isothiocyanate (FITC)-conjugated anti-human CD71 (Transferrin Receptor) (BD Biosciences, USA), cells were 2 times washed and assessed for surface staining in a BD Biosciences FACScan. Data were analyzed using the CellQuest software (BD Biosciences).

Alternatively, they were cytospined in order to access the morphology of individual cells following May-Grunwald-Giemsa staining, using an Olympus Imaging Corp. (Japan) Bx41TF optical microscope. The images were acquired using a digital camera, model C7070WZ, in HQ mode and processed using the Corel Photo-Paint 9 software to adjust brightness/contrast/intensity.

3. RESULTS AND DISCUSSION

As shown in **Table 1**, among fat-derived cell subsets, only the $CD133/1^+$ selected cells were able to form colonies under the influence of hematopoietic cytokines in CFU assays. The colonies were not as abundant as those from UCB-derived $CD34^+$ progenitors (**Figure (1A)**), but showed typical myeloid morphology, comprising white (CFU-GM), red (BFU-E) and mixed (CFU-GEMM) colonies (**Figure (1B)**), with the rate and frequency varying according to the sample (**Table 1**). The aspect of individual cells recovered from fat-derived CFUs and stained with May-Grunwald-Giemsa seemed compatible with blood forming, although, compared with those from UCB-derived CFUs, they presented a higher frequency of eosinophilic granulocytes and macrophage-like morphologies. Also, a percentage of the cells recovered from fat-derived CFUs revealed, under cytofluorometric analysis, a positive staining for the markers of erythroid development Glycophorin-A and CD71 (Transferrin Receptor) (**Figure 2**), the first being expressed on cell surface when proerythroblasts first appear [23]. The observed differentiation bias toward eosinophilic granulocytes and macrophage-like morphologies may reflect the previous influence of fat microenvironment, still under analysis.

Compared to $CD34^+$-UCB-derived CFUs, $CD133/1^+$-fat-derived CFUs took longer to reveal as colonies, three weeks instead of the two required by the former. This suggests that they represent primitive hemogenic stem cells present in the subcutaneous fat, and that they possibly share with the UCB-derived $CD133/1^+$ cells the qui-

Table 1. Colony Forming Unit assays with cell subsets from stromal-vascular fractions (SVF) of human lipoaspirates.

Exp	Crude SVF Cell Number	Number of Selected $CD34^+45^-$ Seeded	Number of Selected $CD140b^+$ Seeded	Number of Selected $CD133/1^+$ Seeded	*Observed CFU Number/Approximate Frequency of Colonies
1	2.5×10^8	1.2×10^5	-	-	None
2	2×10^7	-	2×10^5	-	†None
3	2×10^7	-	1.5×10^5	-	†None
4	5×10^7	-	-	5×10^4	4 BFU-E 1/12.500
5	4.5×10^7	-	-	10^4	3 BFU-E 1/3.300
6	7.5×10^7	-	-	7.5×10^4	2 BFU-E, 1 CFU-GEMM 1/25.000
7	6×10^6	-	-	10^5	4 BFU-E, 2 CFU-GM 1/16.600
8	5×10^6	-	-	10^4	2CFU-GM, 2 BFU-E 1/2.500
9	5.5×10^7	-	-	2×10^5	3CFU-GM, 4 BFU-E 1/28.500

*After 3 weeks of culture. †Grew massively adherent under semisolid medium. BFU-E, erythroid progenitors; CFU-GM, granulocyte-macrophage progenitors; CFU-GEMM, mixed granulocyte, erythroid, macrophage and megakaryocyte progenitors.

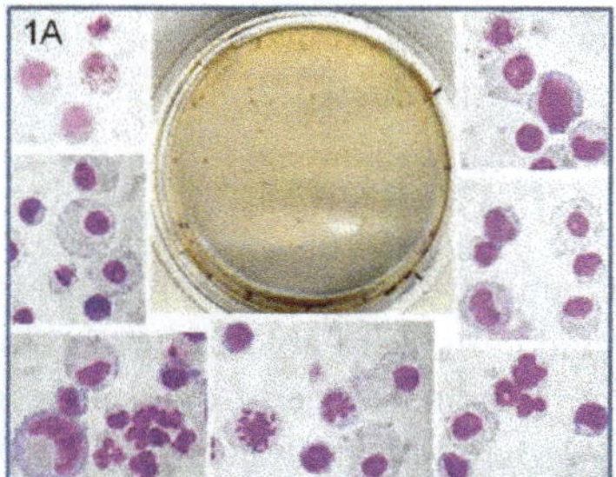

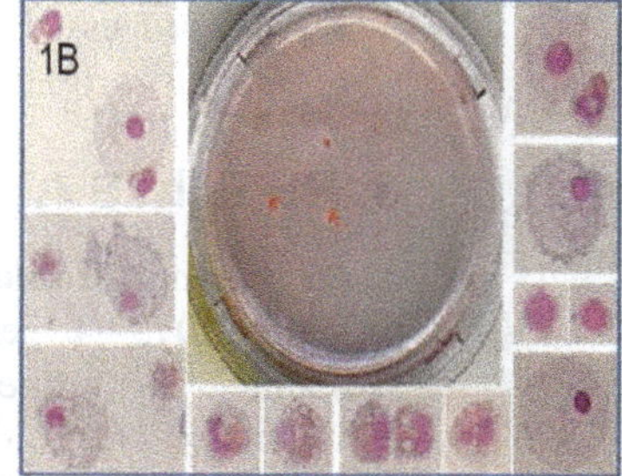

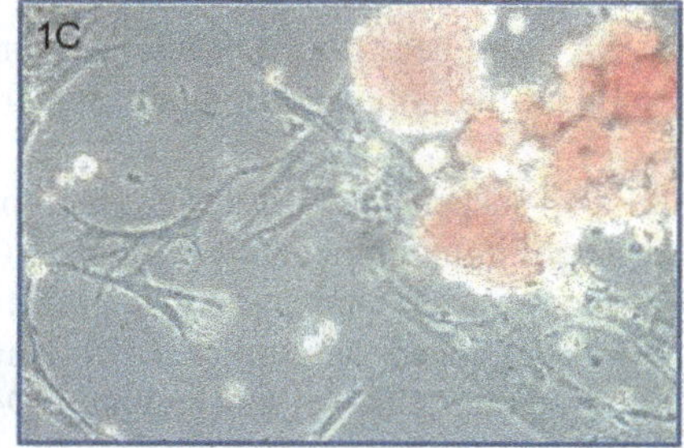

Figure 1. Colony forming unit assay with fat-derived $CD133/1^+$ cells, using umbilical cord blood-derived $CD34^+$ as the positive control. (1A) $CD34^+$ cells from mononuclear fraction of umbilical cord blood, and (1B) $CD133/1^+$ cells from the stromal—vascular fraction of human lipoaspirates, were positively selected and cultured in semisolid medium containing hematopoietic cytokines. After 2 (in 1A) or 3 weeks (in 1B), the colonies were harvested as pools, the cell suspensions were cytospined, and individual cell types were observed following staining with May-Grunwald-Giemsa, using an Olympus Bx41TF optical microscope and a digital camera model C7070WZ in High-Quality mode (original magnification ×400 for individual cells in 1A and 1B). Images were adjusted for brightness/contrast/intensity using the Corel Photo-Paint 9 software. (1C) Using a NIKON TMS-F inverted phase microscope (Japan), some fat-derived $CD133/1^+$ cells were observed adhering to the plates, under the semisolid medium, presenting aspect of mesenchymal cells (original magnification ×300). Shown one experiment typical of six.

escent phenotype [15], thus requiring a longer period of incubation with the cytokines. The presently observed fat-derived primitive progenitors would putatively take part in the long-term hematopoietic reconstitution previously reported in a mouse model [5], besides the committed $CD34^+45^+$ progenitors to which it was ascribed.

Neither $CD34^+45^-$ nor $CD140b^+$ selected cells produced colonies in response to hematopoietic cytokines (**Table 1**). The latter were observed growing massively under the semisolid medium, adherent to the plates, and displayed typical mesenchymal morphology (not shown). Similarly, in the $CD133/1^+$ selected pool, a few adherent cells grew under the semisolid medium (**Figure (1C)**), though their characteristics were not accessed in this work. They could represent either mesenchymal contaminants in the selected suspension or true $CD133/1^+$ cells acquiring an adherent phenotype [19,24]. In this respect, Pozzobon *et al.* [25] reported that BM-derived $CD133^+$ cells possess the ability to adhere to plastic surfaces, acquiring mesenchymal differentiation potentialities, however without the loss of hemogenic or endothelial potential [25]. In contrast, unselected BM-derived mesenchymal cells expanded by adherence did not display hemogenic nor endothelial potential [25], suggesting a mesenchymal commitment not yet achieved by the $CD133^+$ pool, or a hierarchy.

Concluding, in regard to fat-derived cells under the conditions presented, comparison between $CD133/1^+$ and $CD140b^+$ subsets revealed segregation of the hemogenic potential to cells in the $CD133/1^+$ subpopulation, unravelling the ambiguity of potentialities, and pointing to the presence, in adult human fat, of a hemogenic progenitor with a more primitive character than that previously reported. Considering developmental decisions, pericytes

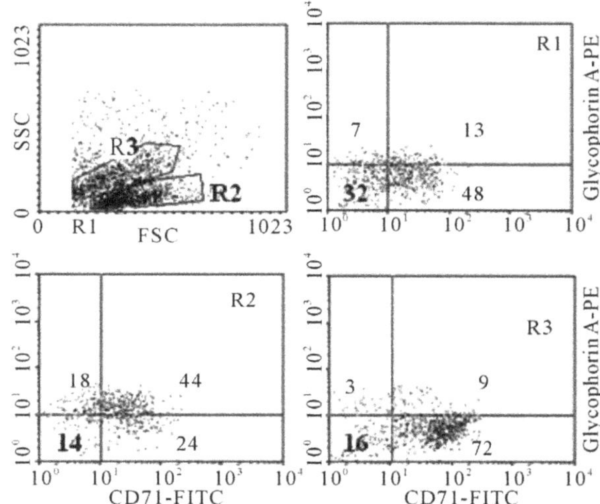

Figure 2. Erythroid development assessed by cytofluorometric analysis of cell suspensions from fat-derived CFUs. Colonies were harvested as pools and washed cell suspensions incubated with FcR Blocking Reagent followed by fluorochrome-conjugated antibodies (anti-Glycophorin A-PE/Gly and anti-CD71-FITC). High left, dot plot shows the analysis windows depicting three cell subpopulations (R1, R2, R3) based on their size (FSC) versus granulosity (SSC). R1, R2 and R3 dot plots show the fluorescence intensity of staining in each subpopulation. R1 (small and smooth cells) comprised Gly negative (neg) cells, either CD71 neg or intermediately (int) positive (pos). R2 (large and smooth cells) comprised mainly Gly pos, CD71 int cells. R3 (both small and large granular cells) comprised mainly Gly neg, CD71 high cells, which probably precedes R2 as an early developmental stage [23]. Shown one of two experiments.

presented commitment to a mesenchymal fate revealed by the unresponsiveness to hemogenic cytokines and massive adherent growth. These findings further punctuate the diversity of stem/progenitor subsets present in adult human fat, still poorly characterized.

4. ACKNOWLEDGEMENTS

FAPERJ, INCA-FIOCRUZ, Laranjeiras Perinatal Clinic Board and Obstetrics Team, Pedro Ernesto Hospital Surgery Team, Experimental Medicine and Pediatric Oncohematology Research Programs of the National Cancer Institute, RJ, Brazil.

REFERENCES

[1] Freitas, C.S. and Dalmau, S.R. (2006) Multiple sources of non-embryonic multipotent stem cells: Processed lipoaspirates and dermis as promising alternatives to bone marrow-derived cell therapies. *Cell and Tissue Research*, **325**, 403-411. doi:10.1007/s00441-006-0172-x

[2] Da Silva Meirelles, L., Chagastelles, P.C. and Nardi, N.B. (2006) Mesenchymal stem cells reside in virtually all post-natal organs and tissues. *Journal of Cell Science*, **119**, 2204-2213. doi:10.1242/jcs.02932

[3] Zuk, P.A., Zhu, M., Ashjian, P., De Ugarte, D.A., Huang, J.Y., *et al.* (2002) Human adipose tissue is a source of multipotent stem cells. *Molecular Biology of the Cell*, **13**, 4279-4295. doi:10.1091/mbc.E02-02-0105

[4] Fraser, J.K., Wulur, I., Alfonso, Z. and Hedrick, M.H. (2006) Fat tissue: An underappreciated source of stem cells for biotechnology. *Trends in Biotechnology*, **24**, 150-154. doi:10.1016/j.tibtech.2006.01.010

[5] Cousin, B., André, M., Arnaud, E., Pènicaud, L. and Casteilla, L. (2003) Reconstitution of lethally irradiated mice by cells isolated from adipose tissue. *Biochemical and Biophysical Research Communications*, **301**, 1016-1022. doi:10.1016/S0006-291X(03)00061-5

[6] Han, J., Koh, Y.J., Moon, H.R., Ryoo, H.G., Cho, C.H., *et al.* (2010) Adipose tissue is an extramedullary reservoir for functional hematopoietic stem and progenitor cells. *Blood*, **115**, 957-964. doi:10.1182/blood-2009-05-219923

[7] Traktuev, D.O., Merfeld-Clauss, S., Li, J., Kolonin, M., Arap, W., *et al.* (2008) A population of multipotent CD34-positive adipose stromal cells share pericyte and mesenchymal surface markers, reside in a periendothelial location, and stabilize endothelial networks. *Circulation Research*, **102**, 77-85. doi:10.1161/CIRCRESAHA.107.159475

[8] Lin, G., Garcia, M., Ning, H., Banie, L., Guo, Y.L., *et al.* (2008) Defining stem and progenitor cells within adipose tissue. *Stem Cells and Development*, **17**, 1053-1063. doi:10.1089/scd.2008.0117

[9] Zimmerlin, L., Donnenberg, V.S., Pfeifer, M.E., Meyer, E.M., Péault, B., *et al.* (2010) Stromal Vascular Progenitors in Adult Human Adipose Tissue. *Cytometry Part A*, **77**, 22-30. doi:10.1002/cyto.a.20884

[10] Sengenes, C., Lolmede, K., Zakaroff-Girard, A., Busse, R. and Bouloumié, A. (2005) Preadipocytes in the human subcutaneous adipose tissue display distinct features from the adult mesenchymal and hematopoietic stem cells. *Journal of Cellular Physiology*, **205**, 114-122. doi:10.1002/jcp.20381

[11] Waller, E.K., Huang, S. and Terstappen, L. (1995) Changes in the growth properties of $CD34^+$, $CD38^-$ bone marrow progenitors during human fetal development. *Blood*, **86**, 710-718.

[12] Florek, M., Haase, M., Marzesco, A.-M., Freund, D., Ehninger, G., *et al.* (2005) Prominin-1/CD133, a neural and hematopoietic stem cell marker, is expressed in adult human differentiated cells and certain types of kidney cancer. *Cell and Tissue Research*, **319**, 15-26. doi:10.1007/s00441-004-1018-z

[13] Gallacher, L., Murdoch, B., Wu, D.M., Karanu, F.N., Keeney, M., *et al.* (2000) Isolation and characterization of human CD34.2Lin2 and CD34.1Lin2 hematopoietic stem cells using cell surface markers AC133 and CD7. *Blood*, **95**, 2813-2820.

[14] Meregalli, M., Farini, A., Belicchi, M. and Torrente, Y. (2010) $CD133^+$ cells isolated from various sources and their role in future clinical perspectives. *Expert Opinion on Biological Therapy*, **10**, 1521-1528.

[15] Summers, Y.J., Heyworth, C.M., de Wynter, E.A., Hart, C.A., Chang, J., *et al.* (2004) $AC133^+$ G0 cells from cord blood show a high incidence of long-term culture-initi-

ating cells and a capacity for more than 100 million-fold amplification of colony-forming cells in vitro. *Stem Cells*, **22**, 704-715. doi:10.1634/stemcells.22-5-704

[16] Aranguren, X.L., Luttun, A., Clavel, C., Moreno, C., Abizanda, G., *et al.* (2007) In vitro and in vivo arterial differentiation of human multipotent adult progenitor cells. *Blood*, **109**, 2634-2642. doi:10.1182/blood-2006-06-030411

[17] Loges, S., Fehse, B., Brockmann, M.A., Lamszus, K., Butzal, M., *et al.* (2004) Identification of the adult human hemangioblast. *Stem Cells and Development*, **13**, 229-242. doi:10.1089/154732804323099163

[18] Yokomizo, T. and Dzierzak, E. (2010) Three-dimensional cartography of hematopoietic clusters in the vasculature of whole mouse embryos. *Development*, **137**, 3651-3661. doi:10.1242/dev.051094

[19] Peichev, M., Naiyer, A.J., Pereira, D., Zhu, Z., Lane, W.J., *et al.* (2000) Expression of VEGFR-2 and AC133 by circulating human $CD34^+$ cells identifies a population of functional endothelial precursors. *Blood*, **95**, 952-958.

[20] Miñana, M.D., Carbonell-Uberos, F., Mirabet, V., Marín, S. and Encabo, A. (2008) IFATS collection: Identification of hemangioblasts in the adult human adipose tissue. *Stem Cells*, **26**, 2696-2704. doi:10.1634/stemcells.2007-0988

[21] Hagedorn, M., Balke, M., Schmidt, A., Bloch, W., Kurz, H., *et al.* (2004) VEGF coordinates interaction of pericytes and endothelial cells during vasculogenesis and experimental angiogenesis. *Developmental Dynamics*, **230**, 23-33. doi:10.1002/dvdy.20020

[22] Amos, P.J., Shang, H., Bailey, A.M., Taylor, A., Katz, A.J., *et al.* (2008) IFATS collection: The role of human adipose-derived stromal cells in inflammatory microvascular remodeling and evidence of a perivascular phenotype. *Stem Cells*, **26**, 2682-2690. doi:10.1634/stemcells.2008-0030

[23] Rogers, C.E., Bradley, M.S., Palsson, B.O. and Koller, M.R. (1996) Flow cytometric analysis of human bone marrow perfusion cultures: Erythroid development and relationship with burst-forming units-erythroid. *Experimental Hematology*, **24**, 597-604.

[24] Handgretinger, R., Gordon, P.R., Leimig, T., Chen, X., Buhring, H.J., *et al.* (2003) Biology and plasticity of $CD133^+$ hematopoietic stem cells. *Annals of the New York Academy of Sciences*, **996**, 141-151. doi:10.1111/j.1749-6632.2003.tb03242.x

[25] Pozzobon, M., Piccoli, M., Ditadi, A., Bollini, S., Destro, R., *et al.* (2009) Mesenchymal stromal cells can be derived from bone marrow $CD133^+$ cells: Implications for therapy. *Stem Cells and Development*, **18**, 497-510. doi:10.1089/scd.2008.0003

27

Characterization of a mesenchymal stem cell line that differentiates to bone and provides niches supporting mouse and human hematopoietic stem cells

Sonal R. Tuljapurkar[1], John D. Jackson[2], Susan K. Brusnahan[3], Barbara J. O'Kane[4], John G. Sharp[1*]

[1]Departments of Genetics, Cell Biology and Anatomy, University of Nebraska Medical Center, Omaha, USA
[2]Pathology and Microbiology, University of Nebraska Medical Center, Omaha, USA
[3]Pharmaceutical Sciences, University of Nebraska Medical Center, Omaha, USA
[4]Creighton University Medical Center, Omaha, USA; [*]Corresponding Author: jsharp@unmc.edu

ABSTRACT

Identification of mouse cell lines with properties of primary multipotential mesenchymal stromal cells (MSC) is required to facilitate the use of mouse models for evaluation of mechanisms in bone formation, hematopoiesis and cellular therapies for regenerative medicine. Primary murine MSC vary between strains, are difficult to grow *in vitro* and have inconsistent properties. The main aim of the study was to establish OMA-AD cells as an appropriate model system to conduct studies on MSC, bone formation and hematopoiesis. OMA-AD cells were isolated by differential trypsinization of C57BL/6J mouse bone marrow (BM) cells. The cells were then repassaged, cloned and characterized. OMA-AD cells were immortal and non-tumorigenic, differentiated readily to all mesenchymal cell types including bone, supported mouse and human hematopoiesis and were immunosuppressive. Our results demonstrated that OMA-AD cells possessed the properties of primary MSC. In addition, these cells grew readily and consistently, thereby facilitating future studies of bone formation, hematopoiesis and mesenchymal cells for regenerative medicine.

Keywords: Bone; Cell Therapy; Hematopoiesis; MSC; Regenerative Medicine; Stem Cells

1. INTRODUCTION

In recent years there has been increased interest in mesenchymal cells, their differentiation to cartilage and bone, their role in stem cell niches [1] and potential utility in regenerative medicine. Although, originally MSC were used therapeutically for skeletal problems [2] and gene therapy [3,4] multiple additional therapeutic applications have been evaluated, including promotion of hematopoietic recovery in stem cell transplant recipients [5,6] severe, acute graft-versus-host disease [7], autoimmune diseases [8], muscle repair [9], skin healing [10], intestine healing following irradiation [11], stroke [12], myocardial ischemia [13,14] as well as other diseases.

MSC were first identified in the bone marrow, where they are present with about ten-fold higher concentrations than the circulation and can be obtained from all tissues with varying frequencies [15,16]. In man, the number of viable, freshly isolated cells is limited due to dispensable bone marrow volume [17].

Consequently, animal studies are a powerful tool for investigations of diverse potential applications for MSC. Apart from the increasing applications of the functional properties of MSC, there is substantial interest in evaluation of the role of these cells in the stem cell niche and mouse models of diseases [18]. The numbers of MSC obtained in murine models are adequate and can be maneuvered to differentiate into several cell types. However, primary MSC from murine sources do not grow readily in culture, and exhibit considerable variability in their biological properties from different strains of mice [19]. Consequently, there is substantial merit in identifying mouse cell populations that grow consistently and at the same time exhibit characteristics of primary mouse MSC.

OMA-AD cells were obtained by differential trypsinization of whole bone marrow cells from C57BL/6J mice. The cells were passaged several times and only rare adherent cells that survived passaging were cloned and characterized further. Briefly, the cells were probed for their doubling time, phenotype and differentiation into various lineages. OMA-AD cells were seeded as the adherent layer in long-term cultures with BM cells and added to mixed lymphocyte reactions. In addition, OMA-

AD cells were injected into non-irradiated and lethally irradiated recipients. A preosteoblast cell line with apparently similar properties to OMA-AD cells has been described (D1 cells) and employed in orthopedic studies [20]. However, the D1 cell line is of Balb/c origin, whereas the OMA-AD cell line is of C57BL/6J origin therefore genetically compatible with most transgenic mouse models. OMA-AD cells have been employed and reported previously [21]. However, the isolation, derivation, differentiation to cartilage and bone, support of mouse and human hematopoiesis and overall properties of these cells have not been described previously and is the primary aim of this report.

2. MATERIALS AND METHODS

2.1. Isolation of OMA-AD Cell Line

C57BL/6J and C57BL/6J-EGFP (enhanced green fluorescent protein) expressing mice were purchased from Jackson Laboratories, or bred in the University of Nebraska Medical Center (UNMC) comparative medicine department. These mice were used in the studies as approved by the UNMC Institutional Animal Care and Use Committee (IACUC). The mice were housed in individual microisolator cages and provided food and water ad libitum. Bone marrow cells were gently aspirated from the femoral diaphysis and maintained in Fisher's medium supplemented with 15% fetal bovine serum (FBS; Hyclone) and 15% horse serum (HS; Hyclone) The cultures were maintained at 33˚C in a mixture of 5% CO_2 and air, as described previously for long term bone marrow cultures [22].

2.2. Cell Line Development

In order to obtain cell lines, the supernatants were discarded and the remaining cells were trypsinized repeatedly until only rare adherent cells remained. Fisher's medium with 15% FBS and 15% HS was added and surviving cells were maintained in culture. The cells were observed for areas (colonies) of outgrowths of cells. Most of the cells in the majority of flasks differentiated and died. However, rare outgrowths were observed. These were trypsinized and re-passaged. The majority of re-passages failed to grow, but a few cells survived passaging. These cells were cloned in microtiter plates and progeny frozen for future studies. One of these clones, with the most robust and consistent patterns of growth, was designated as OMA-AD cell line and the properties of this cell line were characterized in more detail.

2.3. Morphology and Cell Growth Analysis

OMA-AD cells were plated in growth supporting medium [RPMI-1640 (Gibco Inc.), 10% FBS, 10% HS, 1% Penicillin-Streptomycin (Gibco Inc.), 1% L-glutamine (Gibco Inc.)] in T25 cm^2 flasks (Corning Inc.) with a concentration of 1×10^5 cells or 4000 cells/cm^2. For morphological analyses, the flasks were monitored for confluence and photographed using a Nikon phase contrast microscope and Nikon Coolpix P5000 10 MegaPixel camera. For doubling time analyses, at each defined time point, 3 flasks were trypsinized and cell counts were obtained using a cell counter (Beckman Coulter Inc.) The mean of the data points obtained were plotted (Sigmaplot Statistical Software 7.0) Doubling time was calculated from equation $dt = t * \ln 2/\ln(Ct/Co)$, where t = the time point in exponential growth of the plot, Ct = cell count at time "t", Co = cell count when plated or initial time point on the exponential part of the growth curve.

2.4. Surface Phenotype

1×10^6 OMA-AD cells were placed into 12 × 75 mm test tubes, centrifuged for 2 minutes and resuspended in 200 µl staining buffer (Phospaphate Buffered Saline (PBS) with 0.2% Bovine Serum Albumin (BSA) 2 µl (0.4 µg/ml concentration) of antibody was added to cells and vortexed. A 20-minute incubation was performed on ice in the dark. The mixture was washed with 1 ml of staining buffer and centrifuged for 2 minutes using an immufuge (Baxter Corp). The cells were resuspended in 0.5 ml of staining buffer and 50 µl Vitalyse® fixative prior to analysis. Antibodies against mouse CD 3, 4, 8, 11b, 14, 19, 24, 25, 31, 34, 40, 44, 45, 48, 49d, 73, 80, 105, 133, 150, e-cadherin, SDF-1, Oct 3/4, B220, Mac-1, Gr-1, CXCR4, Thy 1.1 and 1.2, were purchased from BD Biosciences (San Jose, CA). Flow cytometric analysis was performed and analyzed using Cell Quest Pro (BD Biosciences) software.

2.5. Differentiation to Adipocytes, Osteoblasts and Chondrocytes

OMA-AD cells were seeded onto 3 - 6 coverslips in a 60 mm petridish with growth supporting medium (RPMI 1640 medium + 10% FBS + 10% HS + 1% Penicillin-Streptomycin + 1% L-glutamine) Upon 60% - 70% confluence, adipocyte differentiation medium (ADM) (DMEM with 10% FBS, dexamethasone 1 µM, isobutylmethylxanthine 0.5 µM, Insulin 1 µg/ml, indomethacin 100 mM) was added (day1) and changed every 2 days up to 2 weeks. The coverslips were mounted on slides using Permount solution on day 7. Adipogenic differentiation was monitored as lipid droplets formed inside the cells and as red droplets after Oil Red O staining at day 7. Osteoblast stimulating medium (OSM) (DMEM with 10% FBS, dexamethasone 100nM, beta-glycerophosphate 10 mM, L-ascorbic-2-phosphate 50 nM, penstrep 1%) was added upon 60% confluence (day1) 0.5 ml medium was added to the culture every 3rd day. After 12 days, coverslips were mounted on a slide and stained for alkaline phosphatase using a kit (Sigma-Aldrich) to identify the osteoblasts. Chondrocyte differentiation was carried out as per the protocol provided by Miltenyi Biotech. Briefly, 1×10^6 OMA-AD cells were centrifuged in a 15 ml conical polypropylene tube and formed into a compact pellet. Chondrocyte differentiation media (Miltenyi Biotech) was added on top of the pellet. The tubes were incubated at 37°C, 5% CO_2. Media was changed every other day for 24 days. The pellets were fixed in 3.7% neutral buffered formalin and subsequently embedded in paraffin. Chondrocytic differentiation was confirmed using Alcian blue-Periodic Schiff Staining. OMA-AD cells maintained undifferentiated in the growth supporting medium, were employed as controls and were confirmed by staining negative for Oil Red O, alkaline phosphatase and Alcian blue-PAS staining. All the slides were counterstained with wright giemsa stain (Fisher Scientific).

2.6. Support of Murine Hematopoiesis

The ability of OMA-AD cells to support mouse hematopoietic cells was evaluated by using OMA-AD cells as an adherent layer for long term bone marrow cultures. OMA-AD cells were seeded at 1×10^6 cells in a T25 culture flask (Greiner Biosciences). Upon 60% confluence, the flasks were seeded with whole bone marrow cells or bone marrow sorted side population (SP) cells from EGFP donors (EGFP expressing on background of C57BL/6J mice) so that any hematopoietic cells maintained and/or generated could be identified by fluorescence microscopy or by flow cytometric analyses. Cultures were maintained at 33°C for 6 months with intermittent change of culture medium.

2.7. Support of Human Hematopoiesis

The ability of OMA-AD cells to maintain human hematopoiesis was determined by evaluating their ability to sustain human hematopoietic cell production and granulocyte-monocyte progenitor cells (GM-CFC) as assayed in a clonal colony forming cell assay. Human cell sources evaluated were monocyte depleted cord blood, T cell depleted cord blood and granulocyte colony stimulating factor (G-CSF) mobilized blood cells. The comparison adherent cells were grown with or without a pre-established, irradiated mouse bone marrow stromal layer. The cord blood cells were obtained from full term deliveries with IRB (Institutional Review Board) approval and informed consent of the donor. The cord blood samples were depleted of monocytes by employing 2 one hour adhesion incubations in culture dishes. After the first adhesion period, the non-adherent cells were removed and placed in the second culture dish. After the second adhesion period, the non-adherent cells were isolated and used in the experiments. T-cells were depleted employing magnetic bead separation. G-CSF mobilized blood depleted of T cells by anti-CD3 antibody were obtained with IRB approval and informed consent of a donor who received five consecutive daily subcutaneous injections of G-CSF (5 μg/kg) (Amgen Inc). The non-adherent cellularities of these co-cultures were determined weekly using an electronic cell counter. The GM-CFC assay was performed, as described previously [23], every two weeks, on non-adherent cells and, at the termination of the co-cultures, on both the non-adherent and adherent cells.

2.8. Precursor Frequency Determination

For the G-CSF mobilized blood cells and human leukemic cell line; OMA-AML1 cells [24], a limiting dilution of cobblestone area formation was employed to determine precursor frequencies.

2.9. Radioprotection

One of two doses of total body irradiation were administered to C57BL/6J EGFP (to track the origin of cells) mice; a lethal dose (10 Gy) or a sub-lethal dose (7.5 Gy). Mice receiving the lethal dose (n = 7) and sub-lethal dose (n = 7) were injected with 1×10^6 OMA-AD cells in 200 μl Hank's Balance Salt Solution (HBSS; Gibco Inc). Controls (mice receiving the sublethal dose) were not injected with OMA-AD cells (n = 7). Circulating blood cell numbers, GFP expression and survival were tracked.

2.10. Tumorigenicity

1×10^5 OMA-AD cells were injected in 200 μl HBSS, subcutaneously (n = 3) and intraperitonealy (n = 3) subcutaneously in the flank (Ip and SQ are switched) of syngeneic C57BL/6J mice. The mice were examined twice weekly for 120 days and the site of injection palpated to detect any tumor growth. Any growths were examined histologically.

2.11. Immunosuppression

Spleen cells were obtained from DBA and C57BL/6J (referred to as B6) mice where DBA spleen cells were stimulators and B6 spleen cells were responders. 1×10^5 cells of each type were added to each well in a 96-well flat bottom plate (Corning Inc). OMA-AD cells were titrated into this assay which employed allogeneic mixtures of mouse spleen cells to generate a mixed lymphocyte reaction (MLR). Samples were run in quadruplicate. Spleen cells from DBA mice, appropriate numbers of spleen cells from B6 mice and OMA-AD cells were irradiated at 20 Gy. Irradiated DBA spleen cells along with non-irradiated B6 cells comprised the "experimental" group. Irradiated B6 cells along with non-irradiated B6 cells were the "control" group. Irradiated OMA-AD cells were plated 24 hrs prior to addition of other cell types to ensure adherence. The wells with OMA-AD cells along with irradiated DBA and non-irradiated B6 cells were termed "Experimental + OMA-AD" or control + OMA-AD (irradiated B6 + non-irradiated B6 + OMA-AD). Cells were grown in RF 10 (RPMI-1640; Gibco, Fetal Bovine Serum 10%; Hyclone, Penicillin/Streptomycin; Gibco) for 4 days. The cells were pulsed at day 3 and day 4 with tritiated thymidine (1 microcurie/well) to measure cell proliferation. Upon 18 - 24 hrs incubation, cells were harvested using cell harvester (PHD cell harvester) and radioactivity determined using a liquid scintillation counter (Perkin Elmer, Shelton, CT). Stimulation of immune response or inhibition of stimulation was determined by measuring cell proliferation. Experimental groups were plotted against cell proliferation (counts/minute) using SigmaPlot (7.0) software. Three sets of independent experiments were conducted and the data obtained was averaged and plotted in **Figure 5**.

2.12. Statistics

The statistical differences amongst groups were analyzed using unpaired Student's t-test. Significance was set at a p-value of less than 0.05.

3. RESULTS

3.1. Morphology and Doubling Time

OMA-AD cells were isolated from a long-term (Dexter) bone marrow cultures by differential trypsinization and limiting dilution cloning. Despite originating from a single cell, cultured unmanipulated OMA-AD cells exhibited morphological heterogeneity (**Figure 1(a)**) with a doubling time of approximate 35 hrs (**Figure 1(b)**).

3.2. Phenotype

The phenotype of unmanipulated OMA-AD cells demonstrated a minor representation of several cell types including mesenchymal, endothelial and even differentiated hematopoietic cells (**Table 1**) but a predominant phenotypic marker was not identified and markers previously noted for MSC (CD 80, CD 90, CD 105) were not expressed at significant levels. Whether these data indicate that OMA-AD cells represent a primitive, entirely undifferentiated multipotential progenitor cell with a capacity to differentiate along various lineages or reflects epigenetically generated variations in progeny of a single cloned precursor cell is unclear. Note that these options are not necessarily exclusive.

3.3. Differentiation into Multiple Lineages

The primary characteristic of a bonafide MSC is their

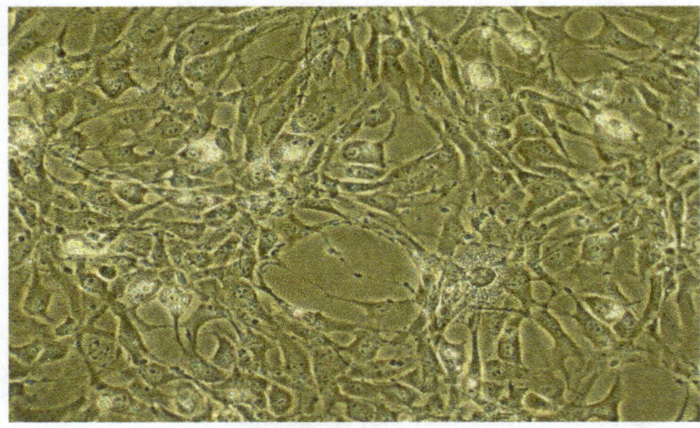

(a)

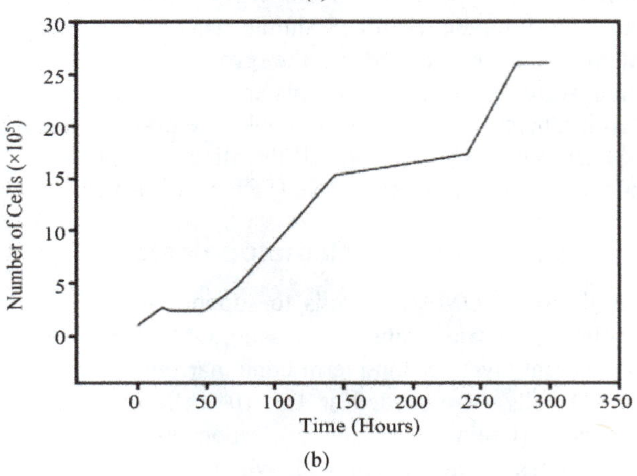

(b)

Figure 1. *In vitro* characterization of OMA-AD cells. (a) OMA-AD cells: Undifferentiated cells, display heterogeneity (Nikon Coolpix P5000, 20× Magnification); (b) Doubling time plot. OMA-AD cells had a doubling time of approximately 35 hours.

Table 1. Phenotypic characterization of OMA-AD cells. Based on the number of events (% positive OMA-AD cells), markers were segregated into biologically likely (>5% gated) and unlikely (<5% gated). The markers that were expressed <1% were considered as background. OMA-AD cells displayed heterogeneity in cell surface marker expression.

Surface Marker	% Positive OMA-AD Cells
CD 11b	12.0
CD 24	10.0
CD 25	6.0
CD 31	6.0
CD 34	5.0
CD 44	5.9
CD 45	8.0
CD 48	18.3
B220	18.4
Gr-1	13.0
CD 48-B220+	17.0
CD 3, 8, 14, 40, 49d, 73, 80, 105, 133, 150, E-cadherin, NK, Oct 3/4 , Mac-1, SDF-1, TCR, Thy 1.2	<5%
CD 4, 19, 90, CXCR4, Thy 1.1	<1% (background)

ability to differentiate into multiple mesenchymal lineages. OMA-AD cells were subjected to various differenttiation conditions to examine their ability to differentiate into adipocytic, osteoblastic and chondrocytic lineages. Upon incubation with ADM for 7 days, OMA-AD cells differentiated into adipocytes, with oil droplet accumulation observed at day 7 and confirmed by Oil Red O staining (**Figures 2(b)** and **(c)**) OMA-AD cells were incubated with OSM for 20 days, alkaline phosphatase staining at 11 days showed presence of osteoblasts, which was confirmed by calcium deposition detected by von Kassa staining at day 20 (**Figures 2(e)** and **(f)**) indicating an ability to form bone. OMA-AD cells were incubated for 24 days in chondrocyte differentiation medium and stained with Alcian blue-PAS to detect presence of chondrocytes (**Figure 2(h)**) OMA-AD cells maintained undifferentiated were confirmed by staining negative for Oil Red O, alkaline phosphatase and Alcian blue-PAS (**Figures 2 (a)**, **(d)** and **(g)**).

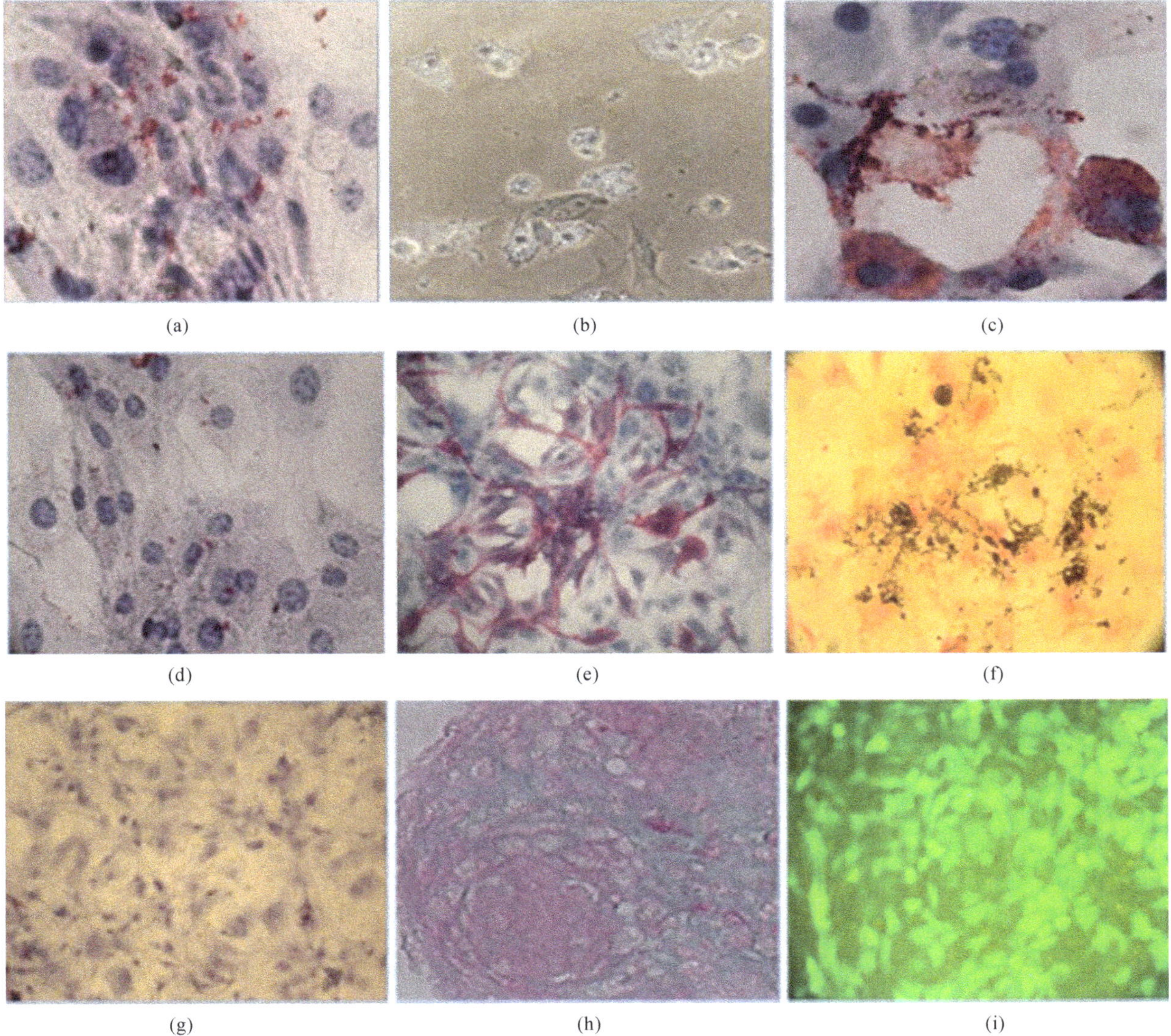

Figure 2. Differentiation and Hematopoietic Support. (a) Differentiation into adipocytes: Undifferentiated OMA-AD cells stain negative for Oil Red O (40× magnification); (b) Intracellular lipid accumulation observed adipocytes at day 7 (20× magnification); (c) Oil Red O positive adipocytes at day 7 (40× magnification); (d) Differentiation into Osteoblasts: Undifferentiated OMA-AD cells stain negative for alkaline phosphatase (20× magnification); (e) On day 11, OMA-AD cells differentiated into alkaline phosphatase positive osteoblasts (20× magnification); (f) Calcium deposition confirmed by von Kassa staining at day 20 (20× magnification); (g) Differentiation into chondroblasts: OMA-AD cells stained negative for Alcian blue-PAS staining (10× magnification); (h) OMA-AD cells differentiated to chondrocytes, Alcian blue-PAS staining (on day 24, 10× magnification); (i) OMA-AD cells support murine hematopoiesis *in vitro*. Bone marrow from GFP + C57BL/6J mouse were seeded upon adherent layer of OMA-AD cells. The cultures were photographed at 11 weeks (10× magnification). All photographs were taken using a Nikon microscope and Nikon Coolpix P5000 10 Megapixel camera.

3.4. Hematopoietic Support

OMA-AD cells promoted survival of mouse hematopoietic stem cells and their differentiation for 3 months (as demonstrated in **Figure 2(i)**) OMA-AD cells provided stromal support to human hematopoietic cells compared to ones grown without stroma or irradiated BM stroma (**Figure 3(a)**) ($p < 0.05$). Similarly, the numbers of granulocytes and macrophages were significantly higher on OMA-AD supported stroma compared to ones grown without a stromal layer (**Figure 3(b)**) ($p < 0.05$) and pre-irradiated stroma (did not reach statistical significance) OMA-AD cells, grown as an adherent layer supported GM-CSF mobilized peripheral blood cells and human leukemic hematopoietic cells in culture (**Figures 3(c)** and **(d)**) OMA-AD cells supported human CFU-GM from T-cell and monocyte depleted cord blood cells (**Tables 2 (a)** and **(b)**) These results demonstrated that OMA-AD cells promoted survival of quiescent mouse pluripotent hematopoietic stem cells, normal and human leukemic cells and permitted determination of hematopoietic precursor frequencies thereby establishing their ability to provide niches for mouse and human stem cells.

3.5. Radioprotection

In preliminary experiments, lethally irradiated mice that received 10^6 OMA-AD cells intravenously survived about 10 days in apparent good health, then succumbed. Since there is no exclusive marker on OMA-AD cells, mice expressing the green fluorescent protein, *i.e.* GFP mice, were employed as the recipients. C57BL/6J mice were irradiated with a lethal (10 Gy) and sub lethal (7.5 Gy) doses of irradiation and subsequently injected intravenously with 1×10^6 OMA-AD cells. Control mice received sub lethal dose of irradiation (7.5 Gy) and were

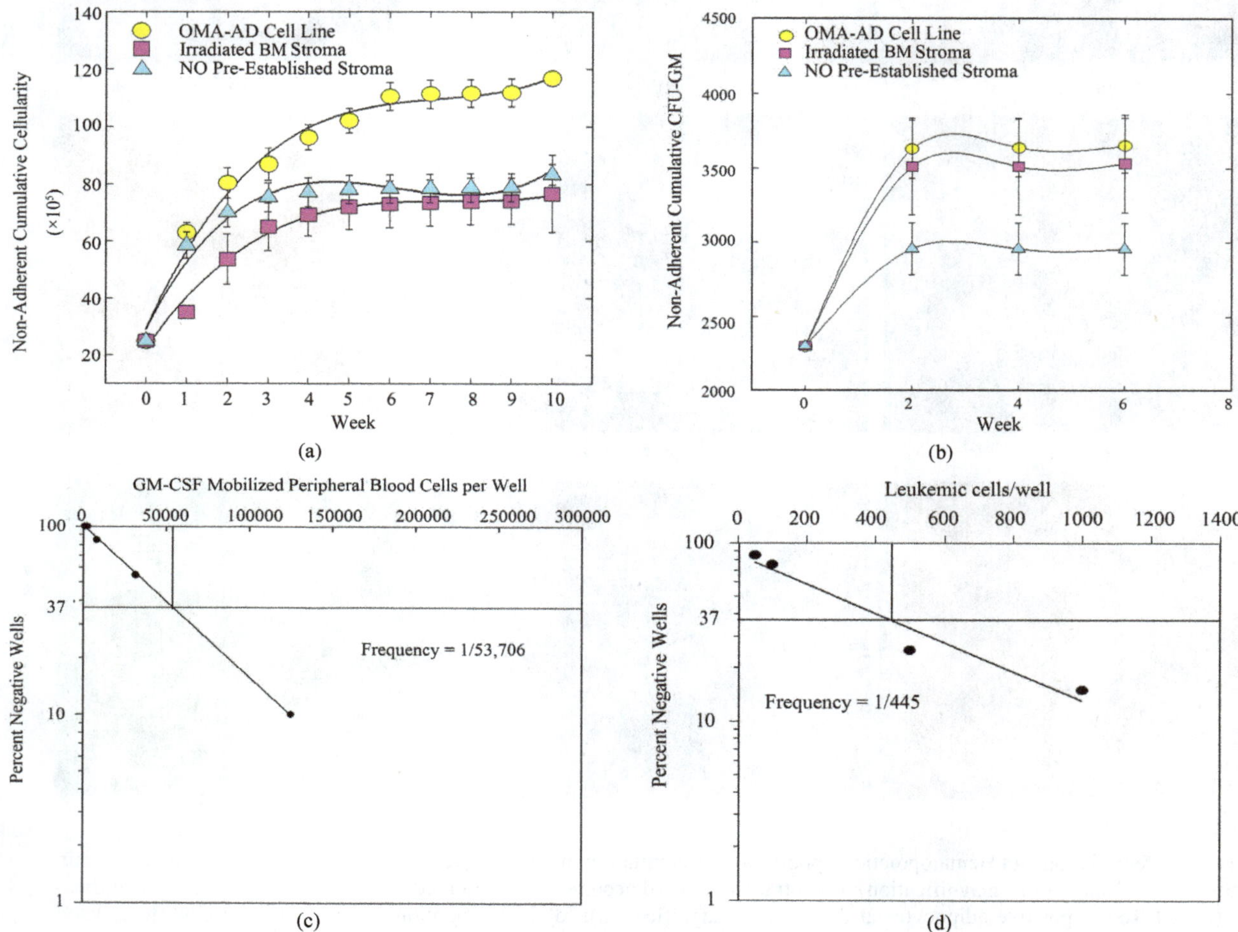

Figure 3. OMA-AD long-term support of human hematopoietic cells and long-term culture initiating cells (LTC-IC). (a) Hematopoietic cells grow better on an OMA-AD adherent layer than irradiated BM stroma ($p < 0.05$) or without stroma ($p < 0.05$); (b) Hematopoietic colony formation is improved in the presence of an OMA-AD adherent layer compared to controls *i.e.* without stroma ($p < 0.05$) and irradiated BM stroma (did not reach statistical significance); (c) Limiting dilution analysis of cobblestone area formation by GM-CSF mobilized blood cells with OMA-AD cells providing stromal support; (d) Limiting dilution analysis of cobblestone area formation by leukemic cells on OMA-AD cells as adherent layer.

Table 2. OMA-AD cells supported human long-term hematopoiesis *in vitro*. (a) OMA-AD supported human CFU-GM from monocyte depleted cord blood. (b) OMA-AD supported CFU-GM from T-Cell depleted cord blood. CFU-GM were maintained for a longer time in the presence of an adherent layer formed by OMA-AD cells compared to controls ($p < 0.05$) OMA-AD long-term support of human granulopoiesis did not require the presence of human T lymphocytes or monocytes. Controls were grown in the absence of OMA-AD as adherent layer.

(a)

Duration of Culture Time (Weeks)	Culture Fraction	OMA-AD Support Colonies/Flask (Mean ± sem)	Control Colonies/Flask (Mean ± sem)
0	Non-adherent	18,700 ± 500	18,700 ± 500
2	Non-adherent	95,370 ± 7480	3040 ± 192
4	Non-adherent	6708 ± 312	3762 ± 154
6	Non-adherent	1280 ± 32	30 ± 8
12	Adherent & Non-adherent	462 ± 44	<2

(b)

Duration of Culture Time (Weeks)	Culture Fraction	OMA-AD Support Colonies/Flask (Mean ± sem)	Control Colonies/Flask (Mean ± sem)
0	Non-adherent	9450 ± 500	9450 ± 500
2	Non-adherent	7514 ± 476	4680 ± 192
4	Non-adherent	1158	255
11	Adherent & Non-adherent	1416 ± 186	46 ± 5

not injected with OMA-AD cells. Despite cell depletion, all mice injected with OMA-AD cells maintained 80% - 90% circulating cells expressing GFP indicating that OMA-AD did not contribute significantly to the circulating cell pool. All lethally irradiated mice died 11 days after irradiation demonstrating that OMA-AD cells were unable to rescue hematopoiesis (**Figure 4**). However, mice receiving sub lethal irradiation and OMA-AD injection, survived several months post irradiation (**Figure 4**) up to 125 days post irradiation but did not have evidence of progeny derived from OMA-AD cells (data not shown).

3.6. Tumorigenicity

No tumors were formed by OMA-AD cells injected subcutaneously or intraperitoneally into 6 syngeneic mice after monitoring them for over 120 days (data not shown). The non-tumorigenic properties of OMA-AD are vital for their use in homing studies as well as regenerative medicine.

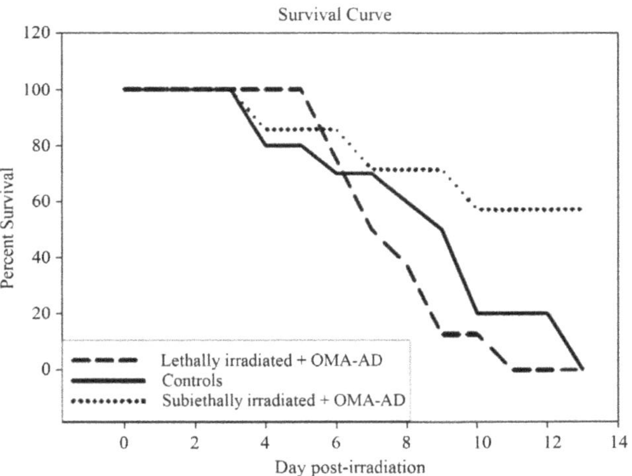

Figure 4. Injection of OMA-AD cells into lethally irradiated recipients for radioprotection. C57BL/6J mice were irradiated with lethal dose (10 Gy) or sub lethal dose (7.5 Gy) and subsequently injected with 1×10^6 OMA-AD cells. Control group received sub lethal irradiation but no OMA-AD injection. All mice receiving lethal dose died by 11 days after irradiation demonstrating that OMA-AD did not rescue hematopoiesis. Mice receiving sub lethal dose had about 50% survival by 13 days, with all mice dead by 125 days post irradiation (not shown).

3.7. Immunosuppression

Irradiated DBA spleen cells stimulated an immune response from non-irradiated B6 cells (experimental group) greater than that in the control group, $p < 0.05$ (irradiated B6 cells with non-irradiated B6 cells) (**Figure 5**). When OMA-AD cells were added to the experimental group (irradiated DBA with non-irradiated B6); termed "Experimental + OMA-AD", there was inhibition of immune response compared to the experimental group alone ($p < 0.05$). Similarly, control + OMA-AD (irradiated B6 + non-irradiated B6 + OMA-AD) suppressed the immune response even further ($p < 0.05$). These data clearly show that OMA-AD cells were immunosuppressive in a mixed lymphocytic reaction (**Figure 5**) making them ideal for *in vivo* studies.

4. DISCUSSION

OMA-AD cells represent a spontaneously immortalized mouse MSC line. OMA-AD cells are capable, under appropriate inductive conditions, of generating all of the primary differentiated cell lineages of mesenchymal (connective) tissue lineages: chondroblasts, osteoblasts and adipocytes. Further, OMA-AD cells not only maintained mouse quiescent pluripotent hematopoietic stem cells *in vitro* [21] but also supported human normal and leukemic cells in culture [24]. In addition to mimicking the properties of primary mouse MSC, this cell population is non-tumorigenic, even though it is immunosup pressive. This is an important component of their function

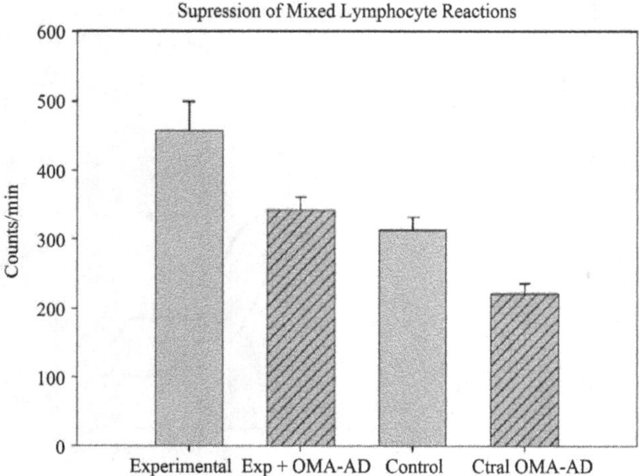

Figure 5. Suppression of Mixed Lymphocyte Reactions (MLR). Spleen cells were obtained from DBA and B6 mice where DBA spleen cells were stimulators and B6 spleen cells were responders. Cell proliferation was measured by thymidine uptake. The presence of OMA-AD cells significantly suppressed the MLR as shown by decreased cell proliferation ($p < 0.05$).

since they are able to ameliorate the consequences of graft versus host disease (GVHD) (data not shown). Although cloned and subsequently re-cloned, OMA-AD cells continued to generate heterogeneous progeny in culture with a doubling time of approximately 35 hours. This is characteristic of MSC and is comparable to primary rat MSC described by Ho *et al.* 2008 [25]. Since OMA-AD cells are clonally derived, generation of such progeny indicates heterogeneity of their differentiation abilities, rather than origins from a heterogeneous collection of progenitor cells. Under appropriate culture conditions, OMA-AD cells were able to differentiate into adipocytes, osteoblasts and chondrocytes. However, when cultured, OMA-AD cells piled up and they differentiated spontaneously to osteoblasts, suggesting the possible involvement of locally acting autocrine or paracrine factors, although a role for cell-cell contact cannot be excluded. OMA-AD cells did not express markers typically associated with primary MSC. The reasons for this are unclear because they differentiated in a manner identical to primary MSC. They did have a low expression of several markers of hematopoietic cells, although they showed no evidence of hematopoietic function (**Table 1**). Potentially, they represent an undifferentiated multipotential stem/progenitor population with either little or no expression of differentiated cell markers.

The primary role of MSC in the hematopoietic microenvironment is support of hematopoietic stem cell survival as well as maintenance of quiescence and differentiation. OMA-AD cells supported hematopoiesis *in vitro* when cultured with BM cells (from green fluorescent mice) for 11 weeks and also supported human hematopoietic cells long term *in vitro* (**Tables 2(a)** and **(b)**). This demonstrated that OMA-AD mimic primary MSC in regulation of hematopoietic progenitors [25] and provision of stem cell niches. MSC can protect the ovaries from chemotherapy induced damage and potentially protect against radiation damage [26] therefore, an approach was devised to test the effects of OMA-AD cells in irradiated mice. Two doses of radiation were employed, one sufficient to eliminate most endogenous hematopoietic stem cells (10 Gy) and a second (7.5 Gy), a sub lethal dose that permits survival of some, albeit low numbers, of endogenous stem cells. In addition to survival, the repopulation of blood cells in these mice, if any, was tracked, as well as the expression of GFP by the nucleated cells to determine the origins of the repopulating cells. No production of blood cells by OMA-AD cells was observed. OMA-AD cell injections into lethally irradiated recipients did not rescue hematopoiesis. This further confirmed that OMA-AD cells represented the nonhematopoietic component of BM and did not possess hematopoietic progenitors, or at least in sufficient numbers, to effect hematopoietic repopulation. However, the observation that a majority of the mice receiving a high sub lethal dose of irradiation and 1×10^6 OMA-AD cells survived for up to 125 days post irradiation, hints that OMA-AD cells might help support endogenous HSC.

This study also demonstrated an approach that can be employed to isolate additional MSC cell lines which can be engineered to express fluorescent cell markers (data not shown).

The MSC component of BM can be tracked and has the ability to give rise to rare types that integrate into injured target tissues [27]. Given that the frequency of cells with such ability is low and because intravenously injected MSC are found for only a short time in lung, liver and bone marrow (in that order) and are mostly undetectable after 72 hours (data not shown), this direct approach which depends on integration and plasticity is unlikely to result in significant tissue repair. More information on the regulation of self renewal and differentiation of MSC is needed as well as the mechanisms that target these cells to sites of tissue injury. Additionally, the relative contribution of these cells to target tissues by "plasticity", as opposed to their ability to promote repair by stimulating endogenous cells and the mechanisms of these effects needs to be probed. Currently, it appears that their ability to immunosuppress and promote repair by tropic factors dominates [18]. Despite these uncertainties, it is clear that MSC can support hematopoietic stem cells and can contribute to repair of tissue injury. OMA-AD cells provide a useful approach to improving our understanding of the mechanisms of these effects in mouse models [18].

5. CONCLUSION

OMA-AD cells are easier to grow and exhibit more consistent properties than primary mouse MSC. Consequently, their use is more efficient and economical than that of primary cells. Most importantly, this consistency presents an opportunity to further investigate the mechanisms of MSC differentiation to bone, support of hematopoietic stem cells, amelioration of GVHD and promotion of tissue repair and regeneration which have previously been challenging given the heterogeneity of primary MSC populations. Consequently, OMA-AD mouse MSC line exhibits all of the properties of primary MSC, is easier to grow, exhibits consistent properties, is non-tumorigenic and immunosuppressive and has significant promise to advance our mechanistic understanding of the role of MSC in tissue repair and regenerative medicine.

6. ACKNOWLEDGEMENTS

The authors would like to thank the following individuals who assisted with or advised these studies: Shantaram Joshi, PhD, Molly Lang, MS, Greg Perry, PhD, Sam Pirruccello, MD, Lisbeth Welniak, PhD and Tami Houdesheldt who typed the manuscript. These studies were supported as a part of assay development by funds from the National Institute on Aging and the State of Nebraska Department of Health and Human Services. This support is gratefully acknowledged.

REFERENCES

[1] Zhang, J., Niu, C., Ye, L., Huang, H., He, X., Tong, W.G., Ross, J., Haug, J., Johnson, T., Feng, J.Q., Harris, S., Wiedemann, L.M., Mishina, Y. and Li, L. (2003) Identification of the haematopoietic stem cell niche and control of the niche size. *Nature*, **425**, 836-841. doi:10.1038/nature02041

[2] Bruder, S.P., Fink, D.J. and Caplan, A.I. (1994) Mesenchymal stem cells in bone development, bone repair, and skeletal regeneration therapy. *Journal of Cellular Biochemistry*, **56**, 283-294. doi:10.1002/jcb.240560303

[3] Pereira, R.F., Halford, K.W., O'Hara, M.D., Leeper, D.B., Sokolov, B.P., Pollard, M.D., Bagasra, O. and Prockop, D.J. (1995) Cultured adherent cells from marrow can serve as long-lasting precursor cells for bone, cartilage, and lung in irradiated mice. *Proceedings of the National Academy of Sciences of the USA*, **92**, 4857-4861. doi:10.1073/pnas.92.11.4857

[4] Horwitz, E.M., Prockop, D.J., Fitzpatrick, L.A., Koo, W.W., Gordon, P.L., Neel, M., Sussman, M., Orchard, P., Marx, J.C., Pyeritz, R.E. and Brenner, M.K. (1999) Transplantability and therapeutic effects of bone marrow-derived mesenchymal cells in children with osteogenesis imperfecta. *Nature Medicine*, **5**, 309-313. doi:10.1038/6529

[5] Koc, O.N., Gerson, S.L., Cooper, B.W., Dyhouse, S.M., Haynesworth, S.E., Caplan, A.I. and Lazarus, H.M. (2000) Rapid hematopoietic recovery after coinfusion of autologous-blood stem cells and culture-expanded marrow mesenchymal stem cells in advanced breast cancer patients receiving high-dose chemotherapy. *Journal of Clinical Oncology*, **18**, 307-316.

[6] Le Blanc, K. and Ringden, O. (2005) Immunobiology of human mesenchymal stem cells and future use in hematopoietic stem cell transplantation. *Biology of Blood and Marrow Transplantation*, **11**, 321-334. doi:10.1016/j.bbmt.2005.01.005

[7] Le Blanc, K., Frassoni, F., Ball, L., Locatelli, F., Roelofs, H., Lewis, I., Lanino, E., Sundberg, B., Bernardo, M.E., Remberger, M., Dini, G., Egeler, R.M., Bacigalupo, A., Fibbe, W., Ringden, O. and Developmental Committee of the European Group for Blood and Marrow Transplantation (2008) Mesenchymal stem cells for treatment of steroid-resistant, severe, acute graft-versus-host disease: A phase II study. *Lancet*, **371**, 1579-1586. doi:10.1016/S0140-6736(08)60690-X

[8] Tyndall, A. and Uccelli, A. (2009) Multipotent mesenchymal stromal cells for autoimmune diseases: Teaching new dogs old tricks. *Bone Marrow Transplant*, **43**, 821-828. doi:10.1038/bmt.2009.63

[9] Kobayashi, N., Yasu, T., Ueba, H., Sata, M., Hashimoto, S., Kuroki, M., Saito, M. and Kawakami, M. (2004) Mechanical stress promotes the expression of smooth muscle-like properties in marrow stromal cells. *Experimental Hematology*, **32**, 1238-1245. doi:10.1016/j.exphem.2004.08.011

[10] Falanga, V., Iwamoto, S., Chartier, M., Yufit, T., Butmarc, J., Kouttab, N., Shrayer, D. and Carson, P. (2007) Autologous bone marrow-derived cultured mesenchymal stem cells delivered in a fibrin spray accelerate healing in murine and human cutaneous wounds. *Tissue Engineering*, **13**, 1299-1312. doi:10.1089/ten.2006.0278

[11] Semont, A., Francois, S., Mouiseddine, M., Francois, A., Sache, A., Frick, J., Thierry, D. and Chapel, A. (2006) Mesenchymal stem cells increase self-renewal of small intestinal epithelium and accelerate structural recovery after radiation injury. *Advances in Experimental Medicine and Biology*, **585**, 19-30. doi:10.1007/978-0-387-34133-0_2

[12] Li, Y., Chen, J., Chen, X.G., Wang, L., Gautam, S.C., Xu, Y.X., Katakowski, M., Zhang, L.J., Lu, M., Janakiraman, N. and Chopp, M. (2002) Human marrow stromal cell therapy for stroke in rat: Neurotrophins and functional recovery. *Neurology*, **59**, 514-523.

[13] Laflamme, M.A. and Murry, C.E. (2005) Regenerating the heart. *Nature Biotechnology*, **23**, 845-856. doi:10.1038/nbt1117

[14] Tang, Y.L. (2005) Autologous mesenchymal stem cells for post-ischemic myocardial repair. *Methods in Molecular Medicine*, **112**, 183-192.

[15] Da Silva Meirelles, L., Chagastelles, P.C. and Nardi, N.B. (2006) Mesenchymal stem cells reside in virtually all post-natal organs and tissues. *Journal of Cell Science*, **119**, 2204-2213. doi:10.1242/jcs.02932

[16] Sudo, K., Kanno, M., Miharada, K., Ogawa, S., Hiroyama, T., Saijo, K. and Nakamura, Y. (2007) Mesenchymal progenitors able to differentiate into osteogenic,

chondrogenic, and/or adipogenic cells *in vitro* are present in most primary fibroblast-like cell populations. *Stem Cells*, **25**, 1610-1617. doi:10.1634/stemcells.2006-0504

[17] Pilgaard, L., Lund, P., Rasmussen, J.G., Fink, T. and Zachar, V. (2008) Comparative analysis of highly defined proteases for the isolation of adipose tissue-derived stem cells. *Regenerative Medicine*, **3**, 705-715. doi:10.2217/17460751.3.5.705

[18] Phinney, D.G. and Prockop, D.J. (2007) Concise review: Mesenchymal stem/multipotent stromal cells: The state of transdifferentiation and modes of tissue repair—Current views. *Stem Cells*, **25**, 2896-2902. doi:10.1634/stemcells.2007-0637

[19] Phinney, D.G., Kopen, G., Isaacson, R.L. and Prockop, D.J. (1999) Plastic adherent stromal cells from the bone marrow of commonly used strains of inbred mice: Variations in yield, growth, and differentiation. *Journal of Cellular Biochemistry*, **72**, 570-585. doi:10.1002/(SICI)1097-4644(19990315)72:4<570::AID-JCB12>3.0.CO;2-W

[20] Shen, F.H., Visger, J.M., Balian, G., Hurwitz, S.R. and Diduch, D.R. (2002) Systemically administered mesenchymal stromal cells transduced with insulin-like growth factor-I localize to a fracture site and potentiate healing. *Journal of Orthopaedic Trauma*, **16**, 651-659. doi:10.1097/00005131-200210000-00007

[21] Klarmann, K., Ortiz, M., Davies, M. and Keller, J.R. (2003) Identification of *in vitro* growth conditions for c-Kit-negative hematopoietic stem cells. *Blood*, **102**, 3120-3128. doi:10.1182/blood-2003-04-1249

[22] Crouse, D.A., Mann, S.L. and Sharp, J.G. (1984) Segregation and characterization of lymphohematopoietic stromal elements. *Kroc Found Ser Journal*, **18**, 211-231.

[23] Kessinger, A., O'Kane Murphy, B., Jackson, J.D. and Sharp, J.G. (2005) An *ex vivo* model of hematopoietic stem cell mobilization. *Cytotherapy*, **7**, 463-469. doi:10.1080/14653240500361418

[24] Pirruccello, S.J., Jackson, J.D., Lang, M.S., DeBoer, J., Mann, S., Crouse, D., Vaughan, W.P., Dicke, K.A. and Sharp, J.G. (1992) OMA-AML-1: A leukemic myeloid cell line with CD34+ progenitor and CD15+ spontaneously differentiating cell compartments. *Blood*, **80**, 1026-1032.

[25] Ho, A.D., Wagner, W. and Franke, W. (2008) Heterogeneity of mesenchymal stromal cell preparations. *Cytotherapy*, **10**, 320-330. doi:10.1080/14653240802217011

[26] Fu, X., He, Y., Xie, C. and Liu, W. (2008) Bone marrow mesenchymal stem cell transplantation improves ovarian function and structure in rats with chemotherapy-induced ovarian damage. *Cytotherapy*, **10**, 353-363. doi:10.1080/14653240802035926

[27] Abe, S., Lauby, G., Boyer, C., Rennard, S.I. and Sharp, J.G. (2003) Transplanted BM and BM side population cells contribute progeny to the lung and liver in irradiated mice. *Cytotherapy*, **5**, 523-533. doi:10.1080/14653240310003576

Bone morphogenetic protein-4 affects both trophoblast and non-trophoblast lineage-associated gene expression in human embryonic stem cells

Margaret L. Shirley[1,2*], Alison Venable[1*], Raj R. Rao[3], Nolan L. Boyd[4], Steven L. Stice[1,5,6], David Puett[1#], Prema Narayan[7#]

[1]Department of Biochemistry and Molecular Biology, University of Georgia, Athens, USA;
[#]Corresponding Author: puett@bmb.uga.edu
[2]Department of Psychiatry, University of California, San Francisco, USA
[3]Department of Chemical and Life Science Engineering, School of Engineering, Virginia Commonwealth University, Richmond, USA
[4]Cardiovascular Innovation Institute, University of Louisville, Louisville, USA
[5]Regenerative Bioscience Center, University of Georgia, Athens, USA
[6]Department of Animal and Dairy Sciences, University of Georgia, Athens, USA
[7]Department of Physiology, Southern Illinois University School of Medicine, Carbondale, USA;
[#]Corresponding Author: pnarayan@siumed.edu

ABSTRACT

Human embryonic stem cells (hESC) can be induced to differentiate to trophoblast by bone morphogenetic proteins (*BMPs*) and by aggregation to form embryoid bodies (EB), but there are many differences and controversies regarding the nature of the differentiated cells. Our goals herein were to determine if BG02 cells form trophoblast-like cells (a) in the presence of *BMP*4-plus-basic fibroblast growth factor (*FGF*-2) and (b) upon EB formation, and (c) whether the *BMP*4 antagonist noggin elicits direct effects on gene expression and hormone production in the cells. Transcriptome profiling of hESC incubated with *BMP4*/*FGF*-2 showed a down-regulation of pluripotency-associated genes, an up-regulation of trophoblast-associated genes, and either a down-regulation or no change in gene expression for many markers of the three embryonic germ layers. Yet, there was up-regulation of several genes associated with mesoderm, ectoderm, and endoderm, strongly suggesting that differentiation to trophoblast-like cells under the conditions used does not yield a homogeneous cell type. Several genes, heretofore unreported, were identified that are altered in hESC in response to *BMP*4-mediated differentiation. The production of human chorionic gonadotropin (hCG), progesterone, and estradiol in the differentiated cells confirmed that trophoblast-like cells were obtained. Gene expression by EB was characterized by an up-regulation of a number of genes associated with trophoblast, ectoderm, endoderm, and mesoderm, and the production of hCG and progesterone confirmed that trophoblast-like cells were formed. These results suggest that, in the presence of *FGF*-2, BG02 cells respond to *BMP*4 to yield trophoblast-like cells, which are also obtained upon EB formation. Thus, *BMP*4-mediated differentiation of hESC represents a viable cell system for studying early developmental events post-implantation; however, up-regulation of non-trophoblast genes suggests a somewhat diverse response to *BMP4*/*FGF*-2. Noggin altered the transcription of a limited number of genes but, not surprisingly, did not lead to secretion of hormones.

Keywords: Human Embryonic Stem Cells; Trophoblasts; Bone Morphogenetic Protein-4; Embryoid Bodies; Noggin

1. INTRODUCTION

In the human blastocyst, the first step of differentiation from the morula, composed of totipotent cells, yields the inner cell mass and trophoblast. The former differentiates into the hypoblast, leading to the extraembryonic endoderm and the epiblast, that differentiates to give the amniotic ectoderm and the primitive ectoderm. The primitive ectoderm, in turn, differentiates into the embryonic

[*]These authors contributed equally to this work.

ectoderm and the primitive streak, the latter giving rise to extraembryonic mesoderm, primitive mesoderm, and embryonic endoderm. The trophectoderm is composed of epithelial cells and differentiates into several lineages. The trophoblast precursor cells begin rapid proliferation into cytotrophoblasts, with some fusing to form multinucleate syncytiotrophoblasts, a terminally differentiated trophoblast cell; in addition, villous and extravillous cytotrophoblasts are formed [1-3]. One of the hallmarks of trophoblast differentiation is the production of the heterodimeric glycoprotein hormone, human chorionic gonadotropin (hCG), that is secreted throughout gestation, being essential for progesterone production by the corpus luteum in the first trimester of human pregnancy [4,5]. There is a paucity of adequate cell models for studying early trophoblast development, and a reliable system will greatly facilitate progress in the area of human reproduction.

Recent studies have shown that human embryonic stem cells (hESCs) can undergo differentiation into trophoblast-like cells spontaneously from colonies [6], growth of the cells beyond confluence [7], or embryoid bodies (EBs) [3,8-12]. Similarly, trophoblast-like cells can be obtained from hESCs via induced differentiation from the bone morphogenetic proteins (*BMP*s) 2, 4, and 7 [13-24]. Fortunately, timely reviews are available [25-28]. Others have reported that RNAi-mediated knockdown of Oct4 in hESCs can also lead to trophoblast-like cells [29,30]. The *BMP*s, members of the transforming growth factor-b (TGFb) superfamily, function to regulate many aspects of development which act by binding to cell surface serine/threonine kinase receptors that, in turn, phosphorylate particular Smads, thus enabling them to enter the nucleus and act as transcriptional regulators [31-34].

These cellular models for trophectoderm differentiation begin to fill a long-awaited need for new systems to study early development, particularly in view of the major differences between human and mouse trophoblast [35-37]. Yet, the characteristics of the human trophoblast cells obtained by *BMP*-mediated differentiation vary, sometimes quite significantly, depending upon the cell type, culture conditions (including the presence or absence of growth factors, particularly *FGF*2), and mode of differentiation [10,18,38]. Moreover, in a number of instances there are considerable differences and controversies regarding the product(s) of differentiation obtained with *BMP*. For example, *BMP*4-mediated differentiation was found to yield little evidence of trophoblast-like cells under standard culture conditions [38]. Another study found that 14 genes were highly up-regulated as determined by microarrays, in addition to many others [21], while another report did not identify six of these particular genes [17]. Also, differences in cell morphology and gene markers have been noted in *BMP*-treated hESCs [18,21]. Explanations for many of these controversial reports were recently provided by two groups. Yu *et al.* [22] reported that b*FGF* (*FGF*-2), which acts via the MEK-ERK pathway, redirects *BMP*4-mediated differentiation from trophectoderm to mesendoderm as judged by the expression of brachyury. The activated MEK-ERK pathway sustains NANOG expression leading to a b*FGF*-independent induction of mesendoderm by *BMP*4. Another recent paper concluded that in the cooperative presence of *FGF*2, *BMP*4 (that acts through brachyury and *CDX*2) leads to the induction of mesoderm, not trophoblast [39].

The present study was undertaken with the goals of: 1) extending the previous reports that were based on a variety of cell lines, different culture conditions, and at times conflicting results, and 2) to critically examine the trophoblast and non-trophoblast *BMP*-regulated genes, particularly since a number of the non-trophoblast *BMP*-regulated genes have been noted in the earlier studies. We chose to use the hESC line, BG02 (karyotype 46, XY), that has not been thoroughly studied in hESC differentiation to trophoblast. This cell line was established from a 6-day embryo with an embryo grade of 3CC [7]. Herein, *BMP*4, in the presence of *FGF*2, was incubated with adherent colonies of BG02 cells to initiate trophoblast differentiation. Identical studies were also done in the presence of the *BMP*4 antagonist noggin, since it has been shown that noggin alters hESC gene expression and morphology, perhaps leading to differentiation toward early neuroectoderm [18]. In addition, trophoblast differentiation was initiated by formation of EBs. Particular emphasis was placed on quantitative profiling of a variety of genes via qRT-PCR, and measurements were made to determine hCG and steroid hormone production by the cells and EBs. Our results have many similarities with the findings of others, including for example the down-regulation of pluripotency genes, the up-regulation of trophoblast genes, and placental hormone production, but there are also notable differences, particularly with the up-regulation of certain genes associated with the three primary germ layers.

2. MATERIALS AND METHODS

2.1. Maintenance of Undifferentiated Cells

In order to ensure pluripotency, the BG02 cells, obtained with proper authorization from Bresagen, Athens, GA, were manually passaged every 2 - 3 days onto mitotically-inactivated mouse embryonic feeder (MEF) layers derived from E13.5 mouse fetuses. The MEF layer was removed from the hESC colony, which was then gently dispersed with the colony pieces being transferred to another 10 cm MEF-containing plate and treated with hESC culture medium: 77% Dulbecco's Modified Eagle Medium (DMEM/F12; Gibco, Carlsbad, CA) supplemented with 15% fetal bovine serum (Hyclone, Logan, UT); 5% knockout serum replacement, 1% non-essential amino acids, 1% penicillin/streptomycin, and 1 mM L-glutamine (all from Gibco); 0.1 mM *β*-mercaptoethanol and 4 ng/mL basic fibroblast growth factor (*FGF*2; Sigma, St. Louis, MO); and 10 ng/mL leukemia inhibitory factor (LIF; Chemicon, Temecula, CA). Cells were passaged every 3 - 4 days. Two days after passage the medium was aspirated and replaced daily.

2.2. *BMP*4-Mediated Differentiation

The cells were passaged by gentle enzymatic digestion using cell dissociation buffer (Gibco) into 10 cm Matrigel-coated dishes (BD Bioscience, Boca Raton, FL). The BG02 cells were cultured in 50% DMEM/F12 medium that was conditioned by MEF layers [21] and then supplemented with 4 ng/mL *FGF*2. Experimental groups included incubation with 100 ng/mL *BMP*-4 (Quest Diagnostics, Lyndberg, NJ) and with 250 ng/mL noggin (Quest Diagnostics), with untreated hESC serving as controls. The medium was collected each day for analysis of secreted hormones. On day 7 the cells were harvested and quick-frozen for RNA extraction

2.3. Formation of Embryoid Bodies

Colonies were sliced into small pieces, then removed gently from the MEF layer where they were allowed to aggregate randomly in suspension on agarose plates. EBs were grown on agarose dishes in 12 mL of the hESC medium described above. Each culture began with ~50 EBs and ended with ~12 EBs of varying sizes. The loss of EB was attributed to aggregation of the individual units and/or to atresia/necrosis. On alternate days the culture plates were swirled to aggregate the EB with 6 mL of medium being removed and frozen. The same volume of fresh medium was added with the EBs then dispersed to prevent clumping.

2.4. Hormone Assays

Media collected from cell cultures and EBs were analyzed for secretion of three placental hormones namely hCG (the assay recognizes both heterodimer and hCG*β*), progesterone, and estradiol using immunofluorescence-based assays. The hormones were measured with an Immulite 1000 with a tri-level internal control in human serum, Con6, being used to standardize all kits (Diagnostic Product Corporation, Los Angeles, CA).

2.5. qRT-PCR

Total RNA was isolated from BG02 (day 0, *i.e.* control, and incubated for 7 days) and from EBs at days 5, 22, and 50 of culture. hESCs were resuspended in 1 mL Trizol (Invitrogen, Carlsbad, CA) and triturated until homogenized. The integrity of isolated RNA isolated from the homogenates (Trizol, Molecular Research Corporation, Albany, NY) was verified and quantified using a RNA 600 Nano Assay (Agilent Technologies, Foster City, CA) and the Agilent 2100 Bioanalyzer. The cDNA Archive Kit (Applied Biosystems, Inc., Foster City, CA) was used to reverse transcribe 5 μg total RNA with the MultiScribe Reverse Transcriptase. Initially, reactions were incubated at 25°C for 10 min and subsequently at 37°C for 120 min. Quantitative PCR (Taqman) assays were selected for the transcripts to be evaluated from Assays-On-Demand (Applied Biosystems, Inc.) and incorporated into 384-well Micro-Fluidic Cards. The cDNA samples and 50 μl of GeneAmp Fast PCR master mix (2×) (Applied Biosystems, Inc.) were loaded in duplicate into respective channels on each microfluidic card and briefly centrifuged.

qRT-PCR and relative quantification were performed with the ABI PRISM 7900 Sequence Detection System (Applied Biosystems, Inc.), with the expression levels of all genes analyzed given relative to 18S rRNA expression. The results for differential expression between the treated and control samples were expressed as means and data with a C_t value greater than 35 were not analyzed. The qRT-PCR data on gene expression of *BMP*4-treated and noggin-treated hESCs on day 7 of culture were analyzed as ddC_t relative to day 0, *i.e.* undifferentiated hESCs. Data were collected for EBs at days 5, 22, and 50 of culture, in all cases using 18S rRNA as the internal reference gene. The values of ddC_t on days 22 and 50 are expressed relative to day 5. In the equations below, std = internal gene standard (18S rRNA), goi = gene of interest under experimental conditions, and con = gene of interest under control conditions. It is assumed that the amplifycation efficiency is identical under all conditions to give the normalized fold-change of the mRNA of interest in treated cells (experimental) relative to that of control cells [40,41].

$$(dC_t)_{goi} = (C_t)_{goi} - (C_t)_{std}, (dC_t)_{con} = (C_t)_{con} - (C_t)_{std}$$

$$ddC_t = (dC_t)_{goi} - (dC_t)_{con}, \text{ Fold-change} = 2^{-ddc_t}$$

As defined, ddC_t is negative if the gene of interest under experimental conditions, *i.e.* BG02 cells plus *BMP*4 or plus noggin on day 7, is expressed at a higher level than the same gene under control conditions, *i.e.* untreated cells at day 0.

2.6. Data Analysis

Most of the PCR experiments were performed in triplicate, although in a few cases n was 2, 4, 5, or 6. Hormone measurements were done in triplicate, and the results are given as mean ± SEM. Data exceeding a fold-change of 2.0 (up-regulated) or –2.0 (down-regulated) were analyzed using a one-way analysis of variance (ANOVA) with the GraphPad Prism software. Results are given for changes with $P < 0.05$ and $P < 0.10$. Although the mean fold-change was large in some cases, significance was at times not reached, often due to n = 2 or to one value in three being particularly different from the others. Outliers were identified using the Grubbs' test (on-line GraphPad software). From over 400 hormone measurements, only about 1% was deemed outliers, and from over 700 qRT-PCR runs, only six and seven outliers were identified in the cell and EB data, respectively.

3. RESULTS

3.1. Effects of *BMP*4 and Noggin on Gene Expression and Hormone Production in hESC

Gene expression: The selection of 177 genes to investigate via qRT-PCR was based on several criteria. For example, it was important to include many that were established markers of pluripotency, trophoblast, ectoderm, endoderm, and mesoderm. In addition to these standard marker genes, others were also screened. Included in this list were genes encoding certain steroidogenic enzymes even if not specific for trophoblast and placenta, e.g. cytochrome P450 side-chain cleavage enzyme (*CYP*11*A*1) and aromatase (*CYP*19*A*1). Other genes encoding proteins for extracellular matrix and various aspects of cell function were monitored.

A heatmap, based on mean values of 2^{-ddc_t} and depicting gene expression of 146 genes in hESCs incubated with either *BMP*4 or with noggin for 7 days, both relative to control cells, is shown in **Figure 1. Table I** provides more information on many of the genes shown in **Figure 1** that are altered by 2-fold or more in response to *BMP*4. It can be seen that a number of genes are up-regulated by *BMP*4, a smaller number down-regulated, and a much larger number exhibit no major change in expression.

*BMP*4 leads to down-regulation of the pluripotency-associated genes: *DNMT3B*, *EBAF*, *FGF*2, *FGF*4, *FGFR*4, *FOXH*1, *GABRB*3, *GBX*2, *LDB*2, *POU5F*1, and *SOX*2, and an up-regulation of genes associated with differentiation to trophoblast or involved in implantation and/or placenta function: *CGB*, *CYP*11*A*1, *CYP*19*A*1, *ENPEP*, *EPAS*1, *GATA*2, *GATA*3, *HEY*1, *INHA*, *KRT*7, *MMP*9, *MSX*2, *PGF*, and *WNT5A*, genes that have also been identified by others (cf. [17,21] and references therein). Moreover, a comparison of *BMP*4-mediated hESC differentiation with human trophectoderm [42] identified

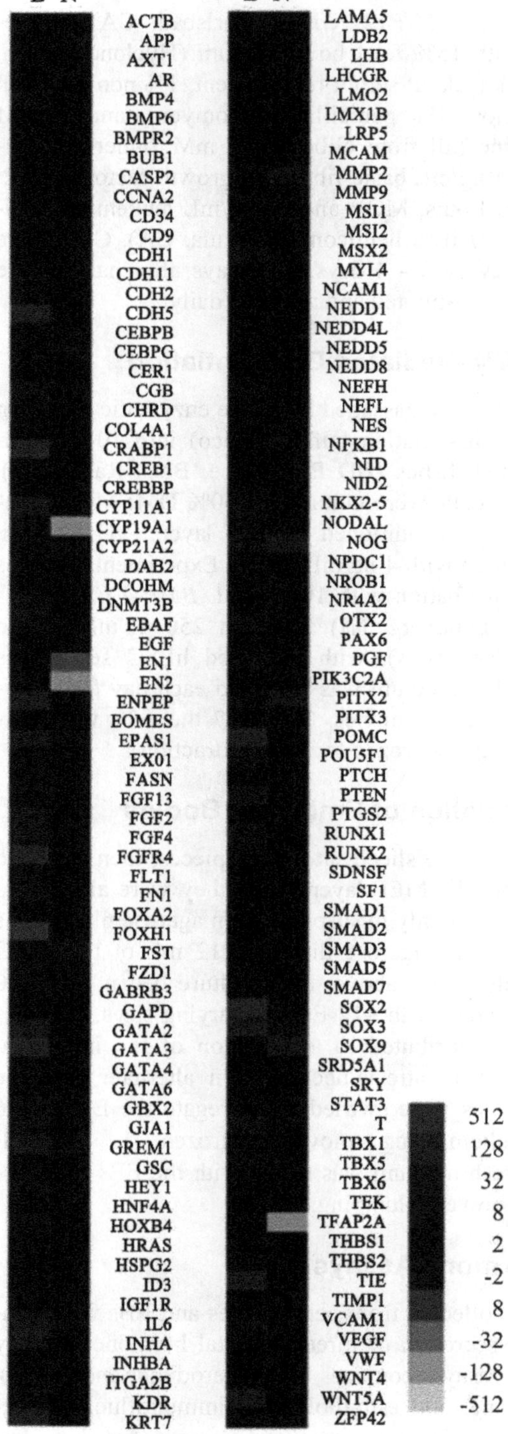

Figure 1. Heatmap showing the alterations in gene expression in hESC after seven days of incubation with either *BMP*4 (B) or noggin (N) relative to control. The data reflect qRT-PCR results given as mean values of 2^{-ddc_t}. The gray bars denote sufficiently low expression that could not be accurately determined, *i.e.* C_t greater than 35.

Table 1. *BMP4*-mediated changes in gene expression of hESCs[a].

Gene	Fold-change	Description
Trophoblast		
CGB	44.9[b]	Chorionic gonadotropin-b
CYP11A1	51.5[c]	Cytochrome P450 family 11, subfamily A
CYP19A1	8.9[b]	Cytochrome P450 family 19, subfamily A
ENPEP	244.6[b]	Glutamyl aminopeptidase
EPAS1	185.6[d]	Endothelial PAS domain protein 1
GATA2	200.2[d]	GATA binding protein 2
GATA3	336.2[d]	GATA binding protein 3
HEY1	18.5[b]	Hairy enhancement of split related with YRPW motif
INHA	89.9[c]	Inhibin a
KRT7	242.2[c]	Keratin 7
MMP9	8.6[c]	Matrix metalloproteinase 9
MSX2	174.1[d]	Msh homeobox 2
PGF	26.5[d]	Placental growth factor
WNT5A	101.8[d]	Wingless-type MMTV integration site family 5A
Pluripotency		
DNMT3B	−3.7[b]	DNA (cytosine-5)-methlytransferase 3 b
EBAF	−4.9[b]	Endometrial bleeding associated factor
FGF2	−5.3[b]	Fibroblast growth factor 2
FGF4	−4.5[b]	Fibroblast growth factor 4
FGFR4	−6.2[d]	Fibroblast growth factor receptor 4
FOXH1	−9.1[d]	Forkhead box protein H1
GBX2	−3.5[b]	Homeobox protein GBX2
POU5F1	−4.8[b]	POU class 5 homoebox 1
SOX2	−26.8[d]	SRY (sex determining region Y)-box 2
Mesoderm		
BMP4	24.1[d]	Bone morphogenetic protein 4
BMPR2	4.4[d]	Bone morphogenetic protein receptor, type II
CDH5	150.2[b]	Cadherin 5, type 2
CDH11	7.1[d]	Cadherin 1, type 2
CHRD	9.1[d]	Chordin
GATA4	13.7[b]	GATA binding protein 4
GJA1	−3.4[d]	Connexin 43, gap junction a3
KDR	−3.4[b]	Kinase insert domain receptor
NKX2-5	15.5[b]	Homeobox protein Nkx 2.5
PITX2	12.4[d]	Paired-like homeodomain transcription factor 2
RUNX1	60.9[d]	Runt-related transcription factor 1
RUNX2	14.3[b]	Runt-related transcription factor 2
SOX9	5.8[c]	SRY (sex determining region Y)-box 9
T	38.1[d]	Brachyury
TBX5	7.6[c]	T box transcription factor
TIE	−11.8[b]	Receptor tyrosine kinase
VEGF	13.2[b]	Vascular endothelial growth factor
Ectoderm		
EN1	2.7[b]	Engrailed homeobox 1
FN1	68.6[c]	Fibronectin 1
HOXB4	24.5[c]	Homeobox protein B4
Gene	**Fold-change**	**Description**
Ectoderm		
MMP2	10.8[d]	Matrix metalloproteinase 2
MSI2	2.6[b]	Musashi homolog 2
MYL4	5.3[b]	Myosin light chain 4
NOG	44.4[c]	Noggin
SOX3	−5.2[d]	SRY (sex determining region Y)-box 3
Endoderm		
GATA6	7.3[b]	GATA binding protein 6
HNF4A	3.5[b]	Hepatocyte nuclear factor 4 a
NODAL	−2.0[b]	Nodal
Others		
AKT1	4.3[d]	Protein kinase B, PKB b
CEBPB	4.3[c]	CCAAT/enhancer binding protein b
CEBPG	3.9[c]	CCAAT/enhancer binding protein g
COL4A1	3.4[c]	Collagen, type IV, a 1
CRABP1	−11.8[c]	Cellular retinoic acid binding protein
DAB2	10.5[c]	Disabled homolog 2
FST	4.7[b]	Follistatin
FZD1	6.3[b]	Frizzled homolog 1
GREM1	−4.8[b]	Gremlin 1
ID3	2.4[b]	Inhibitor of DNA binding 3dominant negative HLH protein
IL6	80.1[b]	Interleukin 6
LAMA5	2.7[b]	Laminin, a 5
NEFH	−5.3[b]	Neurofilament heavy polypeptide
NROB1	6.4[c]	DAX-1 (nuclear receptor subfamily 0, group B, member 1)
OTX2	−13.1[b]	Orthodenticle homeobox 2
POMC	−8.4[b]	Proopiomelenocortin
PTCH	2.6[b]	Protein patched homolog 1
PTGS2	5.2[c]	Prostaglandin enteroperoxide synthase
PTEN	−3.4[b]	Phosphatase and tensin homolog
SMAD3	3.8[b]	Smad 3 (Mad homolog 3)
VCAM1	30.5[b]	Vascular cell adhesion protein 1
WNT4	3.2[c]	Wingless type 4

[a]Genes altered in expression 2-fold or more (see **Figure 1**); [b]$P > 0.10$; [c]$P \leq 0.10$; [d]$P \leq 0$.

many common genes, including ones we also found to be up-regulated: *FST*, *IL*6, and *VCAM*1.

Overall, *BMP*4 resulted either in no increase, and often even a down-regulation, of many genes associated with ectoderm (e.g. *EN*2, *EOMES*, *EXO*1, *FGF*13, *MSI*1, *NEFH*, *NES*, *NR*4*A*2, *PAX*6, *PITX*3, and *SOX*3), endoderm (e.g. *AFP*, *CER*1, and *NODAL*), and mesoderm (e.g. *CD*34, *GJA*1, *GSC*, *KDR*, *LMO*2, *SDNSF*, *TBX*1, and *TIE*). There are, however, important exceptions. Several canonical mesodermal gene markers were up-regulated, *BMP*4, *BMPR*2, *CDH*5, *CDH*11, *CHRD*, *GATA*4, *NKX*2-5, *PITX*2, *RUNX*1, *RUNX*2, *SOX*9, *T*, *TBX*5, and *VEGF*, as were the ectodermal markers, *EN*1, *FN*1, *HOXB*4, *MMP*2, *MSI*2, *MYL*4, and *NOG*, and the endodermal markers, *GATA*6 and *HNF*4*A*. Our transcriptome profiling also revealed the up-regulation of additional genes, including *AKT*1, *CEBPB*, *CEBPG*, *COL*4*A*1, *DAB*2, *FST*, *FZD*1, *IL*6, *LAMA*5, *NROB*1, *PTCH*, *PTGS*2, *SMAD*3, *VCAM*1, and *WNT*4, and the down-regulation of *CRABP*1, *GREM*1, *LHCGR*, *NEFH*, *OTX*2, *POMC*, *PTEN*, and *THBS*2. The regulation of *CEBPB*, *RUNX*2, *SOX*9, and *VEGF* by *BMP*4 has not, to the best of our knowledge, been reported by others.

The results in **Figure 1** demonstrate that noggin alone altered the transcription of several of the 177 genes surveyed. Genes that were up-regulated include *AFP*, *AKT*1 *CDH*5, *CEBPG*, *CER*1, *EBAF*, *EOMES*, *FGF*4, *GBX*2, *GSC*, *HNF*4*A*, *IL*6, *LHCGR*, *OTX*2, *POU*5*F*1, *SOX*2, *T*, *TBX*5, *THBS*2, and *VCAM*1. In addition, noggin down-regulated a number of genes, *CYP*19*A*1, *EN*1, *EN*2, *EPAS*1, *FST*, *GREM*1, *MMP*2, *MMP*9, *NFKB*1, *NOG*, *NROB*1, *PGF*, *PITX*2, *PTGS*2, *SOX*3, *SOX*9, and *TFAP*2*A*. It is worthy of note that the transcription of three of these down-regulated genes, *CYP*19*A*1, *EN*2, and *TFAP*2*A*, fall below the level of detection following treatment with noggin, *i.e.* C_t greater than 35.

Genes highlighted above that were altered similarly by both *BMP*4 and noggin, albeit in some cases to a greater or lesser degree, include, up-regulation: *AKT*1, *CDH*5, *CEBPG*, *IL*6, *TBX*5, *VCAM*1; and down-regulation: *GREM*1 and *SOX*3. These results may imply non-specific action of *BMP*4 and/or direct effects of noggin.

Of the genes surveyed, 31 were not expressed sufficiently to be accurately determined and hence could not be included in **Figure 1**. These genes are listed in the Supplement (**Figure S1**).

Phase-contrast microscopic images of the hESCs are given in the Supplement (**Figure S1**) showing control cells and cells incubated with *BMP*4 and with noggin. Consistent with the transcriptome profiling results, heterogeneity is apparent, but the *BMP*4-treated cells give more the appearance of syncytiotrophoblast while the noggin-treated cells are quite distinct.

Hormone production: The media concentrations of hCG, progesterone, and estradiol were measured daily, up to seven days, for cells incubated with *BMP*4 and with noggin (**Figure 2**). Following incubation with *BMP*4, the three hormones increased on days 6 and 7 relative to control cells. As expected, noggin itself had no effect on hormone production. The concentrations reached on day 7 with *BMP*4 are about 15, 10, and 0.6 ng/mL for hCG, progesterone, and estradiol, respectively.

3.2. Gene Expression and Hormone Production in EB

Gene expression: Expression of 74 genes by EBs is presented as a heatmap (derived from mean values of 2^{-ddc_t}) in **Figure 3** at 22 and 50 days, each relative to day 5. Some of the more prominently expressed genes up-regulated at day 22 and/or day 50 include *AFP*, *CGB*, *CHRD*, *DAB*2, *HSPG*2, *INHBA*, *PGF*, *PTGS*2, *RUNX*1, *TIMP*1, and *VEGF*, only a few of which are trophoblast-associated. Most of the genes shown in **Figure 3** are, however, either down-regulated or exhibit no appreciable change over time. Of the genes surveyed, an arbitrary selection of the 15 most highly expressed at day 5, as assessed by dC_t values, are (in decreasing order):

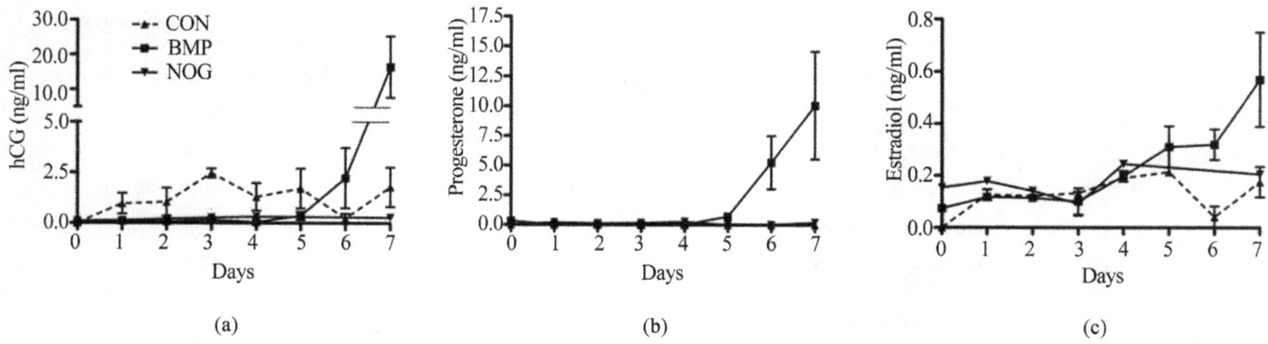

Figure 2. Medium concentrations of hCG (a), progesterone (b), and estradiol (c) of hESC. The cells were incubated in medium alone (CON), in medium containing *BMP*4 (*BMP*), or in medium with noggin (NOG).

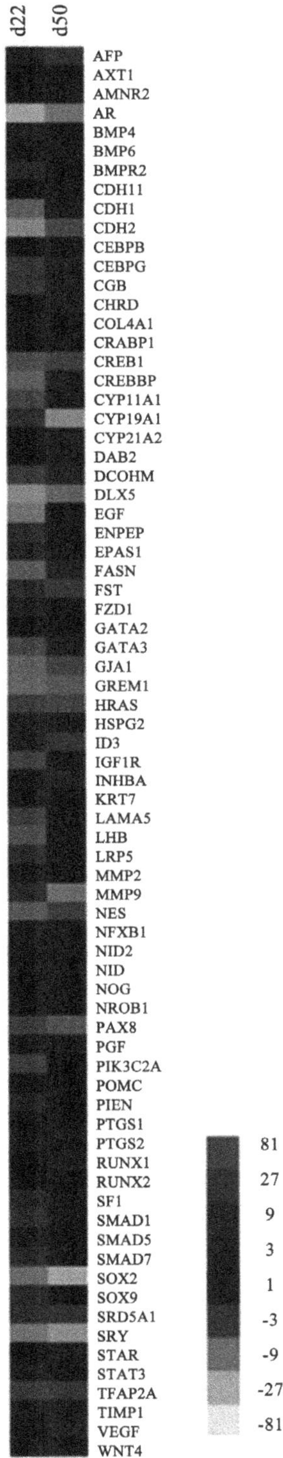

Figure 3. Heatmap showing changes in gene expression of EB at 22 and 50 days, relative to day 5 (mean values of 2^{-ddc_t}). The most prominently altered genes concomitant with time in culture are discussed in the text.

*GJA*1, *CREBBP*, *CDH*2, *ID*3, *CDH*1, *DLX*5, *SOX*2, *CREB*1, *HRAS*, *AR*, *AFP*, *CDH*11, *NES*, *GATA*3, and *GREM1* (data not shown). Supplement **Figure 2** (S. **Figure 2**) shows an H & E stained section of an EB at day 50, and the heterogeneous nature is quite apparent.

Hormone production: **Figure 4(a)** shows the media concentrations of hCG by EBs up to 50 days incubation. Considerable variability was noted in the hormone concentrations, attributed to the different sizes and numbers of EBs in each agarose dish. Moreover, viability may be decreasing after extended culture. hCG begins increasing on about day 18 and reaches a maximum on days 32 - 36 days. Under the conditions of the assay, where 50% of the EB medium is replaced every two days to ensure EB viability, the concentrations measured reflect new synthesis to a large extent, and, to a lesser degree, accumulation. Assuming that hCG is stable in the medium, it is possible to correct the concentrations for the total accumulated values at each two days of measurement. Doing so shows that hCG is continually synthesized between days 20 - 40 and then reaches a plateau of about 660 ng/mL between days 40 - 50. Media concentrations of progesterone follow a similar pattern to that of hCG **Figure 4(b)** and, when concentrations were corrected as described above, reach a plateau of about 1 ng/mL between days 40 - 50. The concentrations of estradiol were also measured (data not shown) and, when corrected as per hCG and progesterone, a maximal concentration of only about 0.04 ± 0.01 ng/mL was achieved. In view of the dynamic nature of EB size and number, quantification of hormone data is precluded.

4. DISCUSSION

4.1. BG02 Cells

This study has shown that, in the presence of *FGF*2, *BMP*4 leads to differentiation of the hESC line, BG02, to trophoblast-like cells, as has been reported by several groups using different cell lines, e.g. H1, H7, H9, H14, HES-2, HES-3 and various culture conditions (cf. [17,19, 21,27]). We have also identified *BMP*4-mediated and specific up-regulation of the genes *AKT*1, *CEBPB*, *RUNX*2, *SOX*9, and *VEGF*. Of these, Xu *et al.* [21] reported only minimal and non-significant changes in *AKT*1 and *CEBPB*. These genes most likely reflect *BMP*4 signaling and are not specific to trophoblast, although *VEGF* is expected to become important in placental formation and development. *AKT*1 encodes an isoform of serine/threonine kinase B (PKBα) involved in cell survival, proliferation, metabolism, and angiogenesis. Its regulation by *BMP*4 and noggin may imply that the *BMP*4-regulated component may be via a non- canonical pathway. The intronless gene *CEBPB* encodes the bZIP transcriptional factor, CCAAT/enhancer binding pro-

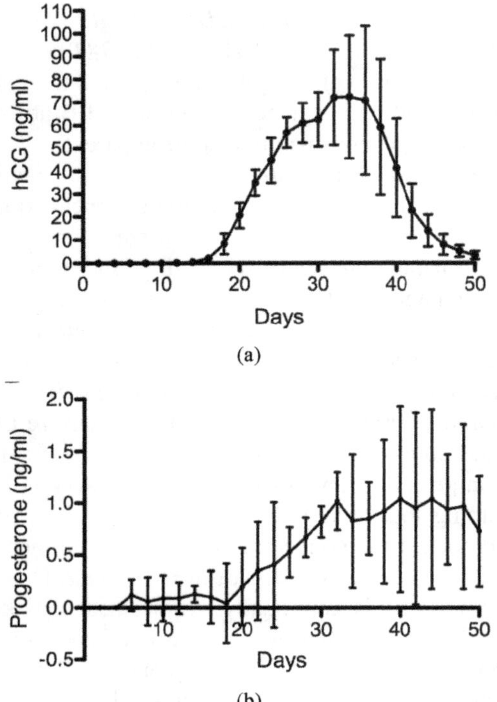

Figure 4. Medium concentration of hCG (a) and progesterone (b) production by EB cultured up to 50 days. The variability at each day is attributable to the dynamic nature of EB, in particular the changing size, number, and possibly atresia and necrosis. As discussed in the text, the conditions are such that new hormone synthesis and secretion is the primary contributor with accumulated prior secretion contributing some as well. A correction for the total accumulated hCG and progesterone, assuming complete stability in the medium, shows that the majority of synthesis occurs between days 20 - 40, after which plateaus of about 660 ng/mL and 1 ng/mL, respectively, are reached. The concentrations of estradiol were also measured and found to be quite low, about 0.04 ± 0.01 ng/mL (data not shown).

tein-b, that forms homodimers or heterodimers with other members of the CEBP family, a, d, and g. *RUNX*2 is regulated by the *BMP* pathway and also encodes a transcriptional factor involved in osteogenesis. Another transcriptional factor, (sex determining region Y)-box 9, is encoded by *SOX*9 and participates in chondrogenesis. Vascular endothelial growth factor, a member of the cystine-knot growth factor family and encoded by *VEGF*, stimulates vasculogenesis and angiogenesis and is expected to function in placental development. The results reported herein demonstrate an effect of noggin on the expression of a number of genes. In some cases *BMP*4 and noggin alter gene expression similarly, suggesting either that the regulation by *BMP*4 may not be via a canonical signaling pathway or that *BMP*4 and noggin may alter transcription similarly. At this time it is not possible to relate the observed changes accompanying treatment with noggin with the early signs of neural differentiation noted by Pera *et al.* [18].

Xu *et al.* [21] first reported that, in the presence of *FGF*2, *BMP*2, *BMP*4, and *BMP*7 promoted differentiation of H1, H7, H9, and H14 cells, cultured in mouse embryonic fibroblast conditioned medium, into trophoblast cells. Later, others found that the induction of trophoblast by *BMP*4 required an inhibition of the Activin/Nodal signaling [43]. The seminal study by Xu *et al.* [21] was followed by other reports confirming *BMP*-mediated hESC differentiation to trophoblast-like cells. Das *et al.* [44], for example, also showed that *BMP*4 directed H1 and H9 cells to trophoblast, while *FGF*2 slowed this differentiation, with oxygen accelerating it and promoting formation of syncytiotrophoblast. Interestingly, it was found that *FGF*2, acting to maintain NANOG levels via the MEK-ERK pathway, is capable of switching *BMP*4-mediated differentiation of hESC to mesendoderm as documented by the expression of brachyury and other primitive streak markers [22]. A similar conclusion was reached by Bernardo *et al.* [39] who showed that differentiation of hESCs by *BMP*4 in the presence of *FGF*2 led to formation of mesoderm and inhibition of endoderm. They also reported that this differentiation was via the ERK pathway and mediated by brachyury and *CDX*2.

In a recent comprehensive study of *BMP*-mediated differentiation of hESC to trophoblast, Marchand *et al.* [17] performed microarray analysis using the Affymetrix Human Gene version 1.0 ST array, along with qRT-PCR on selected genes. H7 and H9 cells were incubated with *BMP*4 for various times, 0, 2, 4, 6, 8, and 10 days, following the removal of *FGF*2. They found that after 2 days *POU5F*1 and *NANOG* were dramatically down-regulated while trophoblast markers were up-regulated. Many new genes were identified and suggested to be involved in trophoblast formation, and pathway analysis provided considerable insight into the myriad signaling systems operative in the differentiation of hESCs to trophoblast. This study was augmented by another report [42] in which the transcriptome of trophectoderm cells obtained from 13 human blastocysts were compared with those of *BMP*4-mediated differentiation of hESCs [17]. Their results documented that *BMP*4-induced differentiation of hESCs offers a good model for studying trophoblasts and contributed significantly to a better delineation of the associated transcriptome.

Our results with *BMP*4 are, by and large, in agreement with the findings from the two major combined microarray and PCR investigations on *BMP*-induced differentiation of hESCs [17,21]. This is somewhat surprising since we and Xu *et al.* [21] maintained *FGF*2 along with

*BMP*4, while Marchand *et al.* [17] removed *FGF*2 from the medium when *BMP*4 was added. A summary of many of the genes found to be altered in the present study compared to other reports is given in the Supplement (S.2). A major difference between our results and those of Marchand *et al.* [17] is in the expression of the mesodermal markers, *BMP*4 and *T*. We observed increased expression of these two genes, while they reported a decrease or no change, attributable to their removal of *FGF*2 during *BMP*-mediated differentiation. Of interest, they found increased expression of *KDR*, while we noted a minimal decrease, albeit not significant. Increased expression of *MMP*9 was found herein, consistent with the findings of Xu *et al.* [21] and Schultz *et al.* [19], but Marchand *et al.* [17] reported down-regulation. With the BG02 cells, we found reduced expression of the pluripotent marker, *FOXH*1, whereas others did not [17,21]. These discrepancies may reflect cell-specific differences, culture differences, e.g. ±*FGF*2, or other factors.

While it has been convincingly documented that members of the *BMP* family lead to differentiation of hESC to trophoblast, there is also considerable evidence that experimental conditions have a profound effect on the type of differentiation obtained. For example, an earlier report on *BMP*4-mediated differentiation of BG02 cells identified the formation and outgrowth of an immature vascular system when the cells are grown in a 3D Matrigel substrate in an endothelial cell growth medium [13]. Further, Pera *et al.* [18] found that, in response to *BMP*2, *BMP*4, or *BMP*2/7, HES-2 and HES-3 hESC differentiated to extra-embryonic endoderm, with only a few percent of the cells having the appearance of the trophoblast precursors described by Xu *et al.* [21]. They also found that the *BMP* antagonist noggin blocks the differentiation to extra-embryonic endoderm and directs differentiation into neural precursors, differentiation that may be mimicked by secretion of gremlin by mouse embryo fibroblast feeder layers. Our results with noggin reflect some type(s) of differentiation, but there is no clear indication for preference of one major pathway. As judged by increased expression of *T*, *MIXL*1, and *WNT*3, others have found that short-term treatment of H1, H7, and H9 hESC with *BMP*4 resulted in the induction of mesoderm progenitor cells that can differentiate into hematopoietic and cardiac lineages [24]. Working with H7 cells, it was reported that *BMP*4 treatment failed to yield trophectoderm using mouse embryonic fibroblasts as a feeder layer; this, however, was overcome by using feeder-free cells on Geltrex-coated plates in StemPro [38]. Lastly, West *et al.* [45] have demonstrated that, in the presence of *BMP*4, the KIT ligand enhances differentiation to germ-like cells. Hence, additional work is needed to clarify the many experimental parameters associated with *BMP*-induced differentiation of hESC.

4.2. EB Derived from BG02 Cells

EB formation by these cells also yielded some degree of differentiation to trophoblast as evidenced by the up-regulation of *CGB* and the production of hCG and progesterone. The most highly expressed genes in EB on day 5 are: *GJA*1, *CREBBP*, *CDH*2, *ID*3, *CDH*1, *DLX*5, *SOX*2, *CREB*1, *HRAS*, *AR*, and *AFP*. Most of these were surveyed in the studies on cells receiving *BMP*4, and none were up-regulated. The results suggest that trophoblast-like cells are not forming to any significant extent by day 5, findings consistent with the absence of hCG and progesterone production until days 18 - 20. These data are consistent with those by Gerami-Naini *et al.* [8] on H1 cell-derived EB growing in Matrigel. They could not detect measureable hormone until about day 20 of culture, and, depending upon the conditions used, maximal production of hCG was reached on days 35 - 40, followed by a decline. In contrast to the results with the Matrigel-embedded EB, they found that in suspension culture EBs were producing hCG, progesterone, and estradiol by 48 h.

In our studies, a comparison of gene expression by EB on days 22 and 50, relative to day 5, with that of hESC receiving *BMP*4 for 7 days, provides additional evidence that differentiation to trophoblast is occurring by day 22, as evidenced by the up-regulation of *CGB*, *PGF*, *PTGS*2, *RUNX*1, and *VEGF*. These results are consistent with the hormone secretion data for hCG and progesterone. In addition to the above genes, there is also up-regulation of *AFP*, *BMP*6, *CHD*11, *CHRD*, DAB2, *HSPG*2, *INHBA*, *PTGS*2, and *TIMP*1. Not surprisingly, the EBs are apparently more heterogeneous in terms of constituent cell types than the *BMP*4-treated hESCs. For example, the early appearance (day 5) of *GJA*1, *CREBBP*, *CDH*2, *ID*3, *CDH*1, *DLX*5, *SOX*2, *CREB*1, *HRAS*, *AR*, *AFP*, *CDH*11, *NES*, *GATA*3, and *GREM*1, followed by the later up-regulation of *AFP*, *BMP*6, *CHD*11, *CHRD*, *DAB*2, *HSPG*2, *INHBA*, *PTGS*2, and *TIMP*1, indicates formation of trophoblast, endoderm, ectoderm, and mesoderm. Consistent with this finding was the observation some years ago that markers for the three embryonic germ layers were expressed in EBs prepared from H9 cells [46].

5. CONCLUSION

Overall, the results presented herein strongly support other reports concluding that, under certain conditions, *BMP*4 directs differentiation of hESCs to trophoblast-like cells. This conclusion notwithstanding, it is clear that experimental conditions, particularly the inclusion or exclusion of *FGF*2 during BMB-mediated differentiation, have a profound effect on the type of differentiation achieved, and, moreover, based on our transcriptome profiling, it is highly likely that other cell types may be forming in response to *BMP*4. On the other hand, it may emerge that some of the other genes we found to have been up-regulated by *BMP*4 function in differentiation to trophectoderm and then to cytotrophoblasts (villous and extravillous) and syncytiotrophoblasts, or be involved in placental formation and function. The heterogeneity of the differentiated cells needs to be carefully established, but the *BMP*-mediated differentiation of hESCs to trophoblast, particularly in the absence of *FGF*2, certainly provides an attractive *in vitro* system for studying early differentiation events and gives a more homogeneous system than that of embryoid bodies. Lastly, our observation that the *BMP*4 antagonist noggin alters gene transcription of a subset of genes investigated may correlate with the morphological changes reported by others; however, more studies are required to map the transcriptional changes to neural differentiation.

6. ACKNOWLEDGEMENTS

We thank Mr. Roger Nilsen of the University of Georgia Functional Genomics Resource Facility for his expert assistance with the RNA analysis. This study was supported by NIH: R01DK033973 (D.P.), R01HD044119 (P.N.), and 5F32HL083741 (N.L.B.).

REFERENCES

[1] Rama, S. and Rao, A.J. (2003) Regulation of growth and function of the human placenta. *Molecular and Cellular Biochemistry*, **253**, 263-268. doi:10.1023/A:1026076219126

[2] Sullivan, M.H. (2004) Endocrine cell lines from the placenta. *Molecular and Cellular Endocrinology*, **228**, 103-119. doi:10.1016/j.mce.2003.03.001

[3] Udayashankar, R., Baker, D., Tuckerman, E., Laird, S., Li, T.C. and Moore, H.D. (2011) Characterization of invasive trophoblasts generated from human embryonic stem cells. *Human Reproduction*, **26**, 398-406. doi:10.1093/humrep/deq350

[4] Jameson, J.L. and Hollenberg, A.N. (1993) Regulation of chorionic gonadotropin gene expression. *Endocrine Reviews*, **14**, 203-221.

[5] Mesiano, S. (2009) The endocrinology of human pregnancy and fetoplacental neuroendocrine development. In: Strauss, J.F. and Barbieri, R.L., Eds., *Yen and Jaffe's Reproductive Endocrinology*. 6th Edition, Physiology, Pathophysiology and Clinical Management, Philadelphia, 249-281.

[6] Thomson, J.A., Itskovitz-Eldor. J., Shapiro, S.S., Waknitz, M.A., Swiergiel, J.J., Marshall, V.S. and Jones, J.M. (1998) Embryonic stem cell lines derived from human blastocysts. *Science*, **282**, 1145-1147. doi:10.1126/science.282.5391.1145

[7] Mitalipova, M., Calhoun, J., Shin, S., Wininger, D., Schulz, T., Noggle, S., Venable, A., Lyons, I., Robins, A. and Stice, S. (2003) Human embryonic stem cell lines derived from discarded embryos. *Stem Cells*, **21**, 521-526. doi:10.1634/stemcells.21-5-521

[8] Gerami-Naini, B., Dovzhenko, O.V., Durning, M., Wegner, F.H., Thomson, J.A. and Golos, T.G. (2004) Trophoblast differentiation in embryoid bodies derived from human embryonic stem cells. *Endocrinology*, **145**, 1517-1524. doi:10.1210/en.2003-1241

[9] Giakoumopoulos, M., Siegfried, L.M., Dambaeva, S.V., Garthwaite, M.A., Glennon, M.C. and Golos, T.G. (2010) Placental-derived mesenchyme influences chorionic gonadotropin and progesterone secretion of human embryonic stem cell-derived trophoblasts. *Reproductive Science*, **17**, 798-808. doi:10.1177/1933719110371853

[10] Golos, T.G., Pollastrini, L.M. and Gerami-Naini, B. (2006) Human embryonic stem cells as a model for trophoblast differentiation. *Semin Reproductive Medicine*, **24**, 314-321. doi:10.1055/s-2006-952154

[11] Harun, R., Ruban, L., Matin, M., Draper, J., Jenkins, N.M., Liew, G.C., Andrews, P.W., Li, T.C., Laird, S.M. and Moore, H.D. (2006) Cytotrophoblast stem cell lines derived from human embryonic stem cells and their capacity to mimic invasive implantation events. *Human Reproduction*, **21**, 1349-1358. doi:10.1093/humrep/del017

[12] Peiffer, I., Belhomme, D., Barbet, R., Haydont, V., Zhou, Y.P., Fortunel, N.O., Li, M., Hatzfeld, A., Fabiani, J.N. and Hatzfeld, J.A. (2007) Simultaneous differentiation of endothelial and trophoblastic cells derived from human embryonic stem cells. *Stem Cells and Development*, **16**, 393-402. doi:10.1089/scd.2006.0013

[13] Boyd, N.L., Dhara, S.K., Rekaya, R., Godbey, E.A., Hasneen, K., Rao, R.R., West, F.D., Gerwe, B.A. and Stice, S.L. (2007) *BMP*4 promotes formation of primitive vascular networks in human embryonic stem cell-derived embryoid bodies. *Experimental Biology and Medicine*, **232**, 833-843.

[14] Chen, G., Ye, Z., Yu, X., Zou, J., Mali, P., Brodsky, R.A. and Cheng, L. (2008) Trophoblast differentiation defect in human embryonic stem cells lacking PIG-A and GPI-anchored cell-surface proteins. *Cell Stem Cell*, **2**, 345-355. doi:10.1016/j.stem.2008.02.004

[15] Kee, K., Gonsalves, J.M., Clark, A.T. and Pera, R.A. (2006) Bone morphogenetic proteins induce germ cell differentiation from human embryonic stem cells. *Stem Cells and Development*, **15**, 831-837. doi:10.1089/scd.2006.15.831

[16] Liu, Y.P., Dovzhenko, O.V., Garthwaite, M.A., Dambaeva, S.V., Durning, M., Pollastrini, L.M. and Golos, T.G. (2004) Maintenance of pluripotency in human embryonic stem cells stably over-expressing enhanced green fluorescent protein. *Stem Cells and Development*, **13**, 636-645. doi:10.1089/scd.2004.13.636

[17] Marchand, M., Horcajadas, J.A., Esteban, F.J., McElroy, S.L., Fisher, S.J. and Giudice, L.C. (2011) Transcriptomic signature of trophoblast differentiation in a human embryonic stem cell model. *Biology of Reproduction*, **84**, 1258-1271. doi:10.1095/biolreprod.110.086413

[18] Pera, M.F., Andrade, J., Houssami, S., Reubinoff, B.,

Trounson, A., Stanley, E.G., Ward-van Oostwaard, D. and Mummery, C. (2004) Regulation of human embryonic stem cell differentiation by *BMP*-2 and its antagonist noggin. *Journal of Cell Science*, **117**, 1269-1280. doi:10.1242/jcs.00970

[19] Schulz, L.C., Ezashi, T., Das, P., Westfall, S.D., Livingston, K.A. and Roberts, R.M. (2008) Human embryonic stem cells as models for trophoblast differentiation. *Placenta*, **29**, S10-S16.

[20] Xu R.H. (2006) In vitro induction of trophoblast from human embryonic stem cells. *Methods in Molecular Medicine*, **121**, 189-202.

[21] Xu, R.H., Chen, X., Li, D.S., Li, R., Addicks, G.C., Glennon, C., Zwaka, T.P. and Thomson, J.A. (2002) *BMP*4 initiates human embryonic stem cell differentiation to trophoblast. *Nature Biotechnology*, **20**, 1261-1264. doi:10.1038/nbt761

[22] Yu, P., Pan, G., Yu, J. and Thomson, J.A. (2011) *FGF*2 sustains NANOG and switches the outcome of *BMP*4-induced human embryonic stem cell differentiation. *Cell Stem Cell*, **8**, 326-334. doi:10.1016/j.stem.2011.01.001

[23] Yu, X., Zou, J., Ye, Z., Hammond, H., Chen, G., Tokunaga, A., Mali, P., Li, Y.M., Civin, C., Gaiano, N. and Cheng, L. (2008) Notch signaling activation in human embryonic stem cells is required for embryonic, but not trophoblastic, lineage commitment. *Cell Stem Cell*, **2**, 461-471. doi:10.1016/j.stem.2008.03.001

[24] Zhang, P., Li, J., Tan, Z., Wang, C., Liu, T., Chen, L., Yong, J., Jiang, W., Sun, X., Du, L., Ding, M. and Deng, H. (2008) Short-term *BMP*-4 treatment initiates mesoderm induction in human embryonic stem cells. *Blood*, **111**, 1933-1941. doi:10.1182/blood-2007-02-074120

[25] Douglas, G.C., Vande-Voort, C.A., Kumar, P., Chang, T.C. and Golos, T.G. (2009) Trophoblast stem cells: Models for investigating trophectoderm differentiation and placental development. *Endocrine Reviews*, **30**, 228-240. doi:10.1210/er.2009-0001

[26] Golos, T.G., Giakoumopoulos, M. and Garthwaite, M.A. (2010) Embryonic stem cells as models of trophoblast differentiation: Progress, opportunities, and limitations. *Reproduction*, **140**, 3-9. doi:10.1530/REP-09-0544

[27] Pera M.F. and Trounson A.O. (2004) Human embryonic stem cells: Prospects for development. *Development*, **131**, 5515-5525. doi:10.1242/dev.01451

[28] Roberts, R.M., Ezashi, T. and Das, P. (2004) Trophoblast gene expression: Transcription factors in the specification of early trophoblast. *Reproductive Biology and Endocrinology*, **2**, 47. doi:10.1186/1477-7827-2-47

[29] Hay, D.C., Sutherland, L., Clark, J. and Burdon, T. (2004) Oct-4 knockdown induces similar patterns of endoderm and trophoblast differentiation markers in human and mouse embryonic stem cells. *Stem Cells*, **22**, 225-235. doi:10.1634/stemcells.22-2-225

[30] Matin, M.M., Walsh, J.R., Gokhale, P.J., Draper, J.S., Bahrami, A.R., Morton, I., Moore, H.D. and Andrews, P.W. (2004) Specific knockdown of Oct4 and beta 2-microglobulin expression by RNA interference in human embryonic stem cells and embryonic carcinoma cells. *Stem Cells*, **22**, 659-668. doi:10.1634/stemcells.22-5-659

[31] Bragdon, B., Moseychuk, O., Saldanha, S., King, D., Julian, J. and Nohe, A. (2011) Bone morphogenetic proteins: A critical review. *Cell Signal*, **23**, 609-620. doi:10.1016/j.cellsig.2010.10.003

[32] Rider, C.C. and Mulloy, B. (2010) Bone morphogenetic protein and growth differentiation factor cytokine families and their protein antagonists. *The Biochemical Journal*, **429**, 1-12. doi:10.1042/BJ20100305

[33] Walsh, D.W., Godson, C., Brazil, D.P. and Martin, F. (2010) Extracellular *BMP*-antagonist regulation in development and disease: Tied up in knots. *Trends in Cell Biology*, **20**, 244-256. doi:10.1016/j.tcb.2010.01.008

[34] Zeng, S., Chen, J. and Shen, H. (2010) Controlling of bone morphogenetic protein signaling. *Cell Signal*, **22**, 888-893. doi:10.1016/j.cellsig.2009.12.007

[35] Malassine, A., Frendo, J.L. and Evain-Brion, D. (2003) A comparison of placental development and endocrine functions between the human and mouse model. *Human Reproduction*, **9**, 531-539. doi:10.1093/humupd/dmg043

[36] Rossant, J. (2001) Stem cells from the mammalian blastocyst. *Stem Cells*, **19**, 477-482. doi:10.1634/stemcells.19-6-477

[37] Smith, A.G. (2001) Embryo-derived stem cells of mice and men. *Annual Reviews of Cell and Developmental Biology*, **17**, 435-462. doi:10.1146/annurev.cellbio.17.1.435

[38] Erb, T.M., Schneider, C., Mucko, S.E., Sanfilippo, J.S., Lowry, N.C., Desai, M.N., Mangoubi, R.S., Leuba, S.H. and Sammak, P.J. (2011) Paracrine and epigenetic control of trophectoderm differentiation from human embryonic stem cells: the role of bone morphogenic protein 4 and histone deacetylases. *Stem Cells Development*, **20**, 1601-1614. doi:10.1089/scd.2010.0281

[39] Bernardo, A.S., Faial, T., Gardner, L., Niakan, K.K., Ortmann, D., Senner, C.E., Callery, E.M., Trotter, M.W., Hemberger, M., Smith, J.C., Bardwell, L., Moffett, A. and Pedersen, R.A. (2011) BRACHYURY and *CDX*2 mediate *BMP*-induced differentiation of human and mouse pluripotent stem cells into embryonic and extra embryonic lineages. *Cell Stem Cell*, **9**, 144-155. doi:10.1016/j.stem.2011.06.015

[40] Livak, K.J. and Schmittgen, T.D. (2001) Analysis of relative gene expression data using real-time quantitative PCR and the 2(-delta delta C(T)) method. *Methods*, **25**, 402-408.

[41] Pfaffl, M.W. (2001) A new mathematical model for relative quantification in real-time RT-PCR. *Nucleic Acids Research*, **29**, e45. doi:10.1093/nar/29.9.e45

[42] Aghajanova, L., Shen, S., Rojas, A.M., Fisher, S.J., Irwin, J.C. and Giudice, L.C. (2012) Comparative transcriptome analysis of human trophectoderm and embryonic stem cell-derived trophoblasts reveal key participants in early implantation. *Biology and Reproduction*, **86**, 1-21. doi:10.1095/biolreprod.111.092775

[43] Wu, Z., Zhang, W., Chen, G., Cheng, L., Liao, J., Jia, N., Gao, Y., Dai, H., Yuan, J. and Xiao, L. (2008) Combinatorial signals of activin/nodal and bone morphogenic protein regulate the early lineage segregation of human embryonic stem cells. *The Journal of Biological Chemistry*,

283, 24991-25002. doi:10.1074/jbc.M803893200

[44] Das, P., Ezashi, T., Schulz, L.C., Westfall, S.D., Livingston, K.A. and Roberts, R.M. (2007) Effects of *fgf* 2 and oxygen in the *bmp*4-driven differentiation of trophoblast from human embryonic stem cells. *Stem Cell Research*, **1**, 61-74. doi:10.1016/j.scr.2007.09.004

[45] West, F.D., Roche-Rios, M.I., Abraham, S., Rao, R.R., Natrajan, M.S., Bacanamwo, M. and Stice, S.L. (2010) KIT ligand and bone morphogenetic protein signaling enhances human embryonic stem cell to germ-like cell differentiation. *Human Reproduction*, **25**, 168-178. doi:10.1093/humrep/dep338

[46] Itskovitz-Eldor, J., Schuldiner, M., Karsenti, D., Eden, A., Yanuka, O., Amit, M., Soreq, H. and Benvenisty, N. (2000) Differentiation of human embryonic stem cells into embryoid bodies compromising the three embryonic germ layers. *Molecular Medicine*, **6**, 88-95.

1. Supplement

1.1. S1. The Following Genes Were Not Expressed Sufficiently to Be Measured in Control and *BMP4*-Mediated Differentiation of hESCs

AMH, *AMHR2*, *BAPX1*, *BMP1*, *BMPR1B*, *DLX5*, *ESR1*, *ESR2*, *FGF5*, *FIGF*, *FSHB*, *FSHR*, *GJA5*, *GJB3*, *IGF1*, *INHBB*, *IPF1*, *LAMR1*, *LY6G6D*, *NKX2-2*, *PAX8*, *PECAM1*, *PGR*, *PP13*, *PROML1*, *PTGS1*, *PTPRC*, *STAR*, *TAL1*, *TITF1*, *TSHB*, and *WT1*.

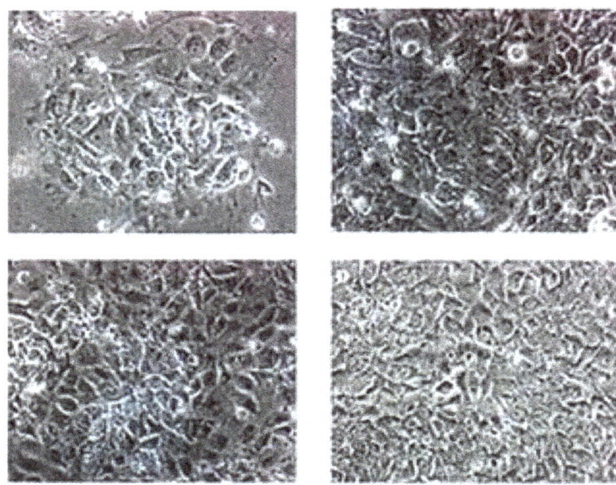

Figure S1. Phase-contrast microscopy of hESCs before and after incubation with *BMP4* or noggin. (A) Cells at day 0 in media; (B) Cells at day 7 in media; (C) Cells at day 7 in media-plus-100 ng/mL *BMP4*; (D) Cells at day 7 in media-plus-250 ng/mL noggin. Cells incubated with *BMP4* and with noggin exhibit distinct morphological changes.

1.2. S2. A Comparison of Our Results with *BMP4*-Induced Differentiation of hESCs and the Results of Others Gives the Following Similarities

We found increased expression of *CDH11*, *CGB*, *ENPEP*, *EPAS1*, *FN1*, *GATA2*, *GATA3*, *HEY1*, *KRT7*, *MSX2*, *PGF*, *PITX2*, and *WNT5A*, as well as decreased expression of *DNMT3B* and *POU5F1*, in agreement with Xu *et al.* [21] and Marchand *et al.* [17]. Consistent with the data of Xu *et al.* [21], we found increased expression of *CDH5*, *DAB2*, *MMP9*, and *WNT4*, along with decreased expression of *SOX3*. Our results and those of Marchand *et al.* [17] show increased expression of *BMPR2*, *COL4A1*, *CYP11A1*, and *CYP19A1*, decreased expression of *CRABP1*, *FGF2*, *GREM1*, *OTX2*, and *SOX2*, and either no changes or minimal changes in a number of other genes, including *AFP*, *GSC*, *NES*, *PAX6*, and others. Schultz *et al.* [19] also found increased expression in *CGB*, *GATA2*, *GATA3*, *KRT7*, and *MSX2*, and decreased expression of *POU5F1* and *SOX2*.

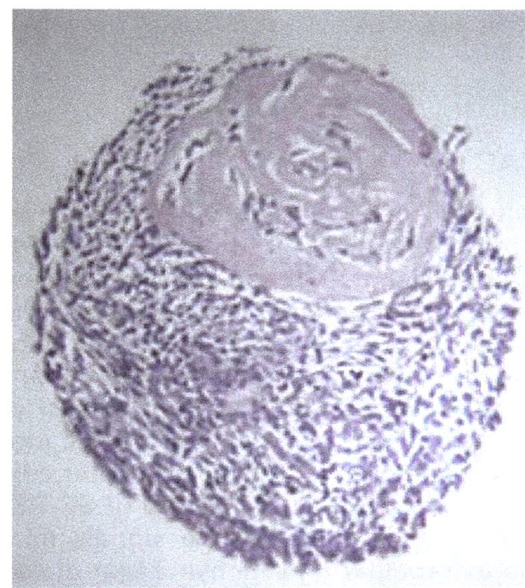

Figure S2. Following formation of embryoid bodies from hESCs and incubation for 50 days (d50), an embryoid body was fixed in formalin, embedded in paraffin, sectioned (5 microns), and stained with H&E.

Low level of activin A secreted by fibroblast feeder cells accelerates early stage differentiation of retinal pigment epithelial cells from human pluripotent stem cells

Heidi Hongisto[1,2*], Alexandra Mikhailova[1,2*], Hanna Hiidenmaa[1,2], Tanja Ilmarinen[1,2], Heli Skottman[1,2#]

[1]Institute of Biomedical Technology, University of Tampere, Tampere, Finland;
[#]Corresponding Author: heli.skottman@uta.fi
[2]Institute of Biosciences and Medical Technology, Tampere, Finland

ABSTRACT

Human pluripotent stem cells (hPSC) differentiated to retinal pigment epithelial cells (RPE) provide a promising tool for cell replacement therapies of retinal degenerative diseases. The *in vitro* differentiation of hPSC-RPE is still poorly understood and current differentiation protocols rely on spontaneous differentiation on fibroblast feeder cells or as floating cell aggregates in suspension. The fibroblast feeder cells may have an inductive effect on the hPSC-RPE differentiation, providing variable signals mimicking the extraocular mesenchyme that directs the differentiation *in vivo*. The effect of the commonly used fibroblast feeder cells on the hPSC-RPE differentiation was studied by comparing suspension differentiation in standard RPEbasic (no bFGF) medium to RPEbasic medium conditioned with mouse embryonic (mEF-CM) and human foreskin (hFF-CM) fibroblast feeder cells. The fibroblast secreted factors were found to enhance early hPSC-RPE differentiation. The onset of pigmentation was faster in the conditioned media (CM) compared to RPEbasic for both human embryonic (hESC) and induced pluripotent (iPSC) stem cells, with the first pigments appearing around two weeks of differentiation. After four weeks of differentiation, CM conditions consistently contained higher number of pigmented cell aggregates. The ratio of *PAX6* and *MITF* positive cells was quantified to be clearly higher in the CM conditions, with mEF-CM containing most positive cells. The mEF cells were found to secrete low levels of activin A growth factor that is known to regulate eye field differentiation. As RPEbasic was supplemented with corresponding, low level (10 ng/ml) of recombinant human activin A, a clear increase in the hPSC-RPE differentiation was achieved. Thus, inductive effect provided by feeder cells was at least partially driven by activin A and could be substituted with a low level of recombinant growth factor in contrasts to previously reported much higher concentrations.

Keywords: Retinal Pigment Epithelial Cell; Human Pluripotent Stem Cell; Conditioned Medium; Human Foreskin Fibroblast; Mouse Embryonic Fibroblast; Activin A; Cell Differentiation

1. INTRODUCTION

Retinal pigment epithelium (RPE) is a highly polarized and specialized monolayer of cells located between the neural retina and choroid at the back of the eye. RPE has several vitally important functions as a part of the blood-retina-barrier and in supporting photoreceptor function and survival [1,2]. RPE degeneration has a major role in pathogenesis of retinal diseases including age-related macular degeneration (AMD) and retinitis pigmentosa. The degeneration of RPE cells leads to the degradation of photoreceptors and as a consequence to either partial or total loss of vision. Currently, functionality of destroyed RPE cells can be restored only with cell transplantation, setting high demands to develop novel cell sources for replacement therapy. Transplantation of RPE cells has been studied extensively in animal models and also in humans [2-5]. Several cell sources have been

[*]Equal contribution.

studied for cell therapy but currently human pluripotent stem cells (hPSCs) are considered to be the most promising cell source of differentiating cells for tissue engineering applications due to their differentiation potential and high replicative capacity. Several research groups have reported successful differentiation of RPE cells from hPSCs [6-10] and first clinical studies using human embryonic stem cell (hESC) derived RPE cells are ongoing [11].

During mammalian development, RPE and neural retina are both derived from optic neuroepithelium and share the same progenitor [12]. The neuroepithelium near the anterior part of the neural tube evaginates laterally to form the optic vesicles. Invagination of the distal part of the optic vesicle leads to the formation of the optic cup in a complex environment affected by many external signals [13]. By the sixth or seventh week of development, the optic cup has differentiated into two epithelial sheets. Of these, the distal layer differentiates into the neural retina and the proximal layer develops into the RPE in interactions with the surrounding extraocular tissue, including the extraocular mesenchyme [12,14,15].

In the absence of external signal molecules, the hPSCs choose the neural differentiation pathway as a default [16]. Most of the published hPSC-RPE differentiation protocols rely on spontaneous differentiation in absence of basic fibroblast growth factor (bFGF). The induction of differentiation is based on confluent overgrowth on feeder cells especially mouse embryonic fibroblasts (mEF) or through embryoid body/neurospehere formation [7, 9,10]. Recently, RPE differentiation efficiency has been enhanced with prolonged culture and growth factor/inhibitor based differentiation strategies. Factors, such as activin A, transforming growth factor $\beta 1$ (TGF$\beta 1$), and nodal antagonist SB431542 [17] as well as Wnt signaling inhibitor CKI-7 together with Dkk-1, Lefty-A, FGF antagonist Y-27632 and SB431542 [18,19] have been used. Regardless of these, many groups are using feeder cell (mEF, foreskin fibroblasts, PA6 cells) containing methods with spontaneous differentiation method [20,21] and first clinical studies are conducted with mEF supported and spontaneously differentiated hESC-RPE cells [11]. It is not clear why the removal of FGFs from feeder cell based hPSC cultures [20] or the use of PA6 stromal feeder cell to promote neural differ- entiation [22-24] is sufficient to produce RPE cells but both of the differentiation strategies suggest important function of external signals provided by mesenchymal fibroblasts/stromal cells.

We hypothesized that fibroblast feeder cells used for the culture of undifferentiated hPSC may have an inductive effect on RPE cell differentiation providing mesenchymal signals necessary for the key cellular decision guiding optic cup differentiation and further cell commitment towards RPE cell fate [25,26]. Moreover we hypothesized that different feeder cells types (mEF and human foreskin fibroblast, hFF) may provide variable mesenchymal signals guiding RPE differentiation. In this study, we studied the inductive effects of feeder cells routinely used for hPSC differentiation towards RPE cells. Human PSCs were differentiated using media conditioned by two types of fibroblasts feeder cells (hFF-CM and mEF-CM) and non-conditioned differentiation medium (RPEbasic).

2. MATERIALS AND METHODS

All cells were cultured in 37°C, 5% CO_2 incubator (Thermo Electron Corp., Waltham, MA, USA) and monitored regularly with Nikon Eclipse TE2000-S phase contrast microscope (Nikon Instruments Europe B.V., Amstelveen, The Netherlands).

2.1. Fibroblast Feeder Cell Culture

Human FF (CRL-2429™, American Type Culture Collection, ATCC, Manassas, VA, USA) were cultured in Iscove's Modified Dulbecco's Medium (IMDM, Life Technologies, Carlsbad, CA, USA) supplemented with 10% FBS (PAA Laboratories GmbH, Pasching, Austria) and 0.5% Penicillin/Streptomycin (Lonza Group Ltd, Basel, Switzerland). P-MEF (EmbryoMax®, Millipore, Billerica, MA, USA) were cultured in Knock-Out Dulbecco's Modified Eagle Medium (KO-DMEM) supplemented with 10% FBS and 1% GlutaMax-I, sterile-filtered prior use. Cell culture flasks for mEF were precoated with 0.1% porcine gelatin (Sigma-Aldrich, St. Louis, MO, USA) for 1 h at room temperature (RT). Both fibroblast cell lines were purchased as frozen stocks and cryopreserved at early passages with 5% - 10% dimethyl sulfoxide (DMSO, Sigma-Aldrich) supplementation.

2.2. Human Pluripotent Stem Cell Culture

The human embryonic stem cell (hESC) line Regea 06/040 was derived at IBT—The Institute of Biomedical Technology (former Regea—Institute for Regenerative Medicine), University of Tampere, Finland. The hESC line was derived on hFF feeder cells and cultured and characterized as described previously [27]. Human induced pluripotent stem cell (iPSC) line FiPS5-7 was established by Professor Otonkoski's research group at University of Helsinki, Finland. It was generated from human fibroblasts using four transcription factors—*OCT*3/4 (*POU5F*1), *SOX*2, *nanog*, and *LIN*28 [28], and transgene silencing was confirmed with qPCR [29]. Prior to the experiments, both pluripotent cell lines were cultured on hFF feeder cells in standard hPSC culture medium consisting of KO-DMEM supplemented with 20%

knock-out serum replacement (KO-SR), 2 mM GlutaMax-I, 0.1 mM 2-mercaptoethanol (all from Life Technologies), 1% Non-Essential Amino Acids (NEAA), 50 U/ml Penicillin/Streptomycin (both from Lonza Group Ltd.) and 8 ng/ml human bFGF (R&D Systems Inc., Minneapolis, MN, USA). The culture medium was changed five times a week and undifferentiated colonies were manually passaged onto new, γ-irradiated (40 Gy) feeder cell layers once a week.

2.3. Collection of Conditioned Media

Both hFF (passage 6 - 11) and mEF (passage 4 - 5) were harvested at confluency with TrypLE™ Select (Life Technologies) at 37°C, 15 min, and mitotically inactivated with γ-radiation (40 Gy). Irradiated fibroblasts were seeded onto 0.1% gelatin-coated culture dishes (cell density $3.6 \times 10^4/cm^2$) and left to adhere overnight. The cells were adapted to serum-free culture conditions by sequential addition of RPE differentiation medium (RPEbasic) the day after irradiation. RPEbasic included the same reagents as described above for hPSC culture medium, but supplemented with 15% KO-SR and lacking bFGF. For a period of 10 days, 2 ml/cm^2 of RPEbasic was collected daily from the culture dishes and replaced with equal amount of fresh medium. Collected media were centrifuged at 1000 rpm, 4 min, transferred to new tubes and stored at −70°C. After collection, CM for each fibroblast type was thawed, pooled, and stored at −70°C in aliquots until used for differentiation experiments. Four different batches of CM were similarly prepared for both fibroblast types.

2.4. Differentiation Culture

Undifferentiated hPSC colonies (Regea06/040 and FiPS5-7) were manually dissected, and the pieces transferred to low cell-bind cell culture plates (Corning Inc., Corning, NY, USA) in RPEbasic, mEF-CM or hFF-CM. The media were changed five times a week. Human ESC line (Regea06/040) was used for differentiation experiments at passage levels 31 - 91 and hiPSC line (FiPS5-7) at passage levels 48 - 117. The differentiation experiments were repeated six times in total. Influence of activin A on RPE differentiation was tested with hESC line (Regea06/040) (passages 37 - 42) using RPEbasic supplemented with 10 ng/ml activin A (Peprotech, London, England). The activin A supplementation test was repeated three times. The workflow of the study and analyses performed are summarized in **Figure 1**.

After six to seven weeks in suspension culture, pigmented areas of cell aggregates were selectively replated to adherent cultures, in order to create purified populations of hPSC-RPE. Pigmented areas were selected, washed with Dulbecco's Phosphate Buffered Saline (DPBS, Lonza Group Ltd.) and dissociated with 1× Trypsin-EDTA (Lonza Group Ltd.) for 20 - 35 min at 37°C with repeated trituration. Trypsin was inactivated with 10% human serum (PAA Laboratories), and cells collected to appropriate culture medium through 40 μm cell strainers. Dissociated cells were plated either on 24-well plate wells (Corning Cellbind, Corning Inc.) coated with 5 μg/cm^2 human placental collagen IV (Sigma-Aldrich) for 3 h at 37°C, or to permeable 0.3 cm^2 BD BioCoat™ mouse collagen IV cell culture inserts (Becton, Dickinson and Company, Franklin Lakes, NJ, USA). Adherent cultures were maintained using appropriate media that were changed three times a week.

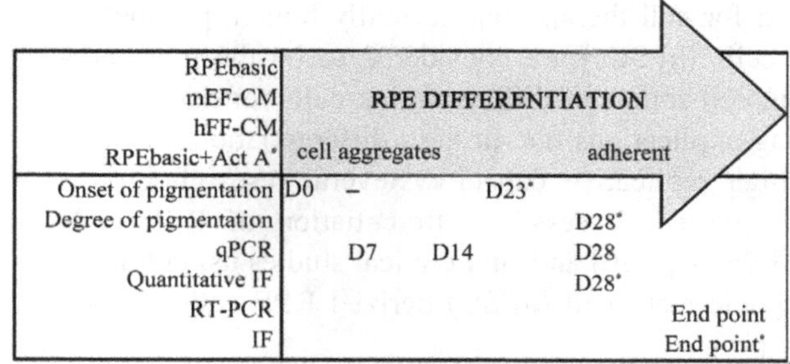

Figure 1. Workflow of the study. RPE differentiation was performed using four test media: RPEbasic, hFF and mEF conditioned media and RPEbasic supplemented with activin A. Analyses performed in different time points are presented.

2.5. Analysis of Pigmentation

The onset of pigmentation was followed daily and the day of appearance of the first pigmented cells in each medium was recorded. The appearance of first pigmentation was recorded from five individual differentiation experiments for hESCs, four experiments for hiPSCs, and three activin A supplementation experiments. To assess the amount of pigmentation after four weeks of differentiation, the ratio of cell aggregates containing pigment in relation to total number of aggregates was counted after 28 days of differentiation. This was done in three individual differentiation experiments for both studied cell lines and for all three activin A supplementation experiments. Results were plotted using Microsoft Excel 2003 and figures edited with Adobe PhotoShop CS4.

2.6. Quantitative Real-Time Polymerase Chain Reaction

Differences in expression levels of genes related to RPE differentiation: retina and anterior neural fold homeobox (*RAX*), paired box gene 6 (*PAX6*) and microphthal-mia-associated transcription factor (*MITF*), were studied with qPCR. Gene expression was evaluated for hPSCs differentiated in the three test media: RPEbasic, mEF-CM and hFF-CM, after 7, 14, and 28 days in differentiation culture. Additionally the expression of neural retina markers ceh-10 homeodomain containing homolog (*CHX*10) and cone-rod homeobox protein (*CRX*) was studied after 28 days of differentiation.

Ten to fifteen differentiated cell aggregates were collected from each test medium. In addition, pieces of undifferentiated colonies of both hPSC lines were collected for control material prior to the beginning of the experiment. Total RNA was extracted using the NucleoSpin RNA XS kit (Macherey-Nagel, GmbH & Co., Düren, Germany), according to the manufacturer's protocol. The RNA quality and concentration were determined using NanoDrop-1000 spectrophotometer (NanoDrop Technologies, Wilmington, DE, USA). Complementary DNA (cDNA) was synthesized from 200 ng of each RNA sample, using MultiScribe Reverse Transcriptase in the presence of RNase inhibitor (High-capacity cDNA RT kit, Applied Biosystems Inc., Foster City, CA, USA), according to the manufacturer's instructions. The synthesis of cDNA was carried out in PCR MasterCycler (Eppendorf AG, Hamburg, Germany): 10 min at 25°C, 120 min at 37°C, 5 min at 85°C, and finally cooled down to 4°C.

FAM-labeled TaqMan® Gene Expression Assays (Applied Biosystems Inc.) were used for qPCR reactions: *RAX* (Hs00429459_m1), *PAX*6 (Hs00240871_m1), *MITF* (Hs01115553_m1), *CRX* (Hs01549131_m1) and *CHX*10 (Hs01584048_m1). Glyceraldehyde 3-phosphate dehydrogenase, *GAPDH* (Hs99999905_m1) was used as endogenous control. Each reaction mixture consisted of 7.5 μl TaqMan® Universal PCR Master Mix (2×), 0.75 μl Gene Expression Assay (20×), 3 μl of cDNA (diluted 1:5 with sterile water) and sterile water to the total volume of 15 μl. All samples and controls were run as triplicate reactions using the 7300 Real-time PCR system (Applied Biosystems Inc.) as follows: 2 min at 50°C, 10 min at 95°C, and 40 cycles of 15 s at 95°C, and 1 min at 60°C. Results were analyzed using 7300 System SDS Software (Applied Biosystems Inc.). Based on the C_T-values given by the software, the relative quantification of each gene was calculated using the $2^{-\Delta\Delta Ct}$ method [30] and Microsoft Excel 2003.

The values for each sample were normalized to expression levels of *GAPDH*. The expression level of undifferentiated hPSC sample was set as the calibrator (fold change equals 1). Results were plotted using Microsoft Excel 2003 and figures edited with Adobe PhotoShop CS4. For visualization of down-regulation, the fold change values <1 are presented as the negative inverse of the value, calculated as –1/(fold change). Standard deviations were calculated for each set of technical replicates, and presented as error bars.

2.7. Immunofluorescence

Differences in protein expression of *PAX*6 and *MITF* after 28 days of differentiation were studied using immunofluorescence. The cell aggregates were dissociated to single cells as described above. Single-cell suspensions containing 1.6 – 3.5 × 10^5 cells/ml were prepared in DPBS, and 150 μl samples were centrifuged onto 15-mm glass cover slips at 600 rpm, 5 min, using Shandon Cytospin 2 cytocentrifuge (Thermo Fisher Scientific, Waltham, MA, USA). Cells were fixed immediately with 4% paraformaldehyde (PFA, Sigma-Aldrich) for 15 min at RT. Cells were permeabilized with 0.1% Triton X-100 (Sigma-Aldrich) in DPBS at RT for 10 min, and unspecific binding blocked with 3% bovine serum albumin (BSA, Sigma-Aldrich) at RT for 1 h. Incubation with primary antibodies was carried out either overnight at 4°C or for 1 h at RT with the appropriate antibody: 1:200 dilution of mouse anti-*PAX*6 (Developmental Studies Hybridoma Bank, University of IOWA, Department of Biology, Iowa City, IA, USA) or 1:350 dilution of rabbit anti-*MITF* (Abcam, Cambridge, UK). Secondary antibodies were diluted 1:1500 in 0.5% BSA-DPBS and cells incubated 1 h at RT in either Alexa Fluor 568-conjugated goat anti-mouse IgG or goat anti-rabbit IgG (both from Molecular probes, Life Technologies). Cell nuclei were stained with VectaShield mounting medium (Vector Laboratories Inc., Burlingame, CA, USA) containing 4', 6'-diamidino-2-phenylidole (DAPI). Cells were imaged with Olympus BX60 microscope (Olympus, Tokyo, Japan) using a 40× objective. The images were captured using same exposure time within each experiment and imaged areas were selected randomly. Minimum 700 cells were counted from each condition. *PAX*6 and *MITF* expression was quantified using Image J Image Processing and Analysis Software [31]. For each experiment, the threshold for positive expression was set by analysing several randomly selected images. Intensity threshold was adjusted for each image within an experiment and label to normalize the levels of background intensity. Cells below the set threshold level were considered negative. The total number of cells in each image was determined by counting nuclei counterstained with DAPI. The numbers of cells expressing *PAX*6 or *MITF* in relation to the total amount of cells were counted for hESC-RPE from two individual experiments and two activin A supplementation experiments. Results were plotted as bar charts using Microsoft Excel 2003 and figures edited with Adobe PhotoShop CS4.

Monolayers of hESC-RPE maturated on mouse collagen IV cell culture inserts were analyzed with immunofluorescence for the expression and correct localization of RPE-related proteins: *MITF*, cellular retinal-dehyde-binding protein (CRALBP), Bestrophin, and tight junction protein zona occludens-1 (ZO-1). Detailed protocol has been published previously [21]. Images were taken either with Olympus BX60 microscope or LSM 700 confocal microscope (Carl Zeiss, Jena, Germany) using a 63× oil immersion objective. All images were edited using ZEN 2009 Light Edition (Zeiss) and Adobe Photoshop CS4.

2.8. Reverse Transcriptase PCR

Monolayers of hPSC-RPE maturated on human collagen IV were analyzed for expression of RPE specific genes by reverse transcription polymerase chain reaction (RT-PCR). Expression of the following genes was assessed: RPE precursor markers *MITF* and orthodenticle homeobox 2 (*OTX*2), and mature RPE-specific markers retinal pigment epihelium-specific protein 65 kDA (*RPE*65), bestrophin (*BEST*1), pre-melanosomal protein 17 (*PMEL* 17), pigment epithelium-derived factor (*PEDF*) and tyrosinase (*TYR*). *GAPDH* was used as endogenous control. Total RNA was extracted and 40 ng was reverse- transcribed to cDNA as described above. Genomic control reactions excluding the reverse transcriptase enzyme (-RT) for each RNA sample were performed. RT-PCR was carried out using 1 μl of cDNA as template. Detailed protocol and primer sequences used have been previously published [21].

2.9. Growth Factor Secretion Analysis

The three differentiation media: RPEbasic, mEF-CM and hFF-CM were analyzed for concentrations of TGF-β1, activin A and bFGF growth factors with enzyme-linked immunosorbent assay (ELISA). The following comercial ELISA kits were used: Human TGF-β1 Immunoassay, Human/Mouse/Rat Activin A Immunoassay, human FGF basic Immunoassay (all from Quantikine®, R&D Systems, Minneapolis, MN, USA). The Human TGF-β1 Immunoassay and human FGF basic Immunoassays have been previously shown to detect the growth factor concentrations also from mEF-CM [32]. All assays were performed according to manufacturer's instructions. All standards and samples were tested in duplicates. For the activin A immunoassay, each sample was diluted 1:5 and 1:25, with the diluent supplied in the kit. Optical densities were measured using Wallac Victor$^{2\text{TM}}$ 1420 Multilabel counter (Perkin Elmer-Wallace, Norton, OH, USA). Using optical densities of the standard series, standard curves were created using Microsoft Excel 2003 and concentrations of the samples calculated accordingly. Standard deviations were calculated from the concentrations of duplicates of each tested sample, and were presented as error bars. The measurements were repeated twice from two different batches of CM.

2.10. Ethical Considerations

The study of human embryos at University of Tampere has been approved by National Authority for Medicolegal Affairs Finland (TEO) (Dnro 1426/32/300/05). We have a supportive statement of Ethical Committee of Pirkanmaa Hospital District to derive, culture, and differentiate hESC lines from surplus human embryos (Skottman/R05116). No new cell lines were derived for this study.

3. RESULTS

3.1. Appearance of Pigmentation Was Accelerated in the Conditioned Media

Human ESCs and iPSCs were differentiated in suspension as floating cell aggregates in three different media: standard RPEbasic, hFF-CM and mEF-CM. Differentiation rate of hPSC-RPE was monitored by recording the appearance of first pigmented cells in each medium. The appearance of pigmented cells was faster in the CM compared to the RPEbasic for both hESCs and iPSCs. On average, the hESCs pigmented fastest in mEF-CM (day 13), next in hFF-CM (day 15) and slowest in RPEbasic (day 16) (**Figure 2(A)**). Human iPSCs generated pigmented cells on average at day 16 in both CM and at day 18 in RPEbasic (data not shown).

3.2. hPSCs Expressed Marker Genes for Eye Field and RPE Precursor Cells during Differentiation

Gene expression of early eye field markers *PAX*6 and *RAX*, and RPE precursor marker *MITF* was analyzed with relative qPCR after 7, 14 and 28 days of differentiation. The gene expression levels were compared to undifferentiated hPSCs. For hESCs, expression of *PAX*6 increased substantially during differentiation, suggesting that differentiation progressed to eye field direction in all studied media (**Figure 2(B)**). Expression levels of *RAX* increased during the first two weeks of differentiation, and decreased by day 28 in cells differentiated in both CM (**Figure 2(C)**). This decrease in *RAX* expression was accompanied by a 10-fold increase in the expression of RPE-specific *MITF* (**Figure 2(D)**) which indicates progress toward RPE fate. In RPEbasic, expression of *RAX* further increased by day 28, but the pattern of *MITF* expression was similar to that of CM. In addition, the expression of neural retina markers *CHX*10 and *CRX* were analyzed at day 28 and found to be substantially decreased for both CM conditions compared to RPEbasic. Especially the early neural retina marker *CHX*10 expression was 15 times higher in the RPEbasic condition compared to mEF-CM and 9 times higher compared to hFF-CM (data not shown). This expression pattern indicated increased differentiation toward neural retina direction in RPEbasic and toward RPE fate in CM. The studied genes showed a similar expression pattern also in

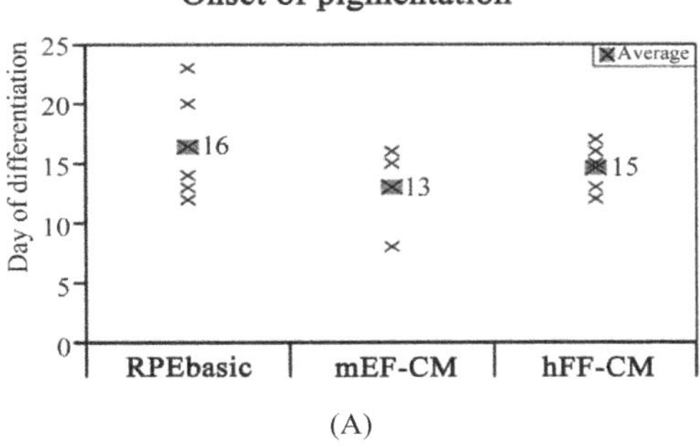

(A)

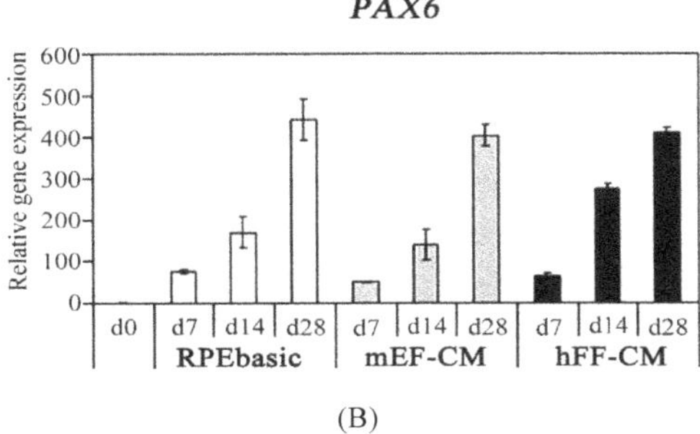

(B)

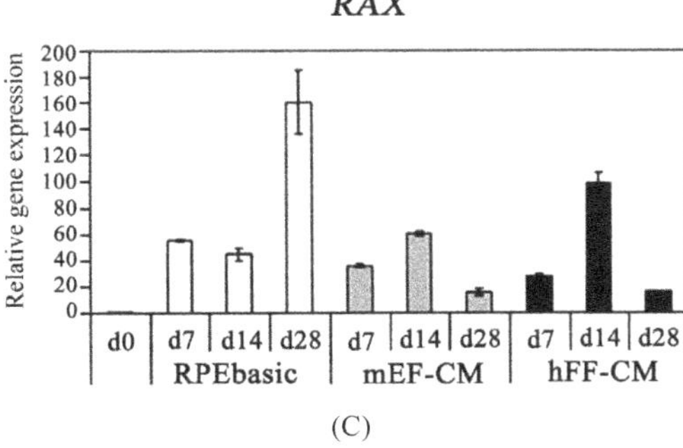

(C)

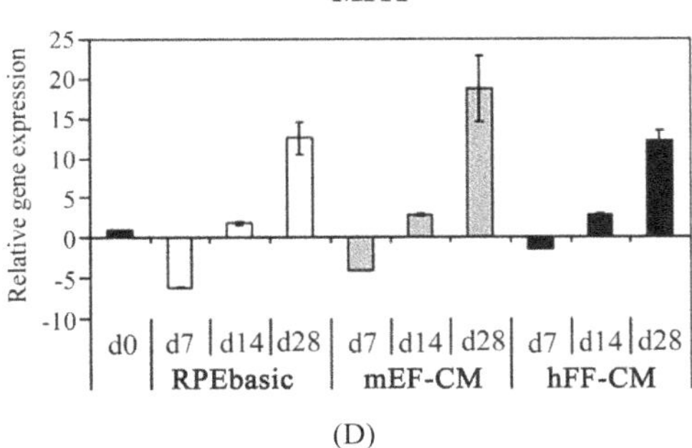

(D)

Figure 2. Analysis of early-stage hESC-RPE differentiation. The day of first pigmentation observed in replicate experiments, as well as the average, shown for each medium (A). Gene expression of the early eye-field markers *PAX*6 (B) and *RAX* (C) as well as early RPE marker *MITF* (D), relative to undifferentiated stem cells (d0) was analysed with qPCR.

hiPSC differentiation but with lower relative expression levels (data not shown).

3.3. Conditioned Media Contained More RPE Cells after Four Weeks of Differentiation

After four weeks of differentiation, the number of pigmented cell aggregates to total number of aggregates was calculated for each medium. CM consistently contained higher percentage of pigmented cell aggregates compared to RPEbasic for both hESCs (**Figure 3(A)**) and hiPSCs (data not shown) in each of the three replicate experiments. Typically, the pigmented areas were also larger in CM compared to RPEbasic (**Figure 3(B)**), indicating higher number of pigmented cells within the areas. In addition, the number of *PAX*6 and *MITF* expressing cells in the differentiated cell aggregates in each medium were quantified at 28 day time point. After dissociation to single cells and immunostaining, the number of positive cells was calculated. In two replicate experiments, the ratios of *PAX*6 and *MITF* positive cells were clearly higher in CM compared to RPEbasic (**Figure 3(C)**) with mEF-CM containing highest percentage of positive cells. On average, over 90% of cells expressed *PAX*6 and *MITF* in both CM, whereas in RPEbasic only 61% (±8%) of cells were positive to *PAX*6 and 74% (±8%) to *MITF*. Representative images of cells immunolabeled for *PAX*6 and the same cells counterstained with DAPI are shown in **Figure 3(D)**.

3.4. Mature hPSC-RPE Cells Possessed RPE Morphology and Expressed RPE-Specific Genes and Proteins

After selective plating of pigmented areas to adherent cultures on collagen IV, pigmentation and RPE-like cell morphology were initially lost. Cells acquired fibroblast-like morphology and proliferated to confluence, after which cobblestone morphology and pigmentation began to reappear within two weeks of culture. Mature cells were pigmented and possessed regular hexagonal arrangement typical to RPE (**Figure 4(A)**).

Expression of RPE-specific markers was studied at the protein level with immunofluorescence. Cells co-expressed *MITF* in the nuclei and CRALBP in the cytoplasm and cell membranes (**Figure 4(B)**). Moreover, expression of Bestrophin (**Figure 4(C)**) and tight junction protein ZO-1 (**Figure 4(D)**) confirm the maturity of hESC-derived RPE cells. The maturated hPSC-RPE cells were analysed for RPE-specific gene expression with RT-PCR. Cells in all three test media were shown to express RPE precursor genes *MITF* and *OTX*2, as well as genes specific to mature RPE, namely *RPE*65, *BEST*1, *PMEL*17, *PEDF* and *TYR*, confirming differentiation to RPE fate. The maturated hESC-RPE (**Figure 4(E)**) and hiPSC-RPE (data not shown) cells showed identical gene expression profile.

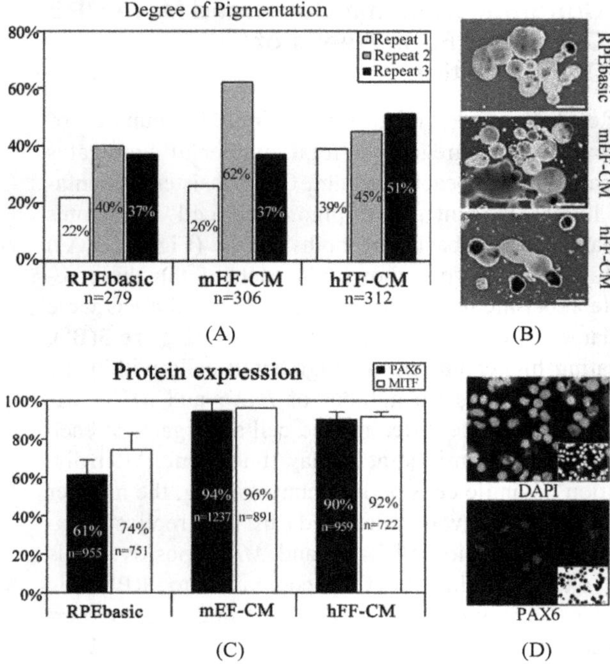

Figure 3. Degree of RPE differentiation at the 28 day time-point. The ratio of pigmented cell aggregates to total number of aggregates in each medium shown for three replicate experiments, n = total number of counted cell aggregates (A). Representative images of pigmented cell aggregates in each medium, scale bars 500 μm (B). Average percentage of cells expressing *PAX6* and *MITF* in two replicate experiments quantified by cell counting. Standard deviations as error bars, n = total number of counted cells (C). Illustrative images of cells labelled with anti-*PAX6* for cell counting before and after thresholding (D).

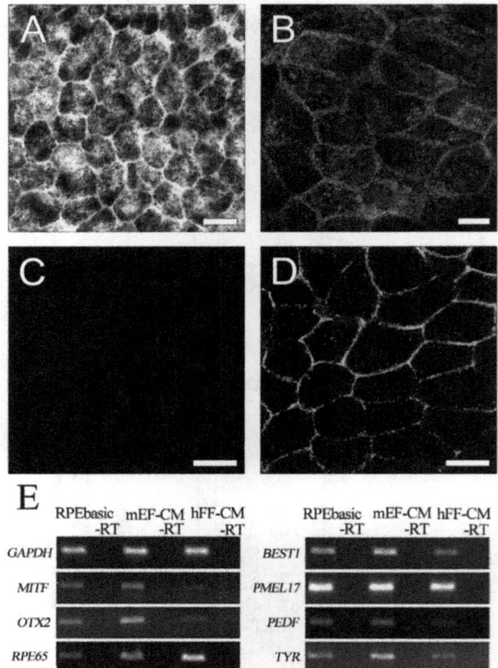

Figure 4. Analysis of mature hESC-RPE cells. Maturated cells possessed appropriate RPE morphology and pigmentation (A). Protein expression of CRALBP (green) and *MITF* (red) (B), Bestrophin (C), and ZO-1 (D) was confirmed with immunofluorescence, Scale bars 10 μm. Similar results were obtained in each test medium. Representative images in (A)-(D) are of cells cultured in mEF-CM. Gene expression profile of several RPE-related genes shown for hESC-RPE differentiated in the three test media, -RT = genomic control (E).

3.5. Feeder Cells Secreted Activin A and TGF-β1

Concentrations of bFGF, activin A and TGF-β1 were measured in both CM and RPEbasic with ELISA. Concentration of bFGF was undetected in all tested media. Concentration of TGFβ in RPEbasic (15% KO-SR) was 67 pg/ml. Both fibroblast types secreted low levels of TGF-β: mEF-CM contained 207 pg/ml and hFF-CM 549 pg/ml. In addition, mEFs secreted substantially more activin A compared to hFFs—mEF-CM contained 7.1 ng/ml of activin A, whereas hFF-CM contained 1.0 ng/ml. Activin A was undetected in RPEbasic, meaning that practically all the activin A present in CM was secreted by the fibroblasts.

3.6. Activin A Supplementation Accelerated hESC-RPE Differentiation

Based on the results of the growth factor analyses, inductive effect of activin A was tested by supplementing RPEbasic with 10 ng/ml of recombinant human activin A. In all three separate repeats, addition of activin A had a pronounced effect on the early-stage RPE differentiation. Activin A accelerated the onset of pigmentation from an average of day 16 to day 11 (**Figure 5(A)**), and by day 28 of differentiation enhanced the degree of pigmentation from 30% to 70% of pigmented cell aggregates (**Figure 5(B)**). Furthermore, differentiation cultures treated with activin A showed higher expression of *PAX6* and *MITF*, quantified from immunofluorescence samples. On average, 96% (±1%) of cells were positive for *PAX6* and 71% (±14%) for *MITF* after activin A treatment, while corresponding values in RPEbasic were 74% (± 16%) and 57% (±13%) (**Figure 5(C)**). After adherent maturation culture, the cells in RPEbasic supplemented with 10 ng/ml activin A showed mature RPE phenotype with corresponding pigmentation, morphology and protein expression (**Figures 5 (D)-(G)**).

4. DISCUSSION

During early eye development, RPE is surrounded by the

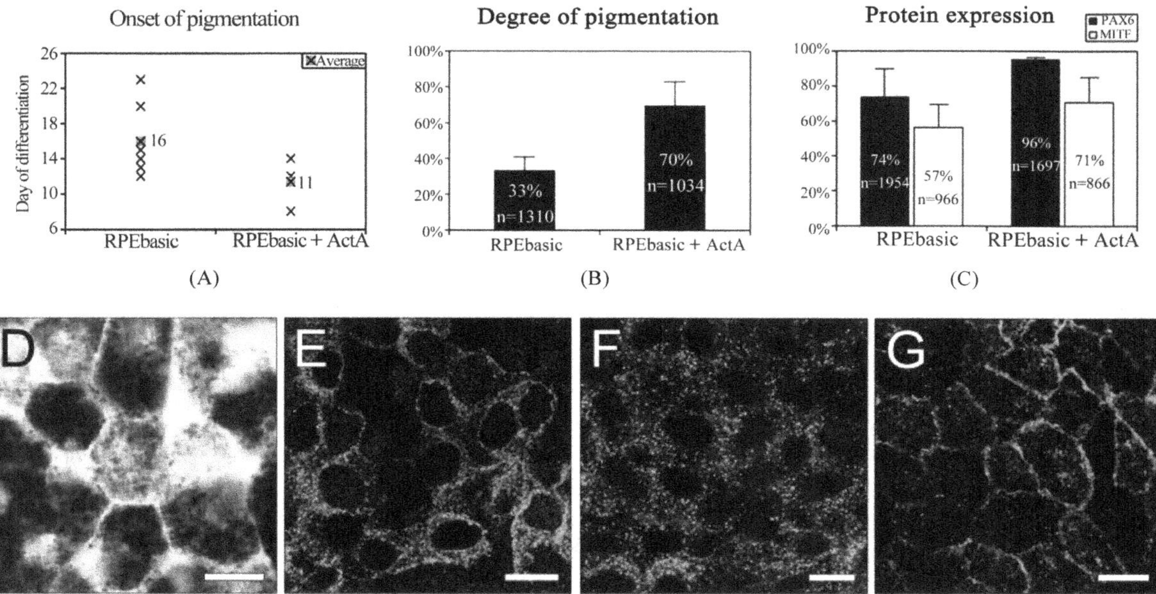

Figure 5. Differentiation efficacy of medium supplemented with activin A. Addition of activin A to the RPEbasic medium had a positive effect on the onset of pigmentation (A). Similarly, ratio of pigmented cell aggregates after 28 days of differentiation was enhanced, n = total number of cell aggregates counted (B). Percentage of *PAX*6 and *MITF* positive cells with and without activin A supplementation (C). Mature hESC-RPE cells cultured in RPEbasic supplemented with activin A possessed appropriate cell morphology and pigmentation (D) and expressed CRALBP (green) and *MITF* (red) (E), Bestrophin (F), and ZO-1 (G). Scale bars 10 μm.

extraocular mesenchyme, while the ectoderm faces the neural retina. RPE cell differentiation is known to be regulated by two key regulatory transcription factors *MITF* and *OTX*2. Expression of these transcription factors is controlled by interactions with the surrounding extraocular tissue, including the extraocular mesenchyime [12].

In the present study we hypothesized that fibroblast feeder cells used for the culture of undifferentiated hPSC may provide variable mesechymal signals having an inductive effect on spontaneous RPE cell differentiation *in vitro*. The results of this study clearly demonstrated the inductive effect of the two most commonly used fibroblast feeder cell types, mEFs and hFFs, on RPE cell differentiation both from hESC and iPSCs. In the presence of soluble factors secreted by feeder cells, both the onset of pigmentation and its rate were clearly enhanced. As expected, there was considerable biological variation in the appearance and amount of pigmentation between the replicate experiments typical for suspension culture methods. However, a clear correlating trend was observed. Along with the appearance of pigmented cells, eye field transcription factor genes *RAX* and *PAX*6 were expressed. After four weeks of differentiation, expression of RPE-specific transcription factor *MITF* was the highest in cells differentiated in mEF-CM, accompanied by decreased expression of *RAX* and a low expression of *CRX* and *CHX*10 demonstrating the early neural precursors' progress towards RPE cell fate instead of neural retina. Similar but moderated effect was seen with cells differentiated in hFF-CM. Most importantly, both of the CM conditions were verified to contain substantially more *PAX*6 and *MITF* expressing cells compared to non-conditioned RPEbasic at the protein level, using quantitative cell counting. After selective plating of pigmented clusters to adherent culture, the cells showed mature RPE morphology and expression of RPE-specific markers, both at gene and protein level. Taken together, the induction of RPE differentiation with feeder cell CM had a positive effect on hPSC-RPE differentiation.

Fibroblast feeder cells in general are known to secrete various factors promoting or inhibiting the growth and differentiation of hPSC cells [33-37]. To elucidate the inductive effect of CM in RPE differentiation, we further studied the secretion of bFGF, TGF-β1 and activin A, known factors regulating eye field differentiation, by the feeder cells. As a result we found that secretion of activin A was substantially higher by mEFs compared to hFFs. In contrast, secretion of TGF-β was higher for hFFs compared to mEFs. This is consistent with our previous studies showing that mEFs secrete more activin A and hFFs secrete more TGFβ [38]. We were not able to detect any measurable levels of bFGF from either CM thus possible effect of difference in bFGF concentration was excluded. Similar trend in fibroblast growth factor secretion has been confirmed by another research group [32]. The extraocular mesenchyme secretes TGF-β1 superfamily growth factors such as activin A, activates the expression of *MITF* and down-regulates *CHX*10 expression directing RPE cell fate differentiation *in vivo*. Similar effects of activin A inducing *MITF* expression have been shown [26]. Activin A has also been shown to induce hESC-RPE differentiation *in vitro,* but only after pretreatment with nicotinamide [17,39]. The superior secretion of activin A by mEF feeder cells could thus be one of the key factors enhancing the early RPE differentiation and reduction of the *RAX*, *CRX*, *CHX*10 expression.

To study the effect of activin A secretion by mEF, we supplemented the RPEbasic medium with 10 ng/ml activin A and concluded that addition of activin A at this low level had a pronounced effect on the early-stage RPE differentiation. In previously published studies, relatively high activin A concentrations of 140 ng/ml between day 14 - 28 of differentiation [17] and 100 ng/ml between day 20 - 40 [40] have been used. On the contrary, we were able to induce early RPE differentiation with substantially lower activin A concentration. However, in addition to activin A both mEF-CM and hFF-CM may contain a pool of other possible factors inducing RPE cell differentiation. Both fibroblast types secrete various ECM components like collagens I and IV, nidogen I, and fibronectin as well as proteins involved in TGFβ, BMP, Wnt and IGF signaling [33]. In addition mEFs secrete the neurotrophic pigment epithelium derived factor (PEDF) [33,34] leaving the field open to identify other important players.

5. CONCLUSION

In this study, we confirmed the inductive effect of commonly used fibroblast feeder cells on hPSC differentiation towards RPE cells. Human PSCs were differentiated using media conditioned by two types of fibroblasts originated from mouse embryos and neonatal human foreskin tissue. Both feeder cell type CM increased RPE differentiation as compared to the non-conditioned medium (RPEbasic). The growth factor activin A, known inductive agent of RPE fate, was concluded to be an important factor present especially in mEF-CM. Consequently, supplementation of RPEbasic medium with a low concentration of activin A increased the differentiation rate of RPE cells to comparative level achieved with CM. Thus, inductive effect provided by feeder cells was at least partially driven by activin A.

6. ACKNOWLEDGEMENTS

We thank Professor Timo Otonkoski's group at University of Helsinki for the kind gift of the hiPSC line FiPS5-7. We thank Outi Melin, Hanna Koskenaho and Elina Konsén for technical assistance. The study was financially supported by Academy of Finland (218050; 133879), The Competitive Research Funding of the Tampere University Hospital (9H114; 9M098), Päivikki and Sakari Sohlberg foundation, Finnish Cultural Foundation and Tampere Graduate Program in Biomedicine and Biotechnology. The *PAX*6 antibody developed by Kawakami A was obtained from the Developmental Studies Hybridoma Bank (DHSB) developed under auspices of the NICHD and maintained by the University of IOWA, Department of Biology, Iowa City, IA, 52242.

REFERENCES

[1] Binder, S., Stanzel, B.V., Krebs, I. and Glittenberg, C. (2007) Transplantation of the RPE in AMD. *Progress in Retinal and Eye Research*, **26**, 516-554. doi:10.1016/j.preteyeres.2007.02.002

[2] Klassen, H., Sakaguchi, D.S. and Young, M.J. (2004) Stem cells and retinal repair. *Progress in Retinal and Eye Research*, **23**, 149-181. doi:10.1016/j.preteyeres.2004.01.002

[3] Binder, S., Krebs, I., Hilgers, R.D., Abri, A., Stolba, U., Assadoulina, A., Kellner, L., Stanzel, B.V., Jahn, C. and Feichtinger, H. (2004) Outcome of transplantation of autologous retinal pigment epithelium in age-related macular degeneration: A prospective trial. *Investigative Ophthalmology & Visual Science*, **45**, 4151-4160. doi:10.1167/iovs.04-0118

[4] Chen, F.K., Uppal, G.S., MacLaren, R.E., Coffey, P.J., Rubin, G.S., Tufail, A., Aylward, G.W. and Da Cruz, L. (2009) Long-term visual and microperimetry outcomes following autologous retinal pigment epithelium choroid graft for neovascular age-related macular degeneration. *Clinical & Experimental Ophthalmology*, **37**, 275-285. doi:10.1111/j.1442-9071.2009.01915.xs

[5] Radtke, N.D., Aramant, R.B., Seiler, M.J., Petry, H.M. and Pidwell, D. (2004) Vision change after sheet transplant of fetal retina with retinal pigment epithelium to a patient with retinitis pigmentosa. *Archives of Ophthalmology*, **122**, 1159-1165. doi:10.1001/archopht.122.8.1159

[6] Carr, A.J., Vugler, A.A., Hikita, S.T., Lawrence, J.M., Gias, C., Chen, L.L., Buchholz, D.E., Ahmado, A., Semo, M., Smart, M.J., Hasan, S., Da Cruz, L., Johnson, L.V., Clegg, D.O. and Coffey, P.J. (2009) Protective effects of human iPS-derived retinal pigment epithelium cell transplantation in the retinal dystrophic rat. *PLoS One*, **4**, e8152. doi:10.1371/journal.pone.0008152

[7] Klimanskaya, I., Hipp, J., Rezai, K.A., West, M., Atala, A. and Lanza, R. (2004) Derivation and comparative assessment of retinal pigment epithelium from human embryonic stem cells using transcriptomics. *Cloning and Stem Cells*, **6**, 217-245.

[8] Lu, B., Malcuit, C., Wang, S., Girman, S., Francis, P., Lemieux, L., Lanza, R. and Lund, R. (2009) Long-term safety and function of RPE from human embryonic stem cells in preclinical models of macular degeneration. *Stem Cells*, **27**, 2126-2135. doi:10.1002/stem.149

[9] Lund, R.D., Wang, S., Klimanskaya, I., Holmes, T., Ramos-Kelsey, R., Lu, B., Girman, S., Bischoff, N., Sauve, Y. and Lanza, R. (2006) Human embryonic stem cell-derived

cells rescue visual function in dystrophic RCS rats. *Cloning and Stem Cells*, **8**, 189-199. doi:10.1089/clo.2006.8.189

[10] Vugler, A., Lawrence, J., Walsh, J., Carr, A., Gias, C., Semo, M., Ahmado, A., Da Cruz, L., Andrews, P. and Coffey, P. (2007) Embryonic stem cells and retinal repair. *Mechanisms of Development*, **124**, 807-829. doi:10.1016/j.mod.2007.08.002

[11] Schwartz, S.D., Hubschman, J.P., Heilwell, G., Franco-Cardenas, V., Pan, C.K., Ostrick, R.M., Mickunas, E., Gay, R., Klimanskaya, I. and Lanza, R. (2012) Embryonic stem cell trials for macular degeneration: A preliminary report. *The Lancet*, **379**, 713-720. doi:10.1016/S0140-6736(12)60028-2

[12] Westenskow, P., Piccolo, S. and Fuhrmann, S. (2009) Beta-catenin controls differentiation of the retinal pigment epithelium in the mouse optic cup by regulating *Mitf* and Otx2 expression. *Development*, **136**, 2505-2510. doi:10.1242/dev.032136

[13] Eiraku, M. and Sasai, Y. (2012) Mouse embryonic stem cell culture for generation of three-dimensional retinal and cortical tissues. *Nature Protocols*, **7**, 69-79. doi:10.1038/nprot.2011.429

[14] Fuhrmann, S. (2008) Wnt signaling in eye organogenesis. *Organogenesis*, **4**, 60-67. doi:10.4161/org.4.2.5850

[15] Yang, X.J. (2004) Roles of cell-extrinsic growth factors in vertebrate eye pattern formation and retinogenesis. *Semin Cell and Developmental Biology*, **15**, 91-103. doi:10.1016/j.semcdb.2003.09.004

[16] Smukler, S.R., Runciman, S.B., Xu, S. and Van Der Kooy, D. (2006) Embryonic stem cells assume a primitive neural stem cell fate in the absence of extrinsic influences. *The Journal of Cell Biology*, **172**, 79-90. doi:10.1083/jcb.200508085

[17] Idelson, M., Alper, R., Obolensky, A., Ben-Shushan, E., Hemo, I., Yachimovich-Cohen, N., Khaner, H., Smith, Y., Wiser, O., Gropp, M., Cohen, M.A., Even-Ram, S., Berman-Zaken, Y., Matzrafi, L., Rechavi, G., Banin, E. and Reubinoff, B. (2009) Directed differentiation of human embryonic stem cells into functional retinal pigment epithelium cells. *Cell Stem Cell*, **5**, 396-408. doi:10.1016/j.stem.2009.07.002

[18] Osakada, F., Jin, Z.B., Hirami, Y., Ikeda, H., Danjyo, T., Watanabe, K., Sasai, Y. and Takahashi, M. (2009) *In vitro* differentiation of retinal cells from human pluripotent stem cells by small-molecule induction. *Journal of Cell Science*, **122**, 3169-3179. doi:10.1242/jcs.050393

[19] Osakada, F., Ikeda, H., Mandai, M., Wataya, T., Watanabe, K., Yoshimura, N., Akaike, A., Sasai, Y. and Takahashi, M. (2008) Toward the generation of rod and cone photoreceptors from mouse, monkey and human embryonic stem cells. *Nature Biotechnology*, **26**, 215-224. doi:10.1038/nbt1384

[20] Rowland, T.J., Buchholz, D.E. and Clegg, D.O. (2012) Pluripotent human stem cells for the treatment of retinal disease. *Journal of Cellular Physiology*, **227**, 457-466. doi:10.1002/jcp.22814

[21] Vaajasaari, H., Imarinen, T., Juuti-Uusitalo, K., Rajala, K., Onnela, N., Narkilahti, S., Suuronen, R., Hyttinen, J., Uusitalo, H. and Skottman, H. (2011) Towards defined and xeno-free differentiation of functional human pluripotent stem cell-derived retinal pigment epithelium cells. *Molecular Vision*, **22**, 558-575.

[22] Clarke, L., Ballios, B.G. and Van Der Kooy, D. (2012) Generation and clonal isolation of retinal stem cells from human embryonic stem cells. *European Journal of Neuroscience*, **36**, 1951-1959. doi:10.1111/j.1460-9568.2012.08123.x

[23] Gong, J., Sagiv, O., Cai, H., Tsang, S.H. and Del Priore, L.V. (2008) Effects of extracellular matrix and neighboring cells on induction of human embryonic stem cells into retinal or retinal pigment epithelial progenitors. *Experimental Eye Research*, **86**, 957-965. doi:10.1016/j.exer.2008.03.014

[24] Okamoto, S. and Takahashi, M. (2011) Induction of retinal pigment epithelial cells from monkey iPS cells. *Investigative Ophthalmology & Visual Science*, **52**, 8785-8790. doi:10.1167/iovs.11-8129

[25] Martinez-Morales, J.R., Rodrigo, I. and Bovolenta, P. (2004) Eye development: A view from the retina pigmented epithelium. *Bioessays*, **26**, 766-777. doi:10.1002/bies.20064

[26] Fuhrmann, S., Levine, E.M. and Reh, T.A. (2000) Extraocular mesenchyme patterns the optic vesicle during early eye development in the embryonic chick. *Development*, **127**, 4599-4609.

[27] Skottman, H. (2010) Derivation and characterization of three new human embryonic stem cell lines in Finland. *In Vitro Cellular & Developmental Biology*: *Animal*, **46**, 206-209. doi:10.1007/s11626-010-9286-2

[28] Rajala, K., Lindroos, B., Hussein, S.M., Lappalainen, R.S., Pekkanen-Mattila, M., Inzunza, J., Rozell, B., Miettinen, S., Narkilahti, S., Kerkela, E., Aalto-Setala, K., Otonkoski, T., Suuronen, R., Hovatta, O. and Skottman, H. (2010) A defined and xeno-free culture method enabling the establishment of clinical-grade human embryonic, induced pluripotent and adipose stem cells. *PLoS One*, **5**, e10246. doi:10.1371/journal.pone.0010246

[29] Hussein, S.M., Batada, N.N., Vuoristo, S., Ching, R.W., Autio, R., Narva, E., Ng, S., Sourour, M., Hamalainen, R., Olsson, C., Lundin, K., Mikkola, M., Trokovic, R., Peitz, M., Brustle, O., Bazett-Jones, D.P., Alitalo, K., Lahesmaa, R., Nagy, A. and Otonkoski, T. (2011) Copy number variation and selection during reprogramming to pluripotency. *Nature*, **471**, 58-62. doi:10.1038/nature09871

[30] Livak, K.J. and Schmittgen, T.D. (2001) Analysis of relative gene expression data using real-time quantitative PCR and the 2(-Delta Delta C(T)) Method. *Methods*, **25**, 402-408.

[31] http://imagej.nih.gov/ij/index.html

[32] Eiselleova, L., Peterkova, I., Neradil, J., Slaninova, I., Hampl, A. and Dvorak, P. (2008) Comparative study of mouse and human feeder cells for human embryonic stem cells. *International Journal of Developmental Biology*, **52**, 353-363. doi:10.1387/ijdb.082590le

[33] Prowse, A.B., McQuade, L.R., Bryant, K.J., Marcal, H.

and Gray, P.P. (2007) Identification of potential pluripotency determinants for human embryonic stem cells following proteomic analysis of human and mouse fibroblast conditioned media. *Journal of Proteome Research*, **6**, 3796-3807. doi:10.1021/pr0702262

[34] Lim, J.W. and Bodnar, A. (2002) Proteome analysis of conditioned medium from mouse embryonic fibroblast feeder layers which support the growth of human embryonic stem cells. *Proteomics*, **2**, 1187-1203. doi:10.1002/1615-9861(200209)2:9<1187::AID-PROT1187>3.0.CO;2-T

[35] Prowse, A.B., McQuade, L.R., Bryant, K.J., Van Dyk, D.D., Tuch, B.E. and Gray, P.P. (2005) A proteome analysis of conditioned media from human neonatal fibroblasts used in the maintenance of human embryonic stem cells. *Proteomics*, **5**, 978-989. doi:10.1002/pmic.200401087

[36] Bendall, S.C., Hughes, C., Campbell, J.L., Stewart, M.H., Pittock, P., Liu, S., Bonneil, E., Thibault, P., Bhatia, M. and Lajoie, G.A. (2009) An enhanced mass spectrometry approach reveals human embryonic stem cell growth factors in culture. *Molecular & Cellular Proteomics*, **8**, 421-432. doi:10.1074/mcp.M800190-MCP200

[37] Bendall, S.C., Stewart, M.H., Menendez, P., George, D., Vijayaragavan, K., Werbowetski-Ogilvie, T., RamosMejia, V., Rouleau, A., Yang, J., Bosse, M., Lajoie, G., and Bhatia, M. (2007) IGF and FGF cooperatively establish the regulatory stem cell niche of pluripotent human cells *in vitro*. *Nature*, **448**, 1015-1021. doi:10.1038/nature06027

[38] Hongisto, H., Vuoristo, S., Mikhailova, A., Suuronen, R., Virtanen, I., Otonkoski, T. and Skottman, H. (2012) Laminin-511 expression is associated with the functionality of feeder cells in human embryonic stem cell culture. *Stem Cell Research*, **8**, 97-108. doi:10.1016/j.scr.2011.08.005

[39] Kokkinaki, M., Sahibzada, N. and Golestaneh, N. (2011) Human induced pluripotent stem-derived retinal pigment epithelium (RPE) cells exhibit ion transport, membrane potential, polarized vascular endothelial growth factor secretion, and gene expression pattern similar to native RPE. *Stem Cells*, **29**, 825-835. doi:10.1002/stem.635

[40] Meyer, J.S., Howden, S.E., Wallace, K.A., Verhoeven, A.D., Wright, L.S., Capowski, E.E., Pinilla, I., Martin, J.M., Tian, S., Stewart, R., Pattnaik, B., Thomson, J.A. and Gamm, D.M. (2011) Optic vesicle-like structures derived from human pluripotent stem cells facilitate a customized approach to retinal disease treatment. *Stem Cells*, **29**, 1206-1218. doi:10.1002/stem.674

Differentiation of human epidermis-derived mesenchymal stem cell-like pluripotent cells into neural-like cells in culture and after transplantation

Min Zhang, Bing Huang*, Kaijing Li, Zhenghua Chen, Jian Ge, Weihua Li, Jianfa Huang, Ting Luo, Shaochun Lin, Jie Yu, Wencong Wang, Liping Lin

State Key Laboratory of Ophthalmology, Zhongshan Ophthalmic Center, Sun Yat-sen University, Guangzhou, China;
*Corresponding Author: huangbing2000@hotmail.com

ABSTRACT

Skin is the largest organ of the human body and a possible source of stem cells for research and cell-based therapy. We have isolated a population of mesenchymal stem cell-like pluripotent cells from human epidermis, termed human (h) EMSCPCs. This preliminary study tested if these hEMSCPCs can be induced to differentiate into neural-like cells. Human EMSCPCs were first cultured for four to seven days in a serum-free neural stem cell (NSC) medium for pre-induction. During pre-induction, hEMSCPCs coalesced into dense spheres that resembled neural rosettes. In the presence of a conditioned differentiation medium, pre-induced cells took on the morphological characteristics of neural cells, including slender projections with inflated or claw-like ends that contacted the soma or projections of other cells as revealed by confocal microscopy. Moreover, these differentiating cells expressed the neural-specific markers β-III tubulin, MAP2, GFAP, and synapsin I as evidenced by immunocytochemistry. Both pre-induced hEMSCPCs and uninduced hEMSCPCs were labeled with CM-Dil and transplanted into the vitreous cavities of nude mice. Transplanted cells were examined four weeks later in frozen eyeball sections by immunofluorescence staining, which demonstrated superior retinal migration and neural differentiation of pre-induced cells. Our study is the first to demonstrate that hEMSCPCs possess the capacity to differentiate into neural-like cells, suggesting potential uses for the treatment of retinal diseases such as age-related macular degeneration.

Keywords: Human Epidermis; Pluripotent Cells; Differentiation; Neural Cells; Cell Therapy

1. INTRODUCTION

Neurological degenerative diseases like Alzheimer's disease, Parkinson's disease, and age-related macular degeneration are a group of chronic, diverse and progressive disorders. Studies have shown heredity, oxidative stress, neurotrophic factor deficiency, dysbolism and other unknown factors could cause a main pathological change of special neurons degeneration and loss, followed by demyelination of nerve fibers [1]. These pathophysiology leads to a decreased activity in the pathway of neural conduction, and results in disturbance of memory, learning, moving and other activities, which causes severe public health burden, particularly in an aging population. Current treatments for these diseases include neuroprotective agents, surgery, physical stimulation, gene therapy, and cell replacement [2-4]. However, pharmacologic, surgical, and physical therapies cannot cure these diseases. Recent reports have shown that gene and cell-replacement therapies are promising alternatives for treating or even curing neurological disorders [5-7]. However, the complexity of the human genome and proteome limits the therapeutic effects of single gene therapy. Indeed, the results of clinical trials testing single gene therapies for Parkinson's disease were less than ideal [8-9].

Theoretically, cell-replacement therapy can cure neurodegenerative diseases by replacing lost cells and reconstructing tissues, leading to functional recovery. Multipotent stem cells are widely used for research on cell-replacement therapy and can be derived from both the embryo (embryonic stem cells, ESCs) and adult tissue (adult stem cells, ASCs). The strong plasticity of ASCs enables directional differentiation into multiple cell types. Numerous studies have revealed that ESCs, neural stem cells (NSCs), bone marrow stem cells (BMSCs), and precursor cells derived from peripheral blood, umbilical cord blood, and fat tissue can differentiate into neural cells [10-17]. However, there are ethical issues surrounding the harvesting of ESCs; moreover, these cells are potentially oncogenic [18-19]. Neural stem cells exist in several adult human tissues but are difficult to isolate [20]. The process of isolating BMSCs is invasive and painful, and the quantities obtained are generally not sufficient for therapeutic applications [21]. Moreover, more accessible peripheral blood and umbilical cord blood contain relatively low numbers of precursor cells, and it is still disputed whether these precursor cells can integrate with the host tissue and differentiate into the appropriate cell types after transplantation [22-24]. Although fat tissue is easily extracted, techniques for the isolation and purification of precursor cells from adipose tissue are still not fully developed [25].

Skin is the largest human organ and its cells are easily harvested. Several groups have isolated pluripotent cells from mammalian skin that can differentiate into neural cells [26-32]. After transplantation into animal models, these skin-derived pluripotent cells were able to promote nerve regeneration and functional improvement after injury [33-36]. It is known that epidermal stem cell-like pluripotent cells are present in the epidermal-basal layer and function in the repair and regeneration of the epidermis [37-38]. We have isolated a population of mesenchymal stem cell-like pluripotent cells from mixed cultures of human epidermal cells that we refer to as human epidermis-derived mesenchymal stem cell-like pluripotent cells (hEMSCPCs) (national patent number: 201010282388.0) [39]. In this exploratory study, we examined whether hEMSCPCs have the capacity to differentiate into neural-like cells. Our data revealed that hEMSCPCs can be induced to differentiate into cells with neural cell characteristics *in vitro* and express some neural cell-specific markers *in vivo* when transplanted into the mouse eye, suggesting the hEMSCPCs may be used for autologous cell-based therapies to treat neurological disorders.

2. MATERIALS AND METHODS

2.1. Isolation of hEMSCPCs and Cultured in Growth Medium

The hEMSCPCs were isolated from foreskin tissue obtained from circumcision surgery. Tissue donors were healthy as defined by normal blood and urine test results, normal liver and lung function, no history of genetic disease, and the absence of current infectious disease. Written informed consent was provided by the participants. The study was approved by the Medical Ethics Committee of Zhongshan Ophthalmic Center, Sun Yat-sen University (No. 2008-30).

Briefly, foreskin tissue was rinsed in phosphate buffered saline (PBS) containing gentamycin (1000 U/ml) for subsequent treatment, the tissue was cut into pieces of 3 mm × 3 mm in size using scalpes and transferred into a sterilized 15 ml centrifugation tube. Then Dispase II (2 U/ml; GIBCO, USA) was added into the tube, incubated at 6°C - 8°C for 15 hours and then 37°C for 1 hour to remove the dermis. The epidermis were transferred into a new sterilized 15 ml centrifugation tube, washed with PBS for 5 times and crushed. Then suspended with PBS containing 0.25% trypsin and gently pippetted, incubated at 37°C for 30 min. Then washed with PBS twice more and centrifugated at 1200 rpm for 5 min, discarded the supernatant. Cell precipitation was suspended in growth medium consisting of 80% DMEM (GIBCO, USA), 18% fetal bovine serum (FBS) (Si Jiqing Ltd., China), 10 ng/ml basic fibroblast growth factor (bFGF) (PERPO-TECH, USA), 2 ng/ml stem cell factor (SCF) (PERPO-TECH, USA), and 1% MEM non-essential amino acids (NEAA) (100 × solution, GIBCO, USA), and plated in T-25 cell culture flask, incubated at 37°C in a 5% CO_2 atmosphere. The flask remained unmoved within 48 hours, then the medium was replaced according to the rate of cell growth, and the un-adherent cells were removed. Ten days later, small hEMSCPCs appeared; three weeks later, they were deplated using 0.25% trypsin-0.02% ethylene diamine tetraacetic acid (EDTA) and passaged at 1:3. They were continuously cultured and passaged over 30 times *in vitro* [39]. The hEMSCPCs from passages 17 to 19 derived from same biopsy (fore-skin of a 21-year-old male) were used for this study.

Cryopreserved hEMSCPCs were resuscitated from liquid nitrogen and suspended in growth medium (mentioned above). Cell suspensions (8 ml of 1.0×10^4 cells/ml) were plated in T-25 cell culture flasks and incubated at 37°C in a 5% CO_2 atmosphere. The medium was replaced according to the rate of cell growth. When cells reached confluence, the hEMSCPCs were deplated using 0.25% trypsin-0.02% EDTA and passaged at 1:3. Cultures were observed and photographed using an inverted microscope (Leica DMIRB, Germany).

2.2. Pre-Induction Culture of hEMSCPCs in NSC Medium

For pre-induction, hEMSCPCs were deplated and suspended in NSC medium consisting of 96% DMEM/F12 (GIBCO, USA), 2% B27 (GIBCO, USA), 20 ng/ml bFGF (PERPOTECH, USA), 20 ng/ml epidermal growth factor (EGF) (PERPOTECH, USA), 2 ng/ml SCF (PERPOTECH, USA), and 1% MEM NEAA (100 × solution, GIBCO, USA). Cell suspensions (8 ml of 1.0×10^4 cells/ml) were replated in T-25 cell culture flasks and incubated at 37°C under 5% CO_2. The medium was replaced everyday. Cultures were observed and photographed as described above.

2.3. Differentiation of hEMSCPCs in Conditioned Differentiation Medium

After 6 days, the NSC medium was replaced with a conditioned differentiation medium consisting of 88% DMEM/F12 (GIBCO, USA), 10% FBS (Si Jiqing Ltd., China), 20 ng/ml bFGF (PERPOTECH, USA), 20 ng/ml EGF (PERPOTECH, USA), and 1% MEM NEAA (100 × solution, GIBCO, USA). Cells were incubated for 1 or 3 weeks depending on the experiment. In addition, hEMSCPCs cultured in growth medium but not pre-induced in NSC medium were cultured in differentiation medium as a control. Cultures were observed and photographed under an inverted microscope (Leica DMIRB, Germany). The hEMSCPCs pre-induced in the NSC medium grew slender projections during differentiation, so some cultures were plated at lower density (1.0×10^3 cells/ml) to aid in morphological observation.

2.4. Subculturing for Immunofluorescence and CM-Dil Staining

To detect the expression of cell-specific markers in hEMSCPCs during differentiation, cells were seeded onto cover slips and immunostained (below). Other cultures were labeled with CM-DiI to observe cell-cell contacts. Seeded cover slips were divided into five groups of 10 slides each. The hEMSCPCs cultured in the growth medium but not pre-induced by NSC medium constituted group A (GM, control). The hEMSCPCs cultured in growth medium and then pre-induced in the NSC medium for six days constituted group B (GM + NSC). Human EMSCPCs cultured in growth medium, pre-induced in NSC medium for six days, and then cultured in the conditioned differentiation medium for three weeks were group C (GM + NSC + CM 3 weeks). Human EMSCPCs cultured in the growth medium but not pre-induced in the NSC medium for six days before culture in the conditioned differentiation medium for three weeks were group D (GM + CM 3 weeks) and served as the control for group C. Group E consisted of hEMSCPCs cultured in growth medium, pre-induced in the NSC medium for six days, and then cultured in the conditioned differentiation medium for one week (GM + NSC + CM 1 week). At the beginning, cell densities of group A and group B were adjusted to 1.0×10^4 cells/ml, while those of groups C, D, and E were adjusted to 1.0×10^3 cells/ml for improved morphological observation of differentiating cells. Human EMSCPCs suspensions were plated onto sterile 22×22 mm^2 cover slips in 35 mm culture dishes. Each culture dish contained one hEMSCPCs cover slip. All cultures were incubated at 37°C under 5% CO_2. After the treatments described above, cover slips were collected for staining. Groups A, B, C, and D cells were stained by immunofluorescence and group E cultures were labeled with CM-DiI.

2.5. CM-Dil Labeling of the Differentiating hEMSCPCs

Cells were labeled with CM-DiI rather than processed for electron microscopy (EM) because EM fixation and processing/staining tend to cause contraction of processes [40,41]. Furthermore, EM is laborious and expensive. In contrast, CM-DiI is a lipid-soluble biomembrane stain that allows for clear visualization of cell morphology and cell-cell contacts [42].

Ten hEMSCPCs-seeded cover slips of group E (defined above) were collected, washed twice in PBS, and stained with 5 μl/ml CM-DiI (Molecular Probes, USA) in 200 μl PBS for 3 min at 37°C. Stained cover slips were washed twice quickly in PBS and then fixed in 4% paraformaldehyde for 40 min. The nuclei were counterstained by Hoechst (Sigma, USA) for 5 min at room temperature (RT). Slides were then treated by an anti-fade solution (Applygen, China) and imaged under a laser confocal scanning microscope (Zeiss, Germany). Ten different visual fields were observed in each cover slip.

2.6. Immunofluorescence Staining of hEMSCPCs Cultured *in Vitro*

Immunofluorescence staining was used to detect the expression of cell-specific antigens in hEMSCPCs cultured *in vitro*. The hEMSCPCs-seeded cover slips of groups A, B, C, and D were collected and fixed in 4% paraformaldehyde for 15 min, permeabilized in 0.3% Triton-X for 15 min, and then incubated at 37°C for 40 min in the following primary antibodies: human nestin, MAP2, synapsin I (Abcam, USA), vimentin (ZSGB-BIO, China), β-III tubulin (Millipore, USA), and GFAP (Eptomics, USA). Slides were then incubated in secondary antibodies, either Cy3-conjugated goat anti-mouse (Millipore, USA) or FITC-conjugated goat anti-rabbit (Southern Biotech, USA) for 30 min at RT. The nuclei were stained by Hoechst (Sigma, USA) for 5 min at RT, and then all slides were treated with an anti-fade solution (Applygen, China) and imaged under a laser confocal scanning microscope (Zeiss, Germany). Ten different visual fields were observed in each cover slip.

2.7. Flow Cytometry

Flow cytometry was used to quantify the expression of cell-specific markers in GM + NSC 4 days and GM hEMSCPCs groups. Both direct labeling and indirect labeling were used. Antibodies used for direct labeling were specific for human CD73 and its PE-iso-type control (BD, USA). Primary antibodies used for indirect labeling were specific for human nestin (Abcam, USA), vimentin (ZSGB-BIO, China), MAP2, and GFAP (Abcam, USA). The secondary antibodies were R-PE-conjugated goat anti-mouse and FITC-conjugated goat anti-rabbit (Southern Biotech, USA). Fix and Perm Cell Permeabilization reagents (Invitrogen, USA) were used for labeling intracellular antigens. Cell suspensions were stained and counted by flow cytometry according to the manufacturer's directions. Cell suspensions treated with secondary antibodies but not primary antibodies served as iso-type controls for indirect labeling. Cell suspendsions were tested immediately by flow cytometry (BD FACSAria^{TM}, USA) using FCS Express V3 software for data analysis. The positive value of iso-type controls was maintained at 0% to 1%.

Prior to cell transplantation *in vivo* (below), the expression levels of immunogenic markers (HLA-I and HLA-DR) in GM + NSC 4 days and GM hEMSCPCs were first detected by direct labeling and flow cytometry. Cell suspensions were treated with antibodies specific for human HLA-I (Invitrogen, USA), HLA-DR, and their FITC-iso-type control (BD, USA). Protocols were in accordance with the manufacturer's directions.

2.8. Transplantation of hEMSCPCs into the Vitreous Cavities of Nude Mice

The retina, an extension of the central nervous system containing a variety of highly differentiated cell types, was chosen to provide the internal microenvironment for hEMSCPCs differentiation. Human EMSCPCs were transplanted into the vitreous cavities of nude mice, and migration and differentiation were observed after four weeks.

The GM + NSC 4 days and GM cultures were termed groups A and B in the transplantation study. Before transplantation, both groups were labeled by CM-DiI (Molecular Probes, USA) according to the manufacturer's instructions. In addition, one 500 μl sample from each cell suspension labeled by CM-DiI was analyzed by flow cytometry to test CM-DiI labeling efficiency. Cell suspensions (1×10^7 cells/ml) with high labeling efficiency were immediately injected into the eyes of nude mice.

Sixteen 6-week-old BLAB/c nude mice of both genders were provided by the Laboratory Animal Center, Sun Yat-sen University (Quality certificate number: 0061839). The mice were cared for in accordance with the Regulations on Administration of Experimental Animals in Guangdong Province, China. They were housed in the specific pathogen-free (SPF) area of the Ophthalmology Animal Experimental Center, ZhongShan Ophthalmic Center, Sun Yat-sen University, with a 12 h light-dark cycle (23°C - 25°C, humidity 55%). These transplantation experiments were approved by the Laboratory Animal Administration and Ethics Committee of Zhongshan Ophthalmic Center, Sun Yat-sen University (No. 2010-024). The 16 nude mice were randomly divided into three groups (group A, B, and C), each with a 1:1 sex ratio. The right eyes of all group A (n = 6) mice were injected with hEMSCPCs that had been pre-induced in the NSC medium for four days, while the right eyes of group B were injected with hEMSCPCs cultured in the growth medium but not pre-induced by NSC medium. The remaining four mice (group C) served as normal controls.

Before transplantation, experimental mice were anesthetized by intraperitoneal injection of 4.3% chloral hydrate (0.01 ml per 1 g body weight) obtained from the Ophthalmologic Hospital, Sun Yat-sen University. Tobramycin eye drops were used to disinfect the experimental eye, followed by dicaine hydrochloride eye drops (both drugs obtained from the Ophthalmologic Hospital, Sun Yat-sen University) for superficial anesthesia. A 1-ml-injector needle was used to pierce the central cornea and drain part of the aqueous humor to lower the intraocular pressure. Under an operating microscopy (Topcon, Japan), a second 1-ml injector containing 10 μl of either cell suspension (pre-induced with NSC medium or untreated) was placed 1 mm outside the corneoscleral junction on the temporal side. The needle penetrated at a 15°C acute angle relative to the eyeball coronal plane. When the needle reached the vitreous cavity, cell suspendsions were injected. The needle was immediately withdrawn at the first signs of eyeball puffing. The experimental eye was then washed with tobramycin eye drops, followed by tobramycin eye ointment. All procedures were performed in the SPF area operating room. Appropriate body temperature was maintained during the operation and intraoperative animal care conformed to institutional guidelines. After mice regained consciousness, they were sent back to the feeding room. To prevent infection, tobramycin eye drops were applied three times daily for three days after the operation.

2.9. Frozen Eyeball Sectioning and Immunofluorescence Staining

Four weeks after cell transplantation, all the mice were anesthetized by intraperitoneal injection of 4.3% chloral hydrate and sacrificed by cervical dislocation. All right eyes were enucleated, frozen in OCT embedding compound (Sakura, USA), and stored at –20°C before cryostat sectioning at 6 μm on a freezing microtome (Leica, Germany). Sections were then processed for immunofluorescence labeling as described (see Immunofluorescence staining of hEMSCPCs cultured *in vitro*). Primary antibodies were specific for human nestin, MAP2, rhodopsin (Abcam, USA), *β*-III tubulin (Sigma, USA), and GFAP (Epitomics, USA). An FITC-conjugated goat anti-rabbit antibody (Southern Biotech, USA) was used for fluorescence tagging. The migration and differentiation of the transplanted hEMSCPCs in nude mice were examined by laser confocal scanning microscopy (Zeiss, Germany). Ten different visual fields were observed in each section.

2.10. Statistical Analysis

Analysis of variance (ANOVA) with repeated measures was used to compare treatment means. A value of $P < 0.05$ was considered statistically different. The SPSS v13.0 software package was used for all statistical analyses.

3. RESULTS

3.1. Morphology of hEMSCPCs Cultured in Growth Medium

When cultured in growth medium, hEMSCPCs appeared as small spindle-shaped cells that adhered to the bottoms of culture flasks in a monolayer arranged in a vortex pattern (**Figures 1(A)** and **(B)**). They proliferated rapidly in growth medium; when seeded at 1.0×10^4 cells/ml × 8 ml in T-25 plastic culture flasks, they reached confluence in two days [39].

3.2. Changes in hEMSCPCs Morphology during Pre-Induction in NSC Medium

To direct hEMSCPCs toward the neuronal lineage, we provided a conducive environment using a neural stem cell (NSC) medium. One day after culture in NSC medium, the hEMSCPCs somata aggregated to form small dense light-reflective spheres that were fully or partly adherent to the bottoms of the flasks. A few small spindle-shaped cells began to stretch out from the edges of the spheres (**Figures 1(C)** and **(D)**). After three days in NSC medium, many spindle-shaped cells stretched out from the edges of the spheres and formed strongly light reflective rosette-shaped clusters at the edges (**Figures 1(E)** and **(F)**). As days went on, the spindle-shaped cells stretched out further and the rosettes enlarged (**Figures 1(G)** and **(H)**).

3.3. Changes in hEMSCPCs Morphology during Culture in Conditioned Differentiation Medium as Revealed by Light Microscopy

At day 6, NSC medium was replaced with a conditioned differentiation medium. Within one day, most cells began to grow one or more slender projections that resembled neurites (**Figures 2(B)- (D)**). Three days later, as these projections became longer and continued to extend, contacts were formed between cells (**Figures 2(E)-(G)**). After one week in conditioned medium, the projections continued to extend and branches emerged at the ends (**Figure 2(H)**). In contrast, hEMSCPCs cultured in the growth medium but not in NSC medium showed no obvious changes in morphology during incubation in the conditioned differentiation medium (**Figure 2(A)**).

3.4. Changes in hEMSCPCs Morphology during Culture in Conditioned Differentiation Medium as Revealed by CM-DiI Labeling

To examine cell morphology and cell-cell contacts in detail, cultures were stained with the membrane dye CM-DiI and viewed under laser confocal scanning microscopy. The profiles of differentiated hEMSCPCs were clearly distinguished by CM-DiI, including cell bodies and slender projections that exhibited inflated ends or even claw-like ends (**Figures 3(A)-(C)**). Many of these CM-DiI-labeled differentiated cells contacted each other, either through projection-soma or projection-projection contacts (**Figures 3(A)-(C)**).

3.5. Immunofluorescence Staining of Cultured hEMSCPCs

Immunofluorescence staining was used to detect the expression of cell-specific markers during culture in the three culture media (growth, NSC, and conditioned differentiation media). When cultured only in the growth medium, hEMSCPCs were positive for the NSC marker nestin as well as the neural precursor cell and mesenchymal cell marker vimentin (**Figures 3(D)** and **(E)**), but negative for neural cell markers β-III tubulin, microtubule-associated protein-2 (MAP2), glial fibrillary acidic protein (GFAP), and the synaptic marker synapsin I (data not shown). After pre-induction in the NSC medium, the expression of these markers was not significantly changed, though cells remained positive for nestin and vimentin (**Figure 3(F)**). Consistent with the marked morphological transformation (**Figures 2** and **3(A)-(C)**), cells cultured in the conditioned differentiation medium following pre-induction in NSC medium expressed neural cell markers β-III tubulin, MAP2, GFAP, and synapsin I (**Figures 3(G)-3(J)**). In contrast, hEMSCPCs cultured in the growth medium but not pre-induced in NSC medium did not express these neural cell markers during culture in conditioned differentiation medium (data not shown).

3.6. Flow Cytometry Analysis

Flow cytometry was used to quantify the different protein expression phenotypes. During culture in growth medium, most hEMSCPCs stably expressed the mesen-

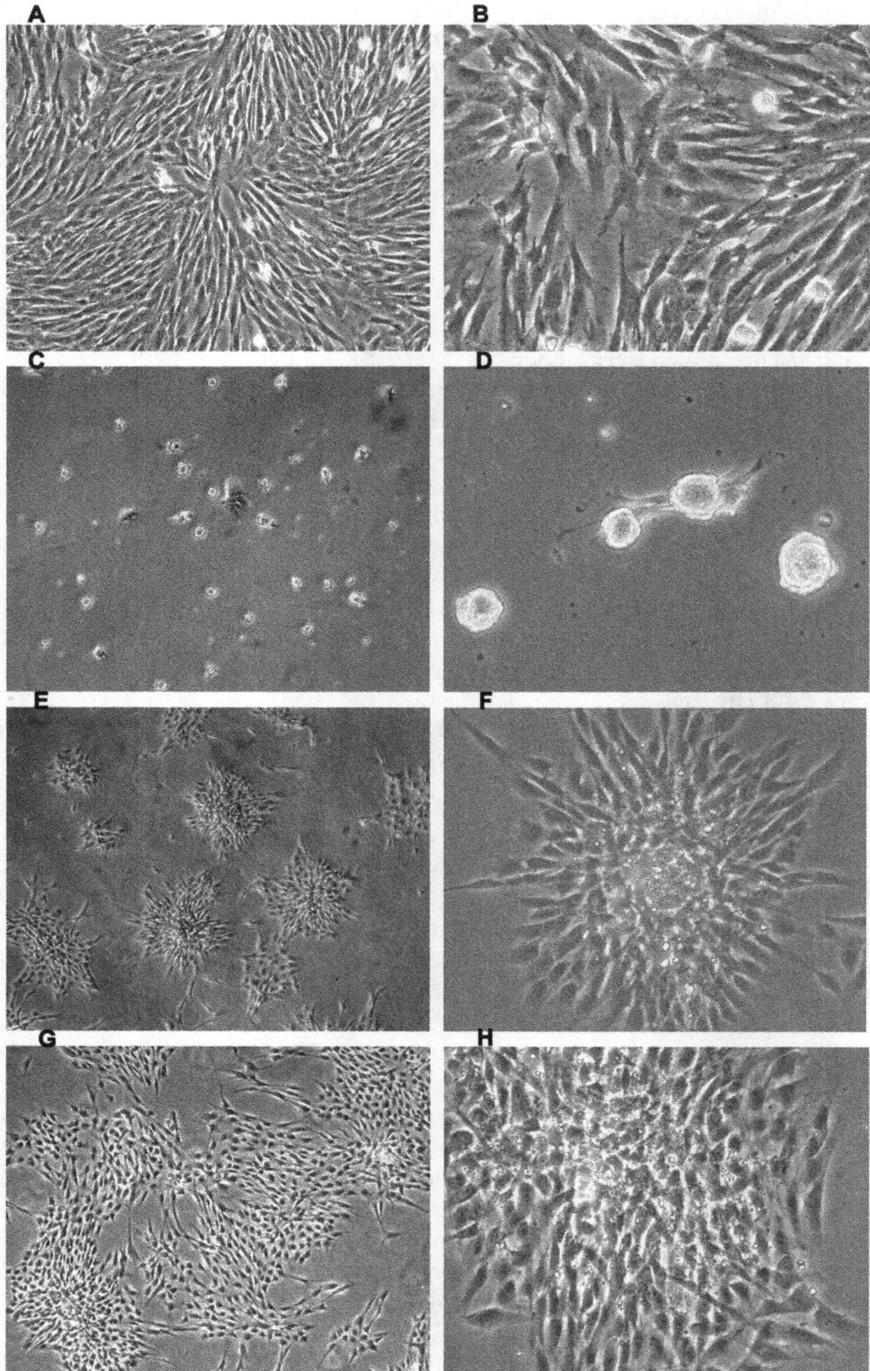

Figure 1. Morphological changes of hEMSCPCs during culture in growth medium and NSC medium. (A) and (B) The morphology of hEMSCPCs cultured in growth medium. Plated cells formed monolayers in a vortex pattern within two days ((A), magnification ×50; (B), magnification ×200). (C)-(H) Change in morphology during pre-induction in NSC medium. One day after changing to the NSC medium, hEMSCPCs formed small dense spheres and a few small spindle-shaped cells began to stretch out from the edges ((C), magnification ×50; (D), magnification ×200). After three days in NSC medium, many spindle-shaped cells stretched out from the spheres ((E), magnification ×50; (F), magnification ×200). After six days, many cells were observed migrating outward ((G), magnification ×50; (H), magnification ×200).

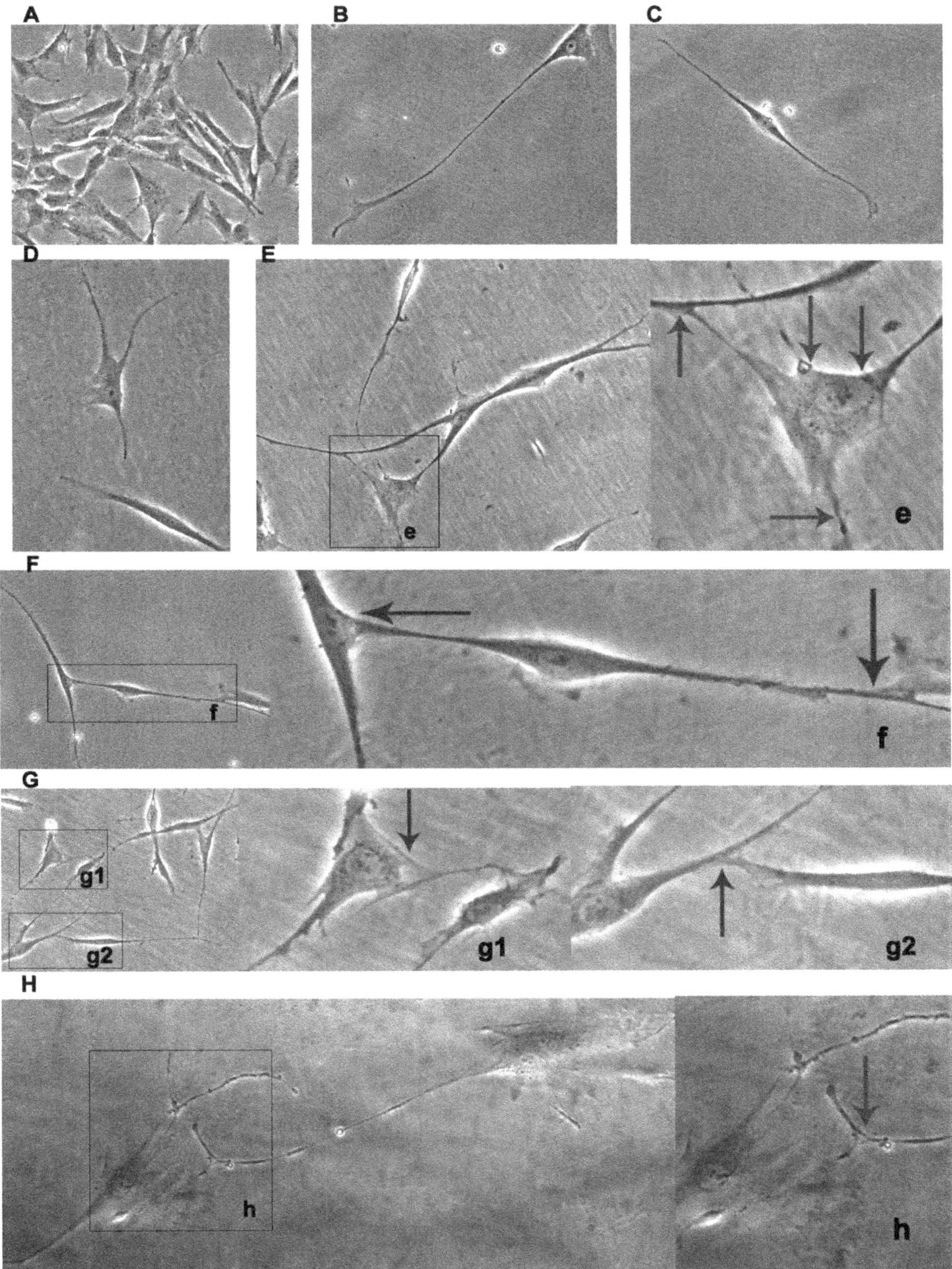

Figure 2. Morphology of hEMSCPCs during culture in conditioned differentiation medium. (A) Human EMSCPCs not pre-induced in NSC medium showed no significant changes in morphology when cultured in the conditioned differentiation medium (magnification ×200). (B)-(H) After one day in the conditioned differentiation medium, hEMSCPCs that were pre-induced began to grow one (B), two (C) or more (D) slender projections (magnification ×200); (E)-(G) After three days in conditioned differentiation medium, these projections were longer and continued to extend toward neighboring cells. Contacts (red arrows) were formed between cells (magnification ×200; (e), (f), (g1), and (g2) are the magnified boxed areas in panels (E), (F), and (G). (H) After one week, the projections continued to extend and branches (red arrows) formed at the ends (magnification ×100, h is the magnified region in (H)).

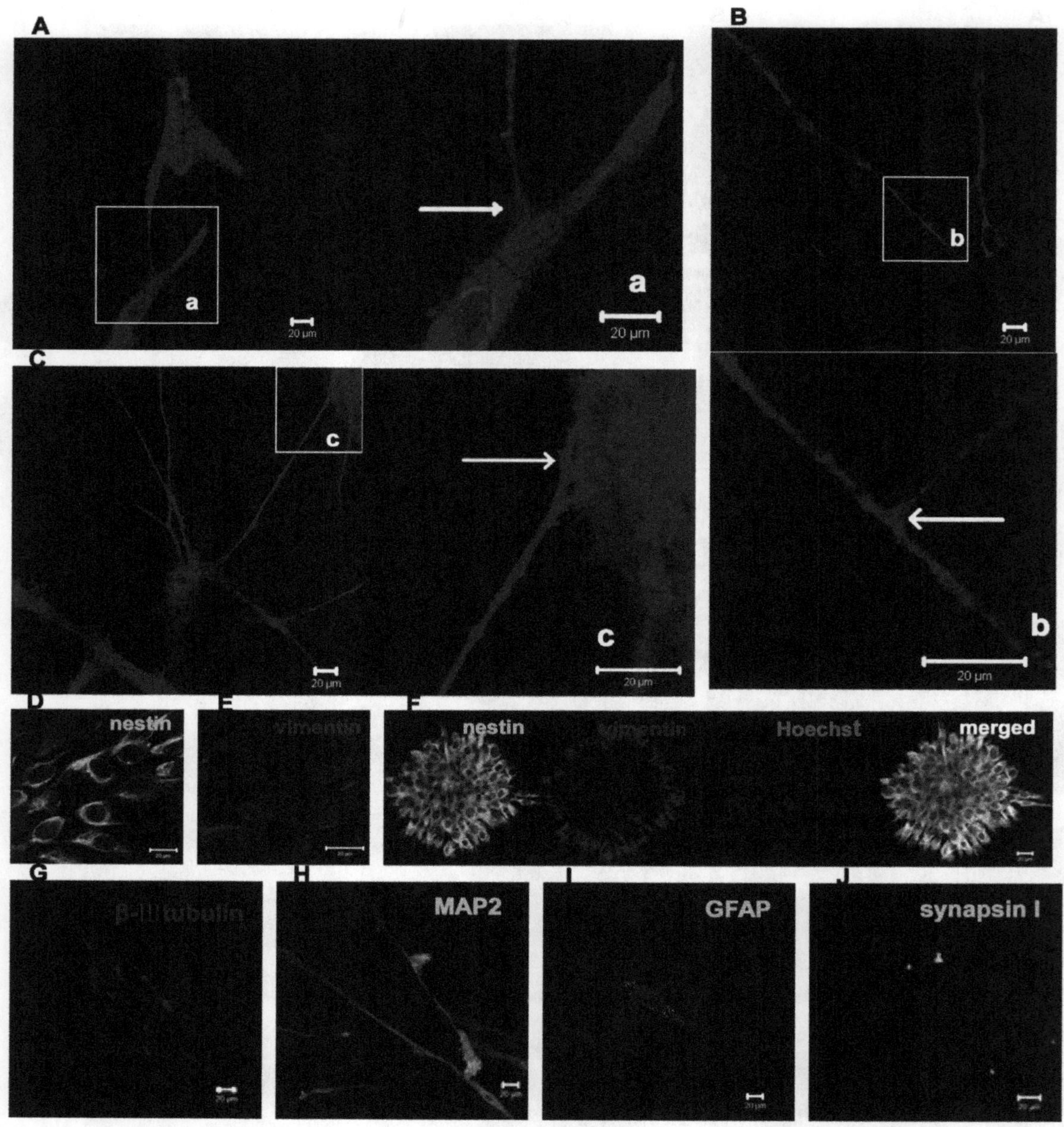

Figure 3. CM-DiI labeling of differentiating hEMSCPCs and immunofluorescence staining of hEMSCPCs cultured *in vitro*. (A)-(C) The profile of differentiated hEMSCPCs labeled by red CM-DiI, showing cell bodies and slender projections with inflated or claw-like ends (white arrows in (C)). These CM-DiI-labeled differentiated cells contacted each other and CM-DiI-labeled cell membranes could be seen between these contacts (white arrows) ((a), (b), and (c) are high magnification zones from panels (A), (B), and (C)). (D)-(E) When cultured in growth medium, many hEMSCPCs were positive for nestin ((D), green) and vimentin ((E), red). (F) After pre-induction in NSC medium, cells were also positive for nestin (green) and vimentin (red). (G)-(J) Cells pre-induced for six days could express the neural cell markers β-III tubulin ((G), red), MAP2 ((H), green), GFAP ((I), green), and the synaptic marker synapsin I ((J), green) during culture in differentiation medium. Nuclei were counterstained with blue Hoechst. All scale bars are 20 μM.

chymal stem cell marker CD73 (94.7%) and the NSC marker nestin (81.4%). A smaller fraction expressed the neural precursor cell and mesenchymal cell marker vimentin (30.8%), while none expressed the neural cell markers MAP2 or GFAP (**Figure 4(A)**). Daily assessment of marker expression during seven days of pre-induction in NSC medium showed that CD73 expression was maintained, while MAP2 and GFAP were still not expressed (**Figure 4(A)**). No statistically significant difference in the expression of CD73, MAP2, and GFAP was found between days in NSC medium (n = 3, $P >$ 0.05) (**Figure 4(A)**). During the first three days of pre-induction, the expression levels of nestin (80.5% ± 0.98% of all cells) and vimentin (34.5% ± 1.08%) were stable (n = 3, $P > 0.05$). From day 3 to day 7, however, the expression of nestin and vimentin fluctuated. Nestin expression was 74.5% ± 0.91% on day 4, 71.2% ± 1.09% on day 5, and 79.6% ± 0.86% on day 6, before decreasing again on day 7 (60.9% ± 1.39%). Vimentin expression first increased from day 3 to 4 (44.5% ± 2.05%), decreased from day 4 to 5 (20.5% ± 1.18%), increased from day 5 to 6 (26.6% ± 1.68%), then decreased again from day 6 to 7 (18.5% ± 0.68%). Changes in expression of both proteins were statistically significant between days (n = 3, $P < 0.001$) **(Figure 4(A))**.

Prior to cell transplantation *in vivo*, the expression of the immunogenic markers HLA-I and HLA-DR were also detected in hEMSCPCs by flow cytometry. When cultured in the growth medium, the hEMSCPCs moderately expressed HLA-I (35.3%) but not HLA-DR (**Figure 4(B)**). After pre-induction for four days, they continued to moderately express HLA-I (38.4%) but not HLA-DR, indicating that hEMSCPCs retained the same immunogenic status in NSC medium (**Figure 4(C)**). In addition, hEMSCPCs were also stained with CM-DiI prior to cell transplantation *in vivo.* Staining efficiency was assessed by flow cytometry and revealed a labeling rate of 99.7% (**Figure 4(D)**).

3.7. Migration and Differentiation of Transplanted hEMSCPCs in the Retinas of Nude Mice

To examine neural differentiation *in vivo*, CM-DiI-stained hEMSCPCs were implanted into the vitreous cavities of nude mice. Two groups of cells were transplanted, hEMSCPCs pre-induced in the NSC medium for four days (group A) and hEMSCPCs cultured in the

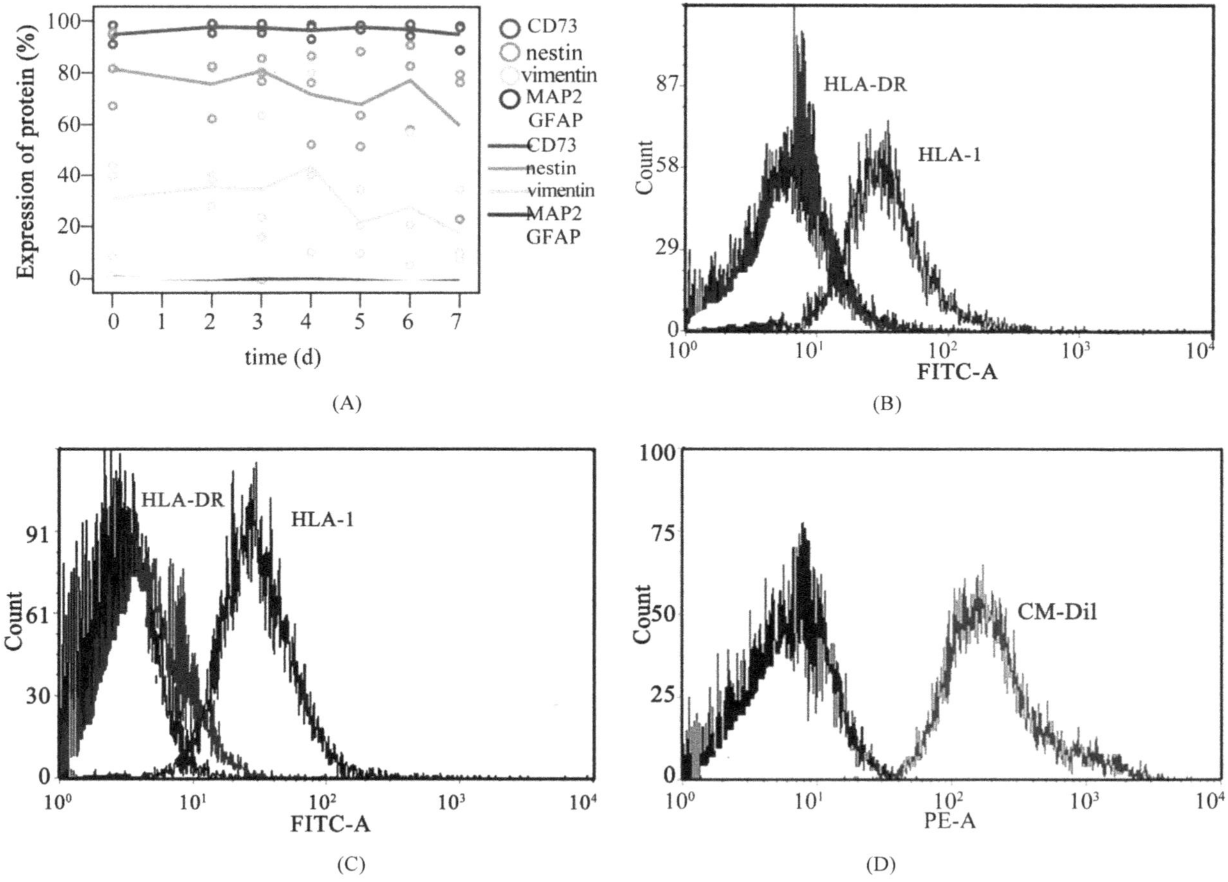

Figure 4. Flow cytometry analysis of cell-specific marker expression. (A) Cell-specific markers (CD73-blue, nestin-cyan, vimentin-gray, MAP2-purple, GFAP-yellow) expressed by hEMSCPCs. During seven days in NSC medium, most hEMSCPCs stably expressed CD73 and nestin, few expressed vimentin, while none expressed MAP2 or GFAP. (B) In growth medium, hEMSCPCs moderately expressed HLA-I (35.3% of cells) but not HLA-DR. (C) After four days in NSC medium, hEMSCPCs still moderately expressed HLA-I (38.4%) but not HLA-DR. (D) The efficiency of CM-DiI labeling prior to transplantation was up to 99.7%.

growth medium but not pre-induced in the NSC medium (group B). Cells of the two groups were separately transplanted into the vitreous cavities of nude mice. Four weeks later, migration and differentiation in the retina were assessed by immunostaining in frozen sections of the eyes. The retinas of normal uninjected nude mice were clear and regular, with no fluorescent (red- or green-labeled) cells (**Figure 5(A)**). In mice injected with group A cells, five of six experimental eyes showed migration of transplanted cells after four weeks (**Figures 5(B)-(F)**). In addition, pre-induced CM-DiI-stained cells expressed the NSC marker nestin and the neural cell markers β-III tubulin and GFAP (**Figures 5(I)-(K)**), but not MAP2 (data not shown). In mice injected with group B cells, however, only one of six experimental eyes showed migration of transplanted cells (**Figures 5(G)** and **(H)**) as well as expression of β-III tubulin (**Figure 5(L)**). No nestin-, MAP2-, or GFAP-positive cells were found (data not shown). Cells of group A exhibited superior migration and differentiation compared to cells of group B. In both experimental groups, no transplanted cells expressed the photoreceptor cell marker rhodopsin (data not shown). The transplanted cells that migrated into the retinas presented as either single cells or as agglomerates (**Figures 5(B)-(H)**). Most cells concentrated in the subretinal cavities, the retinal pigment epithelium (RPE) layer, and other nearby areas (**Figures 5(D)-(F)**, and **5(H)**). Thus, injected cells migrated across all retinal layers to reach the RPE.

4. DISCUSSION

The shear size and reparative capacity of human skin makes it an ideal source of pluripotent cells for research and possible autologous cell-based therapies. As a first step toward utilizing these pluripotent cells for neural regeneration therapy, we developed a two step-culture method that gradually induced the appearance of a neural-like morphology and the expression of several neural-specific cell markers. When introduced into the retina, cells from the first culture step (pre-induction) migrated cross multiple cell layers and expressed neural-specific cell markers. Although they were not functionally integrated into the healthy retina (at least after four weeks), it is possible that these pre-neural-like cells may be induced to replenish lost cells in the degenerating or damage retina, such as photoreceptor cells. The capacity of these hEMSCPCs to express neuron-like and glia-like phenotypes *in vitro* and *in vivo* suggests that these cells are a potential source for neural stem cells to repair damaged neural tissue.

A number of research groups have isolated precursor cells from skin and shown that these cells can differentiate into multiple cell types under appropriate conditions. Miller *et al.* [27,31,43-49] isolated precursors from neonatal mammalian skin that could differentiate into other cell types, and even mediate regeneration after injury in animal models. They retained a normal karyotype and capacity to differentiate even after regular passage for one year *in vitro*, but pluripotency was markedly lower in skin-derived precursors from adult mammals. Furthermore, the biosafety of adult-derived cells is unknown. Katsuoka *et al.* [33-35,50-52] isolated a population of stem cells from mammalian dermal hair-follicles that could also differentiate into other cell types and promote regeneration after injury, but they were difficult to isolate in sufficient quantities for clinical applications. In contrast, the hEMSCPCs that we isolated from adult human epidermis were easily obtained in large quantities, could be continuously passaged over fifty times without changes to the normal karyotype, and demonstrate good biosafety *in vitro* [39].

The growth patterns of hEMSCPCs changed markedly when cultured in NSC medium; individual cells coalesced into dense, highly light-reflective spheres. Spindle-shaped cells educed from these spheres began to spread out so that the aggregates resembled neural rosettes. Once these cells were cultured in a conditioned differentiation medium, many differentiated into cells with a neural phenotype. Some cells grew slender projections with inflated or claw-like ends that contacted the soma or projections of other cells as revealed by the cell tracker CM-DiI, a lipid soluble biomembrane stain that stably labels growing cells for clear imaging of fine morphological features [40-42]. Many also expressed neuronal or glial markers, including β-III tubulin, MAP2, GFAP, and synapsin I. Flow cytometry and immunofluorescence staining showed that hEMSCPCs expressed the NSC marker nestin, the neural precursor and mesenchymal cell marker vimentin, but not the neural cell markers β-III tubulin, MAP2, GFAP, or synapsin I during sequential culture in the growth medium and NSC medium. However, expression of neural cell markers was dependent on pre-induction in NSC medium, as hEMSCPCs cultured only in differentiation medium did not express neural markers (β-III tubulin, MAP2, GFAP, or synapsin I). Moreover, uninduced cells showed inferior migration and differentiation compared to pre-induced cells after transplantation into the vitreous cavities of nude mice. Thus, pre-induction did not markedly alter neural marker expression in hEMSCPCs but was necessary to allow differentiation in a special conditioned medium and in the mouse eye (part of the central nervous system).

Flow cytometry was used to quantify the expression of cell-specific markers. The cell surface glucoprotein CD73 is a marker for mesenchymal stem cells [53]. Nestin is a class VI intermediate filament protein once thought to be a specific marker of NSCs, but recent re-

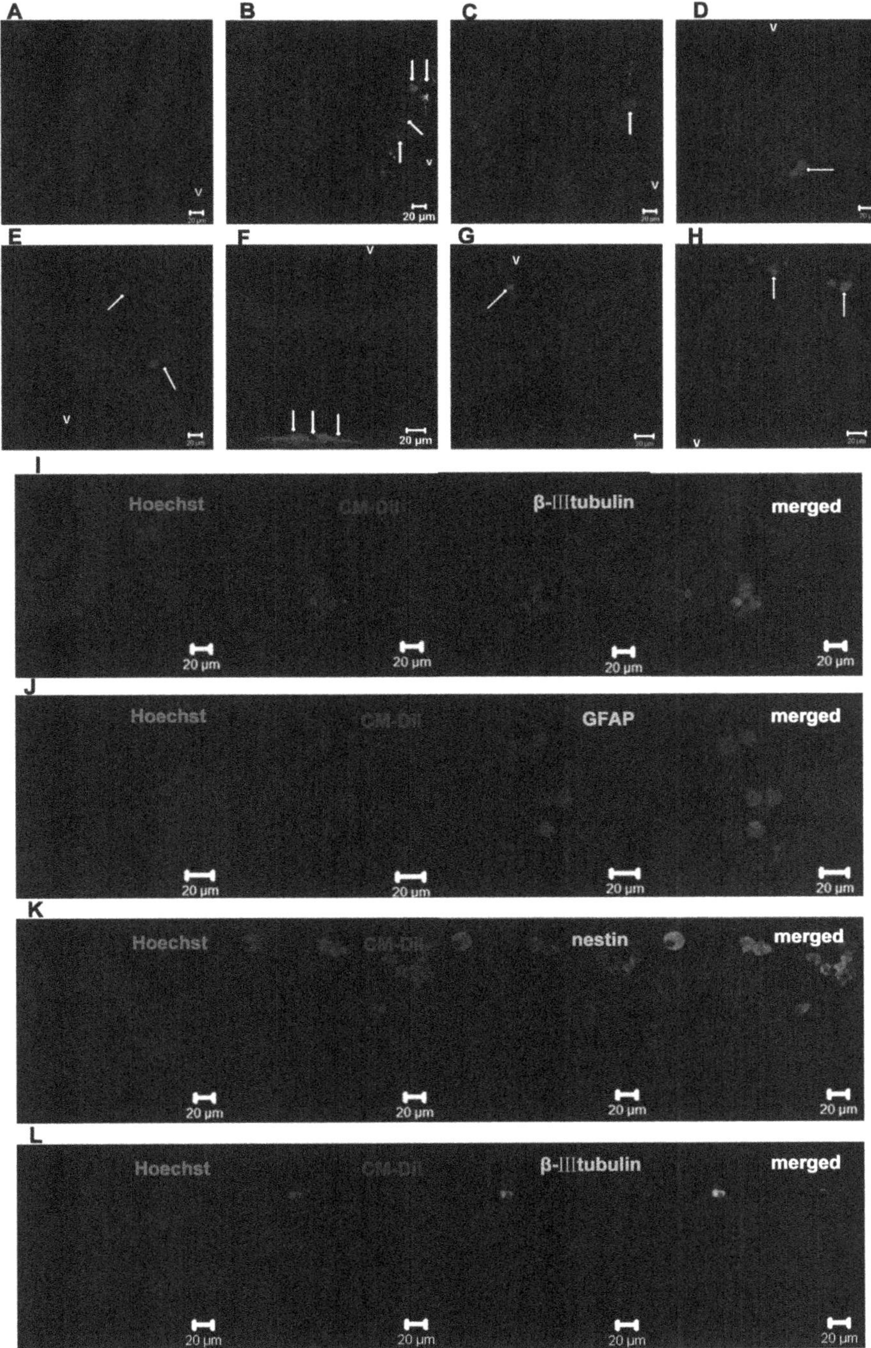

Figure 5. Migration and differentiation of transplanted hEMSCPCs in the retinas of nude mice. (A) The retinas of normal nude mice were clear and regular, and no red- or green-labeled cells were observed. (B)-(L) Four weeks after transplantation into the vitreous cavities of nude mice, many pre-induced hEMSCPCs (white arrows) had migrated into the retinal ganglion cell layer (B), (C), the sub-retinal space (D), (E), and the retinal pigment epithelium layer (E), (F). In addition, pre-induced cells expressed β-III tubulin (I), GFAP (J), and nestin (K). Transplanted cells that had not been pre-induced by NSC medium *in vitro* (white arrows) could migrate into the retinal ganglion cell layer (G) and the sub-retinal space (H), and express β-III tubulin (L). "V" represents the vitreous cavities or nearby areas. Nuclei were counterstained with blue Hoechst. All scale bars represent 20 μM.

ports indicated that it is also expressed by multipotent precursor cells and that expression correlates with the potential for proliferation, migration, and differentiation [54,55]. Vimentin is a class III intermediate filament protein and a marker for neural precursor cells and mesenchymal-derived cells [56-59]. MAP2 is a mature neuronal marker, while the intermediate filament protein GFAP is expressed almost exclusively by astrocytes. Flow cytometry showed that the expression levels of these markers by hEMSCPCs were not significantly changed during culture in growth medium or brief (2 - 3 day) culture in NSC medium. However, from the 3rd to 7th day in NSC medium, expression of nestin and vimentin began to fluctuate, possibly indicating the beginning of a phenotypic transition. However, hEMSCPCs pre-induced in NSC medium grew slender projections that could be easily sheared off the soma during harvesting for flow cytometry, so this fluctuation in expression may reflect variable loss of markers localized to processes. A more accurate determination of marker expression patterns during NSC culture will require the use of alternative methods like real time PCR or Western blotting.

Approximately the same percentage of pre-induced and uninduced hEMSCPCs expressed HLA-I, indicating that these cells have a stable immunogenicity. Nude mice were chosen for hEMSCPC transplantation experiments because they are immunologically defective and so would not generate an immune response to transplanted cells. Four weeks after injection of hEMSCPCs, both induced and uninduced CM-DiI-labeled cells had migrated primarily to the subretinal space, retinal pigment epithetlium layer, and other nearby areas. The reasons for this selective migration are still obscure. Both hEMSCPCs and retinal pigment epithelium originate from the ectoderm, and this homology may have allowed for better survival of transplanted hEMSCPCs. The subretinal cavity may also accumulate transplanted cells even in immunologically active mice because it is an immunoprivileged zone. While both induced and uninduced cells migrated, pre-induced cells showed superior migration and neural differentiation.

There were differences in neural differentiation *in vitro* versus *in vivo*. In contrast to observations *in vitro*, the mature neuron marker MAP-2 was not expressed by either group of transplanted hEMSCPCs, although this might reflect the short transplantation time (four weeks). In addition to common markers like MAP-2, transplanted cells did not express retina-specific markers. For example, rhodopsin, a marker of retinal photoreceptors, was not expressed by transplanted hEMSCPCs that migrated into the retina, possibly because the healthy retina releases no factors that would induce differenttiation. A longer transplantation time or induction of growth factor expression may be required for full expression of neural markers, but these questions require further study.

The epidermis is easily harvested, so hEMSCPCs may be a productive source of cells for autologous cell-based therapy against neurological diseases. Our results show that hEMSCPCs possess the capacity to differentiate into neural-like cells if pre-induced in NSC medium. Whether hEMSCPCs can replenish endogenous neural cells after induction and differentiation requires further study. To reach this goal, further studies are required to understand the neural lineage capacity of these cells, including tests of differentiation efficiency and function *in vitro*, and to assess the biological safety of these cells *in vivo*. Experiments testing the restorative efficacy of these cells in animal models of neurodegenerative diseases are clearly warranted.

5. ACKNOWLEDGEMENTS

We are grateful to members of the State Key Laboratory of Ophthalmology, Zhongshan Ophthalmic Center, Sun Yat-sen University, for discussion and advice. This work was supported by the Science and Technology Projects of Guangdong Province, China (2009B060600002, 2010B060500006).

REFERENCES

[1] Jiang, W. (2010) Neurology. 2nd Edition, People's Medical Publishing House, Beijing.

[2] Carsten, R.B. and Jens, C.S. (2004) Therapeutic strategies for neurodegenerative disorders: Emerging clues from Parkinson's disease. *Biological Psychiatry*, **56**, 213-216. doi:10.1016/j.biopsych.2003.12.025

[3] John, B.S. (2004) Pharmacotherapeutic approaches to the treatment of Alzheimer's disease. *Clinical Therapeutics*, **26**, 615-630. doi:10.1016/S0149-2918(04)90064-1

[4] Zhou, J.W. (2010) Recent progress in neurodegenerative disorder research in China. *Science China Life Sciences*, **53**, 348-355. doi:10.1007/s11427-010-0061-0

[5] Peng, L.S. and Li, C.R. (2009) RNA interference and neural degenerative diseases. *West China Medical Journal*, **21**, 1806-1808.

[6] William, J.M., Raymond, T.B., Joao, S., *et al.* (2010) Gene delivery of AAV2-neurturin for Parkinson's disease: A double-blind, randomised, controlled trial. *The Lancet Neurology*, **9**, 1164-1172. doi:10.1016/S1474-4422(10)70254-4

[7] Wu, J.J., Yu, W.B., Chen, Y., *et al.* (2010) Intrastriatal transplantation of GDNF-engineered BMSCs and its neuroprotection in Lactacystin-induced Parkinsonian Rat Model. *Neurochemical Research*, **35**, 495-502. doi:10.1007/s11064-009-0086-6

[8] William, J.M., Jill, L.O., Leonard, V., *et al.* (2008) Safety and tolerability of intraputaminal delivery of CERE-120 (adeno-associated virus serotype 2-neurturin) to patients with idiopathic Parkinson's disease: An open-label, phase

I trial. *The Lancet Neurology*, **7**, 400-408. doi:10.1016/S1474-4422(08)70065-6

[9] Kerri, S. (2010) Treatment frontiers. *Nature*, **466**, S15-S18. doi:10.1038/nature09476

[10] Jiao, J.W. (2010) Embryonic and adult neural stem cell research in China. *Science China Life Sciences*, **53**, 338-341. doi:10.1007/s11427-010-0070-z

[11] Stefano, P., Lucia, Z., Michela, D. and Gianvito, M. (2005) Neural stem cells and their use as therapeutic too in neurological disorders. *Brain Research Reviews*, **48**, 211-219. doi:10.1016/j.brainresrev.2004.12.011.

[12] Gu, Y., Hu, N., Liu, J., *et al.* (2010) Isolation and differentiation of neural stem/progenitor cells from fetal rat dorsal root ganglia. *Science China Life Sciences*, **53**, 1057-1064. doi:10.1007/s11427-010-4053-x

[13] Keun-Hwa, J., Kon, C., Soon-Tae, L., *et al.* (2008) Identification of neuronal outgrowth cells from peripheral blood of stroke patients. *Annals of Neurology*, **63**, 312-322. doi:10.1002/ana.21303

[14] Sarugaser, R., Ennis, J., Stanford, W.L. and Gianvito, M. (2009) Isolation, propagation, and characterization of human umbilical cord perivascular cells (HUCPVCs). *Methods in Molecular Biology*, **482**, 269-279. doi:10.1007/978-1-59745-060-7-17

[15] Lin-ya, H., Jia-lin, Y., Fang, L., *et al.* (2009) Synapse function of neuron-like cells induced from mesenchymal stem cells by *Salvia miltiorrhiza*. *Acta Academiae Medicinae Militaris Tertiae*, **31**, 144-147. doi:1000-5404(2009)02-0144-04

[16] Shi, Y.F., Hu, G.Z., Su, J.J., *et al.* (2010) Mesenchymal stem cells: A new strategy for immunosuppression and tissue repair. *Cell Research*, **20**, 510-518. doi:10.1038/cr.2010.44

[17] Wu, L., Chen, R.K., Yang, L., *et al.* (2009) Differentiation of adipose-derived stem cells into nerve stem cells across embryonic layer. *Fourth Military Medical University*, **30**, 70-72. doi:1000-2790(2009)01-0070-03

[18] Stefan, A., Helmut, K., Irina, S., *et al.* (2004) Neurally selected embryonic stem cells induce tumor formation after long-term survival following engraftment into the subretinal space. *Investigative Ophthalmology & Visual Science*, **45**, 4251-4255. doi:10.1167/iovs.03-1108

[19] Oscar, H.M. and Angela, N. (2010) Epithelial plasticity, stemness and pluripotency. *Cell Research*, **20**, 1086-1088. doi:10.1038/cr.2010.127

[20] Dengke, K.M., Bonaguidi, M.A., Ming, G.L. and Song, H.J. (2009) Adult neural stem cells in the mammalian central nervous system. *Cell Research*, **19**, 672-682. doi:10.1038/cr.2009.56

[21] Chase, L.G, Lakshmipathy, U, Solchaga, L.A., *et al.* (2010) A novel serum-free medium for the expansion of human mesenchymal stem cells. *Stem Cell Research & Therapy*, **1**, 8. doi:10.1186/scrt8

[22] Raymond, D.L., Shaomei, W., Bin, L., *et al.* (2007) Cells isolated from umbilical cord tissue rescue photoreceptors and visual functions in a rodent model of retinal disease. *Stem Cells*, **25**, 602-611. doi:10.1634/stemcells.2006-0308

[23] Andrew, J.H., Isabel, Z., Henry, H.T., *et al.* (2009) Human umbilical cord blood-derived mesenchymal stem cells do not differentiate into neural cell types or integrate into the retina after intravitreal grafting in neonatal rats. *Stem Cells and Development*, **18**, 399-409. doi:10.1089/scd.2008.0084

[24] Isabel, Z., Andrew, J.H., Faisal, A., *et al.* (2009) Umbilical cord blood mesenchymal stromal cells are neuroprotective and promote regeneration in a rat optic tract model. *Experimental Neurology*, **216**, 439-448. doi:10.1016/j.expneurol.2008.12.028

[25] Xue, G.S., Zhang, Y. and Qi, Z.L. (2008) Current research situation of adipose-derived stem cells and its application in tissue engineering. *Journal of Tissue Engineering and Reconstructive Surgery*, **4**, 174-176.

[26] Hideo, O., Ariane, R., Ce'cile, K., *et al.* (2001) Morphogenesis and renewal of hair follicles from adult multipotent stem cells. *Cell*, **104**, 233-245. doi:10.1016/S0092-8674(01)00208-2

[27] Jean, G.T., Mahnaz, A., Karl, J.L., *et al.* (2001) Isolation of multipotent adult stem cells from the dermis of mammalian skin. *Nature Cell Biology*, **3**, 778-786. doi:10.1038/ncb0901-778

[28] Young, H.E., Steele, T.A., Bray, R.A., *et al.* (2001) Human reserve pluripotent mesenchymal stem cells are present in the connective tissues of skeletal muscle and dermis derived from fetal, adult, and geriatric donors. *Anatomy & Physiology*, **264**, 51-62. doi:10.1002/ar.1128

[29] Shi, C. and Cheng, T. (2003) Effects of acute wound environment on the neonatal dermal multipotent cells. *Cells Tissues Organs*, **175**, 177-185. doi:10.1159/000074939

[30] Shih, D.T. (2005) Isolation and characterization of neurogenic mesenchymal stem cells in human scalp tissue. *Stem Cells*, **23**, 1012-1025. doi:10.1634/stemcells.2004-0125

[31] Jean, G.T., Ian, A.M., Darius, B. and Freda, D.M. (2005) Isolation and characterization of multipotent skin-derived precursors from human skin. *Stem Cells*, **23**, 727-737. doi:10.1634/stemcells.2004-0134

[32] Karl, J.L. Fernandes, I.A. McKenzie, Pleasantine, M. *et al.* (2004) A dermal niche for multipotent adult skin-derived precursor cells. *Nature Cell Biology*, **6**, 1082-1093. doi:10.1038/ncb1181

[33] Yasuyuki, A., Lingna, L., Kensei, K. and Robert, M.H. (2004) Multipotent hair follicle stem cells promote repair of spinal cord injury and recovery of walking function. *Cell Cycle*, **7**, 1865-1869. doi:10.4161/cc.7.12.6056

[34] Yasuyuki, A., Lingna, L., Kensei, K., Sheldon, P. and Robert, M.H. (2005) Multipotent nestin-positive, keratin-negative hair-follicle bulge stem cells can form neurons. *Proceedings of the National Academy of Sciences*, **102**, 5530-5534. doi:10.1073/pnas.0501263102

[35] Yasuyuki, A., Lingna, L., Raul, C., *et al.* (2005) Implanted hair follicle stem cells form Schwann cells that support repair of severed peripheral nerves. *Proceedings of the National Academy of Sciences*, **102**, 17734-17738. doi:10.1073/pnas.0508440102

[36] Patrizia, T., Jeff, W.M., Maria, G.B., *et al.* (2006) Brain

engraftment and therapeutic potential of stem/progenitor cells derived from mouse skin. *The Journal of Gene Medicine*, **8**, 506-513. doi:10.1002/jgm.866

[37] So, P.L. and Epstein, E.H. (2004) Adult stem cells: Capturing youth from a bulge. *Trends in Biotechnology*, **22**, 493-496. doi:10.1016/j.tibtech.2004.08.007

[38] Morasso, M.I. and Omic-Canic, M. (2005) Epidermal stem cells: The cradle of epidermal determination, differentiation and wound healing. *Biology of the Cell*, **97**, 173-183. doi:10.1042/BC20040098

[39] Huang, B., Li, K.J., Yu, J., *et al.* (2011) Generation of Human epidermis-derived mesenchymal stem cell-like pluripotent cells and their reprogramming in mouse chimeras. http://precedings.nature.com/documents/6016/version/1

[40] Yamamoto, N., Higashi, S. and Toyama, K. (1997) Stop and branch behaviors of geniculocortical axons: A time-lapse study in organotypic cocultures. *The Journal of Neuroscience*, **17**, 3653-3663.

[41] Cai, Q., Ji, M., Zhang, J., *et al.* (2011) Comparative study on glutamatergic synaptic connections in rat striatum with laser scanning confocal microscopy and electron microscopy. *Chinese Journal of Histochemistry and Cytochemistry*, **20**, 236-240.

[42] Matsubayashi, Y., Iwai, L. and Kawasaki, H. (2008) Fluorescent double-labeling with carbocyanine neuronal tracing and immunohistochemistry using a cholesterol-specific detergent digitonin. *Journal of Neuroscience Methods*, **174**, 71-81. doi:10.1016/j.jneumeth.2008.07.003

[43] Ian, A.M., Jeff, B., Jean, G.T., *et al.* (2006) Skin-derived precursors generate myelinating Schwann cells for the injured and dysmyelinated nervous system. *Journal of Neuroscience Methods*, **26**, 6651-6660. doi:10.1523/JNEUROSCI.1007-06.2006

[44] Karl, J.L., Fernandes, N.R., Kobayashi, C.J. *et al.* (2006) Analysis of the neurogenic potential of multipotent skin-derived precursors. *Experimental Neurology*, **201**, 32-48. doi:10.1016/j.expneurol.2006.03.018

[45] Jeff, B., Joseph, S.S., Liu, J., *et al.* (2007) Skin-derived Precursors generate myelinating Schwann cells that promote remyelination and functional recovery after contusion spinal cord injury. *Journal of Neuroscience Methods*, **27**, 9545-9559. doi:10.1523/JNEUROSCI.1930-07.2007

[46] Karl, J.L., Jean, G.T. and Freda, D.M. (2008) Multipotent skin-derived precursors: Adult neural crest-related precursors with therapeutic potential. Philosophical *Transactions of the Royal Society B*, **363**, 185-198. doi:10.1098/rstb.2006.2020

[47] Jean-Francois, L., Jeffrey, A.B., Yan, C., *et al.* (2009) Skin-derived precursors differentiate into skeletogenic cell types and contribute to bone repair. *Stem Cells and Development*, **18**, 893-905. doi:10.1089/scd.2008.0260

[48] Jeffrey, B., Maryline, P., Olena, M., *et al.* (2009) SKPs derive from hair follicle precursors and exhibit properties of adult dermal stem cells. *Cell Stem Cell*, **5**, 610-623. doi:10.1016/j.stem.2009.10.019

[49] Hiroyuki, J., Olena, M., Jones, K.L., *et al.* (2010) Convergent genesis of an adult neural crest-like dermal stem cell from distinct developmental origins. *Stem Cells*, **28**, 2027-2040. doi:10.1002/stem.525

[50] Yasuyuki, A., Lingna, L., Kensei, K. and Robert, M.H. (2010) Embryonic development of hair follicle pluripotent stem (hfPS) cells. *Medical Molecular Morphology*, **43**, 123-127. doi:10.1007/s00795-010-0498-z

[51] Yasuyuki, A., Kensei, K., Robert, M.H. (2010) The advantages of hair follicle pluripotent stem cells over embryonic stem cells and induced pluripotent stem cells for regenerative medicine. *Journal of Dermatological Science*, **60**, 131-137. doi:10.1016/j.jdermsci.2010.09.007

[52] Fang, L., Aisada, U., Hiroaki, K., *et al.* (2010) The bulge area is the major hair follicle source of nestin-expressing pluripotent stem cells which can repair the spinal cord compared to the dermal papilla. *Cell Cycle*, **10**, 830-839. doi:10.4161/cc.10.5.14969

[53] Florian, H., Wolf, C.P., David, A., *et al.* (2009) Morphological and immunocytochemical characteristics indicate the yield of early progenitors and represent a quality control for human mesenchymal stem cell culturing. *Journal of Anatomy*, **214**, 759-767. doi:10.1111/j.1469-7580.2009.01065.x

[54] Su, P.H., Wang, T.C., Wong, Z.R., *et al.* (2011) The expression of nestin delineates skeletal muscle differentiation in the developing rat esophagus. *Journal of Anatomy*, **218**, 311-323. doi:10.1111/j.1469-7580.2010.01331.x.

[55] Svachovaa, H., Pour, L., Sana, J., *et al.* (2011) Stem cell marker nestin is expressed in plasma cells of multiple myeloma patients. *Leukemia Research*, **35**, 1008-1013. doi:10.1016/j.leukres.2011.03.001

[56] Frederiksen, K. and McKay, R.D.G. (1988) Proliferation and differentiation of rat neuroepithelial precursor cells *in vivo*. *The Journal of Neuroscience*, **8**, 1144-1151.

[57] Yvan, A., Jean-Guy, V., Jean-Francois, B., *et al.* (2001) Isolation of multipotent neural precursors residing in the cortex of the adult human brain. *Experimental Neurology*, **170**, 48-62. doi:10.1006/exnr.2001.7691

[58] Jahan, A., Saskia, F., Anli, Z. and Melissa, F. (2010) Characterization of neural stem/progenitor cells expressing VEGF and its receptors in the subventricular zone of newborn piglet brain. *Neurochemical Research*, **35**, 1455-1470. doi:10.1007/s11064-010-0207-2

[59] Chanchai, B., Kerstin, K., Sombat B., *et al.* (2011) Fibrosis and evidence for epithelial-mesenchymal transition in the kidneys of patients with staghorn calculi. *British Journal of Urology International*, **107**, 1847. doi:10.1111/j.1464-410X.2011.10350.x

Long-term effect of autologous progenitor cell therapy to induce neo angiogenesis in patients with critical limb ischemia transplantated via intramuscular vs combined intramuscular and distal retrograde intra venous

Luis Padilla[1,2*], Juan Rodriguez-Trejo[3], Ignacio Escotto[3], Manuel López-Hernandez[4], Mauricio González[5], José De Diego[6], Neftaly Rodrgiuez[3], Jesús Tapia[2], Takeshi Landero[1], Carranza Pilar Hazel[1], Horacio Juarez Olguin[1], Mauricio Di Silvio[1,7], Paul Mondragon-Teran[8]

[1]Department of Experimental Surgery, Microsurgery Unit, Centro Medico Nacional "20 de Noviembre" ISSSTE, Mexico City, Mexico; *Corresponding Author: lpadilla@issste.gob.mx
[2]Surgery Department, Faculty of Medicine, Universidad Nacional Autonoma de Mexico, Mexico City, Mexico
[3]Angiology, Vascular and Endovascular Surgery Unit, Centro Medico Nacional "20 de Noviembre" ISSSTE, Mexico City, Mexico
[4]Haematology Unit, Centro Medico Nacional "20 de Noviembre" ISSSTE, Mexico City, Mexico
[5]Bank of Blood Unit, Centro Medico Nacional "20 de Noviembre" ISSSTE, Mexico City, Mexico
[6]Pediatric Hematology Unit Centro Medico Nacional '20 de Noviembre' ISSSTE, Mexico City, Mexico
[7]Department of Research, Hospital General de México OD, Secretaria de Salud México, Mexico City, Mexico
[8]Department of Biomedical Research, Centro Medico Nacional "20 de Noviembre" ISSSTE, Mexico City, Mexico

ABSTRACT

Critical limb ischemia is a medical condition that decreases blood flow and limb oxygen supply; this disease in its late stages of progression leads to only two possible options: either surgical bypass revascularization or limb amputation. We investigated a novel method using autologous transplantation of progenitor cells derived from mobilized peripheral blood bone marrow mononuclear cells to evaluate its long-term effect as a cell therapy to induce neo-angiogenesis and restore blood flow in the affected ischemic limbs. A total of 20 ischemic limbs from critical limb ischemia diagnosed patients, non candidates to surgical revascularization were transplanted with autologous progenitor cells by either intramuscular combined with intravenous (group A) or intramuscular (group B) procedure. Patients were monitored during 31 months. Treatment efficacy was evaluated according to the following parameters: ankle brachial index which increased at a range of 0.29 - 1.0 in group A and 0.40 - 0.90 in group B; pain-free walking distance which increased at a range of 50 - 600 m in group A and 50 - 300 m in group B; and blood perfusion (measured by Laser Doppler) which increased at a range of 48 - 299 in group A and 135 - 225 in group B. We achieved 90% treated ischemic limbs free of amputation in both transplanted groups. Results here described provide a safe, efficient and minimally invasive therapy with progenitor cells to induce angiogenesis and preserve limbs from amputation in CLI diagnosed patients.

Keywords: Neo-Angiogenesis; Cell therapy; Critical Limb Ischemia; Progenitor Cells; Blood Perfusion

1. INTRODUCTION

Peripheral arterial disease (PAD) is a medical problem that comprises the obstruction of blood flow in the arteries causing inadequate oxygen supply to diverse tissues. This disease currently affects approximately 12 million people in the United States of America (USA) [1]. The death risk for people with PAD is 10 to 15 times greater than the death risk for subjects free from this disease as shown in a 10 years follow up study [2]. PAD in lower extremities is mainly expressed with intermittent claudication (IC) which is an early manifestation of pain during ambulation; as disease progresses pain is presented even at rest and patients usually develop a blood flow decrease which leads to ischemic ulcerations and in late stages gangrene requiring minor or major amputations, thus completing the natural story for critical limb ischemia (CLI) [3-5]. Diabetic patients are at a higher risk of developing such CLI condition, since 30% of them will present it earlier in life, compared with non-diabetic population [6,7]; besides, PAD in diabetes mellitus disease is more diffuse and severe, mainly affecting the lower extremities vasculature, while the non-diabetic patients with PAD have a higher aorto-iliac incidence [8,9]. CLI is a growing medical problem and has an estimated incidence of 11% in the general population and 15% in adults over 55 years old; it also has been reported with an incidence of 500 to 1000 individuals per million each year [10]. The reported mortality rates due to CLI has been 20%, 35% 70% and up to 100% for 1, 2, 5 and 10 years respectively and at least 50% of patients will undergo major limb amputation within 6 to 12 months [11-13]. Current treatments for CLI patients include serum lipid levels reduction, antiplatelet (*i.e.* cilostasol) and antihypertensive drugs showing limited efficacy in CLI severe stages [14,15]. Although surgical revascularization remains as the most appropriate CLI therapy aimed to prevent limb loss, it is not suitable for at least 30% of patients because of extent of the disease and the lack of proper non damaged autologous vasculature; which leaves amputation as the only option if CLI has progressed beyond the point of salvage, vascular surgery is too risky or life expectancy is very low [16,17]. Including only USA 100,000 major limb amputations are performed every year due to PAD with an annual cost of more than 13 billion US dollars [18]. Patients with CLI who are not eligible for revascularization have no effective treatment option. Despite there is no Federal Drug Administration (FDA) approved therapy for these CLI patients, there has been several research groups reporting different strategies towards the establishment of progenitor cell therapies to allow the formation of new blood vessels (neo-angiogenesis) as a method to salvage ischemic limbs through autologous transplantation of progenitor cells derived from Bone Marrow-Mononuclear Cells (BM-MNC) [18-23]. At least 40 research groups have obtained promising results with BM-MNC transplantation as progenitor cell therapy treatment for CLI patients, supporting evidence to establish this procedure as an alternative to improve blood perfusion through neo-angiogenesis and to avoid amputation [3, 18]. To reach a maximum local cell concentration, Bartsch *et al.* [21], performed 13 intramuscular and intra-arterial transplantation of BM-MNC obtained from iliac crest bone marrow aspiration and purified through ficoll gradient technique, this procedure resulted in the improvement of the ankle brachial index (ABI); in contrast, the 12 patients in the control group with no cell transplant showed a statistically significant reduction of ABI and venous occlusion plethysmography at rest. Using a rat ischemic limb model we previously demonstrated the induction of effective neo-vascularization after bone marrow mononuclear cell (CD^{34+} and CD^{133+}) transplantation into surgically induced fibrocollagenous tunnels used as scaffolds to enhance cell survival and differentiation [24]. In a second experimental study, our group used dogs as an ischemic limb model confirming that transplantation of mobilized BM-MNC to peripheral blood through the use of Granulocyte Colony-Stimulating Factor (G-CSF) statistically significant increased angiogenesis as compared with cell transplant without G-CSF treatment [25]. Based on the evidence of neo-angiogenesis as a result of mobilized BM-MNC autologous transplantation on these experimental models, we obtained the ethical and research institution committee approval to start a clinical trial in humans for the progenitor cell therapy of CLI patients. In this report we analyze the efficacy of Mobilized BM-MNC transplantation comparing combined procedure intramuscular and distal retrograde-intravenous (saphenous vein) transplantation (IM + IV) versus intramuscular (IM) standard transplantation procedure.

2. MATERIALS AND METHODS

2.1. Trial Profile

The institutional board approved this prospective, controlled, randomized study; all enrolled patients provided written informed consent; all surgical procedures were conducted by senior expert surgeon (PL and RTJ).

2.2. Patient's Inclusion Criteria

Patients older than 18 years old presenting severe lower limb obstructive arterial disease classified as Fontaine stage IIb (Incapacitant intermittent claudication), Fontaine stage III (pain at rest), Rutherford 4, with an ankle-brachial index (ABI) lower than 0.6, and who were non candidates to surgical bypass revascularization nor to endovascular procedure.

2.3. Patient's Exclusion Criteria

Patients with any neoplasia history in the last 10 years, patients with 1 year of life expectancy, patients with severe renal failure, severe malnutrition, or systemic chronic infectious disease at any clinical stage (Hepatitis B, C or HIV infection).

The parameters to evaluate were procedure's safety, treatment efficacy, ABI, blood perfusion and pain-free walking distance evolution. Patients of both experimental and control groups were monitored by measuring those parameters at 0, 3, 12 months after progenitor cell transplant and at 18, 24 and 31 months after cell transplant therapy to evaluate the ratio of patients free of limb amputation.

2.4. Study Design

The study was designed as a randomized prospective controlled clinical trial and its main goal was to improve blood perfusion through neo-angiogenesis and to salvage patient's ischemic limbs. 20 critical ischemic affected limbs (Fontaine II-b, Fontaine III and Rutherford 4) were evaluated in 14 patients non candidates to any form of revascularization who accepted to participate in the study and were included in the trial according to the established inclusion criteria. Limb ischemia diagnosis was based on Laser Doppler blood flow measurements (≤31 perfusion units), ankle brachial index (≤0.6) and pain-free walking distance (≤200 m). Patients were randomly divided into two main groups according to the following transplant strategy (as shown in **Figure 1**):

Group A: 10 ischemic limbs from patients transplanted with progenitor cells using a combination of intramuscular and distal retrograde-intravenous (saphenous vein) transplant. Group A is referred in this report as IM + IV (Intramuscular + Intravenous).

Group B (control group): 10 ischemic limbs from patients with progenitor cell intramuscular transplant. Group B is referred in this report as IM (intramuscular).

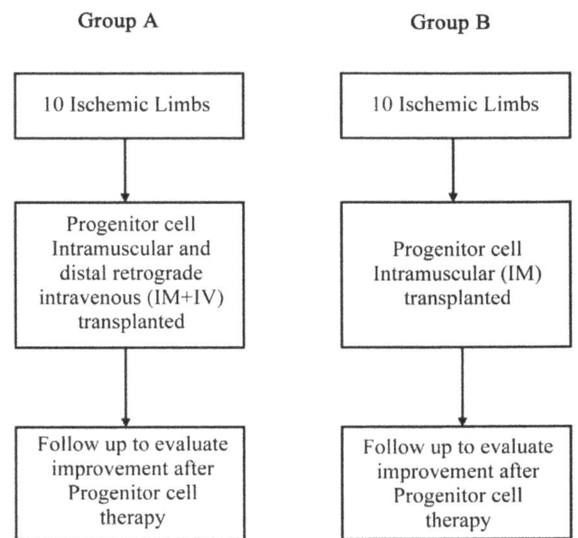

Figure 1. Study design. A total of 14 patients were recruited for this study achieving 10 ischemic limbs per group. Some of the patients presenting both ischemic limbs were included as one of the ischemic limbs in group A and the second ischemic limb in group B.

2.5. Cell Harvest

Mobilization of Bone Marrow-Mononuclear Cells (B-M-MNC) to peripheral blood was achieved by a daily subcutaneous administration of 5 μg of Granulocyte Colony-Stimulating Factor (G-CSF) (Roche) during 5 consecutive days at early morning. Mobilized Peripheral Blood Mononuclear Cells (M-PBMNC) were harvested on the 5th day of treatment by apheresis procedure using a continuous flow COBE-Spectra blood cell automated separator (COBE BCT, Lakewood CO., USA) and a double puncture technique using citrate plus glucose as anticoagulant and physiologic solution as primer. Apheresis was performed as a two-step procedure involving extraction and re-infusion using a Mahurkar or Niagara catheter and extraction/infusion flow speeds between 50 - 55 $mL{\cdot}min^{-1}$. For all patients a 60 mL standard amount of progenitor cell suspension per ischemic limb was obtained at the end of the apheresis procedure.

2.6. Cell Analysis

CD^{34+} (hematopoietic) and CD^{133+} (angioblast) mouse anti human antibody (Beckton Dickinson, Ca, USA) cell marker were used to confirm progenitor cell phenotype-respectively by flowcytometry analysis using a FAC SCalibur and Cell Quest Pro Software (Becton Dickinson, Ca, USA). Cell count was manually obtained using a haemocytometer.

2.7. Surgical Technique

Ultrasound guided punctures on the affected limb muscle compartments were performed under epidural blockade and light sedation using a catheter needle BD Insyte (16GA-1.77IN) (17 × 45 mm). The 60 mL M-PBMN cell suspension per ischemic limb were distributed as follows: 10 mL in the internal vastus compartment, 10 mL in the external vastus compartment, 10 mL in the anterior tibial muscle compartment, 10 mL in the deep posterior muscle compartment and 10 mL in the superficial posterior muscle compartment. For group A, as part of the surgical procedure, the major saphenous vein was localized at the internal malleolus level, at this site a small incision was performed in order to dissect the vein and isolate it using chromic catgut 3 - 0 sutures. Afterwards the vein was temporarily ocluded in a proximal direction and a catheter BD Insyte (16GA-1.77IN) (17 × 45 mm) was placed by direct puncture in order to perform a regional distal retrograde heparinization (1 mL of heparine diluted 1:1000 + 9 mL saline solution). A manual tourniquet was applied to avoid the venous flow to return for 10 minutes followed by the distal retrograde intravenous application of the last 10 mL cell suspension (**Figure 2**). For group B, 12 mL instead of 10 mL of M-PBMN cell suspension were distributed between the 5 muscles compartments as previously mentioned.

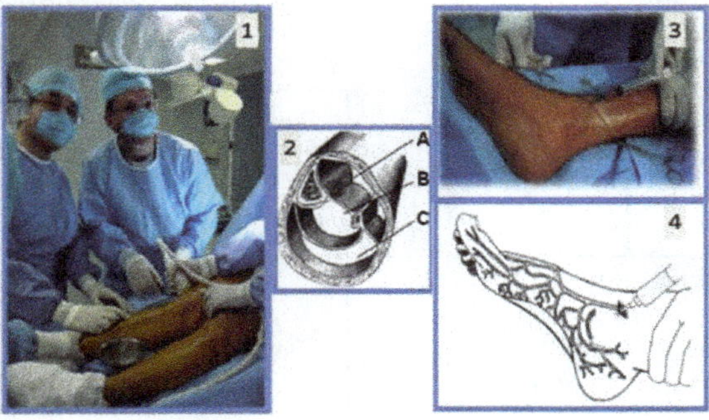

Figure 2. Surgical technique used to induce neo-angiogenesis. Cell transplant was performed ultrasound guided (1), cells were transplanted at different muscle compartments such as: internal and external vastus compartments, anterior tibial muscle compartment (2A), deep posterior muscle compartment (2B), superficial posterior muscle compartment (2C) and at internal malleolus level (3 and 4).

2.8. Lasser Doppler Technique

Blood flow by Laser Doppler measurement is a standard technique for real time measurement of tissue perfusion at micro-vascular level. This technique was first reported in 1964 by Yeh and Cummins [26], and the units of Laser Doppler are given in tissue-Perfusion Units (PU); such PU was standardized through the use of a suspension of latex spheres in movement. This method is non invasive, highly sensitive to local perfusion and useful for continuous monitoring if necessary. A signal proportional to red blood cells (RBC) perfusion is displayed in the screen of the Laser Doppler equipment; this signal represents the transport of RBC through microvasculature [27]. Patient's blood flow measurements were performed by Lasser Doppler technique using a Periflux System 5000 (Perimed Instruments, Stockholm Sweden) prior to the transplant procedure and at 3 and 12 months post transplant in both groups. Lasser Doppler measurements were performed for at least 2 minutes for baseline values prior to temperature increase as stimulus to record RBC perfusion units (See **Figure 3**).

2.9. Statistical Analysis

A database corresponding to quantitative baseline and post treatment values for blood perfusion and ABI per patient was used for statistical analysis. Changes from baseline to 3 and 12 months variables were analyzed by paired t-test according to normal distribution. Statistical significance was assumed for $p < 0.05$ value. All statisticcal analysis was performed with SPSS 16.0 statistical software.

3. RESULTS

3.1. Clinical Characteristics

Fourteen patients with severe CLI (Fontaine IIb, Fontaine III, Rutherford 4) were recruited, transplanted, evaluated and monitored during 31 months. Clinical characteristics from recruited patients are shown in **Table 1(a)** and **Table 1(b)** shows ABI and pain free-walking distance values prior to treatment (defined as time zero—t_0) and post treatment at 12 months (t_{12}).

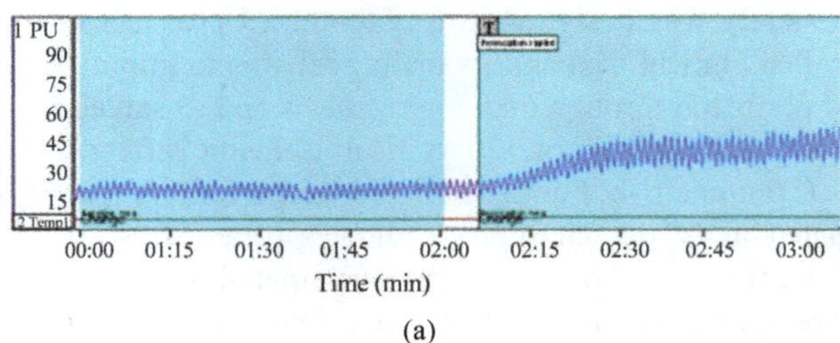

(a)

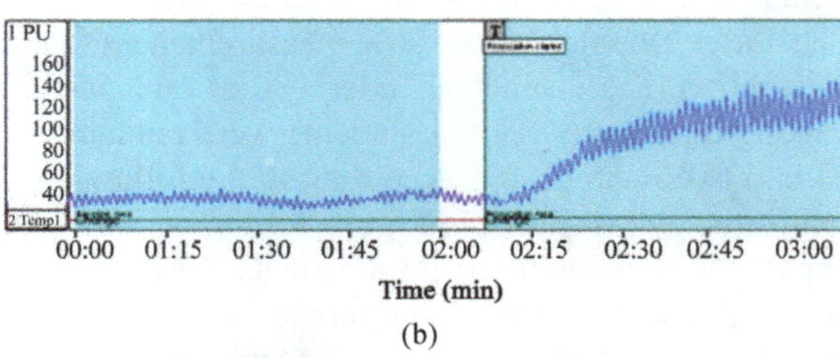

(b)

Figure 3. Representative blood flow measured by Laser Doppler prior to transplant (a) and 12 months post transplant (b).

Table 1. (a) Patient clinical characteristics; (b) Clinical follow up after 12 months post transplantation.

(a)

Clinical Characteristic	Group A (IM + IV) N = 10	Group B (IM) N = 10
Smoking	8	5
Hypercholesterolemia	5	6
Diabetes Mellitus	6	2
Arterial Hypertension	8	6
Myocardial Infarct	2	2

(b)

Parameter	Group A (IM + IV)	Group B (IM)
Limb Amputation	1*	1**
Pain-Free Walking Distance (m) Range (min - max)	50 - 600	50 - 300
ABI Range (min - max)	0.29 - 1.0	0.40 - 0.90
Blood Flow (PU) Range (min - max)	48.82 - 299.02	135.13 - 225.31

*Limb amputation on the 8th month post transplant; **Limb amputation on the 6th month post transplant.

3.2. Transplantated Cell Number

Progenitor cell phenotype was identified by flowcytometry with CD^{34+} and CD^{133+} cell markers (as previously described). The total transplanted cell number per ischemic limb were $17.4 \pm 8 \times 10^6$ CD^{34+} cells for group A, and $15 \pm 5 \times 10^6$ CD^{34+} cells for group B; meanwhile the total transplanted CD^{133+} cells for group A were $2.86 \pm 5.96 \times 10^7$ and $3.01 \pm 5.91 \times 10^7$ for group B.

3.3. Effect of Transplantated Progenitor Cells

Patients were monitored at 0, 3, and 12 months post progenitor cell transplant; parameters evaluated included: Pain free walking distance (reported in meters), ABI, blood flow reported as perfusion units, angiography and ischemic limbs free of amputation (monitored during 31 months post transplant). At 31 months post treatment period it was reported 1 limb amputation in each group, A and B (**Tables 1(b)** and **2**), interestingly both patients were diabetics. Average values for pain-free walking distance parameter increased from 60 ± 39 m pre-transplant to 207 ± 198 m at 12 months post-transplant for group A, and from 87 ± 69 m pre-transplant to 172 ± 127 m at 12 months post-transplant for group B. ABI parameter showed an increase from 0.42 ± 0.14 pre-transplant to 0.70 ± 0.21 at 12 months post-transplant for group A, and from 0.44 ± 0.09 pre-transplant to 0.62 ± 0.15 at 12 months post-transplant for group B. Blood perfusion (measured by Laser Doppler) increased from15.8 ± 9.3 pre-transplant to 205.8 ± 116.7 at 12 months post-transplant for group A, and from 16.6 ± 7 acute myocardial infarction. There were no reported adverse effects due to cell transplant procedure. Blood flow perfusion units

Table 2. Baseline and monitored clinical parameters.

Extremity	Limb	Age (years)	Gender	ABI t_0	ABI t_{12}	Pain free walking distance t_0 (Meters)	Pain free walking $distance_{t12}$ (Meters)	Blood perfusion (t_0)	Blood perfusion (t_3)	Observation
					Group A (IM + IV)					
1	L	77	F	0.70	1	20	100			Salvage
2	R	72	M	0.40	0.50	100	150	6.46	13.53	Salvage
3	U	79	F	0.20	0.80	No data	No data	8.99	30.53	Salvage
4	U	59	M	0.50	0.70	No data	No data	8.23	6.10	Amputate
5	R	67	F	0.86	0.93	100	350	14.07	17.23	Salvage
6	R	54	F	0.50	0.50	50	50	30.60	38.27	Salvage
7	R	63	M	0.26	0.55	10	100	30.56	42.10	Salvage
8	U	70	F	0.40	0.80	No data	No data	10.56	39.20	Salvage
9	R	68	M	0.36	0.70	40	600	20.20	No data	Salvage
10	L	64	F	0.50	0.29	100	100	12.70	31.00	Salvage
					Group B (IM)					
1	R	67	M	0.50	0.50	150	1200	7.4	17.26	Salvage
2	L	67	M	0.50	0.60	150	1200	14.1	31.20	Salvage
3	L	72	M	0.40	0.60	100	150	14.49	16.09	Salvage
4	L	54	F	0.60	0.50	50	50	8.97	52.38	Salvage
5	R	46	F	0.50	0.70	200	400	23.00	61.84	Salvage
6	R	70	F	0.40	0.80	10	50	18.70	37.40	Amputate
7	R	64	F	0.50	0.40	100	100	15.61	24.15	Salvage
8	R	63	M	0.26	0.50	10	100	30.56	42.10	Salvage
9	R	77	F	0.40	0.90	20	100	No data	No data	Salvage
10	R	78	M	0.40	0.70	No data	No data	No data	No data	Salvage

measured by Laser Doppler (as described in Materials and Methods), showed a significant improvement by an average of 14 fold increase ($p < 0.05$) in the case of group A and a 10 fold increase ($p < 0.05$) for group B as compared with the corresponding baseline blood flow measurements for each group. These results suggest that despite both transplant procedures resulted in an important blood flow increase, the effect was higher when progenitor cells were transplanted using a combined intramuscular-intravenous method. **Figure 4** shows blood perfusion from 8 critical ischemic limbs at pre transplant, at 3 and 12 months post transplant as evidence on the increase of blood perfusion after treatment for both groups **Figure 5** shows average perfusion unit values for group A and group B pre and post transplant. Angiographic base line (time zero) index and blood perfusion at 12 months time point, were not performed in all patients due to logistic follow up limitations, however at least 6 patients were subjected to angiography.

Figure 6 shows angiography pre and post transplant for one of the patients included in group A and one in the group B as an example of neo-angiogenesis due to progenitor cell transplant. The neo-angiogenesis process was confirmed with the increase in the blood flow perfusion as shown in **Figures 4** and **5**. Despite ABI, pain free walking distance and blood perfusion parameters were not measured in most of patients at 24 and 31 months, the beneficial effects of treatments were maintained as no limb amputations were performed.

4. DISCUSSION

In this study, we found that CLI diagnosed patients treated by any of both procedures, either A or B progenytor cell transplanted groups, induced neo-angiogenesis improving all clinical parameters and avoiding limb amputation as 90% of limbs in each group were saved. It was found a higher efficiency in terms of blood perfusion, ABI and pain-free walking distance when cell transplant was performed with a combined intra muscular and intra venous procedure; however there was no statistical significant difference between groups. We previously performed the transplant of progenitor cells into surgically induced fibrocollagenous tunnels to a total of 8 ischemic limbs; we initially observed a significant clinical improvement in 5 of the ischemic limbs while the other 3 showed non favorable clinical outcome with improvement in vascular proximal blood perfusion but developed necrosis in toes (non published data). We concluded that for those 3 patients the transplant technique did not allow transplanted cells to reach toe's capillaries. Based on these results, we developed a new protocol in CLI induced rats (Sprague Dawley) as a model in order to allow transplanted cells to reach toe's capillaries; we demonstrated that by adding a distal retrograde-intravenous injection of cells, higher levels of angiogenesis

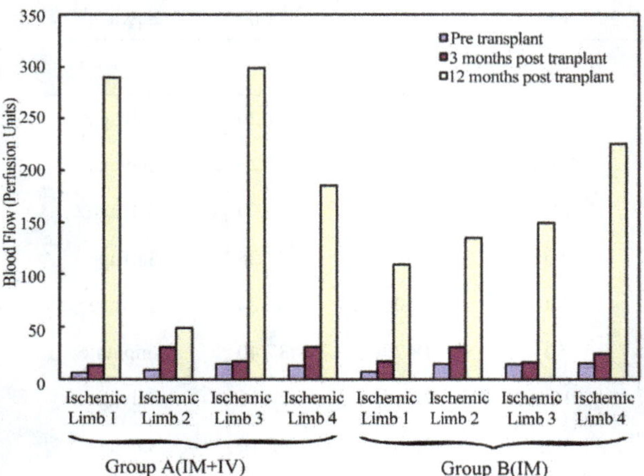

Figure 4. Blood flow given as perfusion units at pre transplant, 3 and 12 months post transplant.

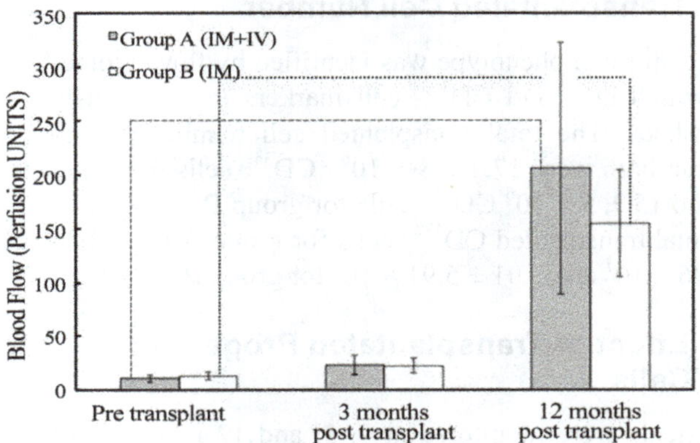

Figure 5. Average PU values for group A and group B. Comparison of blood perfusion between baseline values (pre transplant) and 12 months post transplant resulted in statistically significant differences for (dashed line) group A ($p < 0.05$) and (dotted line) group B ($p < 0.05$).

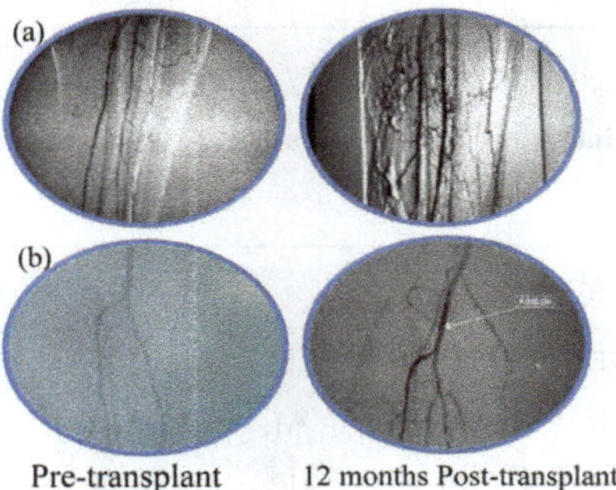

Figure 6. Angiography performed at pre-transplant and 12 months post transplant. Angiography for: (a) one patient from group A and (b) one patient from group B.

were produced as compared with intramuscular cell transplant. We also observed that mononuclear cells attached to the smallest capillary segment used as a scaffold increased survival, proliferation, and cell differentiation towards endothelial cell type [28]. Tepper [29] and Law all [30] demonstrated that angiogenesis or vasculogenesis induction requires the ischemic initial stimulus and the muscle inflammatory response that releases cytokines and growth factors (such as VEGF, bFGF, SDF-1, PDG-BB, IGF-1, TGF-B) that activate proliferation, migration and tubulization of endothelial cells. These findings support the use of muscle as the main target for progenytor cell transplant, however we showed that combined intramuscular and intravenous transplant technique provides a higher transplant efficiency as demonstrated in our previous animal model report [26]. A similar 12 months follow up study reported by Van Tongeren *et al.* [31] demonstrated a higher efficiency when combined intramuscular and intra-arterial transplant strategy was used in comparison with only intramuscular transplant. The main results of our study is the evidence that both transplant procedures increases blood perfusion, ABI and pain free walking distance; showing slightly higher results for combined intramuscular-intravenous group. More importantly, improvements achieved by progenitor cell transplant in this study, were maintained for up to 31 months achieving 90% of the limbs preserved from amputationn.

5. CONCLUSION

Progenitor cell therapy described in this study is a minimally invasive therapeutic option for patients with critical limb ischemia. Both, intramuscular and combined intramuscular-intravenous autologous progenitor cell transplant led to a substantial increase in blood flow perfusion, pain-free walking distance and ankle brachial index. Despite there was no statistical significance between groups, a higher blood perfusion (measured by laser Doppler) was observed when progenitor cells were transplanted combining intramuscular-intravenous as compared with intra muscular procedure. Transplant of progenitor cells described here provides a safe and reliable cell therapy for CLI diagnosed patients who are not candidates for invasive surgical revascularization.

6. ACKNOWLEDGEMENTS

We would like to acknowledge to Reneé Acosta and Paola Lares Juárez for their help on the revision of the manuscript.

REFERENCES

[1] Ouriel, K. (2001) Detection of peripheral arterial disease in primary care. *The Journal of the American Medical Association*, **286**, 1380-1381. doi:10.1001/jama.286.11.1380

[2] Criqui, M.H., Langer, R.D., Fronek, A., Feigelson, H.S., Klauber, M.R., McCann, T.J. and Bronwer, D. (1992) Mortality over a period of 10 years in patients with peripheral arterial disease. *The New England Journal of Medicine*, **326**, 381-386. doi:10.1056/NEJM199202063260605

[3] Aranguren, X.L., Verfaillie, C.M. and Luttun, A. (2009) Emerging hurdles in stem cell therapy for peripheral vascular disease. *Journal of Molecular Medicine*, **87**, 3-16. doi:10.1007/s00109-008-0394-3

[4] Ouriel, K. (2001) Peripheral arterial disease. *The Lancet*, **358**, 1257-1264. doi:10.1016/S0140-6736(01)06351-6

[5] Luther, M., Lepantalo, M., Alback, A. and Mazke, S. (1996) Amputation rates as a measure of vascular surgical results. *British Journal of Surgery*, **83**, 241-244. doi:10.1002/bjs.1800830229

[6] Coffman, J. D. (1991) Intermittent claudication—Be conservative. *The New England Journal of Medicine*, **325**, 577-578.

[7] Beker, G.J., Furguson, J.G., Bakal, C.W., McKinnison, M.G.K., *et al.* (1993) Angioplasty, bypass surgery and amputation for lower extremity peripheral arterial disase in Maryland: A closer look. *Radiology*, **186**, 635-638.

[8] Rutherford, R.B., Flanigon, D.P., Gupta, S.L., Johnsin, K., *et al.* (1986) Suggested standards for reports dealing with lower extremity ischemia. *Journal of Vascular Surgery*, **4**, 80-94.

[9] Deweese, J.A., Leather, R. and Porter, J. (1993) Practice guidelines: Lower extremity revascularization. *Journal of Vascular Surgery*, **18**, 280-294. doi:10.1016/0741-5214(93)90609-P

[10] Norgen, L., Hiatt, W.R., Dormandy, J.A., *et al.* (2007) TASC II working group inter society consensus for the management of pheripheral artherial disease (TASC II). *European Journal of Vascular and Endovascular Surgery*, **33**, 1-75.

[11] Di Stefano, R., Limbruno, U., Barone, D. and Balbarini, A. (2004) Therapeutic angiogenesis of critical lower limb ischemia review of the literature and prospects of research on stem cells. *Italian Heart Journal*, **5**, 1-13.

[12] Boccalon, H., Lehert, P. and Mosnier, M. (2000) Assessment of the prevalence of atherosclerotic lower limb arteriopathy in France as a systolic index in a vascular risk population. *Journal Des Maladies Vasculaires*, **25**, 38-46.

[13] The European Agency for the Evaluation of Medicinal Products, Committee for Proprietary Medicinal Products. (2002) Notes for guidance on clinical investigation of medicinal products for the treatment of peripheral arterial occlusive disease. CPMP/EWP714/98.

[14] Marston, W.A., Davies, S.W., Armstrong, B., Farber, M.A., Mendes, R.C. and Fulton, J.J. (2006) Natural history of limbs with arterial insufficiency and chronic ulceration treated without revascularization. *Journal of Vascular Surgery*, **44**, 108-114. doi:10.1016/j.jvs.2006.03.026

[15] Hilleman, D.E. (1998) Management of peripheral arterial.

Disease. *American Journal of Health Promotion*, **55**, 521-527.

[16] Dormady, J.A. and Rutherford, R.B. (2000) Management of peripheral arterial disease (PAD). TASC working group. *Journal of Vascular Surgery*, **31**, S1-S278.

[17] Aronow, W.S. (2005) Management of peripheral arterial disease. *Cardiology in Review*, **13**, 61-68. doi:10.1097/01.crd.0000126082.86717.12

[18] Franz, R., Parks, A., Shah, K.J., Hankins, T., Hartman, J.F. and Wright, M.L. (2009) Use of autologus bone marrow mononuclear cell implantation therapy as a limb salvage procedure in patients with severe peripheral arterial disease. *Journal of Vascular Surgery*, **50**, 1378-1390. doi:10.1016/j.jvs.2009.07.113

[19] Huang, P.P., Yang, X.F., Li, S.Z., Wen, J.C., Zhang, Y. and Han, Z.C. (2007) Randomised comparison of G-CSF mobilized peripheral blood mononuclear cells versus bone marrow-mononuclear cells for the treatment of patients with lower limb arteriosclerosis obliterans. *Thrombosis and Haemostasis*, **98**, 1335-1342.

[20] Amann, B., Luedeman, C., Ratei, R. and Schmidt-Lucke, A.J. (2009) Autologus bone marrow transplantation increases leg perfusion and reduces amputations in patients with advanced critical limb ischemia due to peripheral artery disease. *Cell Transplantation*, **18**, 371-380. doi:10.3727/096368909788534942

[21] Bartsch, T., Brehm, M., Zeus, T., Kogler, G., Wernet, P. and Strauer, B.E. (2007) Transplantation of autologus mononuclear bone marrow stem cells in patients with periphera arterial disease (The TAM-PAD study). *Clinical Research in Cardiology*, **96**, 891-899. doi:10.1007/s00392-007-0569-x

[22] Powell, R.J., Comerota, A.J., Berceli, S.A., Guzman, R., Henry, D.T., Tzeng, E., Velazquez, O., Marston, W.A., Bartel, R.L., Longcore, A., Stern, T. and Watling, S. (2011) Interim results from the RESTORE-CLI, a randomized, double-blidn multicenter phase II trial comparing expanded autologus bone marrow-derived tissue repair cells and placebo in patients with critical limb ischemia. *Journal of Vascular Surgery*, **54**, 1032-1041. doi:10.1016/j.jvs.2011.04.006

[23] Cobellis, G., Silvestroni, A., Lillo, S., Sica, G., Botti, C., Maione, C., Schiavone, V., Rocco, S., Brando, G. and Sica, V. (2008) Long-term effects of repeated autologus transplantation of bone marrow cells in patients affected by peripheral arterial disease. *Bone Marrow Transplantation*, **42**, 667-672. doi:10.1038/bmt.2008.228

[24] Padilla, L., De la Garza, A.S., Villegas, F., Esperante, S., Rojas, E., Miranda, A., Figueroa, S., Schalch, P., Krotzsch, E. and Di Silvio, M. (2003) Administration of bone marrow cells into surgically induced fibrocollagenous tunnels induces angiogenesis in ischemic rat hindlimb model. *Microsurgery*, **23**, 568-574. doi:10.1002/micr.10208

[25] Padilla, L., Villegas, F., Glennie, G., Escotto, I., Schalch, P., Avila, G., Rodriguez-Trejo, J., Figueroa, S., De la Garza, A.S., Krotzsch, E. and Di Silvio, M. (2007) Bone marrow mononuclear cells stimulate angiogenesis when transplanted into surgically induced fibrocollagenous tunnels: Results from a canine ischemic hinlimb model. *Microsurgery*, **27**, 91-97. doi:10.1002/micr.20289

[26] Yeh, Y. and Cummins, H. (1964) Localized fluid flows measurements with He-Ne laser spectrometer. *Applied Physics Letters*, **4**, 176-178. doi:10.1063/1.1753925

[27] Kvernobo, K. and Slagsvold, C.E. (1998) Laser Doppler flowmetry in evaluation of lower limb resting skin circulation: A study in healthy controls and atherosclerotic patients. *Scandinavian Journal of Clinical & Laboratory Investigation*, **48**, 621-626. doi:10.3109/00365518809085781

[28] Padilla, S.L., Rodriguez, T.J., Escotto, S.L., De Diego, F.J., Rodriguez, R.N., Krötzsch, E., Villegas, A., Landero, T., Carranza, H., Goldberg, J. and Di Silvio, M. (2009) Progenitor mononuclear cell transplantation derived from the bone marrow through distal retrogressive endovenous route in order to induce angiogenesis. *Cirujano General*, **31**, 213-218.

[29] Tepper, O.M., Capla, J.M., Galiano, R.D. and Callaghan, M.J. (2009) Adult vasculogenesis occurs through *in situ* recruitment, proliferation and tubulization of circulating bone marrow derived cells. *Blood*, **105**, 1068-1077. doi:10.1182/blood-2004-03-1051

[30] Lawall, H., Bramage, P. and Amann, B. (2010) Stem cell and progenitor cell therapy in peripheral arterial disease. *Journal of Thrombosis and Haemostasis*, **103**, 696-709.

[31] Van Tongeren, R. and Hamming, J. (2008) Intramuscular or combined intramuscular/intra-arterial administration of bone marrow mononuclear cells; a clinical trial in patients with advanced limb ischemia. *Journal of Cardiothoracic Surgery*, **49**, 51-58.

Permissions

All chapters in this book were first published in SCD, by Scientific Research Publishing; hereby published with permission under the Creative Commons Attribution License or equivalent. Every chapter published in this book has been scrutinized by our experts. Their significance has been extensively debated. The topics covered herein carry significant findings which will fuel the growth of the discipline. They may even be implemented as practical applications or may be referred to as a beginning point for another development.

The contributors of this book come from diverse backgrounds, making this book a truly international effort. This book will bring forth new frontiers with its revolutionizing research information and detailed analysis of the nascent developments around the world.

We would like to thank all the contributing authors for lending their expertise to make the book truly unique. They have played a crucial role in the development of this book. Without their invaluable contributions this book wouldn't have been possible. They have made vital efforts to compile up to date information on the varied aspects of this subject to make this book a valuable addition to the collection of many professionals and students.

This book was conceptualized with the vision of imparting up-to-date information and advanced data in this field. To ensure the same, a matchless editorial board was set up. Every individual on the board went through rigorous rounds of assessment to prove their worth. After which they invested a large part of their time researching and compiling the most relevant data for our readers.

The editorial board has been involved in producing this book since its inception. They have spent rigorous hours researching and exploring the diverse topics which have resulted in the successful publishing of this book. They have passed on their knowledge of decades through this book. To expedite this challenging task, the publisher supported the team at every step. A small team of assistant editors was also appointed to further simplify the editing procedure and attain best results for the readers.

Apart from the editorial board, the designing team has also invested a significant amount of their time in understanding the subject and creating the most relevant covers. They scrutinized every image to scout for the most suitable representation of the subject and create an appropriate cover for the book.

The publishing team has been an ardent support to the editorial, designing and production team. Their endless efforts to recruit the best for this project, has resulted in the accomplishment of this book. They are a veteran in the field of academics and their pool of knowledge is as vast as their experience in printing. Their expertise and guidance has proved useful at every step. Their uncompromising quality standards have made this book an exceptional effort. Their encouragement from time to time has been an inspiration for everyone.

The publisher and the editorial board hope that this book will prove to be a valuable piece of knowledge for researchers, students, practitioners and scholars across the globe.

List of Contributors

Sachiko Takikawa, Akira Iwase and Fumitaka Kikkawa
Department of Obstetrics and Gynecology, Nagoya University Graduate School of Medicine, Nagoya, Japan

Akihito Yamamoto, Kiyoshi Sakai, Ryutaro Shohara and Minoru Ueda
Department of Oral and Maxillofacial Surgery, Nagoya University Graduate School of Medicine, Nagoya, Japan

Cai-Xia Jin
Department of Surgery, University of North Carolina at Chapel Hill, Chapel Hill, USA
Department of Regenerative Medicine and Huadong Stem Cell Bank, Tongji University School of Medicine, Shanghai, China

Lisa Samuelson, Cai-Bin Cui and Yang-Zhong Sun
Department of Surgery, University of North Carolina at Chapel Hill, Chapel Hill, USA

David A. Gerber
Department of Surgery, University of North Carolina at Chapel Hill, Chapel Hill, USA
Lineberger Cancer Center, University of North Carolina at Chapel Hill, Chapel Hill, USA

Manole Corocleanu
Private, Brasov, Romania

Abigail Hielscher
Department of Chemical and Biomolecular Engineering, Johns Hopkins University, Baltimore, USA

Timothy McGuire
School of Pharmacy, University of Nebraska Medical Center, Omaha, USA

Dennis Weisenburger
Department of Pathology, City of Hope Medical Center, Duarte, USA

John Graham Sharp
Department of Cell Biology, Genetics and Anatomy, University of Nebraska Medical Center, Omaha, USA

Keiko Ikemoto
Department of Neuropsychiatry, Fukushima Medical University, School of Medicine, Fukushima, Japan
Department of Psychiatry, Iwaki Kyoritsu General Hospital, Iwaki, Japan

Teruyuki Kajiume, Nobutsune Ishikawa, Norioki Ohno, Yasuhiko Sera, Syuhei Karakawa and Masao Kobayashi
Department of Pediatrics, Graduate School of Biomedical Sciences, Hiroshima University, Hiroshima, Japan

Hamad Ali and Fahd Al-Mulla
Department of Pathology, Human Genetics Unit, Faculty of Medicine, Kuwait University, Kuwait, The State of Kuwait

Nélida Montano, Andrea Quadrelli, Alicia Vaglio and Roberto Quadrelli
Instituto de Genética Médica, Hospital Italiano, Montevideo, Uruguay

Aubrey Milunsky
Center for Human Genetics, Boston University School of Medicine, Boston, USA

Ekaterina Novosadova, Nella Khaydarova, Ekaterina Manuilova, Elena Arsenyeva, Andrey Lebedev, Vyacheslav Tarantul and Igor Grivennikov
Institute of Molecular Genetics, Russian Academy of Sciences, Moscow, Russia

Ma Teresa González-Garza and Jorge E. Moreno-Cuevas
Servicio de Terapia Celular, School of Medicine, Tecnológico de Monterrey, Monterrey, México

Manish Kumar, Renu Singh, Kuldeep Kumar, Pranjali Agarwal, Puspendra Saswat Mahapatra, Bikas C. Das and Sadhan Bag
Division of Physiology and Climatolxcogy, Indian Veterinary Research Institute, Bareilly, India;

Abhisek Kumar Saxena
Division of Surgery, Indian Veterinary Research Institute, Bareilly, India

Ajay Kumar
Division of Biochemistry, Indian Veterinary Research Institute, Bareilly, India

Subrata Kumar Bhanja
Central Avian research Institute, Bareilly, India

Dhruba Malakar
Animal Biotechnology Center, National Dairy Research Institute, Karnal, India

Rajendra Singh
Division of Pathology, Indian Veterinary Research Institute, Bareilly, India

Manabu Akahane and Tomoaki Imamura
Department of Public Health, Health Management and Policy, Nara Medical University School of Medicine, Nara, Japan

Tomoyuki Ueha, Takamasa Shimizu, Yusuke Inagaki, Akira Kido and Yasuhito Tanaka
Department of Orthopedic Surgery, Nara Medical University, Nara, Japan

Kenji Kawate
Department of Artificial Joint and Regenerative Medicine, Nara Medical University, Nara, Japan

Riikka Aanismaa, Jenna Hautala and Susanna Narkilahti
Neuro Group, Institute of Biomedical Technology, University of Tampere, Tampere, Finland

Annukka Vuorinen
Adult Stem Cell Group, Institute of Biomedical Technology, University of Tampere, Tampere, Finland
Finnish Student Health Service, Tampere, Finland

Susanna Miettinen
Adult Stem Cell Group, Institute of Biomedical Technology, University of Tampere, Tampere, Finland

Davide Schiffer, Marta Mellai, Laura Annovazzi, Oriana Monzeglio and Valentina Caldera
Neuro-Bio-Oncology Center, Policlinico di Monza Foundation (Vercelli)/Consorzio di Neuroscienze, University of Pavia, Pavia Italy

Angela Piazzi
Neuro-Bio-Oncology Center, Policlinico di Monza Foundation (Vercelli)/Consorzio di Neuroscienze, University of Pavia, Pavia Italy
Department of Medical Sciences, University of Piemonte Orientale, Novara, Italy

Gautam Kaul
Biochemistry Department, National Dairy Research Institute, Karnal, India
King Edward Memorial Hospital, University of Western Australia, Perth, Australia

Shashi Kumar and Sunita Kumari
Biochemistry Department, National Dairy Research Institute, Karnal, India

Maria Giovanna Scioli, Alessandra Bielli, Roberto Bellini and Augusto Orlandi
Anatomic Pathology, Department of Biomedicine and Prevention, Tor Vergata University, Rome, Italy

Valerio Cervelli and Pietro Gentile
Plastic Surgery, Department of Biomedicine and Prevention, Tor Vergata University, Rome, Italy

Zhicheng Fang, Xiang Zheng, Boyi Liu, Li Chen, Chunfeng Shen, Pei Liu and Yunfei Huang
Department of Intensive Care Unit, Taihe Hospital, Hubei Medicine University, Shiyan, China

Chang'e Zhou
Department of Nephrology, Taihe Hospital, Hubei Medicine University, Shiyan, China

Ana Lucia Miluzzi Yamada, Marcos Jun Watanabe, Carlos Alberto Hussni, Celso Antônio Rodrigues and Ana Liz Garcia Alves
Department of Veterinary Surgery and Anesthesiology, School of Veterinary Medicine and Animal
Science (FMVZ), UNESP, Uni-versidade Estadual Paulista, Botucatu, Brazil

Armando de Mattos Carvalho
Faculty of Veterinary Medicine, Cuiabá University, Cuiabá, Brazil

Andrei Moroz
Department of Morphology, Institute of Biosciences, UNESP, Botucatu, Brazil

Elenice Deffune
Blood Center, School of Medicine, UNESP, Botucatu, Brazil

Ying-Mei Tang, Li-Ying You and Jin-Hui Yang
Hepatology Center, The 2nd Affiliated Hospital of Kunming Medical College, Yunnan Research Center for Liver Diseases, Kun-ming, China

Yun Zhang, Hong-Wei Wang and Xiang Hu
Shenzhen Beike Cell Engineering Research Institute, Shenzhen, China

Wei-Min Bao
Department of General Surgery, Yunnan Provincial 1st People's Hospital, Kunming, China

Daniele Lodi, Giulia Ligabue, Fabrizio Cavazzini, Valentina Lupo, Gianni Cappelli and Riccardo Magistroni
Department of Medicine and Medical Specialties, Division of Nephrology Dialysis and Transplantation, University of Modena and Reggio Emilia, Modena, Italy

Lingling Xian, Xiangwei Wu and Lijuan Pang
Department of Orthopaedic Surgery, School of Medicine, Johns Hopkins University, Baltimore, USA
Shihezi Medical College, Shihezi University, Shihezi, China

Michael Lou, Bing Yu, Frank Frassica, Mei Wan and Xu Cao
Department of Orthopaedic Surgery, School of Medicine, Johns Hopkins University, Baltimore, USA

Chunyi Wen
Department of Orthopaedics, University of Hong Kong, Hong Kong, China

Erik Tryggestad and John Wong
Radiation Oncology Medical Physics, School of Medicine, Johns Hopkins University, Baltimore, USA

Jong S. Rim, Karen L. Strickler, Christian W. Barnes, Lettie L. Harkins and Jaroslaw Staszkiewicz
NuPotential Inc., Baton Rouge, USA

Jeffrey M. Gimble
Stem Cell Biology Laboratory, Pennington Biomedical Research Center, Baton Rouge, USA

Gregory H. Leno
Department of Anatomy & Cell Biology, Carver College of Medicine, University of Iowa, Iowa City, USA

Kenneth J. Eilertsen
NuPotential Inc., Baton Rouge, USA
Stem Cell Biology Laboratory, Pennington Biomedical Research Center, Baton Rouge, USA

S. Gary Brown
Veterinary Orthopedic and Surgery Service, Western University of Health Sciences, Pomona, USA

Robert J. Harman and Linda L. Black
Vet-Stem Inc., Poway, USA

Hitomi Hosoe, Yuri Yamamoto and Yusuke Tanaka
Department of Physical Therapy, Nagoya University School of Health Sciences, Nagoya, Japan

Mami Kobayashi and Nana Ninagawa
Department of Health Sciences, Nagoya University Graduate School of Medicine, Nagoya, Japan

Shigeko Torihashi
Department of Physical Therapy, Nagoya University School of Health Sciences, Nagoya, Japan Department of Health Sciences, Nagoya University Graduate School of Medicine, Nagoya, Japan

Yinda Tang
Department of Pediatric Surgery, School of Medicine, University of Texas, Houston, USA
Center for Stem Cell and Regenerative Medicine, The University of Texas Health Science Center at Houston, Houston, USA
Department of Neurosurgery, Shanghai Xinhua Hospital, School of Medicine, Shanghai Jiao Tong University, Shanghai, China

Wen Xu
Center for Neuroscience, University of Pittsburgh, Pittsburgh, USA

Haiying Pan and Yong Li
Department of Pediatric Surgery, School of Medicine, University of Texas, Houston, USA
Center for Stem Cell and Regenerative Medicine, The University of Texas Health Science Center at Houston, Houston, USA

Shiting Li
Department of Neurosurgery, Shanghai Xinhua Hospital, School of Medicine, Shanghai Jiao Tong University, Shanghai, China

Camila Santos de Moraes and Claudia Sondermann Freitas
Experimental Medicine Program, Research Coordination, National Cancer Institute of Rio de Janeiro, Rio de Janeiro, Brazil

Paulo Roberto Albuquerque Leal
Plastic Surgery, Cancer Hospital I, National Cancer Institute of Rio de Janeiro, Rio de Janeiro, Brazil

Daniel Fabiano Ferreira and Fernando Serra
Pedro Ernesto Hospital, Rio de Janeiro State University, Rio de Janeiro, Brazil

Eliana Abdelhay
Bone Marrow Transplantation Unit, National Cancer Institute of Rio de Janeiro, Rio de Janeiro, Brazil

Sonal R. Tuljapurkar and John G. Sharp
Departments of Genetics, Cell Biology and Anatomy, University of Nebraska Medical Center, Omaha, USA

John D. Jackson
Pathology and Microbiology, University of Nebraska Medical Center, Omaha, USA

Susan K. Brusnahan
Pharmaceutical Sciences, University of Nebraska Medical Center, Omaha, USA

Barbara J. O'Kane
Creighton University Medical Center, Omaha, USA

Margaret L. Shirley
Department of Biochemistry and Molecular Biology, University of Georgia, Athens, USA
Department of Psychiatry, University of California, San Francisco, USA

Alison Venable and David Puett
Department of Biochemistry and Molecular Biology, University of Georgia, Athens, USA

Raj R. Rao
Department of Chemical and Life Science Engineering, School of Engineering, Virginia Commonwealth University, Richmond, USA

Nolan L. Boyd
Cardiovascular Innovation Institute, University of Louisville, Louisville, USA

Steven L. Stice
Department of Biochemistry and Molecular Biology, University of Georgia, Athens, USA
Regenerative Bioscience Center, University of Georgia, Athens, USA
Department of Animal and Dairy Sciences, University of Georgia, Athens, USA

Prema Narayan
Department of Physiology, Southern Illinois University School of Medicine, Carbondale, USA

Heidi Hongisto, Alexandra Mikhailova, Hanna Hiidenmaa, Tanja Ilmarinen and Heli Skottman
Institute of Biomedical Technology, University of Tampere, Tampere, Finland
Institute of Biosciences and Medical Technology, Tampere, Finland

Min Zhang, Bing Huang, Kaijing Li, Zhenghua Chen, Jian Ge, Weihua Li, Jianfa Huang, Ting Luo, Shaochun Lin, Jie Yu, Wencong Wang and Liping Lin
State Key Laboratory of Ophthalmology, Zhongshan Ophthalmic Center, Sun Yat-sen University, Guangzhou, China

Luis Padilla
Department of Experimental Surgery, Microsurgery Unit, Centro Medico Nacional "20 de Noviembre" ISSSTE, Mexico City, Mexico
Surgery Department, Faculty of Medicine, Universidad Nacional Autonoma de Mexico, Mexico City, Mexico

Juan Rodriguez-Trejo, Ignacio Escotto and Neftaly Rodrgiuez
Angiology, Vascular and Endovascular Surgery Unit, Centro Medico Nacional "20 de Noviembre" ISSSTE, Mexico City, Mexico

Manuel López-Hernandez
Haematology Unit, Centro Medico Nacional "20 de Noviembre" ISSSTE, Mexico City, Mexico

Mauricio González
Bank of Blood Unit, Centro Medico Nacional "20 de Noviembre" ISSSTE, Mexico City, Mexico

José De Diego
Pediatric Hematology Unit Centro Medico Nacional '20 de Noviembre' ISSSTE, Mexico City, Mexico

Jesús Tapia
Surgery Department, Faculty of Medicine, Universidad Nacional Autonoma de Mexico, Mexico City, Mexico

Takeshi Landero, Carranza Pilar Hazel and Horacio Juarez Olguin
Department of Experimental Surgery, Microsurgery Unit, Centro Medico Nacional "20 de Noviembre" ISSSTE, Mexico City, Mexico

Mauricio Di Silvio
Department of Experimental Surgery, Microsurgery Unit, Centro Medico Nacional "20 de Noviembre" ISSSTE, Mexico City, Mexico
Department of Research, Hospital General de México OD, Secretaria de Salud México, Mexico City, Mexico

Paul Mondragon-Teran
Department of Biomedical Research, Centro Medico Nacional "20 de Noviembre" ISSSTE, Mexico City, Mexico

www.ingramcontent.com/pod-product-compliance
Lightning Source LLC
Chambersburg PA
CBHW080247230326
41458CB00097B/4005